Cellular, Molecular, and Clinical Aspects of Allergic Disorders

Comprehensive Immunology

Series Editors: ROBERT A. GOOD and STACEY B. DAY
Sloan-Kettering Institute for Cancer Research
New York, New York

Cellular, Molecular, and Clinical Aspects of Allergic Disorders

Edited by
SUDHIR GUPTA, M.D., F.R.C.P.(C), F.A.C.P.
and
ROBERT A. GOOD, Ph.D., M.D.

Sloan-Kettering Institute for Cancer Research
New York, New York

PLENUM MEDICAL BOOK COMPANY
New York and London

Library of Congress Cataloging in Publication Data

Main entry under title:

Cellular, molecular, and clinical aspects of allergic disorders.

(Comprehensive immunology; 6)
Includes index.
1. Allergy. 2. Allergy – Etiology. I. Gupta, Sudhir. II. Good, Robert A., 1922-
III. Series.
RC586.C45 616.9'7'07 79-867

ISBN-13: 978-1-4684-0990-1 e-ISBN-13: 978-1-4684-0988-8
DOI: 10.1007/978-1-4684-0988-8

Softcover reprint of the hardcover 1st edition 1979
227 West 17th Street, New York, N.Y. 10011

Plenum Medical Book Company is an imprint of Plenum Publishing Corporation

Contributors

K. Frank Austen Departments of Medicine, Robert B. Brigham Hospital and Harvard Medical School, Boston, Massachusetts

C. Edward Buckley, III Department of Medicine, Duke University School of Medicine, Durham, North Carolina

Rebecca H. Buckley Departments of Pediatrics and Microbiology and Immunology, Duke University School of Medicine, Durham, North Carolina

Daniel G. Colley The Veterans Administration Hospital, and Department of Microbiology, Vanderbilt University School of Medicine, Nashville, Tennessee

John T. Connell Nasal Diseases Study Center, Holy Name Hospital, Teaneck, New Jersey

A. L. de Weck Institute of Clinical Immunology, Inselspital, Bern, Switzerland

H. F. Dvorak Department of Pathology, Massachusetts General Hospital, and Department of Pathology, Harvard Medical School, Boston, Massachusetts

S. J. Galli Department of Pathology, Massachusetts General Hospital, and Department of Pathology, Harvard Medical School, Boston, Massachusetts

Robert A. Good Memorial Sloan-Kettering Cancer Center, New York, New York

Michael H. Grieco R. A. Cooke Institute of Allergy and the Allergy, Clinical Immunology, and Infectious Disease Division, Medical Service, The Roosevelt Hospital, New York, New York, and Department of Clinical Medicine, Columbia University College of Physicians and Surgeons, New York, New York

Sudhir Gupta Memorial Sloan-Kettering Cancer Center, New York, New York

Philip C. Ho Department of Immunology, The Hospital for Sick Children, University of Toronto, Toronto, Ontario, Canada

Kimishige Ishizaka Department of Medicine and Microbiology, The Johns Hopkins University School of Medicine, Baltimore, Maryland

Teruko Ishizaka Department of Medicine and Microbiology, The Johns Hopkins University School of Medicine, Baltimore, Maryland

Stephanie L. James Department of Medicine, Harvard Medical School, Boston, Massachusetts

Allen P. Kaplan Allergic Diseases Section, Laboratory of Clinical Investigation, National Institute of Allergy and Infectious Diseases, National Institutes of Health, Bethesda, Maryland. Present affiliation: Division of Allergy-Rheumatology, Health Sciences Center, State University of New York, Stony Brook, New York

Reynold M. Karr Clinical Immunology Section, Department of Medicine, Tulane University School of Medicine, New Orleans, Louisiana

T. P. King The Rockefeller University, New York, New York

Robert A. Lewis Departments of Medicine, Robert B. Brigham Hospital and Harvard Medical School, Boston, Massachusetts

Lawrence M. Lichtenstein Department of Medicine, Division of Clinical Immunology, The Johns Hopkins University School of Medicine, Baltimore, Maryland

Charles D. May Department of Pediatrics, National Jewish Hospital and Research Center, and Department of Pediatrics, University of Colorado Medical School, Denver, Colorado

Robert P. Orange Deceased. Department of Immunology, The Hospital for Sick Children, University of Toronto, Toronto, Ontario, Canada

W. E. Parish Environmental Safety Division, Unilever Research, Sharnbrook, Bedfordshire, England

Roy Patterson Allergy Section, Department of Medicine, Northwestern University Medical School, Chicago, Illinois

Robert E. Reisman Departments of Medicine and Pediatrics, State University of New York, Buffalo, New York

John E. Salvaggio Clinical Immunology Section, Department of Medicine, Tulane University School of Medicine, New Orleans, Louisiana

Larry L. Thomas Department of Medicine, Division of Clinical Immunology, The Johns Hopkins University School of Medicine, Baltimore, Maryland

Preface

Impressive progress has been made in the general field of immunology which has made possible new understanding and pragmatic approaches to the patient with allergic disease. Indeed, one working in the field of immunology senses a major revolution of immunobiologic thinking, much of which has relevance to the clinical practice of allergy. To the practicing allergist, pediatrician, or internist who must deal with allergic patients, the surging new information may seem confusing and bewildering. As part of our comprehensive series on modern immunobiology which aims to digest this progress, we believe it is appropriate to devote an entire volume to the fundamental principles, new knowledge, and clinical lore on which the modern practice of allergy must be based.

In the present volume we strive to bring together relevant contributions from leaders in the field of immunobiology with those whose work stands at the forefront of clinical practice. The advancing understanding has in numerous instances reached the point of clinical application, and we have tried to encompass in this volume the entire scope of modern allergy.

The cellular basis of allergic disease and the body's adjustments to allergic reaction are first considered. A chapter on basophils and mast cells deals with the morphological and functional changes and mechanisms of mediator release during reactions of immediate and delayed onset. Basophil-mediated delayed cutaneous hypersensitivity is discussed in detail. Structure and functions of eosinophils in body defense, the clean-up and control of allergic reactions, are also covered. An extensive review of phenotypic and functional properties of lymphocytes, the subpopulations of lymphocytes, and the role of these cells in the various immediate hypersensitivity disorders is included.

Antigenic determinants on several antigens that are important in clinical and experimental allergies have been reviewed. Immunoglobulin E biosynthesis and mechanisms of immunoglobulin-E-mediated hypersensitivity are discussed. The mechanisms involved in the regulation of IgE antibody formation through antigen-specific suppressor T cells, modification of allergens to make them more tolerogenic, and the potentiation of suppressor T-cell development as an approach toward effective immunotherapy are discussed.

Mediators of immediate hypersensitivity are reviewed with regard to their physicochemical characteristics, their mechanisms of generation and release, their pathophysiological effects, and the interactions of the several biologic activities with fundamental effectors such as macrophages and inflammatory reactions. A chapter on genetics of allergy deals especially with aspects of cognitive functions important in immunity. Current knowledge of the genetics of immunity, including consideration of immune response genes, is reviewed, especially as it relates to atopic diseases.

The clinical presentation and current concepts of the pathogenesis and management of various forms of urticaria and angioedema are discussed. This book also includes reviews of the current knowledge of mechanisms of food hypersensitivity, including the role of mucosal immunity; adverse reactions to drugs which are due to immunological mechanisms; allergic reactions due to common stinging insects; and classification and pathogenesis of various forms of nasal hypersensitivity.

An extensive review of the pathogenesis and pathophysiology of bronchial asthma in the light of current understanding of the immunological, physiological, and pathological principles involved has been presented. Immunopathological features of infiltrative pulmonary diseases based on allergic mechanisms and the clinical management of these diseases are covered. Immunodeficiency disorders associated with augmented IgE synthesis, e.g., hyper-IgE syndromes, are discusssed with regard to their presentation and clinical manifestations. The chapter on hypersensitivity vasculitis includes a description of immune-complex-mediated reactions and of immunohistochemical evidence of immunoglobulin and complement deposition in the lesions of the cutaneous vasculitis in man. Special emphasis has been placed on identification of antigens which contribute to these complexes.

Newer laboratory techniques and interpretations of the results obtained with them that are basic to diagnosis and management of hypersensitivity disorders have also been thoroughly covered. Finally, principles of immunological and pharmacological approaches to the management of patients with allergic diseases are discussed.

The aim of this volume is to provide a background for understanding allergic diseases of man and to present information of immediate usefulness to the clinician as well as analyses of value to investigators involved in research on allergic diseases. We hope this volume will serve as a guide for practicing allergists, a source of orientation and information for medical students, and a companion to all physicians concerned with allergy and hypersensitivity, whether they be academicians or practicing physicians.

Contents

Chapter 2
Participation of Eosinophils in Immunological Systems 55
Daniel G. Colley and Stephanie L. James

Chapter 3
Lymphocyte Subpopulations and Functions in Hypersensitivity Disorders 87
Sudhir Gupta and Robert A. Good

Chapter 4
Molecular Properties of Allergens 139
T. P. King

Chapter 5
Immunoglobulin E: Biosynthesis and Immunological Mechanisms of IgE-Mediated Hypersensitivity 153
Kimishige Ishizaka and Teruko Ishizaka

Chapter 6
Mediators of Immediate Hypersensitivity 179
Philip C. Ho, Robert A. Lewis, K. Frank Austen, and Robert P. Orange

Chapter 16

Hypersensitivity Vasculitis: The Acute Phase of Leukocytoclastic (Necrotizing) Lesions 537

W. E. Parish

Chapter 17

Laboratory Diagnosis of Immediate Hypersensitivity Disorders 569

Larry L. Thomas and Lawrence M. Lichtenstein

1

Basophils and Mast Cells: Structure, Function, and Role in Hypersensitivity

S. J. GALLI and H. F. DVORAK

1. Introduction

Several important discoveries of the past few decades have launched a renaissance of research into basophil and mast cell function. These include the discovery of IgE and its affinity for basophils and mast cells and the demonstration of the ability of these cells to elaborate and release not only histamine but also a variety of low-molecular-weight mediators of immediate hypersensitivity. Moreover, the application of modern methods of tissue fixation and processing has permitted confident identification of basophils and mast cells with both the light and electron microscopes in diverse experimental and clinical situations, and has clearly implicated these cells in a variety of delayed-onset immunological phenomena where their participation had been entirely unexpected.

This chapter will selectively review current knowledge regarding basophil and mast cell structure, function, and roles in hypersensitivity phenomena. We will particularly emphasize findings that implicate basophils and mast cells in immunological reactions of delayed onset, because we feel that the study of such phenomena is likely to elucidate the normal immunological functions of these cells. Whenever possible, the data presented will be derived from human studies. However, in many instances, information about human mast cells and basophils is sparse or lacking altogether. For this reason, significant conclusions derived from animal experiments are included when appropriate.

S. J. GALLI and H. F. DVORAK • Department of Pathology, Massachusetts General Hospital, Boston, Massachusetts 02114, and Department of Pathology, Harvard Medical School, Boston, Massachusetts 02115.

2. Origin, Distribution, and Morphology

2.1. Origin and Normal Distribution

Basophils are polymorphonuclear granulocytes that differentiate in the bone marrow and circulate in the blood of most vertebrates, including man (A. Dvorak, 1978). Like other granulocytes, basophils do not normally occur in extravascular sites other than the bone marrow (A. Dvorak, 1978). Mast cells, in contrast, are normally distributed throughout the connective tissue, particularly in the vicinity of blood and lymphatic vessels and peripheral nerves. They may be especially abundant near epithelial surfaces exposed to environmental antigens such as those of the respiratory and gastrointestinal systems and the skin (Riley, 1959; Brinkman, 1968; Trotter and Orr, 1973, 1974; Feltkamp-Vroom *et al.* , 1975; Padawer, 1978). Mast cells occasionally may be found within normal or diseased epithelia (Barnett, 1973; Colvin *et al.*, 1974; Feltkamp-Vroom *et al.*, 1975). In some species, mast cells can be numerous in the fibrous connective tissue capsules of various internal organs and in physiological transudates (Padawer, 1978), and they may occur in the connective tissue of the bone marrow and lymph nodes (Spicer *et al.*, 1975). Although one group (Csaba *et al.*, 1969) claimed that mast cells circulate in the peripheral blood of rats, the number of circulating cells is so small that they cannot be detected by routine methods of examination.

Mast cells are long-lived cells (Padawer, 1974) that apparently may either differentiate *in situ* or undergo mitotic division as morphologically mature cells. Thus Miller's studies (1971) have demonstrated that, during helminth expulsion in the rat, intestinal mast cells can differentiate *in situ* from cells resembling lymphoblasts. These observations are supported by *in vitro* evidence indicating that mononuclear cells in the thymus, spleen, and lymph nodes can give rise to mast cells in the mouse (Ginsburg, 1963; Ginsburg and Lagunoff, 1967) and that both thymus cells and monolayers of embryo cells can give rise to mast cells in the rat (T. Ishizaka *et al.*, 1976). Unlike mature basophils, fully differentiated mast cells can divide locally, particularly in growing animals or in sites of pathology (Fawcett, 1955; Allen, 1962; Blenkinsopp, 1967; A. Dvorak *et al.*, 1976c).

2.2. Morphology

The morphology of basophils and mast cells has recently been reviewed in detail (A. Dvorak, 1978; Lagunoff, 1972b; Anderson *et al.*, 1973; Trotter and Orr, 1973, 1974; Padawer, 1978). The present discussion will emphasize the morphological distinctions between mature human basophils and mast cells.

Basophils (Figure 1) are the smallest of the human granulocytes, with a diameter determined by phase-contrast microscopy of 10–14 μm (Ackerman and Bellios, 1955). In 1-μm Epon-embedded tissue sections, human basophils are polymorphonuclear cells with prominent, brightly metachromatic cytoplasmic granules that are larger, fewer, and more widely separated than those of mast cells. By electron microscopy, human basophil cytoplasmic granules are round to angular, membrane-bound structures up to 1.2 μm in size, over twice that of human mast cell granules. The granule substructure is composed of dense particles in a less dense matrix, and occasionally includes complex membrane figures (A. Dvorak, 1978). A subpopulation of smaller granules that are usually found between the nuclear lobes and that differ from the larger granules both ultrastructurally and histochemically has also been described in human basophils (Ackerman and Clark, 1971; Nichols and Bainton, 1973; Hastie, 1974).

The cytoplasm of mature human basophils also contains abundant glycogen deposits, a small Golgi apparatus, a few mitochondria, ribosomes, strands of rough endoplasmic reticulum, and a complex vesicular system that will be described in detail in the sections on basophil degranulation (Sections 5.2 and 5.3).

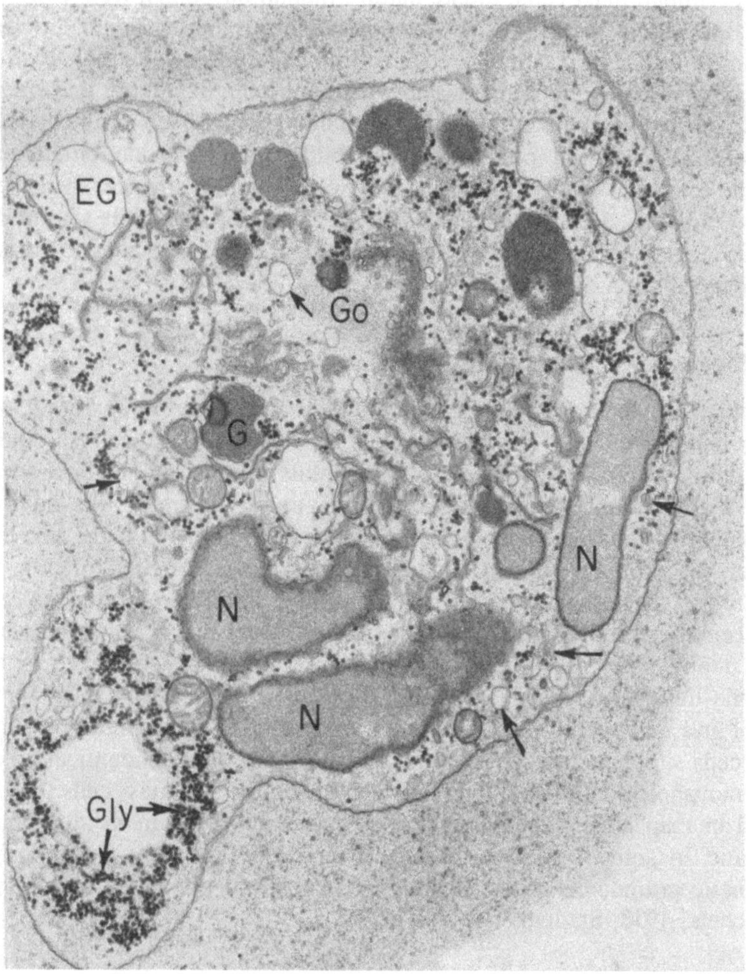

Figure 1. Electron photomicrograph of a typical human basophil present in a skin reaction of contact sensitivity to poison ivy. This partially degranulated cell has a multilobed nucleus (N), numerous cytoplasmic aggregates of glycogen particles (Gly), a Golgi apparatus (Go), several strands of rough endoplasmic reticulum, and mitochondria. Typical intact granules (G) have an electron-dense matrix, whereas depleted granules (EG) appear as large, membrane-bound vacuoles. Numerous cytoplasmic vesicles (arrows) are also present. 15,600×. Reprinted from A. Dvorak (1978), p. 378, by courtesy of Dekker, New York.

Human mast cells (Figure 2) appear in tissue sections as round, oval, or elongated cells, 10–30 μm in diamter, that may have branching processes extending considerable distances between intercellular connective tissue elements (Braunsteiner, 1962; Trotter and Orr, 1973, 1974). In humans, as in experimental animals, mast cell morphology and size vary somewhat depending on the organ or site of origin (Trotter and Orr, 1973, 1974; Pearce *et al.*, 1977). The nucleus usually appears round to oval, with chromatin that becomes progressively more clumped and densely staining as the cell matures. The round, closely packed cytoplasmic granules vary from 0.1 to 0.4 μm in diameter and may have a complex whorled or crystalline (Trotter and Orr, 1973, 1974; Padawer, 1978) substructure by electron microscopy. Human mast cells, unlike mature human basophils, frequently exhibit centrioles, may have a complex system of numerous plasmalemmal ridges and folds, and have little cytoplasmic glycogen. Both basophils (A. Dvorak *et al.*, 1972) and mast cells (Padawer, 1969) may pinocytose particulate material that frequently is then transported to their cytoplasmic granules. It has been claimed that both types of cell may exhibit phagocytic capability under certain circumstances, although the evidence supporting a phagocytic function is stronger in the case of mast cells (Padawer, 1971; Spicer *et al.*, 1975) than for basophils (Sampson and Archer, 1967; A. Dvorak *et al.*, 1972). It is unclear what role phagocytosis plays in the normal function of these cells.

2.3. Phylogenetic Considerations

Basophils are the rarest of human granulocytes, accounting for 0.5–1% of circulating leukocytes and approximately 0.3% of nucleated cells in the bone marrow (Juhlin, 1963). The frequency of basophils in most mammalian species is similar to that in man, although rabbits have up to 10 times this number. In nonmammalian vertebrates basophils are considerably more abundant, and in some reptiles may account for more than half of leukocytes (Michels, 1938). Within different animal species, there is a striking although not invariant inverse relationship between the frequency of basophils and of mast cells. For example, rats, mice, and many fishes, in which basophils are rare or absent, have extremely numerous tissue mast cells. This relation, together with the biochemical similarity of basophil and mast cell granule contents, supports the widespread presumption that these cells supplement each other and have similar or even identical functions. The clear morphological distinctions between basophils and mast cells that can be recognized in man and in many other species are not present in all animals. In chickens and in some lower vertebrates it appears that only a single type of metachromatic granule-bearing cell both circulates and populates the connective tissue (Michels, 1938; Stadecker *et al.*, 1977).

3. Chemical Mediators of Hypersensitivity Reactions

The chemical mediators of immediate hypersensitivity are discussed in detail elsewhere in this volume (Chapter 6). Our remarks will deal primarily with selected aspects of certain mediators that may have relevance to the role of basophils and mast cells in delayed-onset immunological phenomena.

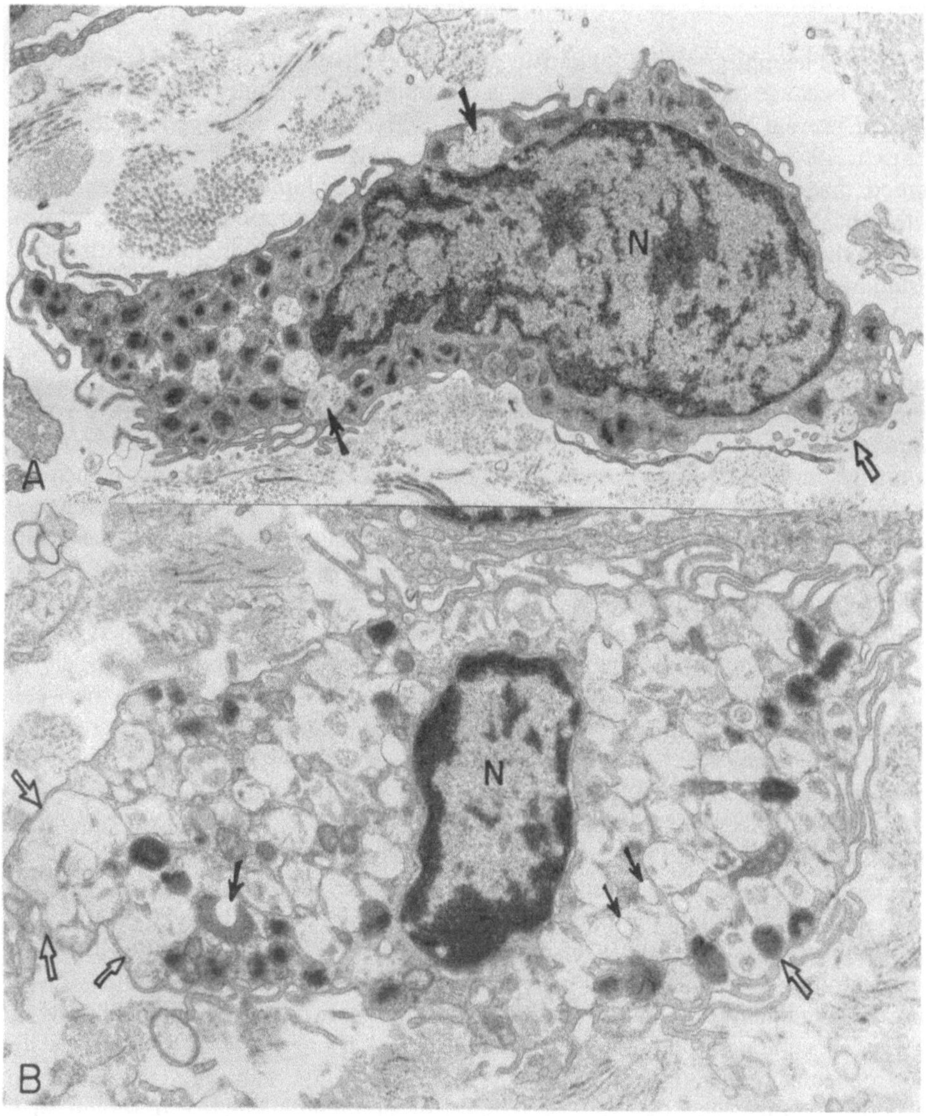

Figure 2. Electron photomicrographs of typical human mast cells in the dermis of normal skin (A) and a 2-day contact reaction to urushiol (B). The normal-appearing mast cell in A has an eccentric, unilobed nucleus (N) with heavily condensed chromatin. A few of the numerous specific cytoplasmic granules appear swollen and have contents of greatly reduced electron density (arrows). The upper arrow marks fusion of adjacent granules. Another granule (open arrow) opens to the extracellular space. In contrast, the mast cell illustrated in B exhibits numerous enlarged granules that have lost most of their normally electron-dense contents. One empty-appearing granule is within the tip of a plasma membrane fold (lower left). Many affected granules intercommunicate to form aggregates (open arrows). Several small vesicles (closed arrows), some of them invaginated into adjacent granules, are present in the cytoplasm. The nucleus (N) has heavily condensed peripheral chromatin. A, 10,000×; B, 11,000×. Reduced 9% for reproduction. Reprinted from A. Dvorak *et al.* (1976c), by courtesy of Williams and Wilkins, Baltimore.

3.1. Histamine and Histamine-Synthesizing Capacity

That basophils might contain a portion of blood histamine has long been inferred because of evidence associating histamine content and basophil frequency both in normal volunteers and in patients with chronic myelogenous leukemia (Ehrich, 1953; Graham *et al.*, 1955; Valentine *et al.*, 1955). It is now generally agreed that virtually all of the histamine present in human blood is contained within basophils. The situation is quite different in the rabbit, however, where, despite their relative frequency, basophils carry only about one-quarter of blood histamine, the remainder being associated with the platelets (Benveniste *et al.*, 1973).

Assuming that, in humans, all blood histamine is associated with basophils, it can be estimated that normal basophils contain 1–2 pg of histamine per cell, whereas basophils from patients with chronic myelogenous leukemia have somewhat less (Graham *et al.*, 1955; Sampson and Archer, 1967). The histamine content of highly purified (50–80%) preparations of normal, mature, circulating guinea pig basophils is also approximately 1 pg/cell (Lipinski and H. Dvorak, unpublished data; Galli, unpublished data). By way of comparison, rat peritoneal mast cells contain about 20–30 pg of histamine (Keller, 1966; T. Ishizaka *et al.*, 1975), and guinea pig lung and mesenteric mast cells contain 3 and 8 pg of histamine, respectively (Pearce *et al.*, 1977).

The histamine present within basophils is thought to be confined largely to their specific cytoplasmic granules. This conclusion is based on analogy between basophils and mast cells and on the fact that nearly all blood histamine is released by immunological reactions that result in basophil degranulation (Lichtenstein, 1968). Moreover, cell disruption studies have revealed that most histamine present within human basophils (Pruzansky and Patterson, 1967), like that of mast cells (Anderson and Uvnäs, 1975), is localized in the granule fraction.

The histamine present within blood basophils is apparently synthesized in these cells by a specific cytoplasmic enzyme, histidine decarboxylase (Galli and Dvorak, 1975; Galli *et al.*, 1976). Hartman *et al.* (1961) and Lindell *et al.* (1961) demonstrated that buffy coat cells from normal volunteers and patients with chronic myelogenous leukemia are able to synthesize histamine. Statistical analysis of Lindell's patients demonstrated that histamine formation was correlated with the frequency of basophils but not with that of any other cell type. We have also recently demonstrated that the circulating, predominantly mature basophils of a patient with chronic myelogenous leukemia retain the ability to synthesize and store histamine *in vitro* (Galli *et al.*, unpublished data). Furthermore, we have provided conclusive evidence that normal, mature, circulating guinea pig basophils synthesize histamine (Galli and Dvorak, 1975; Galli *et al.*, 1976). Purified preparations of guinea pig blood basophils were cultured with [^{3}H]histidine *in vitro* for various periods of time, and the amount of newly synthesized histamine was measured by an isotopic thin-layer chromatographic assay. Cell-associated newly synthesized histamine was detectable as early as 1 hr of culture, was substantially increased at 6 hr, and reached maximal levels at 24 hr when it accounted for approximately 6.5% of total cell histamine. Based on the kinetics of basophil maturation in the bone marrow (H. Dvorak *et al.*, 1974b), maturing bone marrow basophils must synthesize histamine *in vivo* at approximately twice the rate of mature circulating basophils *in vitro*. Although Day *et al.* (1974) have claimed that human basophils take up and store histamine, we found that the uptake of exogenous histamine over 24 hr by mature guinea pig basophils was fifty fold less than histamine synthesis during the same period. The same proportion of both newly synthesized (isotopic) histamine and preformed (nonisotopic) histamine was released from cultured basophils by either antigen or concanavalin A. Values of newly synthesized histamine were substantially reduced by including specific histidine decarboxylase inhibitors in the culture medium.

These results indicate that mature, circulating guinea pig basophils retain some ability to synthesize at least one of their granule-associated mediators. More recently, we have demonstrated that mature guinea pig basophils also retain the ability to synthesize granule proteoglycans (see Section 3.2). Together with extensive morphological evidence that basophils participating in a variety of delayed-onset hypersensitivity reactions can undergo a piecemeal, partial loss of their granule contents (see Section 5.2), these data suggest that the functional repertoire of mature, circulating basophils may be more complex than simply the anaphylactic release of their granule contents in a single, brief, explosive, and, for the cell, terminal event. Whether and to what extent basophils can replenish their histamine stores after maximal anaphylactic degranulation remains an open question. Although basophils generally remain viable after antigen-induced degranulation, one group failed to detect histamine synthesis in human blood basophils cultured after degranulation by antigenic challenge (Drobis and Siraganian, 1976). In that study, total cell-associated histamine was measured using a fluorometric assay. It would be important to reexamine this question using a more sensitive technique for detecting newly formed histamine.

3.2. Proteoglycans

The identification of basophils or mast cells in all mammalian species is dependent on the metachromatic staining of their granules with certain basic dyes (Ackerman, 1963). Proteoglycans, complex macromolecules composed of glycosaminoglycans covalently bound to a protein core, are thought to be responsible for this characteristic granule metachromasia. In many species, including man and the guinea pig, these water-soluble materials are leached from tissues by exposure to aqueous solutions, including the standard aqueous fixatives. As a result, the participation of basophils in the delayed-onset reactions of these species that has been clearly demonstrated by the use of 1-μm Epon-embedded, Giemsa-stained sections cannot even be appreciated in formalin-fixed, paraffin-embedded, and hematoxylin- and eosin-stained material.

By analogy with mast cells, the proteoglycan of basophil granules was long considered to represent a heparin. However, it is now recognized that the sulfated proteoglycans of basophils or mast cells of different species represent a structurally and almost certainly also a functionally heterogeneous family of macromolecules. For example, several groups of investigators have reported that chondroitin sulfate, not heparin, is present in chicken mast cells (Sue and Jaques, 1976) and in human and rabbit basophils (Sue and Jaques, 1974; Horn and Spicer, 1964; Olsson, 1969, 1971; Jaques *et al.*, 1977; Olsson *et al.*, 1968). Unfortunately, these studies were not definitive because they were performed on crude cell mixtures in which mast cells or basophils were a minority population and in which the various types of contaminating cells were neither controlled nor defined. In contrast, recent work has established that highly purified rat peritoneal mast cells (Yurt *et al.*, 1977a) and the mast cells of human lung (Metcalfe *et al.*, 1978) do in fact contain a heparin. By contrast, the majority (approximately 85%) of the sulfated glycosaminoglycans of guinea pig basophils labeled with ^{35}S either *in vivo* or *in vitro* represented a roughly equal mixture of chrondroitin and dermatan sulfates. The remaining 15% was heparan sulfate, not heparin (Orenstein *et al.*, 1977, 1978). Electron microscopic autoradiography demonstrated that ^{35}S inorganic sulfate was incorporated into the cytoplasmic granules of bone marrow and peripheral blood basophils. We presume, therefore, that the majority of basophil glycosaminoglycans are granule associated. A cell membrane localization for the heparan sulfate has not been excluded, however, and would be consistent with what is known about other mammalian cells (Kraemer, 1971; Kraemer and Tobay, 1972; Buonassisi and Root, 1975; Kleinman *et al.*, 1975). Although an anticoagulant substance with several of the physicochemical properties of heparin has been isolated from human leukemic leukocytes containing <10% basophils (Amann and Martin, 1961), the glycosaminoglycans of normal human basophils have yet to be identified unequivocally. We recently characterized the sulfated glycosaminoglycans synthesized *in vitro* by human leukemic granulocytes consisting of 50% mature basophils (Galli *et al.*, 1979). Characterization of this material with highly specific polysaccharidases revealed that the majority (75%) was chondroitin sulfate and 9% was dermatan sulfate. Most of the remainder was resistant to hydrolysis by purified heparinase and, therefore, most probably represented heparan sulfate. It is unlikely that heparin could have accounted for any more than 5% of the total newly synthesized glycosaminoglycans.

Intracellularly, the highly anionic proteoglycans are probably ionically bound to cationic granule proteins such as proteases, forming proteoglycan–protein complexes that in turn are thought to ionically bind zinc, histamine (and, in some species, serotonin), and other pharmacologically active granule constituents such as ECF-A (Thon and Uvnäs, 1966; Uvnäs *et al.*, 1970). On the release of cytoplasmic granules from the cell, or their exposure to the extracellular medium via cytoplasmic channels communicating with the cellular exterior, ion exchange mechanisms are thought to result in the release of these loosely bound small molecules (Åborg and Uvnäs, 1968; Lagunoff, 1972a; Wasserman *et al.*, 1974a). Since both heparin and serotonin, but not histamine, apparently function in the intact mast cell granule of the rat to largely inhibit the enzymatic activity of the granule chymase (Yurt and Austen, 1977), dissociation of granule proteoglycans and cationic enzymes may provide a mechanism for the activation of granule-associated proteases *in vivo*.

There is no question that basophil and mast cell proteoglycans may themselves be released from the cell during degranulation. Yurt *et al.* (1977b) have demonstrated that heparin is released along with histamine by rat mast cells responding to an antigenic challenge. Furthermore, morphological studies have established that virtually intact, metachromatic (i.e., proteoglycan-containing) granules discharged from basophils or mast cells can be widely dispersed in the tissues away from the cells of origin (Higginbotham, 1958, 1963; Clark and Higginbotham, 1968; Wintroub *et al.*, 1978). Extruded granules may be phagocytosed by macrophages, neutrophils, and eosinophils (Higginbotham *et al.*, 1956; Higginbotham, 1958, 1963; Mann, 1969a; Padawer, 1970), fibroblasts (Higginbotham, 1958; Clark and Higginbotham, 1968), and tumor cells (A. Dvorak, unpublished observations).

The fate and functions of the released granule proteoglycans are unknown. Because of the early belief that the metachromasia of all mast cell or basophil granules was due to the presence of heparin, it was thought that these cells might locally interact with the clotting system in certain circumstances. It now seems that mast cell and basophil proteoglycan function can hardly be confined to interactions with the clotting system. As has already been mentioned, the basophils or mast cells of some species, i.e., the guinea pig, rabbit, chicken, and man, contain proteoglycans other than heparin. Furthermore, it is important to emphasize that "heparin" itself is a family of compounds with considerable variation in physical and biological properties. Even a single commercial preparation of heparin represents a mixture of components; variability among the heparins of different species is even more marked (Lasker, 1977). It is not surprising, therefore, that even though the native proteoglycan of rat mast cells is certainly a heparin, in its native form it has only 10% of the anticoagulant activity and 20% of the antithrombin cofactor activity of commercial heparin, at least when tested with human blood (Yurt *et al.*, 1977b).

In vitro studies in several species have suggested that the local release of proteoglycans by basophils or mast cells may result in diverse and potentially important effects independent of any direct influence on the clotting system. Described effects include the stimulation of macrophage pinocytosis (heparin, chondroitin sulfate, and other polyanions) (Cohn and Parks, 1967), inhibition of leukocyte hydrolytic enzymes (heparin) (Brittinger *et al.*, 1968; DeChatelet *et al.*, 1972), and stimulation and/or inhibition of cell proliferation (heparin) (Lippman and Mathews, 1977), to name a few. Furthermore, since chondroitin and dermatan sulfates are both important interstitial ground substance proteoglycans in some species, the release of macromolecules such as these may also influence the evolution of inflammatory reactions indirectly by the local alteration of interstitial physicochemical properties.

The observation that heparin (Stathakis and Mosesson, 1977; Mosesson, 1978) and related substances (Smith and vonKorff, 1957) bind to cold-insoluble globulin (CIg, fibronectin), probably at a site different than that responsible for fibronectin–collagen binding (Engvall and Ruoslahti, 1977; Ruoslahti and Engvall, 1978), may have implications for mast cell and basophil proteoglycan function *in vivo*. For example, it has been suggested that fibronectin functions *in vivo* to promote cell adherence to the extracellular matrix (Klebe, 1974; Pearlstein, 1976; Pearlstein and Gold, 1978). If this hypothesis is correct, proteoglycans released by basophils or mast cells potentially may either enhance adherence, by binding simultaneously to both fibronectin and to the surfaces of other cells, or inhibit adherence, by occupying fibronectin binding sites otherwise available to those proteoglycans, such as heparan sulfate, normally present on many cell surfaces (Kraemer, 1971; Kraemer and Tobay, 1972; Buonassisi and Root, 1975; Kleinman *et al.*, 1975). Although these possibilities remain to be directly investigated, it should be noted that previous attempts to define the effects of commercial preparations of heparin in various inflammatory processes have produced confusing and widely conflicting results (Grant, 1973). The reasons for this are probably diverse but doubtless include both differences in experimental design and variability in different commercial preparations of heparin.

In summary, knowledge of the structure of native proteoglycans, particularly the nature of their protein components, is in a very preliminary state of development. Further, we know little of the fate of these compounds following their discharge from the mast cell or basophil cytoplasm *in vivo*. Finally, it should be recognized that the chemical configuration of the proteoglycan(s) isolated from mast cells or basophils *in vitro* may not necessarily be identical to the configuration that is most active *in vivo*. Proteoglycan structural modification may occur either in the interstitium, by the action of enzymes derived from mesenchymal cells, leukocytes, or perhaps the basophils or mast cells themselves, or intracellularly, as a consequence of granule phagocytosis. For these reasons, great caution must be exercised in extrapolating the results from *in vitro* experiments, particularly those performed with commercial preparations of heterologous proteoglycans or glycosaminoglycans, to *in vivo* phenomena.

4. Role in Immediate Hypersensitivity Reactions

4.1. Introduction

That mast cells and basophils are the source of many chemical mediators of immediate hypersensitivity phenomena is clearly established. In all of these reactions—generally characterized by local or systemic smooth muscle contraction, vascular dilatation, and increased vascular permeability—the initiating event is the interaction of mast cell- and/or basophil-bound IgE (or other homocytotropic antibody) with specific antigen. The particular biological manifestations of such homocytotropic antibody-mediated reactions may be diverse, even within a single species, and are determined by a host of factors. These include dose and route of administration of antigen, class and concentration of circulating or tissue-fixed homocytotropic antibody, presence and concentration of nonhomocytotropic (blocking) antibody of similar antigenic specificity, sensitivity of target cells (basophils and/or mast cells) to the degranulation stimulus produced by the interaction of antigen with specific homocytotropic antibody, serum (or other) factors that modulate the extent of anaphylactic degranulation, and factors that influence the catabolism or inactivation of either antigen or specific antibody. There are also considerable species differences in certain manifestations of immediate hypersensitivity. Thus the most biologically significant features of anaphylaxis in the guinea pig are thought to be caused largely by the effects of a single mast cell/basophil mediator, histamine, on a single target tissue, broncial smooth muscle. By contrast, in other rodents and in man the anaphylactic response involves several different important end organs and tissues and is probably determined by the action of multiple mediators (Stechschulte and Austen, 1974).

Work both in the basophil and in the mast cell has demonstrated that many of the diverse stimuli capable of provoking mediator release (antigen or anti-IgE–IgE interactions, certain complement fragments, neutrophil lysosomal proteins, some venoms, etc.) act by initiating a common sequence of morphological events. In general, degranulation is best regarded as a noncytolytic secretory process analogous to the secretion of insulin from β cells of the pancreas or transmitters from neuronal synapses (Johnson and Moran, 1969a,b; Lichtenstein, 1968; Hastie, 1971; Chan, 1972). In this section, we present a general outline of the biochemical mechanisms responsible for the release of histamine and other mediators from basophils and mast cells. Description of the morphological alterations associated with mediator release is deferred to a later section (5.1).

4.2. Homocytotropic Antibody

Because an entire chapter of this volume (Chapter 5) is devoted to immunoglobulin E (IgE), only certain features of the interaction between basophils or mast cells and IgE will be discussed here.

The studies of Ishizaka and Ishizaka (1966, 1967, 1973, 1976) and Johansson and Bennich (Johansson and Bennich, 1967a,b; Bennich and Johansson, 1967; Stanworth *et al.*, 1967; Bennich *et al.*, 1969) have clearly established that IgE is the "reagin" so long implicated in the pathogenesis of atopic allergy. Only a minor component among circulating immunoglobulins [normal concentrations in man are 0.1–0.4 μg/ml, although atopic individuals may have ten times this amount (T. Ishizaka *et al.*, 1973; Conroy *et al.*, 1977)], IgE is composed of two light and two heavy (ϵ) chains, and is divalent. IgE has a short half-life in the serum of about 2–3 days (Waldmann, 1969, Waldmann *et al.*, 1976); by contrast, the $t_{\frac{1}{2}}$ of IgG is 25 days. IgE does not fix complement when reacted with antigen but is apparently able to activate C3 and later components of the complement sequence by means of the alternative pathway (T. Ishizaka and K. Ishizaka, 1973).

A feature of fundamental importance to IgE function is its ability to bind avidly to basophils and mast cells but not to the surfaces of other leukocytes (K. Ishizaka *et al.*, 1970; Tomioka and K. Ishizaka, 1971; Sullivan *et al.*, 1971). The affinity of IgE for the basophil or mast cell surface is normally very high at physiological pH, on the order of 10^8–10^{10} mole $^{-1}$ for human basophils (T. Ishizaka *et al.*, 1973; Stallman *et al.*, 1977a; Malveáux *et al.*, 1978; Marone and Lichtenstein, 1978) and 10^8 and 10^9 mole^{-1} for mouse (Mendoza and Metzger, 1976) and rat (Conrad *et al.*, 1975) mast cells, respectively, and is probably dependent on noncovalent mechanisms (T. Ishizaka *et al.*, 1973; T. Ishizaka and K. Ishizaka, 1974). The site of IgE that binds to basophils or mast cells is located in the Fc fragment (Stanworth *et al.*, 1968). Heat (56°C, 0.5–2 hr) or reduction can irreversibly destroy the ability of IgE to bind to mast cells or basophils, probably by affecting different regions of the binding site (Dorrington and Bennich, 1978). Various studies have demonstrated that IgE may have either a patchy (Sullivan *et al.*, 1971; Ferrarini *et al.*, 1973; Becker *et al.*, 1973) or a uniform (van Elven *et al.*, 1977) distribution on the nondegranulated basophil surface, perhaps depending on whether or not partial capping has occurred. The nature of the membrane receptors for IgE is a subject of active current research and has been recently reviewed elsewhere (Metzger and Bach, 1978).

Estimates of the number of IgE molecules bound to human basophils vary from 5000–40,000 (T. Ishizaka *et al.*, 1973) to 3000–600,000 (Conroy *et al.*, 1977; Stallman and Aalberse, 1977a; Malveáux *et al.*, 1978), differences that may in part reflect different methods of measuring cell-bound IgE. There is agreement, however, that the basophils of most nonatopic individuals have $\leq$100,000 molecules of

IgE/cell. Such cells are able to bind substantially more IgE during brief exposures to relatively high concentrations (3 μg/ml, Malveáux *et al.*, 1978; 100 μg/ml or more, T. Ishizaka *et al.*, 1973) of this immunoglobulin *in vitro*. By means of such experiments, it appears that only a fraction of the basophil's IgE receptor sites are occupied at normal serum concentrations of IgE. By contrast, basophils from atopic individuals have a much reduced capacity for binding additional IgE molecules, suggesting that their IgE receptors may already be nearly saturated (T. Ishizaka *et al.*, 1973). One group, employing immunofluorescence technique, did not detect increased amounts of IgE on basophils incubated either with an IgE myeloma protein or with serum containing high concentrations of IgE (Stallman *et al.*, 1977a). Why these workers were unable to corroborate the findings of Sullivan *et al.* (1971), T. Ishizaka *et al.* (1973), and Malveáux *et al.* (1978) is not entirely clear but may reflect differences in methodology or patient population between Stallman's study and those of the other workers. Although the correlation between circulating and basophil-bound levels of IgE was initially thought to be poor (Sullivan *et al.*, 1971; T. Ishizaka *et al.*, 1973; Assem, 1974), more recent studies have demonstrated a good general correlation between circulating and basophil-bound IgE (Conroy *et al.*, 1977; Stallman and Aalberse, 1977a,b). Furthermore, both the degree of IgE receptor saturation and also the total number of IgE receptors (15,000–600,000/basophil) apparently are directly correlated with the serum concentration of IgE (Malveáux *et al.*, 1978). Factors other than receptor number and serum concentration of IgE contribute to basophil-bound levels of this immunoglobulin, however. The affinity of IgE for the basophils of individual humans, for example, may vary over more than a fortyfold range, possibly because of heterogeneity of the IgE receptor (T. Ishizaka *et al.*, 1973; Malveáux *et al.*, 1978). IgE receptor heterogeneity may be responsible for the observation that certain atopic patients have more cell-bound IgE than nonatopic individuals even in the face of similar serum concentrations of IgE (T. Ishizaka *et al.*, 1973; Stallman and Aalberse, 1977b; Malveáux *et al.*, 1978).

While IgE combines with basophils from all individuals, not all such passively allergized basophils release histamine with equal facility on subsequent exposure to specific allergens or to anti-IgE sera (T. Ishizaka *et al.*, 1973). Moreover, basophils from different donors with approximately the same amount of cell-bound IgE vary greatly in their ability to release histamine in response to either antigen (T. Ishizaka *et al.*, 1973) or anti-IgE (Conroy *et al.*, 1977). These findings support the concept that individual basophils, in addition to differences in their affinity for IgE, may exhibit intrinsic differences in their sensitivity to degranulation stimuli (T. Ishizaka *et al.*, 1973; Lichtenstein and Conroy, 1977).

The amount of IgE bound to mast cells *in vivo* has been most carefully studied in rats. Normal rat peritoneal mast cells have on the order of $2–10 \times 10^5$ receptors for IgE/cell (Conrad *et al.*, 1975; DeMeyts, 1976; T. Ishizaka *et al.*, 1975; Mendoza and Metzger, 1976), somewhat more than the figure given for human basophils (T. Ishizaka *et al.*, 1973; Conroy *et al.*, 1977; Stallman and Aalberse, 1977a; Malveáux *et al.*, 1978). While only about 10% of the receptors are occupied by IgE *in vivo* in normal rats (Mendoza and Metzger, 1976), the majority of receptors bear IgE when the animals are infected with the parasite *Nippostrongylus brasiliensis* (T. Ishizaka *et al.*, 1975). *N. brasiliensis*-infected rats have circulating IgE levels up to 300 times those of normal rats, indicating that the amount of IgE bound to peritoneal mast cells correlates with serum levels of IgE in this species. Such a relationship cannot always be demonstrated, however, and in both humans (T. Ishizaka *et al.*, 1969) and *Ascaris*-infected dogs (Halliwell, 1973) there is evidence that the correlation between circulating and cutaneous mast cell-bound levels of IgE may be poor in individual cases. There does appear to be, however, a rough correlation between basophil-bound and cutaneous mast-cell-bound specific (T. Ishizaka *et al.*, 1969) and total (Stallman *et al.*, 1977b) IgE in individual humans. As a result, the allergic status of many patients may be estimated about as accurately by either intradermal tests or the measurement of antigen-induced histamine release from basophils *in vitro* (Lichtenstein *et al.*, 1967; Norman *et al.*, 1973). Exceptions to this generalization have been reported (Bernstein *et al.*, 1977; Siraganian, 1977).

Immunofluorescence studies of the subcellular distribution of IgE in cutaneous mast cells in the monkey (Hubscher *et al.*, 1970a,b) and dog (Halliwell, 1973) and in intestinal mast cells in the rat (Mayrhofer *et al.*, 1976) have demonstrated bright staining of cytoplasmic granules, but variable and generally less intense staining of the cytoplasmic membrane. Furthermore, monitoring of the subcellular localization of intradermally injected homologous canine IgE by immunofluorescence microscopy indicated an apparent transfer of IgE from the mast cell surface to intracytoplasmic granules that occurred as early as 1 hr after passive sensitization (Halliwell, 1973). Appropriate controls excluded the possibility of nonspecific binding of immunoglobulin to mast cell granules. (Such controls are particularly important in light of the finding that rat mast cell granules, after certain methods of tissue fixation, apparently bind immunoglobulin of several classes nonspecifically; Simson *et al.*, 1977.) By contrast, an immunofluorescence study of mast cells of human adenoids, tonsils, nasal polyps, and skin has demonstrated a predominantly cytoplasmic membrane distribution of IgE (Feltkamp-Vroom *et al.*, 1975). The relevance of these morphological observations to the immunobiology of mast cells and homocytotropic antibody awaits clarification.

Recent work in man and experimental animals has called attention to the presence of IgG homocytotropic antibodies that differ from IgE in both physicochemical and biological properties. These molecules, in comparison with IgE, are resistant both to heat and to reduction alkylation, have much lower affinities for target cell membranes, have a much longer half-life in the circulation and a much shorter half-life in the skin, and on a molar basis are much less potent activators of antigen-mediated degranulation. Although their biological roles are yet to be clearly established, they conceivably could cause significant mediator release *in vivo* despite their low target cell affinity by virtue of their relatively high concentrations in the serum. Conversely, since in some species they are thought to compete for the same membrane receptor as IgE (Bach *et al.*, 1971b), they could function to block IgE-mediated reactions. Current knowledge of experimental animal (Stechschulte, 1978) and human (Parish, 1978) non-IgE homocytotropic antibody has been recently reviewed.

4.3. Mechanisms of IgE-Mediated Histamine Release

Although certain differences have been noted in the biochemical events associated with IgE-mediated histamine release in basophils and mast cells, many features are shared (Austen *et al.*, 1974; Lichtenstein, 1968; Lichtenstein *et al.*, 1973a; Lichtenstein and Henney, 1974; Plaut and Lichtenstein, 1978). We will therefore present a general outline of these processes as they are thought to occur in both of these cells, calling attention to differences between basophils and mast cells when this seems appropriate. It should be remembered that most studies of basophil or mast cell degranulation have been carried out *in vitro* in relatively simple media without serum and have largely excluded the activity of serum factors that may either enhance (Lichtenstein and Osler, 1966a; Siraganian and Levine, 1975; Ida *et al.*, 1977) or inhibit (Lichtenstein and Osler, 1966b; Lichtenstein *et al.*, 1968) antigen-mediated histamine release. Nevertheless, these studies have provided important information about biochemical mechanisms and are clearly relevant to *in vivo* phenomena. Thus in studies of IgE-mediated histamine release using human peripheral blood leukocyte preparations usually containing about 1% basophils a good correlation was found among the sensitivity of the donors' cells to ragweed antigen *in vitro,* skin test results, and the degree of allergic symptomatology (Lichtenstein, 1968; Lichtenstein *et al.,* 1966, 1973a; Norman *et al.*, 1973; Bruce *et al.*, 1974). Furthermore, basophil histamine release determined in whole blood generally correlates very well both with skin test results and with histamine release from washed leukocytes (Siraganian and Brodsky, 1976; Siraganian, 1977).

Recent studies strongly suggest that the initiation of IgE-mediated degranulation requires the bridging of adjacent molecules of cell-bound IgE to form IgE dimers. Bridging may be produced either by divalent or multivalent antigen or by other mechanisms (e.g., anti-IgE); either of these interactions triggers granule release (T. Ishizaka and K. Ishizaka, 1973). Thus monovalent anti-IgE antibody (incapable of bridging) does not cause histamine release. Moreover, studies performed with IgE–allergen complexes prepared in various proportions indicate that IgE:allergen ratios of 2:1 or greater are required to provoke histamine release, whereas complexes with ratios of 1:2 (both IgE antibody receptors bound to separate antigen molecules) do not release histamine. Although the minimum number of IgE dimers required to initiate degranulation is not known, mast cells or basophils are exquisitely sensitive to specific antigen: picogram quantities of allergen (about 100 molecules per basophil) are often sufficient to provoke substantial histamine release (Lichtenstein, 1968; Lichtenstein *et al.,* 1973a). Release is inhibited in substantial antigen excess.

IgE bridging with consequent histamine release apparently may occur in the absence of an antigen–antibody interaction because nonspecifically aggregated IgE molecules or their aggregated Fc fragments may alone trigger basophil histamine release. However, neither monomeric Fc fragments nor aggregated $F(ab')_2$ release mediators. Segal *et al.* (1977) have demonstrated that preparations of soluble IgE dimers can initiate rat mast cell exocytosis in the absence of antigen, whereas monomers show no activity. Recent work indicates that the cross-linking of the IgE receptor alone, by antireceptor antibody, apparently is sufficient to cause histamine release (T. Ishizaka *et al.,* 1977; Isersky *et al.,* 1978).

Primarily on the basis of studies performed in the mast cell with organophosphorus compounds such as diisopropylfluorophosphate (DFP), it has been postulated that one of the earliest events in IgE-mediated histamine release is the activation of a serine esterase closely associated with the receptor for IgE (Austen and Brocklehurst, 1961; Becker and Austen, 1964, 1966; Becker and Henson, 1973;

Taylor and Sheldon, 1974). Cytoplasmic-membrane-associated, stimulus-activated serine proteases appear to be common to a variety of cells, and such enzymes may have a general role in mediator cell activation (Becker and Henson, 1973; Kaliner and Austen, 1973; Henson, 1974; Musson and Becker, 1977). Based on the sensitivity of mast cell degranulation to various serine esterase inhibitors, all of which inhibit degranulation only if present during esterase activation (e.g., by antigen), it is possible that identical (or very similar) enzymes participate in the mediator release induced by antigen C5a (Becker and Austen, 1966; Austen and Becker, 1966) and a neutrophil lysosomal cationic protein (Ranadive and Cochrane, 1971; Ranadive and Muir, 1972). Certain other mast cell/basophil degranulating agents probably bypass this step (see Section 4.4), although there is disagreement on this point (Van Arsdel and Bray, 1961; Ranadive and Ruben, 1973; Taylor and Sheldon, 1974). It seems likely (Pruzansky and Patterson, 1975) that the activation of a masked or inactive serine esterase also is an important early step in IgE-mediated degranulation of human basophils. Although an earlier study (Lichtenstein and Osler, 1966b) reported that basophils previously treated with DFP *failed* to release histamine on subsequent exposure to antigen, these results may very well have reflected a nonspecific, toxic effect of DFP rather than the presence of active esterase on unstimulated basophils (Lichtenstein, personal communication). It should also be noted that organophosphorus compounds may have biological effects apparently unrelated to their ability to phosphorylate serine esterases (Woodin and Wieneke, 1970) and that such effects have not been rigorously excluded in much of the work done on this problem.

The relationship of any stimulus-activatable surface protease involved in degranulation to the other granule and cytoplasmic-membrane-associated proteases of the mast cell and basophil, especially the IgE-inactivating protease that has been identified in particulate (membrane) fractions of sonicated rat peritoneal mast cells (Bach *et al.*, 1978), remains to be determined.

While it is not known how the early biochemical events at the cell surface initiate the intracellular morphological changes leading to degranulation, it is clear that basophils or mast cells activated to release mediators undergo characteristic alterations in intracellular levels of cyclic AMP (cAMP). The early evidence for this, derived from human peripheral blood leukocytes (Lichtenstein and Margolis 1968; Lichtenstein and DeBernardo, 1971; Bourne *et al.*, 1972; Lichtenstein *et al.*, 1973b) and from mast cells of human (Assem and Richter, 1971; Orange *et al.*, 1971; Wasserman *et al.*, 1974b), guinea pig (Assem and Richter, 1971), and monkey (T. Ishizaka *et al.*, 1970, 1971a) lung, human skin (Assem and Richter, 1971), and rat peritoneal cavity (Johnson and Moran, 1970; Loeffler *et al.*, 1971), was largely circumstantial in that it was based on pharmacological studies with tissues or cell suspensions containing a small minority of mast cells or basophils. This work nevertheless clearly established that many agents that are capable of affecting intracellular levels of cAMP (including certain drugs long used clinically in the treatment of allergic disorders) can significantly modulate antigen-mediated degranulation. For example, mediator release can be inhibited by β-adrenergic agonists, E prostaglandins, cholera enterotoxin, and other agents that stimulate adenylyl cyclase and hence increase the conversion of ATP to cAMP, or by methylxanthines and other agents that inhibit the phosphodiesterase that destroys cAMP. Even histamine itself, via activation of H_2 receptors, leads to both increased intracellular cAMP and inhibition of histamine release *in vitro* and might thereby serve as a feedback mechanism for inhibiting its own release in certain circumstances *in vivo* (Bourne *et al.*, 1971; Lichtenstein and Gillespie, 1973, 1975; Charkin *et al.*, 1974; Plaut *et al.*, 1975). This inhibitory effect of cAMP on the secretion of mediators from basophils, mast cells, and other inflammatory cells is novel in that *elevation* of cAMP facilitates secretion in many other cell types (Bourne *et al.*, 1974; Lichtenstein and Henney, 1974).

More recently, the critical role of cAMP in mediator release has been convincingly established by direct measurements of cAMP levels both in very pure preparations of rat peritoneal mast cells (Sullivan *et al.*, 1975a,b; 1976) and in basophil-rich (77% normal-appearing basophils) leukocyte preparations from a patient with chronic myelogenous leukemia (Lichtenstein *et al.*, 1978). Histamine release in both of these systems, whether initiated by anti-IgE (mast cells, basophils) or by concanavalin A (Con A) or agent 48/80 (mast cells), was first detected after the onset of a striking fall in the intracellular concentration of cAMP. The findings in basophils or mast cells did, however, differ in certain respects. In basophils, anti-IgE produced an initial, very transient (seconds) increase in cAMP, followed by an abrupt and sustained (minutes) fall to below baseline level that in turn was followed by histamine release. The sequence of events in Con-A- or anti-IgE-treated mast cells was similar, with one important exception: although histamine release began during a period of rapidly dropping levels of cAMP, significant histamine release did occur before these levels actually fell below baseline. Agent 48/80 produced only a marked drop in cAMP levels, perhaps because this agent bypasses certain early events in the activation sequence. Other studies have also demonstrated that mast cells may differ from basophils in their response to agents that affect cAMP levels (Norn, 1965; Yamasaki and Saeki, 1967; Johnson *et al.*, 1974). Although the mechanism by which cAMP modulates mediator release is yet to be precisely defined, it has been suggested that reduction in levels of cAMP may permit an influx of Ca^{2+} during the "release" phase of histamine release (Foreman and Mongar, 1975; Foreman *et al.*, 1973, 1975, 1976), perhaps through effects related to the cells' microtubule system (Lichtenstein *et al.*, 1973a; Lichtenstein and Henney, 1974; Gillespie, 1975; Lichtenstein, 1975a, 1976).

The secretory function of mast cells and basophils, like that of many types of cell (Rubin, 1974), is critically dependent on Ca^{2+}. Thus cells may be "activated" for histamine release in the absence of calcium and then washed free of fluid (nonbound) antigen, but histamine release will not follow unless the cells are promptly returned to a medium containing calcium at 37°C. Lanthanum chloride, which blocks calcium flux, inhibits histamine release (Lichtenstein and Henney, 1974), and the fusion of calcium-containing phospholipid vesicles with the mast cell plasma membrane appears to be a sufficient stimulus to initiate exocytosis (Theoharides and Douglas, 1978).

It is of interest that if basophils are held in the "activated" state without Ca^{2+} for too long (beyond 2–4 min at 37°C), the activated state "decays" and the cell becomes unresponsive to further challenges with homologous or non-cross-reacting antigen. (Lichtenstein, 1971; Lichtenstein and DeBernardo, 1971). A similar "desensitization" phenomenon had previously been noted with mast cells (Mongar and Schild, 1957). There is evidence that the net histamine release observed for any given set of conditions reflects a balance between simultaneous activation and desensitization processes, and desensitization may serve to limit mediator release under certain circumstances *in vivo* (Baxter and Adamik, 1975; Foreman *et al.*, 1976). Because desensitization exhibits a certain amount of stimulus specificity, it has been used as an experimental tool in the investigation of the mechanisms by which various agents cause basophil or mast cell degranulation (Morrison and Henson, 1978; Morrison, 1978).

In the basophil, an intact cell-glycolytic pathway is also required for the completion of degranulation, and metabolic antagonists such as fluoride or 2-deoxyglucose inhibit histamine release (Lichtenstein *et al.*, 1973a). Oxidative metabolism, however, is not necessary, and neither cyanide, dinitrophenol, nor incubation in an atmosphere of nitrogen inhibits histamine release. In the mast call, either glycolysis or oxidative phosphorylation may provide the ATP necessary for degranulation (Chakravarty, 1968; Kaliner and Austen, 1974), although it is likely that glycolysis alone is sufficient (Mongar and Perera, 1965; Perera and Mongar, 1965). Both ATP and Ca^{2+} may be required for the formation of the granule–granule and granule–cytoplasmic membrane fusions characteristic of anaphylactic degranulation and/or for the function of the contractile proteins (e.g., microfilaments) implicated in mediator release (see Section 5.1) (Becker and Henson, 1973).

4.4. Other Factors That Induce Degranulation

Whereas immediate-type hypersensitivity reactions, by definition (Gell and Coombs, 1968), are initiated by the interaction of antigen with cell-bound homocytotropic antibody, a variety of chemically and physically diverse stimuli are capable of producing a sequence of morphological changes, accompanied by mediator release, that are indistinguishable from antigen-induced degranulation (Uvnäs and Thon, 1966; Lagunoff, 1972a). Despite the morphological similarity of the final result, it appears likely that individual degranulating agents may react with distinct mast cell/basophil cytoplasmic membrane components. The evidence for this and for the concept that different degranulation stimuli may initiate distinct biochemical pathways has been recently reviewed (Morrison, 1978; Morrison and Henson, 1978).

Anti-IgE antibody in the mast cell (T. Ishizaka *et al.*, 1975) or basophil (Osler *et al.*, 1968; K. Ishizaka and T. Ishizaka, 1969; T. Ishizaka *et al.*, 1971b), or anti-IgG class homocytotropic antibodies in the rat mast cell (Kaliner and Austen, 1974), can produce noncytolytic, complement-independent mediator release, presumably by IgE dimer formation. Antibody to rat immunoglobulin may also cause rat mast cell histamine release by a complement-dependent (Austen and Humphrey, 1961; Keller, 1962; Humphrey *et al.* 1963) although noncytolytic (Johnson and Moran, 1969b) mechanism. By contrast, mediator release occurs concurrently with or as a consequence of the complement-dependent cytotoxicity of anti-rat mast cell (Valentine *et al.*, 1967) or anti-guinea pig basophil (Galli *et al.*, 1978) antisera.

Micromolar concentrations of complement fragments C3a and/or C5a, the so-called anaphylatoxins, are capable of causing noncytolytic mediator release from mast cells (Johnson *et al.*, 1975) and basophils (Grant *et al.*, 1975; Hook *et al.*, 1975; Petersson *et al.*, 1975). Although anaphylatoxin- and IgE-mediated degranulation share certain biochemical features, differences have been reported in the kinetics of release. Thus, compared with antigen-IgE, the kinetics of anaphylatoxin-initiated release may be slower in the rat mast cell (Cochrane and Müller-Eberhard, 1968; Morrison *et al.*, 1975a) but faster in the human basophil (Grant *et al.*, 1975; Siraganian and Hook, 1976). Several other biologically derived substances have also been shown to cause noncytolytic mast cell degranulation when present in relatively low concentrations; any or all of them may function under certain circumstances *in vivo*. These include neutrophil (Janoff *et al.*, 1965; Seegers and Janoff, 1966; Ranadive and Cochrane, 1968, 1970; Keller, 1968) and eosinophil (Archer and Jackas, 1965) lysosomal granule polypeptides and insect and reptile venom polypeptides (Habermann, 1972). A cationic protein isolated from cobra venom, cobra venom activator or CVA protein (Morrison *et al.*, 1975b), is one of the most potent of all mast cell degranulators, promoting noncytolytic mediator release when present in concentrations of 0.025 μM, about a hundredfold less than active concentrations of anaphylatoxins. Chymotrypsin (Uvnäs and Antonsson, 1963; Saeki, 1964; Bach *et al.*, 1971b) and other proteases (Bach *et al.*, 1971b) may cause noncytolytic mast cell degranulation. Whether exogenous proteases affect the same substrate as any endogenous stimulus-activatable serine esterase involved in degranulation has not been determined.

Lectins (e.g., concanavalin A), certain polymers (e.g., Compound 48/80, Dextran), polymyxin B, and certain ionophores can produce noncytolytic degranulation of mast cells and also, in many cases, of basophils. Although all of these agents produce morphological changes similar or identical to those seen with antigen-mediated degranulation, they apparently may do so by different mechanisms. Thus concanavalin A is thought to initiate an early step in the biochemical sequence leading to degranulation, perhaps by cross-linking cell-bound IgE (Siraganian and Siraganian, 1975) or other cell surface glycoproteins and/or glycolipids (Bach and Brashler, 1975), whereas the calcium ionophore (A23187, Eli Lilly, Co.) bypasses this early event and apparently functions indpendently of cAMP to directly promote Ca^{2+} egress into the cell (Foreman *et al.*, 1973, 1975; Lichtenstein, 1975b). Although the effects of these substances have been primarily of experimental interest, certain examples of IgE-independent mast cell and/or basophil degranulation may be clinically important, e.g., the sytemic anaphylaxis occasionally seen after the intravenous administration of radiocontrast dyes and the cold-induced degranulation of the basophils and mast cells of certain patents with cold urticaria (Juhlin and Shelley, 1961).

The frequent participation of basophils and/or mast cells in immunological reactions of delayed onset (see Section 6) and the occurrence of cytoplasmic granule alterations in these cells (Sections 5.2 and 5.4) suggest that lymphocytes or their products may modulate the function of basophils participating in these reactions. Incubation of guinea pig basophils for up to 48 hr with lymphocyte supernatants demonstrating MIF activity does result in a slight but statistically significant increase in the proportion of basophils exhibiting motile configurations by electron microscopy; however, there is no evidence of concomitant histamine release or altered histamine synthesis by these cells (Galli *et al.*, unpublished observations). In contrast, Theuson *et al.* (1977, 1979) have demonstrated that a product of human mononuclear cell cultures does liberate histamine from basophils with rapid kinetics. Preliminary evidence indicates that the factor is a T-cell product recovered from the same gel-exclusion chromatographic fractions of culture supernatants as basophil chemotactic factor. These data offer additional support to the hypothesis that lymphocytes modulate basophil function *in vivo*.

5. Morphological Features of Basophil Degranulation

5.1. Basophil Anaphylactic Degranulation

Exposure of the basophils of atopic patients to specific allergens results in a prompt and explosive discharge of granules along with their contained mediators such as histamine (Shelley and Juhlin, 1961). This anaphylactic process occurs either *in vivo* or *in vitro* and is generally complete within 5–15 min. When observed *in vitro* by phase-contrast microscopy (Hastie, 1971), human basophils exposed to specific antigen at first lose their oriented motility and spread out on the coverglass support, extending active pseudopodia in several directions. Basophils that go on to degranulate suddenly develop several phase-pale cytoplasmic "vesicles," many of which quickly increase in size and coalesce to form large, pale, membrane-bound structures that displace the nucleus to the cell periphery. There is a concomitant reduction in the number of identifiable cytoplasmic granules. Subsequently, the vesicles themselves become fainter and disappear over the course of 1 or 2 sec. The actual discharge of granule contents from human basophils generally cannot be observed with phase-contrast microscopy. Most degranulated basophils subsequently become less spread and recover some ameboid motility, indicating that they remain viable.

The most complete ultrastructural studies of basophil anaphylactic degranulation have been performed with guinea pig basophils (Chan, 1972; A. Dvorak *et al.*, unpublished data). The first morphological change is the formation of zones of reduced electron density between the dense granule matrix and its limiting membrane, with consequent granule swelling and variable loosening of the normally tightly packed matrix; these changes suggest partial granule dissolution. Fusion of such altered granules with each other forms intracytoplasmic "vacuoles" (Figure 3) that then fuse with the plasma membrane, permitting the sudden explosive release of partially dissolved granule content into the extracellular space. Contractile microfilaments may participate in these events, and, compared to controls, degranulating basophils, like degranulating mast cells (Behrendt *et al.*, 1978), appear to have increased numbers of these structures in their cytoplasm.

This sequence of changes closely resembles that associated with anaphylactic degranulation of rat, mouse (Mann, 1969b; Röhlich *et al.*, 1971; A. Dvorak, unpublished data), or human (Trotter and Orr, 1973, 1974; Behrendt *et al.*, 1978) mast cells. However, preliminary evidence suggests that rabbit basophils may not follow this pattern (Benveniste *et al.*, 1973).

The anaphylactic pattern of degranulation may also occur in the absence of known exogenous stimuli. A substantial fraction of circulating mature basophils from a patient with basophilic leukemia and a markedly elevated urine histamine content exhibited changes very similar to those seen in guinea pig basophil anaphylactic degranulation (A. Dvorak *et al.*, 1976a). Extrusion of intact granules was not observed.

5.2. Degranulation of Basophils Participating in Delayed-Onset Hypersensitivity Reactions

Although morphological changes of the type described in anaphylaxis have been reported in basophils participating in certain delayed-onset reactions [e.g., those provoked in guinea pigs by cutaneous (Allen, 1973) and intestinal (Rothwell and Dineen, 1972) parasites], such anaphylactic changes have only rarely been observed in basophils infiltrating most other forms of delayed-onset hypersensitivity [e.g., cutaneous basophil hypersensitivity (CBH) in the guinea pig and comparable lesions in man (H. Dvorak *et al.*, 1970, 1973, 1974a; A. Dvorak *et al.*, 1976b)]. Basophils participating in such reactions do, however, regularly exhibit other

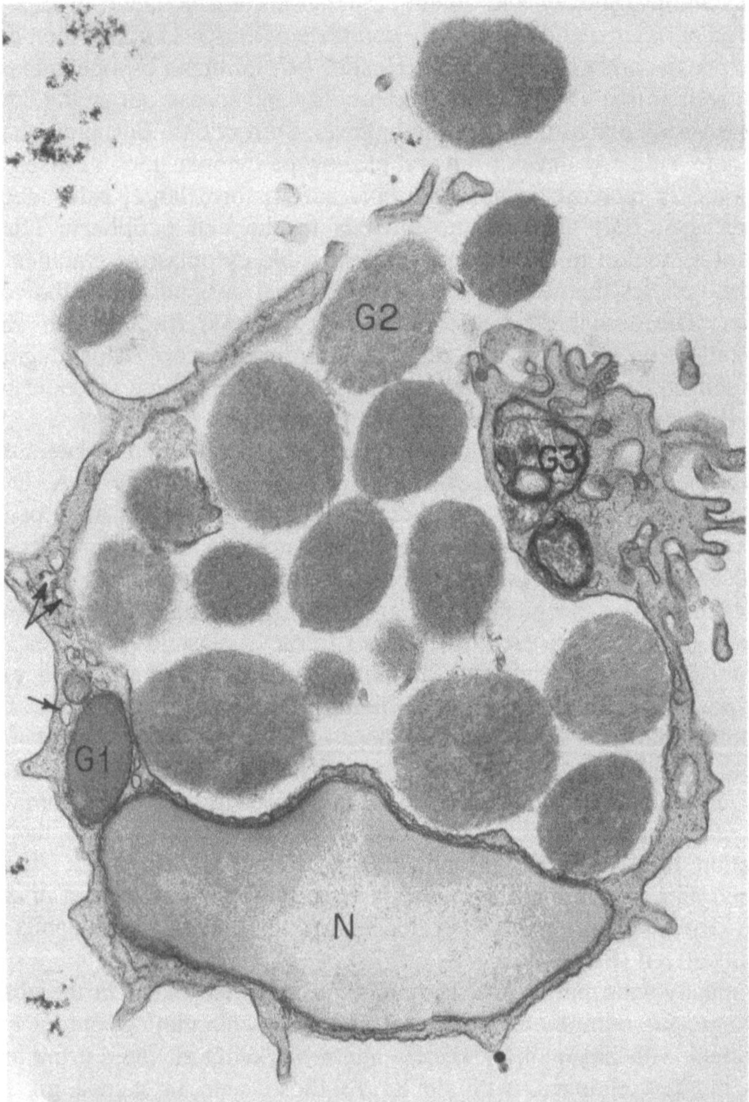

Figure 3. Electron photomicrograph of a guinea pig basophil undergoing anaphylactic-type degranulation induced by concanavalin A. The attenuated cytoplasm contains an intact granule (G1) and numerous vesicles (arrows). Fusion of the majority of granule membranes has formed a large sac open to the cell exterior that permits extrusion of granules (for example, G2) exhibiting loosening of their electron-dense matrix. Some granules (G3) remaining in the cytoplasm contain electron-dense membrane inclusions. 16,800×. Reprinted from A. Dvorak (1978), p. 391, by courtesy of Dekker, New York.

striking alterations in their cytoplasmic granules that are seen progressively over a period of days as the reactions evolve. In human lesions there is a loss of metachromatic granule staining, and many granules, both by light and electron microscopy, appear as lucent vacuoles (Figure 1). In 72-hr reactions of allergic contact dermatitis, 60% of basophils were found to be nearly or completely degranulated by this mechanism, whereas an additional 30% were partly degranulated (A. Dvorak *et al.*, 1976b).

By electron microscopy (H. Dvorak *et al.*, 1974a; A. Dvorak *et al.*, 1976b). The granules of such basophils exhibit localized peripheral zones of diminished electron density (Figure 4A) that may be found in close association or open communication with membrane-bound vesicles fused with the granule membrane (Figure 5). Glycogen particles may be intimately associated with such altered granules, particularly at their points of attachment to vesicles (Figure 5B). More severely affected granules exhibit a diffuse loss of electron-dense granule substance (Figure 4B); in extreme form, such granules appear as slightly enlarged, electron-lucent, membrane-bound vacuoles nearly or completely devoid of particles (Figures 1 and 4D). Basophils undergoing these changes frequently exhibit large accumulations of membranes within both normal-appearing and altered cytoplasmic granules. Fusion of basophil granules with the plasma membrane and extrusion of intact granules from the cell have not been observed in human basophils participating in delayed-onset reaction. Very rarely, several granules fused to form aggregates, a feature of anaphylactic degranulation.

An additional feature of basophils participating in these reactions is the presence in the cytoplasm of numerous 500- to 700-Å membrane-bound vesicles (Figure 4B) of the type seen in guinea pig basophils pinocytosing horseradish peroxidase (A. Dvorak *et al.*, 1972). The majority of these vesicles are free in the cytoplasm and are morphologically indistinguishable from pinocytotic vesicles. Others, however, are found attached to granules or are fused with the plasma membrane in communication with the extracellular space. In basophils exhibiting this nonanaphylactic or "piecemeal" degranulation, some vesicles at all levels of the cytoplasm contain particles similar in structure and electron density to those composing the cytoplasmic granules (Figure 4C); others contain finely granular material similar to that contained in peripheral zones of altered granules. Elongated tubulovesicular structures, possibly derived from the fusion of several contiguous vesicles, are occasionally observed as well. It is therefore possible that some of the vesicles described here represent cross sections taken through continuous serpentine channels. However, if the vesicular structures observed in basophil cytoplasm represent sections through a canalicular system, these channels must either be discontinuous or semipermanent organelles or have some other means of preventing a free interchange between the granules and the cell surface under normal circumstances.

5.3. Model of Basophil Degranulation

The data presented above indicate that basophils either may extrude their granules by anaphylactic mechanisms or may release both granule contents and ingested tracers under conditions in which direct fusion of the granule and plasma membranes apparently does not occur. To explain these findings, a general model of basophil degranulation has been proposed that can account for the varied rates of granule substance release occurring under a variety of physiological and pathological circumstances (A. Dvorak *et al.*, 1972, 1976b; H. Dvorak *et al.*, 1974a; H. Dvorak and A. Dvorak, 1972) and that provides a morphological basis for understanding the roles of basophils both in immediate-type and in certain delayed-type hypersensitivity phenomena. The model holds that loss of granule contents occurs under nonanaphylactic conditions by means of exocytotic vesicles that bud from the granule membrane, carrying with them small quanta of intact or dissolved granule material, and that flow to the cell surface where they fuse with the plasma membrane and discharge their contents into the extracellular space. The glycogen aggregates closely applied to granules at sites of vesicle attachment

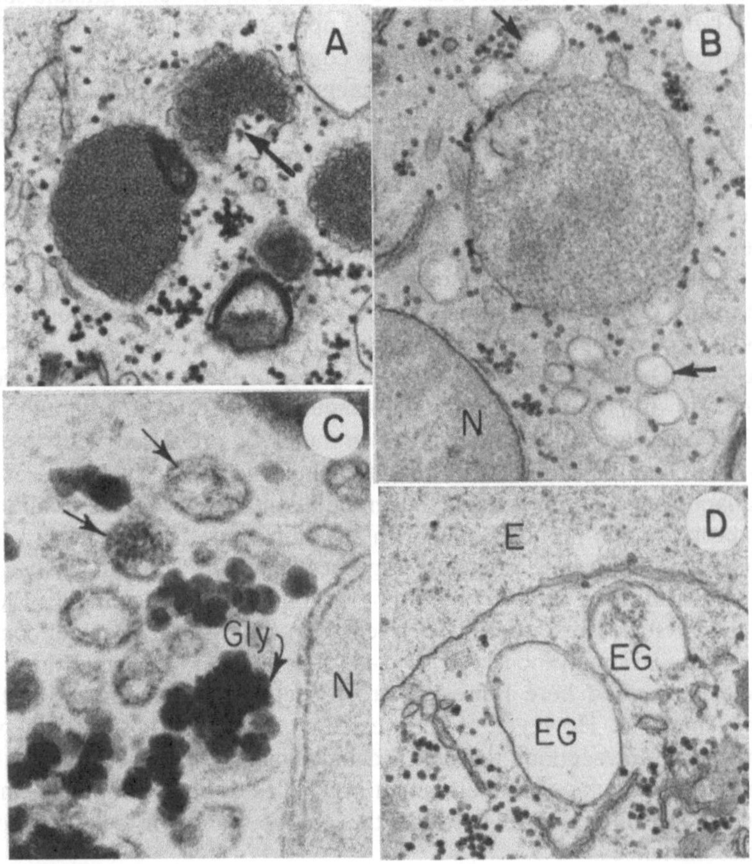

Figure 4. Electron photomicrographs of human basophils in various stages of degranulation in contact allergy. A shows an intact granule with an electron-dense matrix and focal membrane accumulations. An adjacent granule has focal loss of electron-dense content (arrow). In B, a granule exhibits reduced electron-dense content and is surrounded by numerous cytoplasmic vesicles (arrows). C illustrates several cytoplasmic vesicles, two containing what appears to be granule contents (arrows). The densely stained, non-membrane-bound particles are glycogen. Two empty granules (EG) in D have lost almost all their electron-dense contents. A and D, 28,200×; B, 34,800×; C, 98,000×. Reprinted from A. Dvorak (1978), p. 396, by courtesy of Dekker, New York.

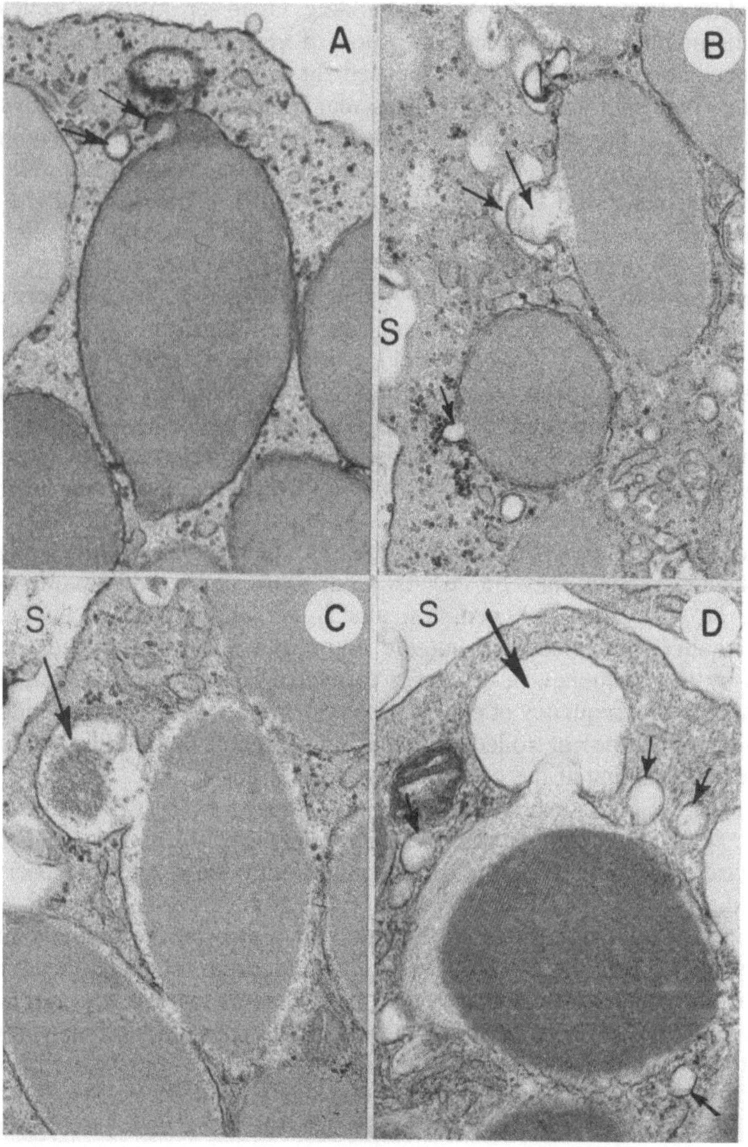

Figure 5. Electron photomicrographs of guinea pig basophils exhibiting features of vesicular degranulation. In A, a structure filled with electron-dense granule matrix material (thin arrow) projects from the surface of a basophil granule; an adjacent vesicle (thick arrow) appears empty. In B, at points oriented toward the cell surface (S), two granules have vesicles budding from their membrane (arrows). The smaller vesicle is intimately related to a cluster of glycogen particles. The larger vesicular outpouching invaginates another vesicle in the cytoplasm (indicated by adjacent arrow). In C, the large membrane-bound outpouching (arrow) from the granule apparently contains electron-dense granule material and approaches the cell surface (S). In D, the granule's electron-dense matrix is surrounded by a rim of looser fibrillar material that protrudes into a large clear vacuole (large arrow). Lucent vacuoles of this type may communicate with the cell surface (S) in another plane of section. The adjacent cytoplasm contains numerous vesicles (small arrows). A and D, 34,000×; B and C, 32,000×. Reprinted from A. Dvorak (1978), p. 394, by courtesy of Dekker, New York.

may afford an energy source for vesicle budding. Once separation of vesicles from the granule membrane is complete, transport of vesicles may proceed at random by Brownian motion, as has been proposed for the movement of similarly sized vesicles involved in transport across vascular endothelial cells (Karnovsky and Shea, 1970). A net flux of granule contents out of the cell will result from random vesicle movement if, for reasons of chemical structure, vesicles are able to fuse only with each other and with the membranes of other granules and the plasma membrane (which behave as absorbing surfaces) but not with the membranes limiting other cell organelles (nucleus, mitochondria, etc.).

Associated with vesicular exocytosis, it is useful to postulate a closely coupled transport of endocytotic (pinocytotic) vesicles migrating from the cell surface to the cytoplasmic granules. Coupled endocytosis is necessary to account for the undiminished (in fact, apparently somewhat increased) size of granules which are releasing their contents and hence are continuously losing portions of their enveloping membranes. The extracellular fluid transported to the granules by endocytotic vesicles may provide solvent for the partial dissolution of granules regularly observed, for example, in the basophils infiltrating the reactions of allergic contact dermatitis. Conceivably, the extra membranes accumulating within these basophil granules may be derived from those of the endocytotic vesicles, indicating an imbalance between vesicular influx and efflux. In our vesicular transport model, the release of granule contents ordinarily proceeds at a rate governed by the frequency of discharge of microvesicles from the granule membrane. Possibly the frequency of exocytosis is determined by the rate of endocytosis which, in turn, may be controlled and modified by agents (antibodies and probably other mediators) acting at the cell surface.

Based on the occasional granule alterations observed in "normal" circulating basophils, it is likely that a slow release of granule substances occurs under physiological conditions (or in the process of isolating these cells for observation). In delayed-type reactions degranulation apparently proceeds at a substantially greater pace. At still faster rates of degranulation a threshold would eventually be reached above which there would be insufficient time between successive discharges to permit complete separation of individual vesicles from the plasma or granule membranes or from each other. Under these conditions, endocytotic and/or exocytotic vesicles budding from the plasma or granule membranes would not form discrete, spherical structures, but rather would coalesce to form continuous channels. In fact, segments of tubulovesicular structures were occasionally observed in the basophils participating in allergic contact dermatitis or endocytosing HRP. Better-developed channels might link the cell surface with granules and/or interconnect neighboring granules, depending on random collisions with either the plasma or granule membranes. Continuous channels of this sort would lead to granule aggregation and fusion of granules with the plasma membrane, characteristic features of anaphylactic degranulation.

While this model adequately accounts for available data concerned with basophil endocytosis and degranulation, particularly as they are observed in the guinea pig, other possible explanations for these data do exist (A. Dvorak *et al.*, 1976b). The model, therefore, must be regarded as tentative until it can be more rigorously tested by methods that permit kinetic analysis of the movement of tracers and granule contents within individual basophils.

5.4. Mast Cell Degranulation

The kinetics and morphological features of rat mast cell degranulation in response to specific antigen, compound 48/80, and other agents are very similar to those already described in basophils (Röhlich *et al.*, 1971; Anderson *et al.*, 1973). Thus exocytosis occurs by the fusion of cytoplasmic granule membranes with each other and with the plasmic membrane, permitting either the release of granules from the cell or their exposure to extracellular medium by a complex series of cytoplasmic channels and vesicles. A very similar sequence of alterations has been described in degranulating human mast cells from several anatomical locations (Trotter and Orr, 1973, 1974; Behrendt *et al.*, 1978). A controversy concerns whether individual mast cell granules in unstimulated cells are always individually membrane bound or whether they may occur in sets of several granules invested by a common membrane (Padawer, 1978). Some investigators feel that such intergranule membrane fusions usually represent an early phase of granule exocytosis (Anderson *et al.*, 1973).

There has been relatively little investigation of the anatomical features of mast cells participating in delayed-onset immunological reactions. An ultrastructural study of allergic contact dermatitis in man (A. Dvorak *et al.*, 1976b) showed that, by the second or third day of the reaction, cutaneous mast cells exhibited striking granule alterations, including granule swelling, fusion between the membranes of adjacent granules and between granules and the plasma membrane, and loss of electron-dense granule content. These changes are similar to those seen in mast cells undergoing anaphylactic, IgE-mediated degranulation (Anderson *et al.*, 1973), even though the immunization procedures that were employed in Dvorak's study are thought to produce an entirely cell-mediated form of hypersensitivity. Extrusion of intact mast cell granules from the cells was not seen. At later intervals (beyond day 3), mast cells appeared increased in number and more immature, and occasional mast cell mitoses were observed. Bursztajn *et al.* (1978) have recently reported that mast cells participating in delayed hypersensitivity reactions in the mouse also exhibit a delayed-onset, progressive alteration of granule morphology unaccompanied by granule extrusion.

6. Roles in Hypersensitivity Reactions of Delayed Onset

6.1. Introduction

Morphological studies, employing modern methods of tissue fixation and processing, have provided conclusive evidence that basophils and/or mast cells participate in diverse delayed-onset immunological reactions in both man and experimental animals. It is important to emphasize that in this discussion we are using the designation "delayed onset" to imply only that a reaction becomes manifest hours to days after the organism experiences the inciting stimulus [usually antigen(s)]. Such reactions are pathogenetically heterogeneous and include at one extreme the delayed sequelae of classical immediate, homocytotropic antibody-mediated reactions, and, at the other extreme, classical T-cell-mediated delayed hypersensitivity. We will use the terms "delayed-type hypersensitivity" and "cell-mediated hypersensitivity" to refer to immunological reactions thought to be mediated by T cells without the participation of antibody.

There is no lack of speculation (some of it reasonably supported by experimental data) about the roles of basophils and mast cells in delayed-onset reactions. It must be stated at the outset, however, that much work remains to be done before our understanding of these cells' functions approaches our knowledge of other inflammatory cells such as the neutrophil, lymphocyte, or macrophages. In this section, we will review the evidence that mast cells and basophils participate in delayed-onset immunological phenomena and review current thinking about the roles of these cells in such reactions.

6.2. Homocytotropic Antibody-Mediated Reactions with Delayed Components

It has long been recognized that immediate IgE-dependent reactions may have late sequalae that are partially or largely mediated by vasoactive amine-facilitated deposition of immune complexes (Cochrane, 1971; Cochrane and Koffler, 1973). Polymorphonuclear leukocytes play a prominent role in these reactions, and appropriate immunofluorescence studies demonstrate the interstitial and/or vascular deposition of both immunoglobulins and complement components. Probable clinical examples of this phenomenon may be demonstrable in certain patients with bronchopulmonary aspergillosis or bird fancier's extrinsic allergic alveolitis. In these patients the intracutaneous injection of appropriate antigens produces the immediate wheal and flare of classical IgE-mediated hypersensitivity, followed by a complete resolution of the wheal and flare, and, 2–4 hr later, an erythematous, edematous reaction that is most intense at 6–12 hr. Histological studies (Pepys *et al.*, 1968) confirm the Arthus-like features of this phenomenon: edema, a prominent infiltrate of neutrophils with lesser numbers of mononuclear cells and some eosinophils, and the deposition of IgG, IgM, and complement components in vessel walls.

In contrast to the Arthus-like sequela of immediate cutaneous hypersensitivity, a second phenomenon has been described that apparently differs both in clinical evolution and in pathogenesis (Dolovich *et al.*, 1973; Solley *et al.*, 1976). These reactions are characterized by a response to intracutaneous antigen injection consisting initially of a typical wheal and flare that is followed by the gradual development of a pruritic, erythematous, indurated, and tender lesion that reaches maximal intensity at 6–12 hr and usually completely resolves by 24 hr. In contrast to the Arthus-like late reaction, this late phenomenon is not preceded by a complete resolution of the initial wheal-and-flare response, and histological studies of the reactions have failed to demonstrate significant deposition of either immunoglobulin or complement. Such reactions have been convincingly demonstrated to be mediated by IgE by passive transfer, and they may be duplicated by injecting the mast cell degranulating agent compound 48/80. That their development depends on mast cell or basophil mediators in addition to histamine is suggested by the inability of intradermal injection of histamine alone to produce any late reaction whatsoever, although histamine does provoke the initial wheal-and-flare response. Some studies have reported prominent perivascular infiltrates of mononuclear cells, neutrophils, and lesser numbers of eosinophils and basophils (Dolovich *et al.*, 1973; Solley *et al.*, 1976); others have emphasized the participation of eosinophils (Atkins *et al.*, 1973; Zweiman *et al.*, 1976). In contrast, a recent detailed study of the histology of these reactions (de Shazo *et al.*, 1979), employing histological methods that permit unambiguous identification of mast cells, basophils, and other leukocytes, has demonstrated a variable but generally sparse mixed cellular infiltrate predominantly composed of mononuclear cells but including variable numbers of neutrophils, basophils, and eosinophils (Figure 6). Of additional interest, the latter study, unlike previous work, also demonstrated significant interstitial fibrin deposition (Figure 6). This finding is not unexpected in view of the important role of fibrin in producing the induration characteristic of cutaneous delayed-type hypersensitivity (H. Dvorak and Mihm, 1972; Colvin *et al.*, 1973a; Colvin and H. Dvorak, 1975). As in previous studies, no deposition of immunoglobulins or complement was detected by immunofluorescence. The role of the mixed leukocytic infiltrate in these reactions in uncertain, particularly in view of the fact that identical sparse infiltrates may be observed at 6-hr antigen injection sites whether or not a macroscopically identifiable late reaction follows the initial wheal-and-flare response. Although mast cells (or basophils) can directly or indirectly generate several potentially important inflammatory mediators, the specific mechanisms by which IgE-triggered events lead to delayed cutaneous reactions are not yet clear (Soter and Austen, 1976).

In summary, it appears incontrovertible that certain late cutaneous reactions to intradermal antigens are initiated by IgE-dependent mast cell degranulation. The lack of detectable immunoglobulin or complement components in some of these reactions, and the inconsistent demonstration of a significant neutrophilic response, suggests that they are mediated without the participation of immune complexes and are not Arthus reactions. It should be remembered, however, that factors such as rapid local degradation can result in an inability to histologically identify immune complexes even in conditions known to have an immune-complex pathogenesis (McCluskey *et al.*, 1978). The mast cell mediators responsible for these phenomena have not been identified, although it is very unlikely that histamine alone could account for all the clinical and histological findings. Furthermore, although histamine effects could result in the extravascular leakage of fibrinogen, other as yet unknown factors, such as a failure of local fibrinolytic mechanisms, must be postulated to explain the deposition of fibrin in these reactions. Newball *et al.* (1975) have described the IgE-mediated release of a kallikrein-like activity from human leukocyte preparations containing approximately 1% basophils. Intradermal administration of kallikrein does produce a prolonged inflammatory response similar in some respects to IgE-mediated late reactions, and kallikrein also exhibits chemotactic activity for mononuclear cells and granulocytes. A kallikrein activity has not yet been demonstrated in mast cells, however.

Although the biological significance of these reactions is uncertain, it would certainly be worth investigating the role of similar mechanisms in certain dermatological conditions such as the chronic urticarias and in certain late asthmatic responses.

6.3. Basophils in Delayed-Onset Immunological Reactions

6.3.1. Cutaneous Basophil Hypersensitivity: Occurrence and Pathogenesis

In addition to their participation in immediate hypersensitivity phenomena, basophils have been clearly implicated in a variety of delayed-onset immune

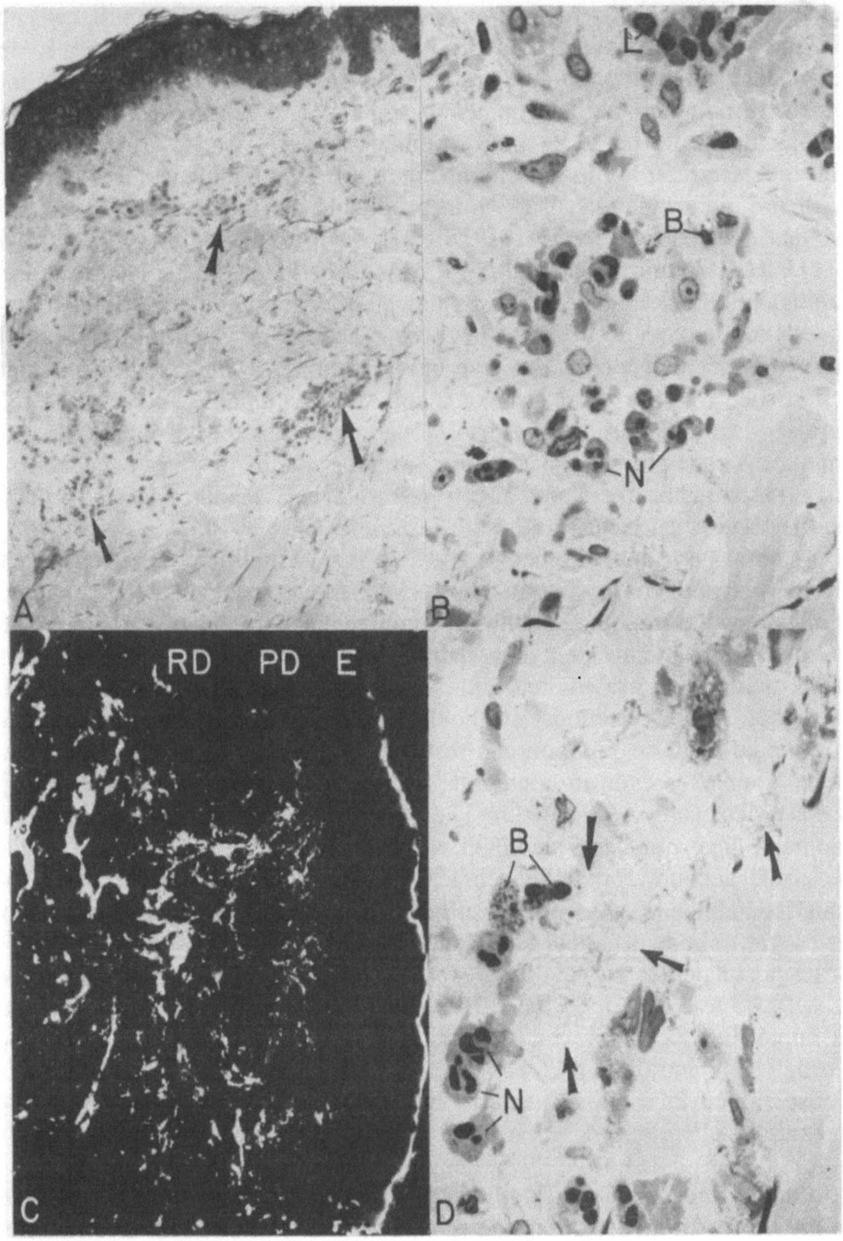

Figure 6. Six-hour late-phase reactions induced with ragweed and studied in 1-μm-thick, Epon-embedded, Giemsa-stained sections (A,B,D) or by immunofluorescence (C). A: Low-power overview indicating slight, largely perivenular inflammatory cell infiltrate (arrows) about vessels of the reticular dermis. B: Higher-magnification view illustrating the mixed cellular infiltrate characteristic of these reactions. L, Lymphocyte; B, basophil; N, neutrophil. C: Fresh-frozen cryostat section stained with anti-human fibrinogen/fibrin (Fib). Note extensive Fib deposits scattered in intervascular zones of the reticular dermis (RD), with relative sparing of papillary dermis (PD). Epidermis (E) is unstained except for artifactual linear staining of superficial stratum corneum. D: Intervascular reticular dermis illustrating meshwork of fibrin strands (arrows) as well as basophils (B) and neutrophils (N). A, 175×; B and D, 800×; C, 235×. Reduced 25% for reproduction. Reprinted from de Shazo *et al.* (1979), by courtesy of Williams and Wilkins, Baltimore.

reactions. Guinea pigs immunized by procedures that avoid the use of mycobacterial adjuvants develop a systemic form of delayed-onset reactivity termed "cutaneous basophil hypersensitivity" (CBH) (Richerson *et al.*, 1969, 1970; H. Dvorak *et al.*, 1970, 1971; H. Dvorak and Hammond, 1978). In contrast to classic, tuberculin-type delayed hypersensitivity (DH), CBH skin reactions are relatively nonindurated and are characterized by extensive infiltrations of basophilic leukocytes in addition to mononuclear cells. CBH reactions also lack extensive fibrin deposits, and, with many antigens, can be elicited only at early intervals after immunization. While most efficiently induced by the intradermal route with a few micrograms of protein, a similar state of reactivity may occur when larger doses of antigen are administered intravenously (Richerson, 1971). Similar reactivity may be induced in guinea pigs to biologically important antigens such as contact allergens (H. Dvorak *et al*, 1971; Medenica and Rostenberg, 1971), vaccinia virus (H. Dvorak and Hirsch, 1971), allogeneic tumor cells (H. Dvorak *et al.*, 1973), schistosomes (Askenase *et al.*, 1975a), ticks (Allen, 1973; Bagnall, 1975), and skin allografts (H. Dvorak, 1971; H. Dvorak *et al.*, 1977c). Although the expression of CBH has been most carefully studied in the skin of guinea pigs, delayed-onset reactions rich in basophils also occur in other organs and species, including the peritoneal rejection of ascites tumor cells (H. Dvorak *et al.*, 1973), the immune expulsion of intestinal metazoan parasites (Rothwell and Dineen, 1972; Rothwell, 1974; Rothwell and Love, 1975), ocular reactions to protein antigens (Freidlaender and Dvorak, 1977), and colonic contact hypersensitivity reactions to DNCB (Askenase *et al.*, 1978a) in guinea pigs; allergic contact dermatitis (H. Dvorak and Mihm, 1972; H. Dvorak *et al.*, 1974a, 1976) and skin (H. Dvorak *et al.*, 1977c) and renal (Colvin and Dvorak, 1974) allograft rejection in man; experimental allergic encephalomyelitis in rats (Hoenig and Levine, 1974); the response to Rous sarcoma virus (Burton and Higginbotham, 1966) and to a mitogen (Stadecker *et al.*, 1977) in chickens; and hypersensitivity reactions to protein antigens and *Staphylococcus aureus* in rabbits (Clark *et al.*, 1976) and to protein antigens and schistosomes in monkeys (H. Dvorak and Colvin, unpublished data).

Significant species differences exist in the frequency with which basophils participate in delayed-onset reactions, and, in some instances, the distinction between CBH and DH is blurred. Basophil infiltration, both absolute and relative, is substantially greater in the guinea pig and rabbit than in any other species thus far studied. In typical guinea pig CBH reactions, basophils are present in concentrations of 300–600/linear mm skin surface and comprise 20–60% of infiltrating cells (Figure 7). This concentration is the more remarkable in that basophils normally account for less than 1% of circulating leukocytes, a fraction not significantly altered by usual techniques of immunization and skin testing. Basophils also account for nearly 60% of cells infiltrating certain delayed-onset reactions in the rabbit (Clark *et al.*, 1976). However, this species may have up to 10 times as many circulating basophils as the guinea pig. In contrast, mature lesions of allergic contact dermatitis in man contain basophils, but these seldom exceed 200/linear mm and comprise $<15\%$ (often $<5\%$) of the infiltrate (H. Dvorak *et al.*, 1974a). Nevertheless, as would be predicted from guinea pig experiments, basophils are more numerous in allergic contact dermatitis in man than they are in classic delayed hypersensitivity reactions to microbial antigens (H. Dvorak *et al.*, 1974a; Askenase and Atwood, 1976).

Considerable work has been done in an attempt to define the role of antibodies as opposed to sensitized lymphocytes in the immunobiology of CBH reactions. CBH reactivity persists for a variable period of time depending on whether or not a significant antibody response ensues. In the case of antigens that induce a strong antibody response, such as most foreign proteins and sheep erythrocytes, CBH reactivity occurs only for 1–2 weeks after sensitization and is thereafter superseded

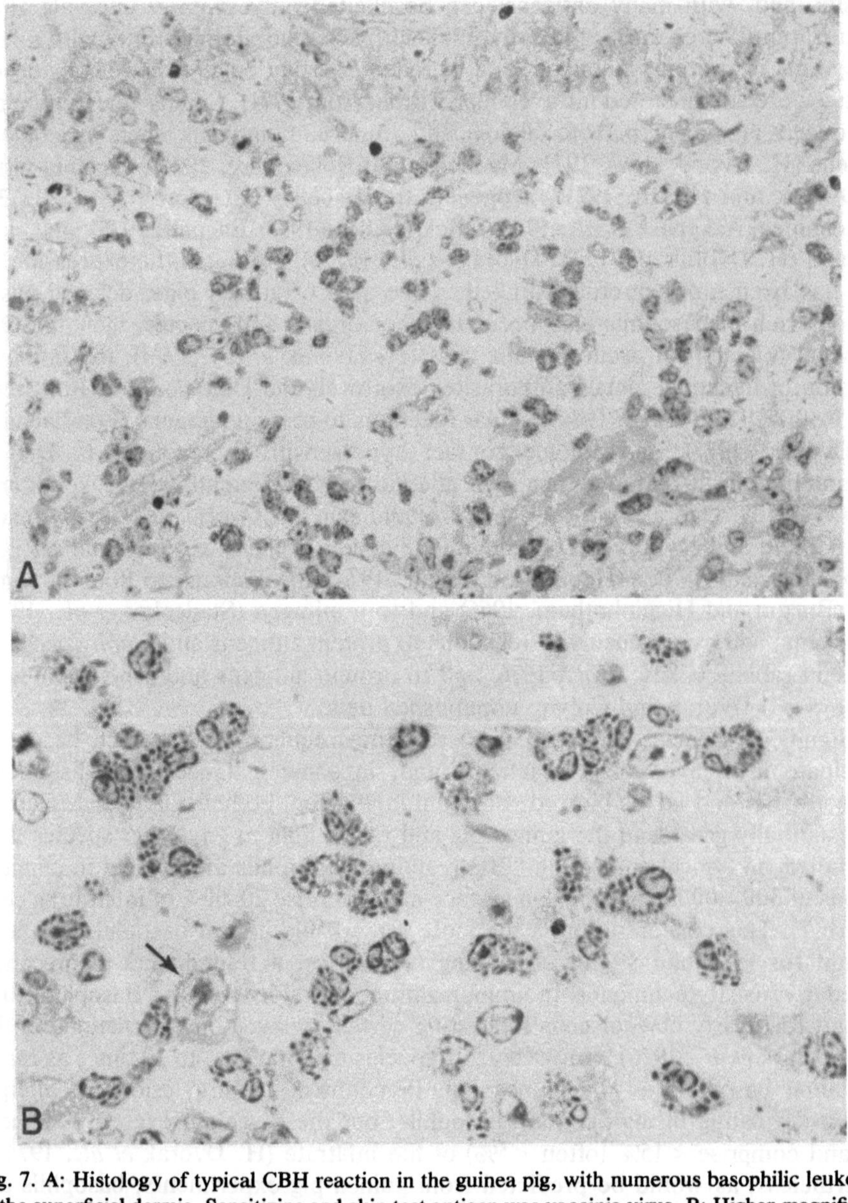

Fig. 7. A: Histology of typical CBH reaction in the guinea pig, with numerous basophilic leukocytes in the superficial dermis. Sensitizing and skin test antigen was vaccinia virus. B: Higher-magnification photomicrograph better illustrating basophils as polymorphonuclear leukocytes with prominent cytoplasmic granules. Arrow indicates a large activated mononuclear cell. A, 400×; B, 1000×. Both 1-μm Epon-embedded, Giemsa-stained sections. Reprinted from H. Dvorak and Hirsch (1971), by courtesy of Williams and Wilkins, Baltimore.

by the appearance of "late reactions," complex lesions composed of sequential but overlapping components of cutaneous anaphylaxis, Arthus reactivity, and a residual basophil component (Colvin *et al.*, 1973b). It is important to emphasize, however, that CBH reactions need not be transient and may persist indefinitely following immunization with antigens which do not initiate a significant antibody response. For example, the delayed-onset, basophil-rich responses to vaccinia virus (H. Dvorak and Hirsch, 1971), dinitrochlorobenzene (H. Dvorak *et al.*, 1971), and syngeneic tumor cells (H. Dvorak *et al.*, 1973) may be elicited many weeks or months after the onset of immunization.

While basophils are a prominent component of CBH reactions, there is no doubt that in many of these reactions T lymphocytes are essential to the induction and expression of this form of hypersensitivity just as they are in classical DH. Animals primed for CBH exhibit an expansion of the thymus-dependent paracortical zones of draining lymph nodes (A. Dvorak *et al.*, 1971), and reactivity may be inhibited by antilymphocyte serum (Richerson *et al.*, 1970). A highly specific anti-T-lymphocyte serum strikingly inhibits the expression of CBH *in vivo* (Stadecker and Leskowitz, 1976), and reactions may be passively transferred to normal recipients by viable sensitized lymph node cells (H. Dvorak *et al.*, 1971) or by peritoneal exudate cells, over 90% of which are T cells (Askenase, 1976). Katz *et al.* (1974) have presented evidence that the expression of both CBH and DH is determined by a balance between cyclophosphamide-sensitive "suppressor," presumably B cells, and cyclophosphamide-insensitive "effector" populations of lymphocytes. Recently, Stashenko *et al.* (1977) established that local transfer of CBH reactivity could be achieved about as effectively by intradermal injection of either purified T or B cells ($1–5 \times 10^6$) from the lymph nodes of guinea pigs primed for CBH reactivity. In contrast, classical DH reactivity to tuberculin could be transferred with as few as 0.5×10^6 T cells, whereas B cells could not transfer DH reactivity unless used in doses of $2–3 \times 10^6$. (Such "B-cell" transfer of DH reactivity was attributed to small numbers of contaminating T cells.) Locally transferred CBH reactions had relatively few basophils (about 6%, whether B or T cells were used) compared to CBH reactions elicited in systemically primed animals, which contain up to 60% basophils. Even fewer basophils (2–3%) were seen in locally transferred DH reactions, however. It is of interest that the purified T cells of guinea pigs primed for classical tuberculin DH, when administered systemically, may transfer reactions that closely resemble CBH (Askenase, 1976). Thus, although delayed skin reactions to tuberculin in donor animals contained only 1% basophils, reactions in recipient animals had 14–18% basophils. This study indicates that a factor(s) may exist that suppresses the infiltration of basophils into the delayed reactions of guinea pigs primed for classical DH. Further experimentation with defined populations of T and B lymphocytes will be required to determine the respective roles and possible interactions of each cell type, as well as other factors that enhance or suppress basophil infiltration, such as chemotactic molecules (see Section 6.3.2), in both CBH and DH.

In contrast to earlier workers, Askenase and associates have passively transferred basophil-rich reactions by means of serum from animals primed for CBH 7–8 days earlier (Askenase, 1973; Haynes *et al.*, 1974, 1975, 1978; Askenase *et al.*, 1975b, 1976). This has been accomplished both with certain hapten-specific CBH reactions and with CBH to certain protein antigens and contact allergens. While several milliliters of serum were required in earlier studies with adult animals, as little as 0.12 ml was effective in transferring reactivity to newborn recipients. Purification studies, including the use of immunoadsorbent columns, revealed that the active serum factor was a specific 7 $S\gamma_1$ antibody (Haynes *et al.*, 1978). Antibody-mediated CBH reactions have kinetics of onset and duration similar to those of T-cell-mediated CBH (or DH) but differ from cell-mediated CBH in certain respects. For example, when CBH reactions are passively transferred with cells, the reactions to intracutaneous challenge in the recipient always contain basophils (although in variable numbers), whether the sensitized lymphocytes are transferred systemically or locally (Stashenko *et al.*, 1977). In contrast, the sera that transfer CBH reactions, when administered systemically, transfer a passive cutaneous anaphylaxis-like reaction rich in eosinophils and devoid of basophils when administered locally (Askenase, 1977). This finding and the observation that the passive transfer of antibody-mediated CBH or PCA reactions may be blocked by normal immunoglobulins or by antibodies of heterologous antigenic specificity suggest to these workers that such reactions may be mediated in part by cutaneous mast cells and may be analogous to the IgE-mediated late reactions to cutaneous antigens described in humans (Askenase, 1977). Whatever the genesis of antibody-mediated CBH reactions, the reasons for the differences in the composition of the cellular infiltrates elicited by the systemic or local transfer of active sera have not been established.

Whether antibodies have any role in the pathogenesis of those CBH reactions that are transferable with T cells is not settled. Typical CBH reactions may be elicited at 4 days after sensitization, before antibodies can be detected by systemic passive or active cutaneous anaphylaxis or by routine serological methods. In fact, animals primed for CBH with certain antigens develop little or no detectable antibody at any interval after immunization. Moreover, intravenous or local injections of sensitizing antigens in guinea pigs bearing mature (24-hr) basophil-rich CBH reactions to human serum albumin (HSA) or to ovalbumin failed to induce vascular permeability alterations characteristic of histamine release, nor did they lead to overt basophil degranulation (H. Dvorak *et al.*, 1971; H. Dvorak, unpublished data). The situation may be different, however, in CBH reactions elicited to certain other antigens. For example, the injection of specific antigen into mature CBH reactions elicited to hemocyanin, an antigen that may produce antibody-dependent CBH and in any event induces a strong homocytotropic antibody response in guinea pigs, provokes both basophil degranulation and histamine release (DeBernardo *et al.*, 1975; Askenase *et al.*, 1978b).

In order to determine whether non-histamine-releasing antibodies might be present on the surface of basophils participating in CBH, direct interactions between basophils and antigen were studied by means of a sensitive rosetting technique (H. Dvorak *et al.*, 1975). Basophils were isolated from the blood or teased from skin reactions of CBH-primed animals and exposed to appropriate specific cell-bound antigens. Under these conditions, the overwhelming majority of basophils circulating in the blood or accumulating in skin reactions of CBH failed to form rosettes (less than 2%, 8%, and 1% of basophils recovered in guinea pigs sensitized to sheep erythrocytes, HSA, and allogeneic tumor cells, respectively). By contrast, nearly 80% of circulating basophils from hyperimmunized animals and one-third of basophils teased from "late reactions" formed specific rosettes. Finally, a substantial proportion of basophils teased from CBH reactions was able to acquire rosetting capacity following exposure to immune serum *in vitro*.

In summary, it appears that delayed-onset immunological reactions containing basophils may be passively transferred in the guinea pig by sensitized T (or possibly B) cells, or, in some cases, by IgG_1 antibodies. The extent to which antibodies are involved in the pathogenesis of the various forms of basophil-rich delayed reactions, particularly those examples of CBH transferable by T cells, remains to be determined. There is suggestive evidence, however, that some varieties of delayed reactivity containing basophils may depend on the participation of both sensitized cells and serum factors, perhaps antibody. For example, when large doses of specific antigen are administered *parenterally* to guinea pigs sensitized to manifest CBH, a delayed-onset diffuse maculopapular rash is produced that is histologically similar to locally elicited CBH (H. Dvorak *et al.*, 1977a). Although neither cells nor serum alone transferred this systemic CBH reactivity, some attempts to transfer reactivity with both cells and serum were successful. Furthermore, studies of basophil-rich skin reactions to the tick *Ixodes holocyclus* in immune guinea pigs suggest that, although passive transfer of protection is better achieved with immune cells than with serum, transfer of both produces maximal effect (Bagnall, 1975). Wikel and Allen (1976), by contrast, found that resistance to the tick *Dermacentor andersoni* could be transferred by immune cells from sensitized guinea pigs but not by immune serum. It should be remembered that the roles of antibodies in such reactions are potentially complex and probably involve much more than merely their relationship to the presence and/or function of basophils.

6.3.2. Basophil Chemotaxis

Recent studies measuring chemotactic migration have provided some insight into the mechanisms by which basophils may be attracted to delayed-type skin reactions and to inflammatory sites in general. Chemotaxis is measured *in vitro* by studying the migration of cells toward various soluble test substances along a chemical gradient across micropore filters of defined pore size in Boyden chambers (Ward *et al.*, 1971). It has been found that macromolecular products (so-called lymphokines) elaborated by sensitized lymphocytes cultured with either specific antigen or B- or T-cell mitogens, as well as products of complement activation, are chemotactic for normal human and guinea pig basophils (Boetcher and Leonard, 1973; Lett-Brown *et al.*, 1976; Ward *et al.*, 1975). In addition, diffusates from lung fragments challenged with allergen, the plasma enzyme kallikrein, and the complement factor complex C567 have been found to be weakly chemotactic for human leukemic basophils (Kay and Austen, 1972). Guinea pig basophils are also attracted weakly by products present in bacterial culture supernatant (Ward *et al.*, 1975). These various serum and bacterial factors are not specifically chemotactic for basophils since neutrophils and/or monocytes also respond to these agents, and in some instances (e.g., bacterial factor) more strongly. However, the kinetics of the basophil's chemotactic response is distinctive, reaching plateau levels as early as 1 hr, whereas neutrophils and monocytes do not achieve such levels for 2 and 3–5 hr, respectively. A human lymphocyte-produced factor chemotactic for basophils has a molecular weight of about 15,000 and may be identical to a factor chemotactic for monocytes (Lett-Brown *et al.*, 1976).

Modification of the basophil's chemotactic response has been achieved by incubation of these cells with appropriate agents prior to assay. Boetcher and Leonard (1973) have shown that the chemotactic response of human basophils to C5a may be augmented five- to tenfold by preincubation with lymphokine-containing fluids. On the other hand, Ward *et al.* (1975) have found that chemotaxis of guinea pig basophils to both lymphocyte culture supernatants and to the C5 fragment is substantially reduced by previous exposure to antigens to which these basophils had specificity. Under the conditions employed, exposure of basophils to antigen was not associated with histamine release or overt degranulation; moreover, antigen alone did not affect the migration of basophils isolated from the hyperimmunized animals used in these experiments. Lett-Brown and Leonard (1977) have demonstrated that histamine, in concentrations as low as 10^{-8} M, inhibits the chemotactic response of normal human basophils to C5a but has no effect on basophil chemotaxis to a leukocyte-derived factor. The inhibition is probably mediated through an effect on basophil H_2 histamine receptors.

The relevance of these chemotactic data to the accumulation of basophils in various inflammatory lesions in man and animals is worthy of brief consideration. Although basophils can respond to some of the neutrophil chemotactic factors, basophils are relatively rare in immunological reactions triggered by immune complexes or in sites of bacterial infection. This may be attributed, at least in part, to the relative paucity of basophils as compared with neutrophils in circulating blood and, in the case of bacterial infection, to the weaker chemotactic response of basophils, *vis-à-vis* neutrophils, to bacterial products. In contrast, the substantial accumulation of basophils that occurs in certain delayed-type reactions in both man and animals probably reflects the fact that the lymphokine(s) chemotactic for basophils lacks significant attraction for the much more numerous neutrophils. Similarly, the preferential accumulation of basophils over monocytes in certain delayed skin reactions may reflect the participation of additional factors (basophil chemotaxis augmentation factor: Lett-Brown *et al.*, 1976). The observation that C5a and T-cell products have a synergistic effect on basophil chemotaxis (Boetcher and Leonard, 1973) may also have relevance to the pathogenesis of certain delayed-onset basophil-rich reaction *in vivo*. Finally, the finding that interaction with specific antigen or histamine substantially reduces the chemotactic response of sensitized basophils provides a possible explanation for the well-known transience of CBH reactivity and for its decline associated with the appearance of circulating antibodies and of basophils that have absorbed such antibodies (Colvin *et al.*, 1973b; H. Dvorak *et al.*, 1975).

6.4. Mast Cells in Delayed-Onset Immunological Reactions

A possible explanation for the large differences in the extent of basophil infiltration into delayed-onset reactions that occur in various species may reside in the tissue mast cell. The similarity of mast cell and basophil granule contents and immunological properties, and the inverse relation between basophil and mast cell frequency in various species, has already been discussed. Further, mast cell hyperplasia is associated with lymphocyte infiltration in many forms of chronic inflammation, parasite infestation, and neoplasia. Taken together, these data suggest that basophils and mast cells are supplementary cells with similar functions and that either or both may participate in delayed-onset immunological reactions, depending on the species and, perhaps, on the site of antigenic challenge. Thus the old finding of increased histamine concentration in classic DH reactions in rats and guinea pigs would suggest increased activity and/or numbers of fixed tissue mast cells (Inderbitzin, 1956; Goldman *et al.*, 1973). Basophils, which are quickly mobilized and short-lived cells, may be an appropriate initial response of the sensitized host to immunogens, particularly in species or organs relatively poor in mast cells. In more chronic processes involving prolonged interaction between the host and foreign antigens, basophils may give way as new mast cells arise by a process of differentiation or replication.

Evidence supporting this general hypothesis comes from morphological studies of delayed-type skin reactions in man in which delayed-onset, partial mast cell degranulation was observed (Figure 2B), particularly within edematous zones of the papillary dermis and about the superficial microvasculature (H. Dvorak *et al.*, 1974a, A. Dvorak *et al.*, 1976b). At later times, some mast cells underwent mitosis and immature mast cells appeared in the dermis. Moreover, during the process of rejection, renal allografts in man are infiltrated by basophils at early intervals after grafting, but striking mast cell hyperplasia occurs later (Colvin and H. Dvorak, 1974). Circumstantial evidence suggests that in many of these instances lymphocytes, probably T lymphocytes, influence the arrival of basophils, the differentiation and/or replication of mast cells, and the degranulation or other function(s) of both basophils and mast cells (H. Dvorak and A. Dvorak, 1972, 1974).

In certain delayed-onset immunological reactions, both cell-mediated and homocytotropic antibody-dependent mechanisms may operate together with other factors to modulate basophil or mast cell function. Such a situation may obtain in certain forms of experimental intestinal helminthiasis in which the interaction of locally shed antigens and cell-bound homocytotropic antibody, as well as the direct action of certain parasite-derived products, probably contributes to basophil and mast cell degranulation (Dineen, 1978).

6.5. Role of Basophils and Mast Cells in Delayed-Onset Immunological Reactions

The precise roles of basophils and mast cells in delayed-onset immunological phenomena are largely unknown; however, there is every reason to believe, on both biochemical and morphological grounds, that these roles are complex. The list of mediators of inflammation that are synthesized or generated by basophils and/or mast cells is long (Lewis and Austen, 1977) and continues to grow (Henderson and Kaliner, 1978; Roberts *et al.*, 1978): their established or suggested effects include smooth muscle and vascular endothelial contraction, vascular dilatation and increased vascular permeability with subsequent effects on local blood flow and shifts of fluid and solutes from intravascular to extravascular compartments, attraction of eosinophils and neutrophils, activation of platelets, activation (or inhibition) of clotting mechanisms, promotion of fibrinolysis, generation of kallikrein activity, and interactions with fibronectin that may influence cell adherence phenomena. Recent work suggests additional, potentially important effects that may be mediated by the granule-associated chymotrypsin and trypsin-like proteases that have been described in both mast cells (Lagunoff and Benditt, 1963; Perera and Mongar, 1963, Yurt and Austen, 1977) and basophils (Orenstein *et al.*, 1976; H. Dvorak *et al.*, 1977b). For example, Werb and Aggeler (1978) have demonstrated that certain proteases, including trypsin and chymotrypsin, stimulate fibroblasts to release collagenase and plasminogen activator *in vitro*. Plasmin is also effective. These findings suggest that granule-derived enzymes of basophils and mast cells may participate in the modulation of tissue remodelling in delayed-type reactions *in vivo*. Because many of the basophils that are observed infiltrating the interstitium of delayed reactions exhibit little or no evidence of degranulation, it is of interest that the recently recognized plasminogen activator of basophils (H. Dvorak *et al.*, 1978) is expressed by intact, nondegranulated cells. This activity, which appears to be associated with the plasma membrane, thus may facilitate the movement of basophils through fibrin (via activation of plasmin) and may also effect changes in the interstitium (via stimulation of fibroblast collagenase secretion).

The diverse mediators, once released, collectively have an almost limitless potential to influence the progression of an individual immunological reaction. Histamine, to take only the most extensively studied example, may promote local inflammation by its effects on smooth muscle and vascular endothelium, but may also directly inhibit a variety of phenomena associated with immediate or delayed hypersensitivity reactions, including MIF production (Rocklin, 1975, 1976), IgE-mediated histamine release from basophils (Bourne *et al.*, 1971), neutrophil lysosomal enzyme release (Zurier *et al.*, 1974), and T-cell-mediated allogeneic cytotoxicity (Plaut *et al.*, 1973). Histamine also may stimulate fibroblast proliferation (Russell *et al.*, 1977). Histamine may be partially responsible both for the attraction of eosinophils to sites of immunological reactivity (Clark *et al.*, 1975) and also, via direct effects (Clark *et al.*, 1977) or via effects on antigenically stimulated lymphocytes (Kownatzki *et al.*, 1978), for the inhibition of their movement once they have arrived. Eosinophils, in turn, may dampen inflammatory processes by a variety of mechanisms (Goetzl and Austen, 1977). Histamine may be inactivated locally by the histaminases of tissues and certain leukocytes, including the eosinophil (Zeiger *et al.*, 1976a,b). These data establish that a single granule-derived mediator has the potential to significantly modulate the progression of either immediate- or delayed-type hypersensitivity reactions.

The specific consequences of basophil or mast cell participation probably vary in different hypersensitivity phenomena, and these cells may have multiple roles in even a single immunological reaction. In rodents, for example, certain cutaneous or intestinal parasites provoke delayed-onset reactions that apparently are composed of elements of both cell-mediated and immediate-type hypersensitivity (Dineen, 1978). The numerous basophils or mast cells participating in such reactions probably function both to discharge amines and perhaps other mediators that manifest direct toxicity to the parasites (Jones *et al.*, 1974; Rothwell *et al.*, 1974a,b) and to promote immune resistance through effects on vascular and/or intestinal mucosal permeability by facilitating the local efflux of antibodies, complement components, and other intravascular factors (Dineen, 1978).

The roles of basophils and mast cells in delayed-onset reactions that appear to be mediated entirely by T cells are particularly obscure. It has long been believed, especially in the case of mast cells, that these cells normally function by regulating properties of the local microenvironment, particularly vascular tone and permeability. Evidence supporting such a role for mast cells in delayed-type reactions has been derived from studies in mice. Certain delayed-onset reactions in this species resemble Jones-Mote reactions in that they occur only at early intervals after immunizations that avoid CFA and wane with the appearance of circulating antibody: Such reactions may be mediated by a short-lived subset of T cells (Askenase *et al.*,1977). Classic DH-type reactions also occur following immunizations with mycobacterial products (Crowle, 1975). As noted above, mice have very few if any circulating basophils, and so their mast cells might be expected to assume added importance. Generally, it has been difficult to elicit delayed reactions in mouse flank skin, but indurated reactions having a delayed onset may be readily elicited in the ear and footpad, sites at which mast cells are particularly numerous. Gershon *et al.* (1975) have reported, moreover, that reserpine, which depletes mouse mast cell granules of 5-hydroxytryptamine, also suppresses both the evanescent and classical form of delayed-type reactivity in this species. These workers agree with our hypothesis that T lymphocytes trigger the release of vasoactive amines from mast cells and that such amines have an important role in the pathogenesis of cell-mediated reactions. The abundant body of related evidence suggesting that mast cells, possibly through effects on the microvasculature, have an important role in the pathogenesis of cell-mediated reactions has been extensively reviewed by Askenase (1977).

Although the evidence is largely circumstantial (Sections 5.2 and 5.4), it appears probable that a relatively slow, sustained release of mediators occurs during the course of delayed-type, as opposed to immediate-type, hypersensitivity reactions. Thus extensive discharge of mast cell granule contents, as in cutaneous anaphylaxis, leads to only a sparse cellular infiltrate, consisting largely of neutrophils, that develops long after normal vascular permeability has been restored (Ovary, 1968).

Finally, it is important to emphasize that basophil and mast cell mediators may, at times, function to dampen rather than to enhance inflammatory processes. As has been discussed, histamine, for example, may inhibit a variety of phenomena associated with immediate- or delayed-type hypersensitivity. Our *in vivo* studies with a heterologous antibasophil serum have provided results consistent with an antiinflammatory role for basophils (Galli *et al.*, 1978). Guinea pigs sensitized to manifest both CBH reactivity to ovalbumin and classical delayed-type hypersensitivity to PPD were selectively depleted of bone marrow and circulating basophils by the intravenous administration of a potent rabbit antibasophil serum (ABS). CBH reactions elicited in these animals contained 63–88% fewer basophils than those elicited in normal rabbit serum (NRS)-treated controls, whereas there were no differences between these two groups in the number of any other leukocytes in CBH sites. Although the CBH reactions of both NRS- and ABS-treated animals appeared macroscopically similar (i.e., flat, nonindurated, erythematous macules), ABS-treated animals had lesions that were significantly *more* erythematous than those of NRS-treated controls. By contrast, the delayed reactions to PPD in ABS- and NRS-treated animals exhibited no significant differences in either cellular composition or gross appearance.

7. Summary

The role of basophils and mast cells as the source of many important mediators of immediate hypersensitivity is widely appreciated. In these reactions, which may be either systemic or local, basophils and/or mast cells undergo rapid granule exocytosis in response to the interaction of antigen with specific cell-bound homocytotropic antibody. *In vitro* studies and clinical observation of patients with disorders of immediate hypersensitivity strongly suggest that such anaphylactic degranulation may be modulated *in vivo* by agents affecting intracellular levels of cyclic nucleotides including certain hormones, E prostaglandins, histamine, a variety of drugs, and possibly interferon. Rapid granule exocytosis also may occur independently of antigen–homocytotropic antibody interactions in response to complement fragments, neutrophil lysosomal proteins, proteases, venom polypeptides, and enzymes and certain drugs.

In addition to their role in immediate hypersensitivity, recent morphological evidence in several different species including man has clearly demonstrated that basophils and/or mast cells also participate in a variety of biologically important hypersensitivity phenomena of delayed onset. These include the reactions to skin and renal allografts, contact allergens, some tumors, many protein antigens, schistosomes, ticks, and vaccinia virus, and the immune expulsion of certain intestinal metazoan parasites.

Much work remains to be done in elucidating the mechanisms responsible for controlling basophil and mast cell accumulation and function in delayed-onset immunological reactions *in vivo*. The relative importance of lymphoid cells and antibody in the expression of these reactions is of particular interest. It appears certain, in the guinea pig at least, that experimental delayed-onset reactions containing both mononuclear cells and basophils may be passively transferred either with lymphocytes (T cells definitely, and possibly also B cells) or with immunoglobulin (IgG_1). It is as yet unclear whether both T cells and antibody participate to some extent in the expression of all experimental and naturally occurring immunologically specific reactions containing basophils; however, the investigation of this question may provide important insights into the role of antibody in delayed-type hypersensitivity responses in general.

Because the functions of basophils and mast cells in delayed-onset immunological reactions, whatever these may be, must be largely mediated by the pharmacologically active contents of their cytoplasmic granules, it becomes critical to understand the nature of the mechanisms promoting the liberation of granule contents in delayed reactions. In some instances, such as the immune expulsion of intestinal parasites, antigen may act (along with other stimuli) to produce anaphylactic degranulation of basophils and/or mast cells: such mechanisms would rapidly provide high local mediator concentrations. In other reactions, antigen probably affects basophils and mast cells indirectly, perhaps through factors liberated from specific T cells. Morphological evidence suggests that, in these reactions, loss of granule contents may occur by mechanisms that are both morphologically and kinetically different from those of classical homocytotropic antibody-mediated anaphylactic granule exocytosis. Mediators would thus be released slowly and over a longer time frame, a process that would reasonably be expected to have biological effects different from those of massive anaphylactic discharge. Some immunological phenomena may exhibit overlapping components of both of these mediator release mechanisms. Furthermore, many of the homocytotropic antibody- or T-cell-independent factors known to produce degranulation *in vitro*, such as complement fragments and proteases, may also function in some delayed-onset reactions *in vivo*.

Still best known as important effector cells in clinically significant immediate-hypersensitivity phenomena, basophils and mast cells are now recognized as prominent participants in diverse forms of protective immunity of delayed onset. The elucidation of their roles in these reactions remains an important goal of current research.

ACKNOWLEDGMENT

We thank Michele Angelo for her excellent secretarial assistance.

8. References

Åborg, C.-H., and Uvnäs, B., 1968, Mode of binding of histamine and some other biogenic amines to a protamine–heparin complex *in vitro*, *Acta Physiol. Scand.* **74**:552–567.

Ackerman, G. A., 1963, Cytochemical properties of the blood basophilic granulocytes, *Ann. N.Y. Acad Sci.* **103**:376–393.

Ackerman, G. A., and Bellios, N.C., 1955, A study of the morphology of the living cells of blood and bone marrow in vital films with the phase microscope. I. Normal blood and bone marrow, *Blood* **10**:3–16.

Ackerman, G. A., and Clark, M. A., 1971, Ultrastructural localization of peroxidase activity in human basophil leukocytes, *Acta Haematol.* **45**:280–284.

Allen, A. M., 1962, Deoxyribonucleic acid synthesis and mitosis in mast cells of the rat, *Lab. Invest.* **11**:188–191.

Allen, J. R., 1973, Tick resistance: Basophils in skin reactions of resistant guinea pigs, *Int. J. Parasitol.* **3**:195–200.

Amann, R., and Martin, H., 1961, Blutmastzellen und Heparin, *Acta Haematol.* **25**:209–219.

Anderson, P., and Uvnäs, B., 1975, Selective localization of histamine to electron dense granules in antigen-challenged sensitized rat mast cells and to similar granules isolated from sonicated mast cells. An electron microscope autoradiographic study, *Acta Physiol. Scand.* **94**:63–73.

Anderson, P., Slorach, S. A., and Uvnäs, B., 1973, Sequential exocytosis of storage granules during antigen-induced histamine release from sensitized mast cells *in vitro*. An electron microscopic study, *Acta Physiol. Scand.* **88**:359–372.

Archer, G. T., and Jackas, M., 1965, Disruption of mast cells by a component of eosinophil granules, *Nature (London)* **205**:599–600.

Askenase, P. W., 1973, Cutaneous basophil hypersensitivity in contact-sensitized guinea pigs. I. Transfer with immune serum, *J. Exp. Med.* **138**:1144–1155.

Askenase, P. W., 1976, Cutaneous basophil hypersensitivity uncovered in the cell transfer of classical tuberculin hypersensitivity, *J. Immunol.* **117**:741–747.

Askenase, P. W., 1977, The role of basophils, mast cells and vasoamines in hypersensitivity reactions with a delayed time course, *Prog. Allergy* **23**:199–320.

Askenase, P. W., and Atwood, J. E., 1976, Basophils in tuberculin and "Jones-Mote" delayed reactions of humans, *J. Clin. Invest.* **58**:1145–1154.

Askenase, P. W., Hayden, B., and Higashi, G., 1975a, Cutaneous basophil hypersensitivity (CBH) and macrophage migration inhibition (MMI) in guinea pigs with schistosomiasis, *J. Allergy Clin. Immunol.* **55**:111.

Askenase, P. W., Haynes, J. D., Tauben, D., and DeBernardo, R., 1975b, Specific basophil hypersensitivity induced by skin testing and transferred using immune serum, *Nature (London)* **256**:52–54.

Askenase, P. W., Haynes, J. D., and Hayden, B. J., 1976, Antibody-mediated basophil accumulations in cutaneous hypersensitivity reactions in guinea pigs, *J. Immunol.* **117**:1722–1730.

Askenase, P. W., Hayden, B., and Gershon, R. K., 1977, Evanescent delayed-type hypersensitivity: Mediation by effector cells with a short life span, *J. Immunol.* **119**:1830–1835.

Askenase, P. W., Boone, W. T., and Binder, H. J., 1978a, Colonic basophil hypersensitivity, *J. Immunol.* **120**:198–201.

Askenase, P. W., DeBernardo, R., Tauben, D., and Kashgarian, M., 1978b, Cutaneous basophil anaphylaxis. Immediate vasopermeability increases and anaphylactic degranulation of basophils at delayed hypersensitivity reactions challenged with additional antigen, *Immunology* **35**:741–755.

Assem, E. S. K., 1974, Leukocyte-bound IgE and cell reactivity in asthma, *Allerg. Immunopathol.* **2**:41–46.

Assem, E. S. K., and Richter, A. W., 1971, Comparison of *in vivo* and *in vitro* inhibition of the anaphylactic mechanism by β-adrenergic stimulants and disodium cromoglycate, *Immunology* **21**:729–739.

Atkins, P., Green, G. R., and Zweiman, B., 1973, Histologic studies of human eosinophil and mast cell responses to ragweed, compound 48/80 and histamine, *J. Allergy Clin. Immunol.* **51**:263–273.

Austen, K. F., and Becker, E. L., 1966, Mechanisms of immunologic injury of rat peritoneal mast cells. II. Complement requirement and phosphonate ester inhibition of release of histamine by rabbit anti-rat gamma globulin, *J. Exp. Med.* **124**: 397–419.

Austen, K. F., and Brocklehurst, W. E., 1961, Anaphylaxis in chopped guinea pig lung. I. Effect of peptidase substrates and inhibitors, *J. Exp. Med.* **113**:521–539.

Austen, K. F., and Humphrey, J. H., 1961, Release of histamine from rat peritoneal mast cells by antibody against rat γ-globulin, *J. Physiol. (London)* **158**:36P–37P.

Austen, K. F., Lewis, R. A., Stechschulte, D. J., Wasserman, S. I., Leid, R. W., Jr., and Goetzl, E. J., 1974, Generation and release of chemical mediators of immediate hypersensitivity, in: *Progress in Immunology II*, Vol. 2 (L. Brent and J. Holborow, eds.), pp. 61–71, North-Holland, Amsterdam.

Bach, M. K., and Brashler, J. R., 1975, Inhibition of IgE and compound 48/80 induced histamine release by lectins, *Immunology* **29**:371–386.

Bach, M. K., Bloch, K. J., and Austen, K. F., 1971a, IgE and IgGa antibody-mediated release of histamine from rat peritoneal cells. II. Interaction of IgGa and IgE at the target cells, *J. Exp. Med.* **133**:772–784.

Bach, M. K., Brashler, J. R., Bloch, K. J., and Austen, K. F., 1971b, Studies on the receptor site for IgE antibody on the peritoneal mast cell of the rat, in: *Biochemistry of the Acute Allergic Reactions* (K. F. Austen and E. L. Becker, eds.), pp. 65–89, Blackwell, Oxford.

Bach, M. K., Bach, S., Brashler, J. R., Ishizaka, T., and Ishizaka, K., 1978, On the nature of the presumed receptor for IgE on mast cells. V. Enhanced binding of ^{125}I labeled IgE to cell-free particulate fractions in the presence of protease inhibitors, *Int. Arch. Allergy Appl. Immunol.* **56**:1–13.

Bagnall, B. G., 1975, Cutaneous immunity to the tick *Ixodes holocyclus*, thesis, University of Sydney, Australia, as cited by Askenase, 1977.

Barnett, M. L., 1973, Mast cells in the epithelial layer of human gingiva, *J. Ultrastruct. Res.* **43**:247–255.

Baxter, J. H., and Adamik, R., 1975, Control of histamine release: Effect of various conditions on rate of release and rate of cell sensitization, *J. Immunol.* **114**:1034–1041.

Becker, E. L., and Austen, K. F., 1964, A comparison of the specificity of inhibition by phosphonate esters of the first component of complement and the antigen-induced release of histamine from guinea pig lung, *J. Exp. Med.* **120**:491–506.

Becker, E. L., and Austen, K. F., 1966, Mechanisms of immunologic injury of rat peritoneal mast cells. I. The effects of phosphonate inhibitors on the homocytotropic antibody-mediated histamine release and the first component of rat complement, *J. Exp. Med.* **124**:379–395.

Becker, E. L., and Henson, P. M., 1973, *In vitro* studies of immunologically induced secretion of mediators from cells and related phenomena, *Adv. Immunol.* **17**:93–193.

Becker, K. E., Ishizaka, T., Metzger, H., Ishizaka, K., and Grimely, P. M., 1973, Surface IgE in human basophils during histamine release, *J. Exp. Med.* **138**:394–409.

Behrendt, H., Rosenkranz, U., and Schmutzler, W., 1978, Ultrastructure of isolated human mast cells during histamine release induced by ionophore A23187, *Int. Arch. Allergy Appl. Immunol.* **56**:188–192.

Bennich, H., and Johansson, S. G. O., 1967, Studies on a new class of human immunoglobulins. II. Chemical and physical properties, in: *Nobel Symposium 3. Gamma Globulin, Structure and Control of Biosynthesis* (J. Killander, ed.), p. 199, Almqvist and Wiksell, Stockholm.
Bennich, H., Ishizaka, K., Ishizaka, T., and Johansson, S. G. O., 1969, A comparative antigenic study of γE-globulin and myeloma-IgND, *J. Immunol.* **102**:826–831.
Benveniste, J., Henson, P. M., and Cochrane, C. G., 1973, A possible role for IgE in immune complex disease, in: *The Biological Role of the Immunoglobulin E System* (K. Ishizaka and D. H., Dayton, eds.), pp. 187–205, U. S. Government Printing Office, Washington.
Bernstein, I. L., Vijay, H. M., and Perelmutter, L., 1977, Non-responder basophils in highly ragweed-sensitive subjects, *Int. Arch. Allergy Appl. Immunol.* **55**:215–216.
Blenkinsopp, W. K., 1967, Mast cell proliferation in adult rats, *J. Cell Sci.* **2**:33–37.
Boetcher, D. A., and Leonard, E. J., 1973, Basophil chemotaxis: Augmentation by a factor from stimulated lymphocyte cultures, *Immunol. Commun.* **2**:421–429.
Bourne, H. R., Melmon, K. L., and Lichtenstein, L. M., 1971, Histamine augments leukocyte cyclic AMP and blocks antigenic histamine release, *Science* **173**:743–745.
Bourne, H. R., Lichtenstein, L. M., and Melmon, K. L., 1972, Pharmacologic control of allergic histamine release *in vitro*: Evidence for an inhibitory role of 3′,5′-adenosine monophosphate in human leukocytes, *J. Immunol.* **108**:695–705.
Bourne, H. R., Lichtenstein, L. M., Melmon, K. L., Henney, C. S., Weinstein, Y., and Shearer, G. M., 1974, Modulation of inflammation and immunity by cyclic AMP, *Science* **184**:19–28.
Braunsteiner, H., 1962, Mast cells and basophilic leukocytes, in: *The Physiology and Pathology of Leukocytes* (H. Braunsteiner and D. Zucker-Franklin, eds.), Ch. 2, Grune and Stratton, New York.
Brinkman, G. L., 1968, The mast cell in normal human bronchus and lung, *J. Ultrastruct. Res.* **23**:115–123.
Brittinger, G., Hirschhorn, R., Douglas, S. D., and Weissmann, G., 1968, Studies on lysosomes. XI. Characterization of a hydrolase-rich fraction from human lymphocytes, *J. Cell Biol.* **37**:394–411.
Bruce, C. A., Rosenthal, R. R., Lichtenstein, L. M., and Norman, P. S., 1974, Diagnostic tests in ragweed-allergic asthma, *J. Allergy Clin. Immunol.* **53**:230–239.
Buonassisi, V., and Root, M., 1975, Enzymatic degradation of heparin-related mucopolysaccharides from the surface of endothelial cell cultures, *Biochim. Biophys. Acta* **385**:1–10.
Bursztajn, S., Askenase, P. W., Gershon, R. K., and Gershon, M. D., 1978, Role of vasoactive amines during early stages of delayed-type hypersensitivity skin reactions, *Fed. Proc.* **37**:590.
Burton, A. L., and Higginbotham, R. D., 1966, Response of blood basophils to Rous sarcoma virus infection in chicks and its significance, *J. Reticuloendothel. Soc.* **3**:314–326.
Chakravarty, N., 1968, Respiration of rat peritoneal mast cells during histamine release induced by antigen–antibody reaction, *Exp. Cell Res.* **49**:160–168.
Chan, B. S. T., 1972, Ultrastructural changes in guinea-pig bone marrow basophils during anaphylaxis, *Immunology* **23**:215–224.
Charkin, L. W., Krell, R. D., Mengel, J., Young, D., Zaher, C., and Wardell, J. R., 1974, Effect of a histamine H_2-receptor antagonist on immunologically induced mediator release *in vitro*. *Agents Actions* **4**:297–303.
Clark, J. M., and Higginbotham, R. D., 1968, Significance of the mast cell response to a lysosomal protein, *J. Immunol.* **101**:488–499.
Clark, J. M., Altman, G., and Fromowitz, F. B., 1976, Basophil hypersensitivity response in rabbits, *Infect. Immunun.* **15**:305–312.
Clark, R. A. F., Gallin, J. I., and Kaplan, A. P., 1975, The selective eosinophil chemotactic activity of histamine, *J. Exp. Med.* **142**:1462–1476.
Clark, R. A. F., Sandler, J. A., Gallin, J. I., and Kaplan, A. P., 1977, Histamine modulation of eosinophil migration, *J. Immunol.* **118**:137–145.
Cochrane, C. G., 1971, Mechanisms involved in the deposition of immune complexes in tissues, *J. Exp. Med.* **134**:75S–89S.
Cochrane, C. G., and Koffler, D., 1973, Immune complex disease in experimental animals and man, *Adv. Immunol.* **16**:185–264.
Cochrane, C. G., and Müller-Eberhard, H. J., 1968, The derivation of two distinct anaphylatoxin activities from the third and fifth components of human complement, *J. Exp. Med.* **127**:371–386.
Coffey, R. G., and Middleton, E., Jr., 1973, Release of histamine from rat mast cells by lysosomal cationic proteins, *Int. Arch. Allergy Appl. Immunol.* **45**: 593–611.

Cohn, Z. A., and Parks, E., 1967, The regulation of pinocytosis in mouse macrophages. II. Factors inducing vesicle formation, *J. Exp. Med.* **125**:213–232.

Colvin, R. B., and Dvorak, H. F., 1974, Basophils and mast cells in renal allograft rejection, *Lancet* **1**:212–214.

Colvin, R. B., and Dvorak, H. F., 1975, Role of the clotting system in cell-mediated hypersensitivity. II. Kinetics of fibrinogen/fibrin accumulation and vascular permeability. Changes in tuberculin and cutaneous basophil hypersensitivity reactions, *J. Immunol.* **114**:377–387.

Colvin, R. B., Johnson, R. A., Mihm, M. C., Jr., and Dvorak, H. F., 1973a, Role of the clotting system in cell-mediated hypersensitivity. I. Fibrin deposition in delayed skin reactions in man, *J. Exp. Med.* **138**:686–698.

Colvin, R. B., Pinn, V. W., Simpson, B. A., and Dvorak, H. F., 1973b, Cutaneous basophil hypersensitivity. IV. The "late reaction": Sequel to Jones-Mote type hypersensitivity. Comparison with rabbit Arthus reaction. Effect of passive antibody on induration and expression of Jones-Mote hypersensitivity, *J. Immunol.* **110**:1279–1289.

Colvin, R. B., Dvorak, A. M., and Dvorak, H. F., 1974, Mast cells in the cortical tubular epithelium and interstitium in human renal disease, *Hum. Pathol.* **5**:315–326.

Conrad, D. H., Bazin, H., Sehon, A. H., and Froese, A., 1975, Binding parameters of the interaction between rat IgE and rat mast cell receptors, *J. Immunol.* **114**:1688–1691.

Conroy, M. C., Adkinson, N. F., Jr., and Lichtenstein, L. M., 1977, Measurement of IgE on human basophils: Relation to serum IgE and anti-IgE-induced histamine release, *J. Immunol.* **118**:1317–1321.

Crowle, A. J., 1975, Delayed hypersensitivity in the mouse, *Adv. Immunol.* **20**:197–264.

Csaba, G., Hodinka, L., and Surján, L., Jr., 1969, Transport of mast cells by the blood circulation, *Experientia* **25**:735–736.

Day, R. P., Dolovich, J., and Bienenstock, J., 1974, Characteristics of tritiated histamine uptake and release by human basophils, *Fed. Proc.* **33**:752.

DeBernardo, R., Askenase, P., Tauben, D., and Douglas, J., 1975, Augmented anaphylaxis at sites of cutaneous basophil hypersensitivity, *J. Allergy Clin. Immunol.* **55**:112.

DeChatelet, L. R., McCall, C. E., and Cooper, M. R., 1972, Inhibition of leukocyte acid phosphatase by heparin, *Clin. Chem.* **18**:1532–1534.

DeMeyts, P., 1976, Cooperative properties of hormone receptors in cell membranes, in: Proceedings of the 1975 ICN-UCLA Winter Conference on Cell and Molecular Biology, *J. Supramol. Struct.* **4**:241–258.

de Shazo, R. D., Levinson, A. I., Dvorak, H. F., and Davis, R. W., 1979, The late phase skin reaction: Evidence for activation of the coagulation system in an IgE-dependent reaction in man, *J. Immunol.* **122**:692–698.

Dineen, J., 1978, The role of homocytotropic antibodies in immunity and pathology of helminthiasis with special reference to the induction and potentiation of IgE production, in: *Immediate Hypersensitivity: Modern Concepts and Developments* (M. K. Bach, ed.), pp. 211–257, Dekker, New York.

Dolovich, J., Hargreave, F. E., Chalmers, R., Sheir, K. J., Gauldie, J., and Bienenstock, J., 1973, Late cutaneous allergic responses in isolated IgE-dependent reactions, *J. Allergy Clin. Immunol.* **52**:33–46.

Dorrington, K. J., and Bennich, H. H., 1978, Physicochemical and conformational properties of immunoglobulin E, in: *Immediate Hypersensitivity: Modern Concepts and Developments* (M. K. Bach, ed.), pp. 47–71, Dekker, New York.

Drobis, J. D., and Siraganian, R. P., 1976, Histamine release from cultured human basophils: Lack of histamine resynthesis after antigenic release, *J. Immunol.* **117**:1049–1053.

Dvorak, A. M., 1978, Biology and morphology of basophilic leukocytes, in: *Immediate Hypersensitivity: Modern Concepts and Developments* (M. K. Bach, ed.), pp. 369–405, Dekker, New York.

Dvorak, A. M., Bast, R. C., Jr., and Dvorak, H. F., 1971, Morphologic changes in draining lymph nodes and in lymphocyte cultures after sensitization with complete or incomplete Freund's adjuvant. Correlation with immunologic events *in vivo* and in culture, *J. Immunol.* **107**:422–435.

Dvorak, A. M., Dvorak, H. F., and Karnovsky, M. J., 1972, Uptake of horseradish peroxidase by guinea pig basophilic leukocytes, *Lab. Invest.* **26**:27–39.

Dvorak, A. M., Dickersin, G. R., Connell, A., Carey, R. W., and Dvorak, H. F., 1976a, Degranulation mechanisms in human leukemic basophils, *Clin. Immunol. Immunopathol.* **5**:235–246.

Dvorak, A. M., Mihm, M. C., Jr., and Dvorak, H. F., 1976b, Degranulation of basophilic leukocytes in allergic contact dermatitis reactions in man, *J. Immunol.* **116**:687–695.
Dvorak, A. M., Mihm, M. C., Jr., and Dvorak, H. F., 1976c, Morphology of delayed-type hypersensitivity reactions in man. II. Ultrastructural alterations affecting the microvasculature and the tissue mast cells, *Lab. Invest.* **34**:179–191.
Dvorak, H. F., 1971, Role of the basophilic leukocyte in allograft rejection, *J. Immunol.* **106**:279–281.
Dvorak, H. F., and Dvorak, A. M., 1972, Basophils, mast cells, and cellular immunity in animals and man, *Hum. Pathol.* **3**:454–456.
Dvorak, H. F., and Dvorak, A. M., 1974, Cutaneous basophil hypersensitivity, in: *Progress in Immunology II*, Vol. 3 (L. Brent and J. Holborow, eds.), pp. 171–181, North-Holland, Amsterdam.
Dvorak, H. F., and Hammond, M. E., 1978, Cutaneous basophil hypersensitivity, in: *Immediate Hypersensitivity: Modern Concepts and Developments* (M. K. Bach, ed.), pp. 659–692, Dekker, New York.
Dvorak, H. F., and Hirsch, M. S., 1971, Role of basophilic leukocytes in cellular immunity to vaccinia virus infection, *J. Immunol.* **107**:1576–1582.
Dvorak, H. F., and Mihm, M. C., Jr., 1972, Basophilic leukocytes in allergic contact dermatitis, *J. Exp. Med.* **135**:235–254.
Dvorak, H. F., Dvorak, A. M., Simpson, B. A., Richerson, H. B., Leskowitz, S., and Karnovsky, M. J., 1970, Cutaneous basophil hypersensitivity. II. A light and electron microscopic description, *J. Exp. Med.* **132**:558–582.
Dvorak, H. F., Simpson, B. A., Bast, R. C., Jr., and Leskowitz, S., 1971, Cutaneous basophil hypersensitivity. III. Participation of the basophil in hypersensitivity to antigen–antibody complexes, delayed hypersensitivity and contact allergy. Passive transfer, *J. Immunol.* **107**:138–148.
Dvorak, H. F., Dvorak, A. M., and Churchill, W. H., 1973, Immunologic rejection of diethylnitrosamine induced hepatomas in strain 2 guinea pigs: Participation of basophilic leukocytes and macrophage aggregates, *J. Exp. Med.* **137**:751–775.
Dvorak, H. F., Mihm, M. C., Jr., Dvorak, A. M., Johnson, R. A., Manseau, E. J., Morgan, E., and Colvin, R. B., 1974a, Morphology of delayed-type hypersensitivity reactions in man. I. Quantitative description of the inflammatory response. *Lab. Invest.* **31**:111–130.
Dvorak, H. F., Selvaggio, S. S., Dvorak, A. M., Colvin, R. B., Lean, D. B., and Rypysc, J., 1974b, Purification of basophilic leukocytes from guinea pig blood and bone marrow, *J. Immunol.* **113**:1694–1702.
Dvorak, H. F., Colvin, R. B., and Churchill, W. H., 1975, Specificity of basophils and lymphocytes in cutaneous basophil hypersensitivity, *J. Immunol.* **114**:507–511.
Dvorak, H. F., Mihm, M. C., Jr., and Dvorak, A. M., 1976, Morphology of delayed-type hypersensitivity reactions in man, *J. Invest. Dermatol.* **67**:391–401.
Dvorak, H. F., Hammond, M. E., Colvin, R. B., Manseau, E. J., and Goodwin, J., 1977a, Systemic expression of cutaneous basophil hypersensitivity, *J. Immunol.* **118**:1549–1557.
Dvorak, H. F., Orenstein, N. S., Dvorak, A. M., Hammond, M. E., Roblin, R. O., Feder, J., Schott, C. F., Goodwin, J., and Morgan, E., 1977b, Isolation of the cytoplasmic granules of guinea pig basophilic leukocytes: Identification of esterase and protease activities, *J. Immunol.* **119**:38–46.
Dvorak, H. F., Mihm, M. C., Jr., Dvorak, A. M., and Barnes, B. A., 1977c, First set skin allograft rejection in man, *Fed. Proc.* **36**:1071.
Dvorak, H. F., Orenstein, N. S., Rypysc, J., Colvin, R. B., and Dvorak, A. M., 1978, Plasminogen activator of guinea pig basophilic leukocytes: Probable localization to the plasma membrane, *J. Immunol.* **120**:766–773.
Ehrich, W. E., 1953, Histamine in mast cells, *Science* **118**:603.
Engvall, E., and Ruoslahti, E., 1977, Binding of soluble form of fibroblast surface protein, fibronectin, to collagen, *Int. J. Cancer* **20**:1–5.
Fawcett, D. W., 1955, An experimental study of mast cell degranulation and regeneration, *Anat. Rec.* **121**:29–52.
Feltkamp-Vroom, T. M., Stallman, P. J., Aalberse, R. C., and Reerink-Brongers, E. E., 1975, Immunofluorescence studies on renal tissue, tonsils, adenoids, nasal polyps, and skin of atopic and non-atopic patients with special reference to IgE, *Clin. Immunol. Immunopathol.* **4**:392–404.
Ferrarini, M., Munro, A., and Wilson, A. B., 1973, Cytophilic antibody: Correlation of its distribution with activation of basophils and macrophages, *Eur. J. Immunol.* **3**:364–370.

Foreman, J. C., and Mongar, J. L., 1975, Calcium and the control of histamine secretion from mast cells, in: *Calcium Transport in Contraction and Secretion* (E. Carafoli, ed.), p. 175, North-Holland, Amsterdam.

Foreman, J. C., Mongar, J. L., and Gomperts, B. D., 1973, Calcium ionophores and movement of calcium ions following the physiological stimulus to a secretory process, *Nature (London)*, **245**:249–251.

Foreman, J. C., Mongar, J. L., Gomperts, B. D., and Garland, L. G., 1975, A possible role for cyclic AMP in the regulation of histamine secretion and the action of cromoglycate, *Biochem. Pharmacol.* **24**:538–540.

Foreman, J. C., Garland, L. G., and Mongar, J. L., 1976, The role of Ca^{2+} in secretory process-model studies in mast cells, in: *Calcium in Biological Systems* (C. J. Duncan, ed.), Cambridge University Press, Cambridge.

Friedlaender, M. H., and Dvorak, H. F., 1977, Morphology of delayed-type hypersensitivity reactions in the guinea pig cornea, *J. Immunol.* **118**:1558–1563.

Galli, S. J., and Dvorak, H. F., 1975, Histamine synthesis by guinea pig basophils in short term tissue culture, *Fed. Proc.* **34**:1045.

Galli, S. J., Galli, A. S., Dvorak, A. M., and Dvorak, H. F., 1976, Metabolic studies of guinea pig basophilic leukocytes in short-term tissue culture. I. Measurement of histamine-synthesizing capacity by using an isotopic-thin layer chromatographic assay, *J. Immunol.* **117**:1085–1092.

Galli, S. J., Colvin, R. B., Verderber, E., Galli, A. S., Monahan, R., Dvorak, A. M., and Dvorak, H. F., 1978, Preparation of a rabbit anti-guinea pig basophil serum: *in vitro* and *in vivo* characterization, *J. Immunol.* **121**:1157–1166.

Galli, S. J., Orenstein, N. S., Gill, P. J., Silbert, J. E., Dvorak, A. M., and Dvorak, H. F., 1979, Sulfated glycosaminoglycans synthesised by basophil-enriched human leukaemic granulocytes *in vitro*, in: *The Mast Cell, Proceedings of the Conference Held in Davos, Switzerland, April, 1979*, Pitman Medical Publishing, Kent, England.

Gell, P. G. H., and Coombs, R. R. A., 1968, *Clinical Aspects of Immunology*, 2nd ed., F. A. Davis, Philadelphia.

Gershon, R. K., Askenase, P. W., and Gershon, M. D., 1975, Requirement for vasoactive amines for production of delayed-type hypersensitivity skin reactions, *J. Exp. Med.* **142**:732–747.

Gillespie, E., 1975, Microtubules, cyclic AMP, calcium, and secretion, *Ann. N.Y. Acad. Sci.* **243**:771–779.

Ginsburg, H., 1963, The *in vitro* differentiation and culture of normal mast cells from the mouse thymus, *Ann. N.Y. Acad. Sci.* **103**:20–39.

Ginsburg, H., and Lagunoff, D., 1967, The *in vitro* differentiation of mast cells. Cultures of cells from immunized mouse lymph nodes and thoracic duct lymph on fibroblast monolayers, *J. Cell Biol.* **35**:685–697.

Goetzl, E. J., and Austen, K. F., 1977, Generation, function and disposition of chemical mediators of the mast cell in immediate hypersensitivity, in: *Immunopharmacology* (J. W. Hadden, R. G. Coffey, and F. Spreafico, eds.), pp. 113–124, Plenum, New York.

Goldman, M. A., Simpson, B. A., and Dvorak, H. F., 1973, Histamine and basophils in delayed-type hypersensitivity reactions, *J. Immunol.* **110**:1511–1517.

Graham, H. T., Lowry, O. H., Wheelwright, F., Lenz, M. A., and Parrish, H. H., 1955, Distribution of histamine among leukocytes and platelets, *Blood* **10**:467–481.

Grant, J. A., Dupree, E., Goldman, A. S., Schultz, D. R., and Jackson, A. L., 1975, Complement mediated release of histamine from human leukocytes, *J. Immunol.* **114**:1101–1106.

Grant, L., 1973, The sticking and emigration of white blood cells in inflammation, in: *The Inflammatory Process*, Vol. 2, 2nd ed. (B. W. Zweifach, L. Grant, and R. T. McCluskey, eds.) pp. 205–249, Academic, New York.

Habermann, E., 1972, Bee and wasp venoms, *Science* **177**:314–322.

Halliwell, R. E. W., 1973, The localization of IgE in canine skin: An immunofluorescent study, *J. Immunol.* **110**:422–430.

Hartman, W. J., Clark, W. G., and Cyr, S. D., 1961, Histidine decarboxylase activity of basophils from chronic myelogenous leukemic patients. Origin of blood histamine, *Proc. Soc, Exp. Biol. Med.* **107**:123–125.

Hastie, R., 1971, The antigen-induced degranulation of basophil leukocytes from atopic subjects studied by phase-contrast microscopy, *Clin. Exp. Immunol.* **8**:45–61.

Hastie, R., 1974, A study of the ultrastructure of human basophil leukocytes, *Lab. Invest.* **31**:223–231.

Haynes, J. D., Hayden, B. J., and Askenase, P. W., 1974, Cutaneous basophil hypersensitivity (CBH) in neonatal guinea pigs immunized for Jones-Mote reactions (JMR): Active sensitization and passive transfer with immune serum, *Fed. Proc.* **33:**733.

Haynes, J. D., Kantor, F. S., and Askenase, P. W., 1975, Hapten specific cutaneous basophil hypersensitivity (CBH) transferred with small amounts of 7S IgG_1 antibody, *Fed. Proc.* **34:**1039.

Haynes, J. D., Rosenstein, R. W., and Askenase, P. W., 1978, A newly described activity of guinea pig IgG_1 antibodies: Transfer of cutaneous basophil reactions, *J. Immunol.* **120:**886–894.

Henderson, W. R., and Kaliner, M., 1978, Immunologic and nonimmunologic generation of superoxide from mast cells and basophils, *J. Clin. Invest.* **61:**187–196.

Henson, P. M., 1974, Mechanisms of activation and secretion by platelets and neutrophils, in: *Progress in Immunology II*, Vol. 2 (L. Brent and J. Holborow, eds.) p. 95, American Elsevier, New York.

Higginbotham, R. D., 1958, Studies on the functional interrelationship of fibroblasts and ground substance mucopolysaccharides, *Ann. N.Y. Acad. Sci.* **73:**186–203.

Higginbotham, R. D., 1963, in: Round Table Discussion, Conference on Mast Cells and Basophils (J. Padawer, mod.), *Ann. N.Y. Acad. Sci.* **103:**441–492.

Higginbotham, R. D., Dougherty, T. F., and Jee, W. S. S., 1956, Fate of shed mast cell granules, *Proc. Soc. Exp. Biol. Med.* **92:**256–261.

Hoenig, E. M., and Levine, S., 1974, Three localized forms of experimental allergic encephalomyelitis: An ultrastructural comparison, *J. Neuropathol. Exp. Neurol.* **33:**251–259.

Hook, W. A., Siraganian, R. P., and Wuhl, S. M., 1975, Complement induced histamine release from human basophils. I, *J. Immunol.* **114:**1185–1190.

Horn, R. G., and Spicer, S. S., 1964, Sulfated mucopolysaccharide and basic protein in certain granules of rabbit leukocytes, *Lab. Invest.* **13:**1–15.

Hubscher, T., Watson, J. I., and Goodfriend, L., 1970a, Target cells of human ragweed-binding antibodies in monkey skin. I. Immunofluorescent localization of cellular binding, *J. Immunol.* **104:**1187–1195.

Hubscher, T., Watson, J. I., and Goodfriend, L., 1970b, II. Immunoglobulin nature of ragweed-binding antibodies with affinity for monkey skin mast cells, *J. Immunol.* **104:**1196–1204.

Humphrey, J. H., Austen, K. F., and Rapp, H. J., 1963, *In vitro* studies of reversed anaphylaxis with rat cells, *Immunology* **6:**226–245.

Ida, S., Hooks, J. J., Siraganian, R. P., and Notkins, A. L., 1977, Enhancement of IgE-mediated histamine release from human basophils by viruses: Role of interferon, *J. Exp. Med.* **145:**892–906.

Inderbitzin, T., 1956, The relationship of lymphocytes, delayed cutaneous allergic reactions, and histamine, *Int. Arch. Allergy Appl. Immunol.* **8:**150–159.

Isersky, C., Taurog, J. D., Poy, G., and Metzger, H., 1978, Triggering of cultured neoplastic mast cells by antibodies to the receptor for IgE, *J. Immunol.* **121:**549–558.

Ishizaka, K., and Ishizaka, T., 1966, Physicochemical properties of reaginic antibody. I. Association of reaginic activity with an immunoglobulin other than γA- or γG-globulin, *J. Allergy* **37:**169–185.

Ishizaka, K., and Ishizaka, T., 1967, Identification of γE antibodies as a carrier of reaginic activity, *J. Immunol.* **99:**1187–1198.

Ishizaka, K., and Ishizaka, T., 1969, Immune mechanisms of reversed type reaginic hypersensitivity, *J. Immunol.* **103:**588–595.

Ishizaka, K., and Ishizaka, T., 1976, Immunoglobulin E, *Arch. Pathol. Lab. Med.* **100:**289–292.

Ishizaka, K., Tomioka, H., and Ishizaka, T., 1970, Mechanisms of passive sensitization. I. Presence of IgE and IgG molecules on human leukocytes, *J. Immunol.* **105:**1459–1467.

Ishizaka, T., and Ishizaka, K., 1973, Biological function of immunoglobulin E, in: *The Biological Role of the Immunoglobulin E System* (K. Ishizaka and D. H. Dayton, eds.), pp. 33–46, U.S. Government Printing Office, Washington.

Ishizaka, T., and Ishizaka, K., 1974, Mechanisms of passive sensitization. IV. Dissociation of IgE molecules from basophil receptors at acid pH, *J. Immunol.* **112:**1078–1084.

Ishizaka, T., Ishizaka, K., Johansson, S. G. O., and Bennich, H., 1969, Histamine release from human leukocytes by anti-γE antibodies, *J. Immunol.* **102:**884–892.

Ishizaka, T., Ishizaka, K., Orange, R. P., and Austen, K. F., 1970, The capacity of human immunoglobulin E to mediate the release of histamine and slow reacting substance of anaphylaxis (SRA-A) from monkey lung, *J. Immunol.* **104:**335–343.

Ishizaka, T., Ishizaka, K., Orange, R. P., and Austen, K. F., 1971a, Pharmacologic inhibition of the antigen-induced release of histamine and slow reacting substance of anaphylaxis (SRS-A) from monkey lung tissues mediated by human IgE, *J. Immunol.* **106:**1267–1273.

Ishizaka, T., Tomioka, H., and Ishizaka, K., 1971b, Degranulation of human basophil leukocytes by anti-γE antibody, *J. Immunol.* **106:**705–710.

Ishizaka, T., Soto, C. S., and Ishizaka, K., 1973, Mechanisms of passive sensitization. III. Number of IgE molecules and their receptor sites on human basophil granulocytes, *J. Immunol.* **111:**500–511.

Ishizaka, T., Konig, W., Kurata, M., Manser, L., and Ishizaka, K., 1975, Immunologic properties of mast cells from rats infected with *Nippostrongylus brasiliensis, J. Immunol.* **115:**1078–1083.

Ishizaka, T., Okudaira, H., Manser, L. E., and Ishizaka, K., 1976, Development of rat mast cells *in vitro*. I. Differentiation of mast cells from thymus cells, *J. Immunol.* **116:**747–754.

Ishizaka, T., Chang, T. H., Taggart, M., and Ishizaka, K., 1977, Histamine release from rat mast cells by antibodies against rat basophilic leukemia cell membrane. *J. Immunol.* **119:**1589–1596.

Janoff, A., Schaefer, S., Scherer, J., and Bean, M. A., 1965, Mediators of inflammation in leukocyte lysosomes. II. Mechanism of action of lysosomal cationic protein upon vascular permeability in the rat, *J. Exp. Med.* **122:**841–851.

Jaques, L. B., Mahadoo, J., and Riley, J. F., 1977, The mast cell/heparin paradox, *Lancet* **1:**411–414.

Johansson, S. G. O., and Bennich, H., 1967a, Immunological studies of an atypical (myeloma) immunoglobulin, *Immunology* **13:**381–394.

Johansson, S. G. O., and Bennich, H., 1967b, Studies on a new class of human immunoglobulins. I. Immunological properties, in: *Nobel Symposium 3, Gamma Globulins, Structure and Control of Biosynthesis* (J. Killander, ed.), p. 193, Almqvist and Wiksell, Stockholm.

Johnson, A. R., and Moran, N. C., 1969a, Selective release of histamine from rat mast cells by compound 48/80 and antigen, *Am. J. Physiol.* **216:**453–489.

Johnson, A. R., and Moran, N. C., 1969b, Release of histamine from rat mast cells: A comparison of the effects of 48/80 and two antigen–antibody systems, *Fed. Proc.* **28:**1716–1720.

Johnson, A. R., and Moran, N. C., 1970, Inhibition of the release of histamine from rat mast cells: The effect of cold and adrenergic drugs on release of histamine by compound 48/80 and antigen, *J. Pharmacol. Exp. Ther.* **175:**632–640.

Johnson, A. R., Moran, N. C., and Mayer, S. E., 1974, Cyclic AMP content and histamine release in rat mast cells, *J. Immunol.* **112:**511–519.

Johnson, A. R., Hugli, T. E., and Müller-Eberhard, H. J., 1975, Release of histamine from rat mast cells by the complement peptides C3a and C5a, *Immunology* **28:**1067–1080.

Jones, W. O., Rothwell, T. L. W., Dineen, J. K., and Griffiths, D. A., 1974, Studies on the role of histamine and 5-hydroxytryptamine in immunity against the nematode *Trichostrongylus colubriformis*. II. Amine levels in the intestine of infected guinea-pigs, *Int. Arch. Allergy Appl. Immunol.* **64:**14–27.

Juhlin, L., 1963, Basophil leukocyte differential in blood and bone marrow. *Acta Haematol.* **29:**89–95.

Juhlin, L., and Shelley, W. B., 1961, Role of mast cell and basophil in cold urticaria with associated systemic reactions, *J. Am. Med. Assoc.* **177:**371–377.

Kaliner, M., and Austen, K. F., 1973, A sequence of biochemical events in the antigen-induced release of chemical mediators from sensitized human lung tissue, *J. Exp. Med.* **138:**1077–1094.

Kaliner, M., and Austen, K. F., 1974, Cyclic AMP, ATP, and reversed anaphylactic histamine release from rat mast cells, *J. Immunol.* **112:**664–674.

Karnovsky, M. J., and Shea, S. M., 1970, Transcapillary transport by pinocytosis, *Microvasc. Res.* **2:**353–360.

Katz, S. I., Parker, D., Sommer, G., and Turk, J. L., 1974, Suppressor cells in normal immunization as a basic homeostatic phenomenon, *Nature (London)* **248:**612–614.

Kay, A. B., and Austen, K. F., 1972, Chemotaxis of human basophil leukocytes, *Clin. Exp. Immunol.* **11:**557–563.

Keller, R., 1962, Effect of antibodies against rat γ-globulin or rat albumin on isolated peritoneal rat mast cells, *Nature (London)* **193:**282–283.

Keller, R., 1966, *Tissue Mast Cells in Immune Reactions*, American Elsevier, New York.

Keller, R., 1968, Interrelations between different types of cells. II. Histamine-release from mast cells of various species by cationic peptides of polymorphonuclear leukocyte lysozymes and other cationic compounds, *Int. Arch. Allergy Appl. Immunol.* **34:**139–144.

Klebe, R. J., 1974, Isolation of a collagen-dependent cell attachment factor, *Nature (London)* **250:**248–251.

Kleinman, H. K., Silbert, J. E., and Silbert, C. K., 1975, Heparan sulfate of skin fibroblasts grown in culture, *Connect. Tissue Res.* **4**:17–23.
Kownatzki, E., Till, G., and Gemsa, D., 1978, Lymphocytes are stimulated by histamine to release an inhibitor of eosinophil chemotactic migration, *Z. Immunitaetsforsch.* **154**:330.
Kraemer, P. M., 1971, Heparan sulfates of cultured cells. II. Acid-soluble and precipitable species of different cell lines, *Biochemistry* **10**:1445–1451.
Kraemer, P. M., and Tobay, R. A., 1972, Cell cycle dependent desquamation of heparan sulfate from the cell surface, *J. Cell Biol.* **55**:713–717.
Lagunoff, D., 1972a, The mechanism of histamine release from mast cells. *Biochem. Pharmacol.* **21**:1889–1896.
Lagunoff, D., 1972b, Contributions of electon microscopy to the study of mast cells, *J. Invest. Dermatol.* **58**:296–311.
Lagunoff, D., and Benditt, E. P., 1963, Proteolytic enzymes of mast cells, *Ann. N.Y. Acad. Sci.* **103**:185–198.
Lasker, S. E., 1977, The heterogeneity of heparins, *Fed. Proc.* **36**:92–97.
Lett-Brown, M. A., and Leonard, E. J., 1977, Histamine-induced inhibition of normal human basophil chemotaxis to C5a, *J. Immunol.* **118**:815–818.
Lett-Brown, M. A., Boetcher, D. A., and Leonard, E. J., 1976, Chemotactic responses of normal human basophils to C5a and to lymphocyte-derived chemotactic factor, *J. Immunol.* **117**:246–252.
Lewis, R. A., and Austen, K. F., 1977, Non-respiratory functions of pulmonary cells: The mast cell, *Fed. Proc.* **36**:2676–2683.
Lichtenstein, L. M., 1968, Mechanisms of allergic histamine release from human leukocytes, in: *Biochemistry of the Acute Allergic Reactions* (K. F. Austen and E. L. Becker, eds.), pp. 153–171, F. A. Davis, Philadelphia.
Lichtenstein, L. M., 1971, The immediate allergic response: *In vitro* separation of antigen activation, decay, and histamine release, *J. Immunol.* **107**:1122–1130.
Lichtenstein, L. M., 1975a, Sequential analysis of the allergic response: Cyclic AMP, calcium and histamine, *Int. Arch. Allergy Appl. Immunol.* **49**:143–154.
Lichtenstein L. M., 1975b, The mechanism of basophil histamine release induced by antigen and by the calcium ionophore A23187, *J. Immunol.* **114**:1692–1698.
Lichtenstein, L. M., 1976, Hormone receptor interaction in the control of allergic and inflammatory reactions, in: *The Role of Immunological Factors in Infectious, Allergic, and Autoimmune Processes* (R. F. Beers and E. G. Bassett, eds.), p. 339, Raven, New York.
Lichtenstein, L. M., and Conroy, M. C., 1977, The "releasability" of mediators from human basophils and granulocytes, in: *Ninth International Congress of Allergology, Buenos Aires* (E. Mathov, ed.), pp. 109–115, Excerpta Medica, Amsterdam.
Lichtenstein, L. M., and DeBernardo, R., 1971, The immediate allergic response: *In vitro* action of cyclic AMP-active and other drugs on the two stages of histamine release, *J. Immunol.* **107**:1131–1136.
Lichtenstein, L. M., and Gillespie, E., 1973, Inhibition of histamine release by histamine is controlled by an H_2 receptor, *Nature (London)* **244**:287–288.
Lichtenstein, L. M., and Gillespie, E., 1975, The effects of the H_1 and H_2 antihistamines on "allergic" histamine release and its inhibition by histamine, *J. Pharmacol. Exp. Ther.* **192**:441–450.
Lichtenstein, L. M., and Henney, C. S., 1974, Adenylate cyclase-linked hormone receptors: An important mechanism for the immunoregulation of leukocytes, in: *Progress in Immunology II*, Vol. 2 (L. Brent and J. Holborow, eds.) pp. 73–83, North-Holland, Amsterdam.
Lichtenstein, L. M., and Margolis, S., 1968, Histamine release *in vitro:* Inhibition by catecholamines and methylxanthines, *Science* **161**:902–903.
Lichtenstein, L. M., and Osler, A. G., 1966a, Studies on the mechanisms of hypersensitivity phenomena. XI. The effect of normal human serum on the release of histamine from human leukocytes by ragween pollen antigen, *J. Immunol.* **96**:159–168.
Lichtenstein, L. M., and Osler, A. G., 1966b, Studies on the mechanisms of hypersensitivity phenomena. XII. An *in vitro* study of the reaction between ragweed pollen antigen, allergic human serum and ragweed-sensitive human leukocytes, *J. Immunol.* **96**:169–179.
Lichtenstein, L. M., Norman, P. S., Winkenwerder, W. L., and Osler, A. G., 1966, *In vitro* studies of human ragweed allergy: Changes in cellular and humoral activity associated with specific desensitization, *J. Clin. Invest.* **45**:1126–1136.

Lichtenstein, L. M., Norman, P. S., and Connell, J. T., 1967, Comparison between skin-sensitizing antibody titers and leukocyte sensitivity measurements as an index of the severity of ragweed hay fever, *J. Allergy* **40:**160–167.

Lichtenstein, L. M., Holtzman, N. A., and Burnett, L. S., 1968, A quantitative *in vitro* study of the chromatographic distribution and immunoglobulin characteristics of human blocking antibody, *J. Immunol.* **101:**317–324.

Lichtenstein, L. M., Gillespie, E., and Bourne, H., 1973a, Studies on the biochemical mechanisms of IgE-mediated histamine release, in: *The Biological Role of the Immunoglobulin E System* (K. Ishizaka and D. H. Dayton, eds.), pp. 165–180, U.S. Government Printing Office, Washington.

Lichtenstein, L. M., Henney, C. S., Bourne, H. R., and Greenough, W. B., 1973b, III. Effects of cholera toxin on *in vitro* models of immediate and delayed hypersensitivity. Further evidence for the role of cyclic adenosine 3′,5′-monophosphate, *J. Clin. Invest.* **52:**691–697.

Lichtenstein, L. M., Sobotka, A. K., Malveaux, F. J., and Gillespie, E., 1978, IgE-induced changes in human basophil cyclic AMP levels, *Int. Arch. Allergy Appl. Immunol.* **56:**473–478.

Lindell, S. E., Rorsman, H., and Westling, H., 1961, Histamine formation in human blood, *Acta Allergol.* **16:**216–227.

Lippman, M. M., and Mathews, M. B., 1977, Heparins: Varying effects on cell proliferation *in vitro* and lack of correlation with anticoagulant activity, *Fed. Proc.* **36:**55–59.

Loeffler, L. J., Lorenberg, W., and Sjoerdsma, A., 1971, Effects of dibutyryl-3′-5′ cyclic adenosine monophosphate, phosphodiesterase inhibitors and prostaglandin E_1 on compound 48/80-induced histamine release from rat peritoneal mast cells *in vitro*, *Biochem. Pharmacol.* **20:**2287–2297.

Malveaux, F. J., Conroy, M. C., Adkinson, N. F., Jr., and Lichtenstein, L. M., 1978, IgE receptors on human basophils: Relationship to serum IgE concentration, *J. Clin. Invest.* **62:**176–181.

Mann, P. R., 1969a, An electron microscopic study of the degranulation of rat peritoneal mast cells brought about by four different agents, *Br. J. Dermatol.* **81:**926–936.

Mann, P. R., 1969b, An electron microscopic study of the relations between mast cells and eosinophil leukocytes, *J. Pathol.* **98:**183–186.

Marone, G., and Lichtenstein, L. M., 1978, Adenosine–adenosine deaminase modulation of histamine release, *J. Allergy Clin. Immunol.* **61:**131.

Mayrhofer, G., Bazin, H., and Gowans, J. L., 1976, Nature of cells binding anti-IgE in rats immunized with *Nippostrongylus brasiliensis*: IgE synthesis in regional nodes and concentrations in mucosal mast cells, *Eur. J. Immunol.* **6:**537–545.

McCluskey, R. T., Hall, C. L., and Colvin, R. B., 1978, Immune complex mediated diseases, *Hum. Pathol.* **9:**71–84.

Medenica, M., and Rostenberg, A., 1971, A comparative light and electron microscopic study of primary irritant contact dermatitis and allergic contact dermatitis, *J. Invest. Dermatol.* **56:**259–271.

Mendoza, G., and Metzger, H., 1976, Disparity of IgE binding between normal and tumor mouse mast cells, *J. Immunol.* **117:**1573–1578.

Metcalfe, D. D., Lewis, R. A., Silbert, J. E., Rosenberg, R. D., Wasserman, S. I., and Austen, K. F., 1978, Isolation, identification, and characterization of heparin from human lung, *Fed. Proc.* **37:**1776.

Metzger, H., and Bach, M. K., 1978, The receptor for IgE on mast cells and basophils: Studies on IgE binding and on the structure of the receptor, in: *Immediate Hypersensitivity: Modern Concepts and Developments* (M. K. Bach, ed.), pp. 561–588, Dekker, New York.

Michels, N. A., 1938, The mast cells, in: *Handbook of Hematology,* Vol. 1 (H. Downey, ed.), pp. 232–372, Hoeber, New York. Reprinted in *Ann. N.Y. Acad. Sci.* **103:** Appendix, 1–372, 1963.

Miller, H. R. P., 1971, Immune reaction in mucous membranes. II. The differentiation of intestinal mast cells during helminth expulsion in the rat, *Lab. Invest.* **24:**339–347.

Mongar, J. L., and Perera, B. A. V., 1965, Oxygen consumption during histamine release by antigen and compound 48/80, *Immunology* **8:**511–518.

Mongar, J. L., and Schild, H. O., 1957, Effect of temperature on the anaphylactic reaction, *J. Physiol. (London)* **135:**320–338.

Morrison, D. C., 1978, Receptor modulation and mast cell secretion, *J. Invest. Dermatol.* **71:**85–91.

Morrison, D. C., and Henson, P. M., 1978, Release of mediators from mast cells and basophils induced by different stimuli, in: *Immediate Hypersensitivity: Modern Concepts and Developments* (M. K. Bach, ed.), pp. 431–502, Dekker, New York.

Morrison, D. C., Roser, J. F., Cochrane, C. G., and Henson, P. M., 1975a, Two distinct mechanisms for the initiation of mast cell degranulation, *Int. Arch. Allergy Appl. Immunol.* **49**:172–178.

Morrison, D. C., Roser, J. F., Henson, P. M., and Cochrane, C. G., 1975b, Isolation and characterization of a noncytotoxic mast cell activator from cobra venom, *Inflammation* **1**:103–115.

Mosesson, M. W., 1978, Structure of human plasma cold-insoluble globulin and the mechanism of its precipitation in the cold with heparin or fibrin-fibrinogen complexes, *Ann. N.Y. Acad. Sci.* **312**:11–30.

Musson, R. A., and Becker, E. L., 1977, The role of an activatable esterase in immune-dependent phagocytosis by human neutrophils, *J. Immunol.* **118**:1354–1365.

Newball, H. H., Talamo, R. C., and Lichtenstein, L. M., 1975, Release of leukocyte kallikrein mediated by IgE, *Nature (London)* **254**:635–636.

Nichols, B. A., and Bainton, D. F., 1973, Differentiation of human monocytes in bone marrow and blood: Sequential formation of two granule populations, *Lab. Invest.* **29**:27–40.

Norman, P. S., Lichtenstein, L. M., and Ishisaka, K., 1973, Diagnostic tests in ragweed hay fever, *J. Allergy Clin. Immunol.* **52**:210–224.

Norn, S., 1965, Influence of anti-rheumatic agents on the release of histamine from rat peritoneal mast cells after an antigen–antibody reaction, *Acta Pharmacol. Toxicol.* **22**:369–378.

Olsson, I., 1969, The intracellular transport of glycosaminoglycans (mucopolysaccharides) in human leukocytes, *Exp. Cell Res.* **54**:318–324.

Olsson, I., 1971, Mucopolysaccarides of rabbit bone marrow cells, *Exp. Cell Res.* **67**:416–426.

Olsson, I., Gardell, S., and Thunell, S., 1968, Biosynthesis of glycosaminoglycans (mucopolysaccarides) in human leukocytes, *Biochim. Biophys. Acta* **165**:309–323.

Orange, R. P., Austen, W. G., and Austen, K. F., 1971, Immunologic release of histamine and slow reacting substance of anaphylaxis from human lung. I. Modulation by agents influencing cellular levels of cyclic 3′,5′-adenosine monophosphate, *J. Exp. Med.* **134**:163S–148S.

Orenstein, N. S., Hammond, M. E., Dvorak, H. F., and Feder, J., 1976, Esterase and protease activity of purified guinea pig basophil granules, *Biochem. Biophys. Res. Communun.* **72**:230–235.

Orenstein, N. S., Galli, S. J., Hammond, M. E., Smith, G. N., Silbert, J. E., and Dvorak, H. F., 1977, Mucopolysaccharides synthesized by guinea pig basophilic leukocytes, *Fed. Proc.* **36**: 1329.

Orenstein, N. S., Galli, S. J., Dvorak, A. M., Silbert, J. E., and Dvorak, H. F., 1978, Sulfated glycosaminoglycans of guinea pig basophilic leukocytes. *J. Immunol.* **121**:586–592.

Osler, A. G., Lichtenstein, L. M., and Levy, D. A., 1968, *In vitro* studies of human reaginic allergy, *Adv. Immunol.* **8**:183–231.

Ovary, Z., 1968, Histology of PCA reactions in guinea pigs. A comparison of reactions produced by guinea pig γG1 and rabbit antibodies, *J. Immunol.* **100**:159–168.

Padawer, J., 1969, Uptake of colloidal thorium dioxide by mast cells, *J. Cell Biol.* **40**:747–760.

Padawer, J., 1970, The reaction of rat mast cells to polylysine, *J. Cell Biol.* **47**:352–372.

Padawer, J., 1971, Phagocytosis of particulate substances by mast cells, *Lab. Invest.* **25**:320–330.

Padawer, J., 1974, Mast cells: Extended lifespan and lack of granule turnover under normal *in vivo* conditions, *Exp. Mol. Pathol.* **20**:269–280.

Padawer, J., 1978, The mast cell and immediate hypersensitivity, in: *Immediate Hypersensitivity: Modern Concepts and Developments* (M. K. Bach, ed.), pp. 301–367, Dekker, New York.

Parish, W. E., 1978, Evidence for human IgG antibodies anaphylactically sensitizing man, in: *Immediate Hypersensitivity: Modern Concepts and Developments* (M. K. Bach, ed.), pp. 277–299, Dekker, New York.

Pearce, F. L., Behrendt, H., Blum, U., Poblete-Freund, G., Pult, P., Stang-Voss, C., and Schmutzler, W., 1977, Isolation and study of functional mast cells from lung and mesentery of the guinea pig, *Agents Actions* **7**:45–56.

Pearlstein, E., 1976, Plasma membrane glycoprotein which mediates adhesion of fibroblasts to collagen, *Nature (London)* **262**:497–500.

Pearlstein, E., and Gold, L. I., 1978, High-molecular-weight glycoprotein as a mediator of cellular adhesion, *Ann. N.Y. Acad. Sci.* **312**:278–292.

Pepys, J., Turner-Warwick, M., Dawson, P. L., and Hinson, K. R. W., 1968, in: *Allergology,* No. 162 (E. Rose, R. Richter, A. Shehon, and A. W. Frankland, eds.), p. 221, Excerpta Medica Foundation, Amsterdam.

Pepera, B. A. V., and Mongar, J. L., 1963, The role in anaphylaxis of a chymotrypsin-like enzyme in rat mast cells, *Immunology* **6:**478–483.

Perera, B. A. V., and Mongar, J. L., 1965, Effect of anoxia, glucose and thioglycollate on anaphylactic and compound 48/80-induced histamine release in isolated rat mast cells, *Immunology* **8:**519–525.

Petersson, B. A., Nilsson, A., and Stalenheim, G., 1975, Induction of histamine release and desensitization in human leukocytes—Effect of anaphylatoxin, *J. Immunol.* **114:**1581–1584.

Plaut, M., and Lichtenstein, L. M., 1978, Pharmacologic control of mediator release, in: *Immediate Hypersensitivity: Modern Concepts and Developments* (M. K. Bach, ed.), pp. 503–532, Dekker, New York.

Plaut, M., Lichtenstein, L. M., Gillespie, E., and Henney, C. S., 1973, Studies on the mechanism of lymphocyte-mediated cytolysis. IV. Specificity of the histamine receptor on effector T-cells, *J. Immunol.* **111:**389–394.

Plaut, M., Lichtenstein, L. M., and Henney, C. S., 1975, Modulation of immediate hypersensitivity and cell-mediated immunity: The role of histamine, in: *Immunopharmacology* (M. Rosenthale and H. Mansmann, eds.), p. 57, Spectrum, Holliswood, New York.

Pruzansky, J. J., and Patterson, R., 1967, Subcellular distribution of histamine in human leukocytes, *Proc. Soc. Exp. Biol. Med.* **124:**56–59.

Pruzansky, J. J., and Patterson, R., 1975, The diisopropylfluorophosphate inhibitable step in antigen-induced histamine release from human leukocytes, *J. Immunol.* **114:**939–943.

Ranadive, N. S., and Cochrane, C. G., 1968, Isolation and characterization of permeability factors from rabbit neutrophils, *J. Exp. Med.* **128:**605–622.

Ranadive, N. S., and Cochrane, C. G., 1970, Basic proteins in rat neutrophils that increase vascular permeability, *Clin. Exp. Immunol.* **6:**905–911.

Ranadive, N. S., and Cochrane, C. G., 1971, Mechanism of histamine release from mast cells by cationic protein (band 2) from neutrophil lysosomes, *J. Immunol.* **106:**506–516.

Ranadive, N. S., and Muir, J. D., 1972, Similarities in the mechanism of histamine release induced by cationic protein from neutrophils and by complement dependent Ag-Ab reaction, *Int. Arch. Allergy Appl. Immunol.* **42:**236–249.

Ranadive, N. S., and Ruben, D. H., 1973, Mechanism of histamine release from rat mast cells by compound 48/80: Comparison with the release induced by cationic protein, *Int. Arch. Allergy Appl. Immunol.* **44:**745–758.

Richerson, H. B., 1971, Cutaneous basophil (Jones-Mote) hypersensitivity after "tolerogenic" doses of intravenous ovalbumin in the guinea pig, *J. Exp. Med.* **134:**630–641.

Richerson, H. B., Dvorak, H. F., and Leskowitz, S., 1969, Cutaneous basophilic hypersensitivity: A new interpretation of the Jones-Mote reaction, *J. Immunol.* **103:**1431–1434.

Richerson, H. B., Dvorak, H. F., and Leskowitz, S., 1970, Cutaneous basophil hypersensitivity. I. A new look at the Jones-Mote reaction, general characteristics, *J. Exp. Med.* **132:**546–557.

Riley, J. F., 1959, *The Mast Cells,* Livingstone, Edinburgh.

Roberts, L. J., II., Lewis, R. A., Hansbrough, R., Austen, K. F., and Oates, J. A., 1978, Biosynthesis of prostaglandins, thromboxanes, and 12-hydroxy-5,8,10,14-eicosatetraenoic acid by rat mast cells, *Fed. Proc.* **37:**284.

Rocklin, R. E., 1975, Regulation of migration inhibitory factor (MIF) production by histamine receptor-bearing lymphocytes, *Fed. Proc.* **34:**977.

Rocklin, R. E., 1976, Modulation of cellular-immune responses *in vivo* and *in vitro* by histamine receptor-bearing lymphocytes, *J. Clin. Invest.* **57:**1051–1058.

Röhlich, P., Anderson, P., and Uvnäs, B., 1971, Electron microscopic observations on compound 48/80 induced degranulation in rat mast cells. Evidence for sequential exocytosis of storage granules, *J. Cell Biol.* **51:**465–483.

Rothwell, T. L. W., 1974, Studies of the responses of basophil and eosinophil leukocytes and mast cells to the nematode *Trichostrongylus colubriformis*. I. Observations during the expulsion of first and second infections by guinea pigs, *J. Pathol.* **116:**51–60.

Rothwell, T. L. W., and Dineen, J. K., 1972, Cellular reactions in guinea pigs following primary and challenge infection with *Trichostrongylus colubriformis* with special reference to roles played by eosinophils and basophils in rejection of the parasite, *Immunology* **22:**733–745.

Rothwell, T. L. W., and Love, R. J., 1975, Studies of the responses of basophil and eosinophil leucocytes and mast cells to the nematode *Trichostrongylus colubriformis,* II. Changes in cell numbers following infection of thymectomised and adoptively or passively immunised guinea pigs, *J. Pathol.* **116:**183–194.

Rothwell, T. L. W., Jones, W. O., and Love, R. J., 1974a, Studies on the role of histamine and 5-hydroxytryptamine in immunity against the nematode *Trichostrongylus colubriformis*, III. Inhibition of worm expulsion from guinea pigs by treatment with reserpine, *Int. Arch. Allergy Appl. Immunol.* **47**:875–886.

Rothwell, T. L. W., Prichard, R. K., and Love, R. J., 1974b, Studies on the role of histamine and 5-hydroxytryptamine in immunity against the nematode *Trichostrongylus colubriformis*. I. *In vivo* and *in vitro* effects of the amines, *Int. Arch. Allergy Appl. Immunol.* **46**:1–13.

Rubin, R. P., 1974, *Calcium and the Secretory Process*, Plenum, New York.

Ruoslahti, E., and Engvall, E., 1978, Immunochemical and collagen-binding properties of fibronectin, in: *Fibroblast Surface Protein* (A. Vaheri, E. Ruoslahti, and D. Mosher, eds.), *Ann. N.Y. Acad. Sci.* **312**:178–191.

Russell, J. D., Russell, S. B., and Trupin, K. M., 1977, The effect of histamine in the growth of cultured fibroblasts isolated from normal and keloid tissue, *J. Cell Physiol.* **93**:389–394.

Saeki, K., 1964, Effects of compound 48/80, chymotrypsin and anti-serum on isolated mast cells under aerobic and anaerobic conditions, *Jpn. J. Pharmacol.* **14**:375–390.

Sampson, D., and Archer, G. T., 1967, Release of histamine from human basophils, *Blood* **29**:722–736.

Seegers, W., and Janoff, A., 1966, Mediators of inflammation in leukocyte lysosomes. VI. Partial purification and characterization of a mast cell-rupturing component, *J. Exp. Med.* **124**:833–849.

Segal, D. M., Taurog, J. D., and Metzger, H., 1977, Dimeric immunoglobulin E serves as a unit signal for mast cell degranulation, *Proc. Natl. Acad. Sci. USA.* **74**:2933–2997.

Shelley, W. B., and Juhlin, L., 1961, New test for detecting anaphylactic sensitivity: Basophil reaction, *Nature (London)* **191**:1056–1058.

Simson, J. A. V., Hintz, D. S., Munster, A. M., and Spicer, S. S., 1977, Immunocytochemical evidence for antibody binding to mast cell granules, *Exp. Mol. Pathol.* **26**:85–91.

Siraganian, R. P., 1977, Automated histamine analysis for *in vitro* allergy testing. II. Correlation of skin test results with *in vitro* whole blood histamine release in 82 patients, *J. Allergy Clin. Immunol.* **59**:214–222.

Siraganian, R. P., and Brodsky, M. J., 1976, Automated histamine analysis for *in vitro* allergy testing. I. A method utilizing allergen induced histamine release from whole blood, *J. Allergy Clin. Immunol.* **57**:525–540.

Siraganian, R. P., and Hook, W. A., 1976, Complement-induced histamine release from human basophils. II. Mechanism of the histamine release reaction, *J. Immunol.* **116**:639–646.

Siraganian, R. P., and Levine, B. B., 1975, Unique serum requirement for histamine release from human basophils, *Int. Arch. Allergy Appl. Immunol.* **48**:530–536.

Siraganian, R. P., and Siraganian, P. A., 1975, Mechanism of action of concanavalin A on human basophils, *J. Immunol.* **114**:886–893.

Smith, R. T., and vonKorff, R. W., 1957, A heparin-precipitable fraction of human plasma. I. Isolation and characterization of the fraction, *J. Clin. Inves.* **36**:596–604.

Solley, G. O., Gleich, G. J., Jordan, R. E., and Schroeter, A. L., 1976, The late phase of the immediate wheal and flare skin reaction, *J. Clin. Invest.* **58**:403–420.

Soter, N. A., and Austen, K. F., 1976, The diversity of mast cell-derived mediators: Implications for acute, subacute, and chronic cutaneous inflammatory disorders, *J. Invest. Dermatol.* **67**:313–319.

Spicer, S. S., Simson, J. A. V., and Farrington, J. E., 1975, Mast cell phagocytosis of red blood cells, *Am. J. Pathol.* **80**:481–498.

Stadecker, M. J., and Leskowitz, S., 1976, The inhibition of cutaneous basophil hypersensitivity reactions by a heterologous anti-guinea pig T cell serum, *J. Immunol.* **116**:1646–1651.

Stadecker, M. J., Lukic, M., Dvorak, A. M., and Leskowitz, S., 1977, The cutaneous basophil response to phytohemagglutinin in chickens, *J. Immunol.* **118**:1564–1568.

Stallman, P. J., and Aalberse, R. C., 1977a, Estimates of basophil-bound IgE by quantitative immunofluorescence microscopy, *Int. Arch. Allergy Appl. Immunol.* **54**:9–18.

Stallman, P. J., and Aalberse, R. C., 1977b, Quantitation of basophil-bound IgE in atopic and monotopic subjects, *Int. Arch. Allergy Appl. Immunol.* **54**:114–120.

Stallman, P. J., Aalberse, R. C., Brühl, P. C., and van Elven, E. H., 1977a, Experiments in the passive sensitization of human basophils, using quantitative immunofluoresence microscopy, *Int. Arch. Allergy Appl. Immunol.* **54**:364–373.

Stallman, P. J., Wagenaar, S. S., Sevierenga, J., van der Wal, R. J., and Feltkamp-Vroom, T. M.,

1977b, Cell-bound IgE on human mast cells and basophilic granulocytes in atopic and non-atopic subjects, *Int. Arch Allergy Appl. Immunol.* **54:** 443–450.

Stanworth, D. R., Humphrey, J. H., Bennich, H., and Johansson, S. G. O., 1967, Specific inhibition of the Prausnitz–Küstner reaction by an atypical human myeloma protein, *Lancet* **2:**330–332.

Stanworth, D. R., Humphrey, J. H., Bennich, H., and Johansson, S. G. O., 1968, Inhibition of Prausnitz–Küstner reaction by proteolytic cleavage fragments of a human myeloma protein of immunoglobulin class E, *Lancet* **2:**17–18.

Stashenko, P. P., Bhan, A. K., Schlossman, S. F., and McCluskey, R. T., 1977, Local transfer of delayed hypersensitivity and cutaneous basophil hypersensitivity, *J. Immunol.* **119:**1987–1993.

Stathakis, N. E., and Mosesson, M. W., 1977, Interactions among heparin, cold-insoluble globulin, and fibrinogen in formation of the heparin precipitable fraction of plasma, *J. Clin. Invest.* **60:**855–865.

Stechschulte, D. J., 1978, Non-IgE homocytotropic antibody in animals, in: *Immediate Hypersensitivity: Modern Concepts and Developments* (M. K. Bach, ed.), pp. 259–276, Dekker, New York.

Stechschulte, D. J., and Austen, K. F., 1974, Anaphylaxis, in: *The Inflammatory Process,* Vol. 3, 2nd ed. (B. W. Zweifach, L. Grant, and R. T. McCluskey, eds.), pp. 237–276, Academic, New York.

Sue, T. K., and Jaques, L. B., 1974, Sulfated mycopolysaccharides and basophilic leukocytes in rabbits on a high cholesterol/oil diet, *Proc. Soc. Exp. Biol. Med.* **146:**1006–1013.

Sue, T. K., and Jaques, L. B., 1976, Susceptibility to experimental atherosclerosis: Relation to mast cells and heparin, *Atherosclerosis* **25:**137–139.

Sullivan, A. L., Grimley, P. M., and Metzger, H., 1971, Electron microscopic localization of immunoglobulin E on the surface membrane of human basophils, *J. Exp. Med.* **134:**1403–1416.

Sullivan, T. J., Parker, K. L., Stenson, W., and Parker, C. W., 1975a, Modulation of cyclic AMP in purified rat mast cells. I. Responses to pharmacologic, metabolic, and physical stimuli, *J. Immunol.* **114:**1473–1479.

Sullivan, T. J., Parker, K. L., Eisen, S. A., and Parker, C. W., 1975b, Modulation of cyclic AMP in purified rat mast cells. II. Studies on the relationship between intracellular cyclic AMP concentrations and histamine release, *J. Immunol.* **114:**1480–1485.

Sullivan, T. J., Parker, K. L., Kulczycki, A., Jr., and Parker, C. W., 1976, Modulation of cyclic AMP in purified rat mast cells. III. Studies on the effects of concanavalin A and anit-IgE on cyclic AMP concentrations during histamine release, *J. Immunol.* **117:**713–716.

Taylor, W. A., and Sheldon, D., 1974, Mast cell degranulation: A comparison of the inhibitory actions of disodium cromoglycate, drugs known to influence the level of intracellular cyclic nucleotide and diisopropylfluorophosphate (DFP), *Int. Arch. Allergy Appl. Immunol.* **47:**696–707.

Theoharides, T. C., and Douglas, W. W., 1978, Secretion in mast cells induced by calcium entrapped within phospholipid vesicles, *Science* **201**:1143–1145.

Theuson, D. O., Speck, L., and Grant, J. A., 1977, Histamine-releasing activity produced by human mononuclear cells, *Fed. Proc.* **36:**1300.

Theuson, D. O., Lett-Brown, M. A., and Grant, J. A., 1979, Histamine release from basophils by mononuclear cell culture supernatants, *Fed. Proc.* **38**:1459.

Thon, I. L., and Uvnäs, B., 1966, Mode of storage of histamine in mast cells, *Acta Physiol. Scand.* **67:**455–470.

Tomioka, H., and Ishizaka, K., 1971, Mechanisms of passive sensitization. II. Presence of receptors for IgE on monkey mast cells, *J. Immunol.* **107:**971–978.

Trotter, C. M., and Orr, T. S. C., 1973, A fine structure study of some cellular components in allergic reactions. I. Degranulation of human mast cells in allergic asthma and perennial rhinitis, *Clin. Allergy* **3:**411–425.

Trotter, C. M., and Orr, T. C. S., 1974, A fine structure study of some cellular components in allergic reactions. II. Mast cells in normal and atopic human skin, *Clin. Allergy* **4:**421–433.

Uvnäs, B., and Antonsson, J., 1963, Triggering action of phophatidase A and chymotrypsins on degranulation of rat mesentery mast cells, *Biochem. Pharmacol.* **12:**867–873.

Uvnäs, B., and Thon, I., 1966, A physico-chemical model of histamine release from mast cells, in: *Mechanisms of Release of Biogenic Amines,* Proceedings of the International Wenner-Gren Symposium, Stockholm 1965, pp. 361–370, Pergamon, Oxford.

Uvnäs, B., Åborg, C.-H., and Bergendorff, A., 1970, Storage of histamine in mast cell. Evidence for an ionic binding of histamine to protein carboxyls in the granule heparin–protein complex, *Acta Physiol. Scand.* **78:** *Suppl.***336:**3–26.

Valentine, M. D., Bloch, K. J., and Austen, K. F., 1967, Mechanisms of immunologic injury of rat peritoneal mast cells. III. Cytotoxic histamine release, *J. Immunol.* **99:**98–110.

Valentine, W. N., Lawrence, J. S., Pearce, M. L., and Beck, W. S., 1955, The relation of the basophil to blood histamine in man, *Blood* **10:**154–159.

Van Arsdel, P. P., Jr., and Bray, R. E., 1961, On the release of histamine from rat peritoneal mast cells by compound 48/80: Effects of metabolic inhibitors, *J. Pharmacol. Exp. Ther.* **133:**319–324.

van Elven, E. H., Stallman, P. J., and Brühl, P. C., 1977, Electron microscopic studies on human basophils from atopic and nonatopic subjects, using horse radish peroxidase labelled anti-IgE, *Int. Arch. Allergy Appl. Immunol.* **54:**560–567.

Waldmann, T. A., 1969, Disorders of immunoglobulin metabolism, *New Engl. J. Med.* **281:**1170–1177.

Waldmann, T. A., Iio, A., Ogawa, M., McIntyre, O. R., and Strober, W., 1976, The metabolism of IgE. Studies in normal individuals and in a patient with IgE myeloma, *J. Immunol.* **117:**1139–1144.

Ward, P. A., Offen, C. D., and Montgomery, J. R., 1971, Chemoattractants of leukocytes, with special reference to lymphocytes, *Fed. Proc.* **30:**1721–1724.

Ward, P. A., Dvorak, H. F., Cohen, S., Yoshida, T., Data, R., and Selvaggio, S. S., 1975, Chemotaxis of basophils by lymphocyte-dependent and lymphocyte-independent mechanisms, *J. Immunol.* **114:**1523–1531.

Wasserman, S. I., Goetzl, E. J., and Austen, K. F., 1974a, Preformed eosinophil chemotactic factor of anaphylaxis (ECF-A), *J. Immunol.* **112:**351–358.

Wasserman, S. I., Goetzl, E. J., Kaliner, M., and Austen, K. F., 1974b, Modulation of the immunological release of the eosinophil chemotactic factor of anaphylaxis from human lung, *Immunology* **26:**677–684.

Werb, Z., and Aggeler, J., 1978, Proteases induce secretion of collagenase and plasminogen activator by fibroblasts, *Proc. Natl. Acad. Sci. USA* **75:**1839–1843.

Wikel, S. K., and Allen, J. R., 1976, Acquired resistance to ticks. I. Passive transfer of resistance, *Immunology* **30:**311–316.

Wintroub, B. U., Mihm, M. C., Jr., Goetzl, E. J., Soter, N. A., and Austen, K. F., 1978, Morphologic and functional evidence for release of mast-cell products in bullous pemphigoid, *New Engl. J. Med.* **298:**417–421.

Woodin, A. M., and Wieneke, A. A., 1970, Action of DFP on the leukocyte and the axon, *Nature (London)* **227:**460–463.

Yamasaki, H., and Saeki, K., 1967, Inhibition of mast cell degranulation by anti-inflammatory agents, *Arch. Int. Pharmacodyn. Ther.* **168:**166–179.

Yurt, R., and Austen, K. F., 1977, Preparative purification of the rat mast cell chymase: Characterization and interaction with granule components. *J. Exp. Med.* **146:**1405–1419.

Yurt, R. W., Leid, R. W., Jr., Spragg, J., and Austen, K. F., 1977a, Native heparin from rat peritoneal mast cells, *J. Biol. Chem.* **252:**518–521.

Yurt, R. W., Leid, R. W., Jr., Spragg, J., and Austen, K. F., 1977b, Immunologic release of heparin from purified rat peritoneal mast cells, *J. Immunol.* **118:**1201–1207.

Zeiger, R. S., Twarog, F. J., and Colten, H. R., 1976a, Histaminase release from human granulocytes, *J. Exp. Med.* **144:**1049–1061.

Zeiger, R. S., Yurdin, D. L., and Colten, H. R., 1976b, Histamine metabolism. II. Cellular and subcellular localization of the catabolic enzymes, histaminase and histamine methyl transferase, in human leukocytes, *J. Allergy Clin. Immunol.* **58:**172–179.

Zurier, R. B., Hoffstein, S., Kammerman, S., and Tai, H. H., 1974, Mechanisms of lysozomal enzyme release from human leukocytes. II. Effects of cAMP and cGMP, autonomic agonists, and agents whigh affect microtubule function, *J. Clin. Invest.* **53:**297–309.

Zweiman, B., Slott, R. I., and Atkins, P., 1976, Factors in the tissue eosinophil response in human immediate hypersensitivity reactions, *Int. Arch. Allergy Appl. Immunol.* **52:**48–52.

2

Participation of Eosinophils in Immunological Systems

DANIEL G. COLLEY and STEPHANIE L. JAMES

1. Introduction

The eosinophil is a polymorphonuclear leukocyte which is characterized by the high affinity of its cytoplasmic granules for acid analine dyes, most commonly eosin. Investigations and interest have been focused on eosinophils for approximately 100 years. Various aspects of this cell have been the topics of a recent book and several current reviews (Beeson and Bass, 1977; Lukens, 1972; Speirs *et al.*, 1974; Zucker-Franklin, 1974; Ottesen, 1976; Butterworth, 1977; Goetzl and Austen, 1977; Kay, 1977; Gupta, 1977, and personal communication; Phillips and Colley, 1978). It would seem that their phylogenetic credentials, tracing back to all but the most primitive vertebrates, and their unique lineage, life cycle, tissue distribution, morphology, and biochemical activities might have earned the eosinophils a distinct position in the biomedical realm. However, most often, the eosinophil is still known through its associations with a variety of other situations, such as infections with certain tissue-dwelling helminths, atopic disorders, and some immune-complex-related disorders. The occurrence of eosinophils in a given environment thus remains relegated to the position of an epiphenomenon. The explanation of why the eosinophil continues to earn only this "associated with" status seems clearly to be based on an inability to assign a functional role to this cell. Most of the current information available continues to deal with the governance of eosinophils by other systems. There are, however, several different eosinophil-related activities which are now being examined as possible functional roles for eosinophils. This chapter will attempt to describe the eosinophil, discuss

DANIEL G. COLLEY • The Veterans Administration Hospital, and Department of Microbiology, Vanderbilt University School of Medicine, Nashville, Tennessee 37203. STEPHANIE L. JAMES • Department of Medicine, Harvard Medical School, Boston, Massachusetts 02115.

its various associations with immune responses, and examine the nature of its activities as an integral component of some of these systems.

2. Description of the Eosinophilic Leukocyte

2.1. History

The eosinophil was probably first identified as a distinct cell type in the blood by the presence of prominent, coarse, refractory granules in the cytoplasm of unstained cells (Samter, 1965). Later, Ehrlich (1879) described the particular eosin-staining property which could be utilized to readily identify these cells, leading to the appellation "eosinophil." By the early part of this century, much work had been done in describing the presence of eosinophils in various animal species and in correlating the presence of eosinophils with numerous disease states. However, no distinct biological activities for these cells, apart from those shared with other leukocytes, could be proven. Eosinophil functions appeared similar to, although possibly less efficient than, those of neutrophils.

Eosinophils exhibit ameboid movement and are able to engulf particles (Archer and Hirsch, 1963a) and kill microorganisms (Baehner and Johnston, 1971; Cline, 1972; Mickenberg *et al.*, 1972). However, their appearance at a reaction site seems to be more closely associated with various types of immune responses than that of neutrophils. In accordance with this observation, several theories have been proposed for the function of eosinophils, including inactivation of histamine and other mediators at sites of anaphylactic reactivity (Archer, 1963), ingestion of antigen–antibody complexes (Litt, 1964), and transport of antigenic complexes between lymphocytes and macrophages (Speirs *et al.*, 1974). In recent years, interest in eosinophils has been renewed, with application of more sophisticated methods of biochemically and immunologically oriented research. Much current investigation is centering on clarification of the role of eosinophils in allergic reactions and helminthic infections, both states in which tissue or peripheral blood eosinophilia is frequently observed, and in an effort to define the relationship of eosinophils with immune response.

2.2. Structure

In adults, most eosinophils appear to be produced in the bone marrow (Rytömma, 1960). There is some argument over whether all granulocytes share a common undifferentiated precursor cell, the theoretical myeloblast (see Section 3.1). However, after some degree of differentiation, nongranulated, committed eosinophil precursors divide and mature through the same developmental stages observed in other granulocytic lines, with progressive condensation of chromatin and lobulation of the nucleus. On ultrastructural examination, the eosinophilic promyelocyte contains large, spherical, homogeneously dense granules. In myelocytes, crystalloids appear in some of these large granules, and as the cells mature these internal opaque bodies become more distinct. Smaller granules are formed at the metamyelocyte stage, and the number of these granules also appears to increase with maturity (Breton-Gorius and Reyes, 1976). Eosinophil enzymes appear to follow the general pathway for intracellular protein transport, being synthesized on ribosomes and transferred through the rough endoplasmic reticulum. Segregation and packaging of enzymes into eosinophil granules are accomplished by the Golgi apparatus (Bainton and Farquhar, 1970).

Mature eosinophils in the blood tend to be slightly larger than neutrophils; human cells appear approximately 13–18 μm in diameter in smears (Tanaka and Goodman, 1972). In man the eosinophil nucleus has a less markedly lobular configuration than that of the neutrophil, generally exhibiting two or sometimes three lobes. In the rat and mouse the eosinophil has a distinctive "doughnut-shaped" nucleus. On maturation, eosinophils, like other granulocytes, lose their capacity to replicate DNA (Breton-Gorius and Reyes, 1976). However, they are still metabolically active and retain cytoplasmic organelles such as mitochondria and Golgi apparatus (Polliack and Douglas, 1975). By far the most distinctive structures in the mature eosinophils are the cytoplasmic granules. The larger granules (0.3–1.2 μm in diameter) contain the characteristic electron-dense core or "internum" (Miller *et al.*, 1966). By transmission electron microscopy at high magnification Miller *et al.* (1966) discerned the core to be crystalloid in nature, with a periodic array ranging from about 28 Å in the mouse to 40 Å in man. However, using freeze-etch techniques, Burns and Hoak (1975) placed the periodicity at approximately 78 Å in human cells. This core has been identified as a low molecular weight (approximately 11,000) basic protein which is rich in arginine and comprises as much as 50% of the granular protein content (Gleich *et al.*, 1973, 1974). This material shows a tendency to form disulfide-linked aggregates and can inactivate heparin and the slow-reacting substance of anaphylaxis (SRS-A) (Gleich, 1977), but its efficacy in these or other roles has yet to be established (Gleich, 1977). The core is surrounded by a homogeneous matrix containing a variety of hydrolytic enzymes (Archer and Hirsch, 1963b), and the granule as a whole is surrounded by a membrane (Miller *et al.*, 1966). The smaller eosinophil granules (0.1–0.5 μm in diameter) appear uniformly dense in the electron microscope and have been determined to be lysosomal in nature (Parmley and Spicer, 1974). Using scanning electron microscopy, Polliack and Douglas (1975) have observed that human peripheral blood eosinophils exhibit surface structures reminiscent of lymphocytes, being spherical with various degrees of microvilli and surface blebs or ruffles. Mahmoud and Warren (1977) and Mahmoud *et al.* (1975a) have reported antigenic differences between mature and immature eosinophils which can be discerned by anti-mature eosinophil sera and anti-precursor eosinophil sera. These exciting studies emphasize the potential advantages of some day subdividing eosinophils not only within their maturational spectrum but possibly even with regard to their functions and characteristics.

2.3. Enzyme Content

Studies on the enzyme content of eosinophils have been hampered by the difficulty of obtaining pure cell populations because these cells normally represent only approximately 3% of the total circulating leukocytes. In a relatively early study, Archer and Hirsch (1963b) examined the content of horse blood and rat peritoneal eosinophil granules and found a variety of enzymes similar to those found in neutrophils. In both horse and rat eosinophils, granules held approximately half the total cellular protein. They contained the enzymes peroxidase, acid phosphatase, β-glucuronidase, arylsulfatase, ribonuclease, and cathepsin. Unlike neutrophils, they lacked the two antibacterial agents lysozyme and phagocytin (Archer and Hirsch, 1963b). In a more recent study, West *et al.* (1975) compared the enzyme content of human eosinophils with neutrophils and found that eosinophils contain 2.65 times as much peroxidase, and at least twice as much β-glucuronidase and β-glycerophosphatase activity. While others have reported detection of some alkaline phosphatase activity in eosinophils, West and his group found none.

Eosinophil peroxidase has been shown to be distinct from the corresponding myeloperoxidase found in neutrophils with respect to histochemical properties (Rytömma and Teir, 1961), absorption spectrum (Archer *et al.*, 1965), and molecular weight. At 65,000, the molecular weight of guinea pig eosinophil peroxidase is only approximately half that of myeloperoxidase (Desser *et al.*, 1972). In addition, the two enzymes are apparently produced under separate genetic control in man (Lehrer and Cline, 1969; Salmon *et al.*, 1970). Eosinophil peroxidase does not appear to participate in the type of peroxide–peroxidase bactericidal system described in neutrophils (Klebanoff, 1968; McRipley and Sbarra, 1967). Bujak and Root (1974) found that human eosinophils have a high resting iodination activity of trichloracetic-acid-precipitable protein, and eosinophils have been shown to produce large amounts of peroxide on phagocytosis (Baehner and Johnston, 1971; Mickenberg *et al.*, 1972). However, iodination activity failed to increase in eosinophils following phagocytosis of *Staphylococcus aureus*. Furthermore, addition of sodium azide, which inhibits peroxidase-catalyzed reactions, impaired neutrophil staphylocidal activity but actually increased eosinophil activity. Eosinophil peroxidase is located in the matrix of the large specific granules (Rogovine *et al.*, 1975), and on disruption by freezing and thawing, enzyme activity has been found to remain associated with the insoluble granule residue (Archer and Hirsch, 1963b). Takenaka *et al.* (1977) have reported extracellular release of peroxidase from human eosinophils on ingestion of immune complexes, particularly those containing IgE. Rate and amount of enzyme release correlated with the amount of complex ingested and extent of granule lysis.

Arylsulfatase has been found within the small granules in human eosinophil granules (Parmley and Spicer, 1974). By analyses of substrate specificities, molecular weight (60,000), and pH optimum, this enzyme has been identified as a type II B arylsulfatase (Wasserman *et al.*, 1975). Eosinophil arylsulfatase has been found to be capable of inactivating SRS-A *in vitro* (Wasserman *et al.*, 1975) and can be released when eosinophils interact with noningestible particles or surfaces capable of activating the alternate complement pathway (Metcalf *et al.*, 1977). A phospholipase D with properties similar to those of plant enzyme has also been isolated from human eosinophils and found to inactivate rat platelet-activating factor in a time- and dose-dependent reaction *in vitro* (Kater *et al.*, 1976). Zeiger and colleagues (Zeiger *et al.*, 1976; Zeiger and Colten, 1977) have reported that the presence of opsonized zymosan or calcium ionophore induces noncytotoxic release of histaminase by eosinophils. The discovery of these three enzymes in eosinophils has generated much speculation regarding the role of these cells in immediate hypersensitivity reactions *in vivo* (see Section 5.1.1). In addition to these enzymatic activities, Hubscher (1975a,b) has reported an eosinophil-derived inhibitor of histamine release (EDI) produced by human eosinophils in response to mechanical or immunological stimuli which is believed to be a mixture of prostaglandins E_1 and E_2.

Intense acid phosphatase activity has been demonstrated in the smaller homogeneous eosinophil granules (Parmley and Spicer, 1974) and within the matrix of the specific granules (Ghidoni and Goldberg, 1966). Although this enzyme is readily apparent in immature specific granules of developing cells (Bainton and Farquhar, 1970), it is evidently found in a latent state in mature cells (Seeman and Palade, 1967). The alkaline phosphatase found in eosinophils by some investigators appears to be similar by several physicochemical criteria to that in neutrophils (Cao *et al.*, 1973) and has been observed only in granules other than the eosinophil-specific granules (Nakatsui *et al.*, 1972). Collagenase has also been found in amounts similar to those in neutrophils (Basset *et al.*, 1976). Eosinophils have been reported to display a more potent oxidative response during phagocytosis of zymosan particles and staphylococci than do neutrophils. This may be due primarily to increased activity of the granule enzyme, NADPH oxidase, leading to greater production of intracellular hydrogen peroxide (Baehner and Johnston, 1971; Iverson *et al.*, 1977).

2.4. Surface Receptors

Gupta *et al.* (1976) have recently reported an extensive study of surface receptors on eosinophils obtained from normal subjects as well as patients with eosinophilia. Using rosetting techniques with sheep erythrocyte–rabbit antibody–complement complexes (EAC) prepared with purified human complement components, they found that these eosinophils shared a common immune adherence receptor for C3b and C4 and possessed a distinct receptor for C3d. These receptors were generally present on approximately 30–60% of the cells examined. Even when high amounts of C4 were used to prepare the complexes, only 25–53% of the eosinophils formed EAC 1–4 rosettes. The receptors for C3d could not be blocked by either C4- or C3b-containing complexes, and, reciprocally, the immune adherence receptor was not blocked by C3d. However, C4-containing complexes prevented rosetting by EAC 1–3b, and *vice versa*. They also found that a small proportion of eosinophils (< 20%) bound aggregated IgG, and some appeared to have phagocytized the material. Eosinophils did not form rosettes with Ripley-coated human erythrocytes and were therefore determined to lack "high-affinity" Fc receptors. Nor were receptors for uncoated or γG- or γM-coated sheep erythrocytes observed by this group. However, using a more sensitive indicator system of OX RBC–rabbit anti-OX RBC IgG complexes, Fc receptors could be detected on 60–90% of eosinophils (Gupta, personal communication). With EA γMC 1–4–EA γMC 1–3d complexes, Gupta *et al.* (1976) observed that approximately 50% of the eosinophils formed complement-mediated rosettes but ingestion was negligible unless the antibody complexes were of the IgG class. It was determined, therefore, that human eosinophils resemble lymphocytes and monocytes in that they have two distinct complement receptors, and differ from neutrophils in possessing a C3d receptor and in their lesser degree of sensitivity for C4 (Gupta *et al.*, 1976; Gupta, 1977, and personal communication). In general, Tai and Spry (1976), Anwar and Kay (1977a), and Ottesen *et al.* (1977) have also demonstrated that approximately 10–20% of normal human peripheral blood eosinophils express receptors for IgG (either rabbit or human) and 30–40% of the eosinophils have complement receptors (C4, C3, C3b, or C3d). The optimal conditions for receptor demonstration seem similar for eosinophils and neutrophils (Ottesen *et al.*, 1977). Under these conditions, 80–90% of the neutrophils are positive for C3 and IgG receptors. Sher and Glover (1976) have reported that up to 20% of eosinophils obtained from the peripheral blood of patients with parasitic infections, allergic disorders, or undiagnosed eosinophilias formed spontaneous rosettes with sheep erythrocytes. Neither Gupta *et al.* (1976) nor Anwar and Kay (1977a) have observed such E rosettes. Hubscher and Eisen (1971) and Hubscher (1975a), using fluorescent autoradiographic techniques and triggering by the use of anti-IgE antisera, have reported IgE of the surface of human eosinophils and basophils.

Butterworth *et al.* (1976) examined guinea pig eosinophils using a rosetting assay and reported that these cells possess Fc receptors for homologous immunoglobulin, so that guinea pig antibody was recognized but rabbit antibody was not. With sheep erythrocytes coated with guinea pig antisera, they observed strong rosetting with a 7 S fraction of sera and no selective difference between recognition of IgG_1 and IgG_2 when the sera were further purified. No rosetting was observed when sheep cells were coated with a 19 S fraction of antisera. Using mouse eosinophil colony cells from bone marrow culture, Rabellino and Metcalf (1975) found receptors for 7 S antibody but not 19 S antibody. No EAC-complement receptors were demonstrated on these immature cells.

It is clear that surface receptors on eosinophils differ in various species. More interesting are recent reports (Spry and Tai, 1976; Tai and Spry, 1976; Anwar and Kay, 1977a; Ottesen *et al.*, 1977) which, although occasionally conflicting, indicate that eosinophil receptors may be altered during various conditions. Tai and Spry (1976) and Spry and Tai (1976) have reported that increased percentages of eosinophils from patients with eosinophilia express receptors for rabbit IgG. However, when those patients with transient eosinophilia recovered, this abnormality disappeared. Furthermore, while the percent of EAC-rosette-forming eosinophils did not rise, the patient eosinophils phagocytosed EAC much more actively than did those from normal individuals. These changes in membrane characteristics were accompanied by observable vacuolation and loss of some of their specific granules. These observations suggest that eosinophils may become altered or "activated" on maturity or in response to certain stimuli. Ottesen *et al.* (1977) have observed increases in the percentages of C3-receptor- and IgG-receptor-bearing eosinophils in patients with eosinophilia associated with helminthic infections. However, in patients with eosinophilias due to a variety of mainly atopic-associated illnesses, Anwar and Kay (1977a) have demonstrated decreases in the percentage of eosinophils which express either C4 or C3b receptors. There were no changes in the expression of receptors for rabbit IgG. Anwar and Kay (1977b) have also demonstrated a potential mechanism for some of these reported alterations in eosinophil membrane receptors. They have shown that, *in vitro*, either the tetrapeptides of eosinophil chemotactic factor of anaphylaxis (ECF-A) or histamine (see Sections 4.2.1 and 4.2.2) could increase the expression by eosinophils of C3 receptors. The percent EAC-3b-positive eosinophils rose from 30% to 65% over a period of about 1 hr. Eosinophil IgG receptors were not altered by these substances, nor were the receptors on neutrophils or lymphocytes. The implications of subpopulations of eosinophils, defined by surface membrane receptors, and potential links with functional qualifications (Anwar and Kay, 1977b; Ottesen *et al.*, 1977) clearly hold great promise for furthering our understanding of eosinophils.

3. Eosinophilopoiesis

3.1. Normal Production and Distribution of Eosinophils

The actual progenitor of the eosinophil in the bone marrow is unknown. Likewise, it is not clear whether eosinophils and other polymorphonuclear cells share such a stem cell in common. As discussed above (Section 2.2), increasing evidence concerning genetic and biochemical distinctions indicates that eosinophils and neutrophils probably develop from separate precursor cells. Thus eosinophil peroxidase is not spectrally, enzymatically, or antigenically similar to neutrophil myeloperoxidase (Archer *et al.*, 1965; Archer and Broome, 1963; Salmon *et al.*, 1970), and genetic anomalies exist in which either neutrophil myeloperoxidase deficiency is accompanied by normal eosinophil peroxidase content (Lehrer and Cline, 1969; Salmon *et al.*, 1970) or eosinophil peroxidase is lacking in the concomitant presence of normal levels of neutrophil myeloperoxidase (Presentey and Szapiro, 1969). Furthermore, both congenital and drug-induced agranulocytosis have been reported in patients with normal or even enhanced numbers of eosinophils (Connell, 1969; Gilman *et al.*, 1970). Either the cell lines do not share a common precursor, or it must be hypothesized that these distinctions in differentiation or mutation must occur subsequent to the early promyelocyte stage.

The mechanism which governs eosinophil production and release during normal situations is not known. Presumably there is a homeostatic method of controlling the normal level of eosinophils which is either augmented or assisted by auxillary mechanisms in times of increased eosinophilopoiesis. A study by Mahmoud *et al.* (1977) may indicate one such possible regulatory mechanism. They have shown that after the induction of an eosinopenia by the administration of antieosinophil serum (AES) there occurs a subsequent peripheral blood eosinophilia. Serum from such eosinophil-depleted mice was shown to be capable of inducing eosinophilia on passive transfer, and the active component in the serum was demonstrated to be peptidelike, with a molecular weight of approximately 1000. It is possible that this substance normally regulates eosinophilopoiesis and that it exerts its influence in an inverse proportion to the level of eosinophils in the host. The source of this circulating material has not yet been determined. A similar factor is currently under investigation in human sera (Mahmoud, personal communication). The human factor has characteristics in common with the murine factor and can be assayed for eosinophilopoietic activity in the mouse.

An understanding of the kinetics of the life cycle of the eosinophil must consider the production, release, tissue distribution, and fate of these cells. Relatively little information is available regarding these aspects of the eosinophil under normal conditions. In the normal rat eosinophil, maturation requires 30 hr (Spry, 1971a) to 2–3 days (Foot, 1965), and mature cells remain in the "marrow reserve" for 41 hr (Spry, 1971a). After release from the marrow, the cells remain in the circulation with a half-life of 6.7 hr (Spry, 1971a). The body compartment distribution ratio of eosinophils in the rat, estimated on equal quantities of marrow:tissues:blood, is 200:200:1 (Rytömma, 1960). In the guinea pig (Hudson, 1968), the same ratio is 400:300:1, respectively, and the resident time which mature eosinophils spend in the marrow reserve is estimated to be 60 hr. On the basis of cell turnover kinetics, a study in normal human subjects (Parwaresch *et al.*, 1976) proposed the existence of two populations of eosinophil precursors. One was slowly dividing but resulted in a cell which left the marrow rapidly on maturation and was long-lived in the blood. The other was rapidly dividing, had an extended marrow reserve time, and remained in the blood for only a short time. The tissue-blood ratio in man is estimated to be 100:1 (Stryckmans *et al.*, 1968).

The removal of ^{51}Cr-labeled eosinophils from the blood of patients with hypereosinophilic syndrome (Herion *et al.*, 1970; Greenberg and Chikkappa, 1971; Dale *et al.*, 1976) has indicated the existence of complex patterns of removal and reappearance of these cells in the circulation. Dale *et al.* (1976) delineated a biphasic kinetic pattern in which the eosinophils left the blood within the first 3 hr, reappeared in the circulation during the remainder of the first day, and then again disappeared, this time with a blood half-life of 44 hr. Two of the six patients had splenomegaly, and concomitantly with the first exit from the blood they exhibited increased spleen surface counts. However, no essential role for spleen localization was indicated because three patients with normal-sized spleens and one who had been splenectomized displayed the same biphasic pattern of disappearance, reappearance, and redistribution. It is difficult to estimate how much the hypereosinophilic state of the patients may have contributed to the patterns obtained in these studies, but they varied distinctly from the uniform blood half-life time of 12 hr obtained for neutrophils in control subjects.

The estimates concerning the actual life cycle and kinetics of eosinophils obviously suffer from a paucity of studies in this area. Until more definitive studies are completed in a variety of species and under various conditions, observations of the activities of eosinophils must always be thought of in relationship to the possible effects of tissue compartmentalization or margination, reserve pools, and transit times. Clearly this cell is primarily a resident of the marrow and the tissues, and studies which delineate or depend on peripheral blood eosinophil levels must always consider this parameter as an indicator system and consider the cells involved as being in an "in transit" state.

3.2. T-Lymphocyte Involvement in Accelerated Eosinophilopoiesis and Eosinophilia

During the early 1970s several situations which involved accelerated eosinophilopoiesis were clearly linked to T-lymphocyte-mediated immune responses. Two independent groups, one associated with Beeson and the other with Speirs, were the primary contributors to these efforts (Beeson and Bass, 1977; Speirs *et al.*, 1974).

Using a model in which peripheral blood eosinophilia was induced in rats by sensitization to *Trichinella spiralis* larvae, Basten and Beeson (1970), Basten *et al.* (1970), and Boyer *et al.* (1970) showed that first exposure to larvae resulted in a primary peripheral blood eosinophilia and that a subsequent challenge yielded an increased secondary eosinophilia. This response was independent of the circulating titer of antilarval antibody but could be passively transferred by the use of sensitized thoracic duct lymphoid cells. Eosinophilia could not develop in rats which had received whole-body irradiation but could develop if the animals were reconstituted with sensitized lymphocytes and normal bone marrow. Neonatal thymectomy, prolonged thoracic duct drainage, or the administration of antilymphocyte serum all greatly decreased the ability to mount an eosinophilia. In extensions of these studies, T-lymphocyte-depleted mice were observed to respond to acute bacterial infections by a normal neutrophilic response, but exposure to *T. spiralis* larvae failed to stimulate the dramatic eosinophilia observed in immunologically intact or thymus-reconstituted mice (Walls *et al.*, 1971). Similar situations have since been observed in T-lymphocyte-depleted or congenitally athymic (nude) mice exposed to *Schistosoma mansoni* (Fine *et al.*, 1973; Hsu *et al.*, 1976; Phillips *et al.*, 1977), *Ascaris suum* (Nielsen *et al.*, 1974), and *T. spiralis* (Ruitenberg *et al.*, 1977).

The rat–*T. spiralis* intravenous larvae model was also used effectively to analyze the kinetics of the production of eosinophils and their release from the bone marrow into the circulation under accelerated conditions. It was determined that after stimulation by the lodging of larvae in the pulmonary vascular bed the normal cell cycle time of 30 hr was decreased to only 9 hr, and the precursor cells were stimulated to undergo five or six additional divisions. The 41-hr resident time which a mature eosinophil normally remained in the marrow was also decreased, to a period of only 18 hr (Spry, 1971a,b). In the guinea pig, stimulation resulted in a decreased time in the marrow reserve of from 60 to 29 hr (Hudson, 1968). Thus at least a portion of the T-lymphocyte regulation of peripheral blood eosinophilia was seen to be exercised at the level of medullary eosinophilopoiesis.

Independently, Speirs *et al.* (1974) demonstrated that appropriate secondary exposure of mice to alum-precipitated tetanus toxoid resulted in a peritoneal eosinophilia. Further analysis of this system indicated that, to produce a secondary eosinophilia to antigenic challenge, irradiated mice required a source of normal stem cells and a specifically sensitized lymphoid population (McGarry *et al.*, 1971). The eosinophilia occurred independently of antibody formation, and based on several approaches both peritoneal eosinophilia and accelerated eosinophilopoiesis in the bone marrow were seen to require sensitized T lymphocytes but not B lymphocytes (Jenkins *et al.*, 1972; Speirs *et al.*, 1973; Ponzio and Speirs, 1973, 1975); similar data were derived using an *Ascaris* antigen system (Walls, 1976). In another model system using rats and pulmonary embolization of antigen-coated latex beads, Schriber and Zucker-Franklin (1975) demonstrated that peripheral blood eosinophilia correlated well with the development of T-lymphocyte responsiveness to the antigen.

Neither the mechanism by which stimulated T lymphocytes might accelerate eosinophilopoiesis nor what regulates whether this occurs during any given immune response is known. The passive transfer of the stimulation of peripheral blood eosinophilia by sensitized lymphocytes in millipore cell-tight chambers (Basten and Beeson, 1970) suggested the possibility that a soluble mediator might be responsible. McGarry and Miller (1974) and Miller and McGarry (1976) have utilized peritoneally implanted diffusion chambers (quadrachambers), which separate spleen cells from marrow cells by cell-impermeable membranes, to study eosinophilopoiesis. They have shown that antigen-stimulated, sensitized spleen cells produce a soluble product which will stimulate accelerated eosinophilopoiesis in adjacent (but membrane-separated) bone marrow cells. Miller *et al.* (1976) and McGarry *et al.* (1977) have pursued this system in the mouse–*S. mansoni* model and have presented evidence that *in vitro* stimulation of spleen cells from infected mice resulted in the production of a soluble factor which, when administered to eosinopenic mice in a concentrated form, preferentially stimulated eosinophilopoiesis. Ruscetti *et al.* (1976) have shown that supernatant fluids from activated lymphocytes are able to stimulate eosinophil colony formation in an *in vitro* colony-forming assay.

The involvement of the T-lymphocyte activation in eosinophilopoiesis appears established. Yet it remains unclear why this has been detected as yet only in certain situations involving cell-mediated immune responses. It is evident that there is no inherent need for an antigen to be helminthic of origin to be able to stimulate eosinophilopoiesis. However, such antigens appear to be more potent in this regard. The observations that particulate forms of antigens may be required to induce the proper sequence or combinations of responses to result in eosinophilia (Walls and Beeson, 1972; discussed in Butterworth, 1977) may lead to some elucidation of the regulations involved.

Furthermore, the above data regarding T-lymphocyte control of eosinophilopoiesis should not be interpreted to mean that there is only one mechanism which regulates accelerated eosinophil production. As will be discussed later, immune complexes can induce both local and systemic eosinophilia, IgE antibody involvement (perhaps via T-lymphocyte interactions) is correlated with eosinophilia, and a wide variety of totally nonimmunological conditions affect eosinophils (Beeson and Bass, 1977). Factors included in this category range from diurnal variation (Halberg and Visscher, 1950; Colley, 1974) to a sudden deprivation of magnesium in the diet (Kashiwa and Hungerford, 1958). Some of these situations may be related to stress–corticosteroid–eosinophil interactions (Speirs and Meyer, 1949), but most are not readily explicable based on currently known mechanisms. Actual inhibition of eosinophilopoiesis has been demonstrated by Bass (1975a,b, 1977) during acute inflammatory processes (see Section 5.5.1).

4. Regulation of Eosinophil Migration and Localization

As previously detailed, the eosinophil is primarily a tissue cell. It seems likely that any functional role which might be ascribed to this cell would thus be accomplished in localized tissue sites. It is therefore of importance to determine when and how eosinophils might be attracted to, or retained within, certain tissue reactions, and to define under what conditions this occurs. A wide variety of substances have been shown to be chemotactic for eosinophils. Most such agents appear to be related to immunological phenomena, and they have been studied under a multitude of *in vivo* and *in vitro* conditions. Furthermore, the specific nature of their chemotactic activities for eosinophils, i.e., in perference to attracting other cell types, is most often a matter of relativity. It remains clear that any attempts to extrapolate artificially designed chemotaxis studies to explain *in vivo*, naturally occurring observations must take into account a wide range of tissue-related variables, and must be considered conjectural. We will discuss the agents which appear to be chemotactic for eosinophils in relationship to the immunological situations in which each has been described.

4.1. Complement-Generated Factors

Activation of the complement cascade by either the classical or the alternate pathway leads to the production of three materials which exert chemotactic activity: C3a, C5a, and C567. These substances can attract both neutrophils and eosinophils (Ward *et al.*, 1965; Ward, 1969; Keller and Sorkin, 1969; Lachmann *et al.*, 1970). *In vitro* studies in the guinea pig system emphasize the relative importance of C5a as a chemotactic mediator and suggest that it is preferentially active in regard to eosinophils (Kay, 1970b). Kay *et al.* (1973) have reported on another aspect of these systems which serves to emphasize the complexity of the reactions. They have demonstrated a synergistic chemotactic effect on eosinophils when they are simultaneously exposed to both C5a and ECF-A (eosinophil chemotactic factor of anaphylaxis; see below). Thus the mixed activities of some agents may not be simply the sum of the individual component parts. This is of importance in understanding *in vivo* eosinophil responses where the mechanisms are often mixed and/or overlapping.

The *in vivo* eosinophilia observed in a variety of experimental (Litt, 1964; Cohen *et al.*, 1964; Kay, 1970a; Parish, 1970, 1972a) and certain clinical (Marcussen, 1974; Person and Rogers, 1977) (see Section 5) situations may be explained by the above *in vitro* studies demonstrating the potential chemotactic activities of C3a, C5a, and C567 for eosinophils.

4.2. Mast-Cell-Derived Factors

4.2.1. Eosinophil Chemotactic Factor of Anaphylaxis (ECF-A)

Anaphylactic triggering of mast cells, by the binding of antigen to mast cell surface membrane-associated specific IgE-type antibody, results in the release of the various pharmacological mediators of immediate hypersensitivity. The long-standing association of reaginic antibody sensitization and eosinophilia prompted Kay *et al.* (1971) to examine the products of sensitized and challenged mast cells for substances which might be chemotactic for eosinophils. Such an activity was found and was termed "eosinophil chemotactic factor of anaphylaxis" (ECF-A). The activity was specific for eosinophils and was expressed by a 500–600 dalton peptide. Continued studies have demonstrated that ECF-A-like activity is preformed in the mast cells and basophils of guinea pigs, humans, and rats (Parish, 1972b; Goetzl and Austen, 1975, 1977; Mann and Cruickshank, 1975). Goetzl and Austen (1975) have purified human ECF-A and obtained two acidic tetrapeptides with amino acid sequences of Ala-Gly-Ser-Glu and Val-Gly-Ser-Glu. When prepared, the synthetic peptides displayed activity comparable to that of the purified tetrapeptides (Goetzl and Austen, 1977). Kay (1977) has found that in the human system an analogue, Val-Glu-Asp-Glu, behaves similarly to the other two tetrapeptides described, but of the three only Ala-Gly-Ser-Glu had even a modicum of activity in regard to guinea pig eosinophils (Kay, 1977). There is considerable variability in the dose-response curves obtained using the tetrapeptides as eosinophil chemotactic agents on eosinophils from different donors (Goetzl and Austen, 1977; Turnbull *et al.*, 1977). The optimal molar ranges were usually quite narrow and were sometimes further complicated by bi- or even triphasic optima.

Prior exposure of eosinophils to very low concentrations of the tetrapeptides rendered the cells "deactivated" or unresponsive to the activity of the homologous chemotactic agents. The effect was not altered by washing the cells. Furthermore, the ECF-A COOH-terminal tripeptide (Gly-Ser-Glu) can mediate this inhibition of the cell. The NH_2-terminal tripeptides also reduced the cells' ability to respond to the tetrapeptides, but their effect appeared to be a reversible inhibition which was thought to be due to competitive binding characteristics (Goetzl and Austen, 1976, 1977). Such inhibitory capabilities could serve to immobilize the once-summoned cells within a local tissue site. Anwar and Kay (1977b) have implicated this process in the actual alteration of expression of eosinophil C3 and C4 receptors (see Section 2.4).

4.2.2. Histamine

The ability of histamine to mediate systemic and local eosinophilia was at one time assumed by the correlative atopic associations of histamine and eosinophils and then subsequently discredited by an inability to consistently demonstrate *in vitro* or *in vivo* eosinophil chemotaxis toward histamine gradients (Beeson and Bass, 1977; Parish, 1970). More recently, Clark *et al.* (1975, 1977) have revived interest in histamine-mediated chemotaxis of human eosinophils. They obtained positive *in vitro* results by using wide dose ranges and found that greater than 10^{-6} M concentrations were inhibitory. Turnbull and Kay (1976) have extended these reports to show that histamine and imidazoleacetic acid, a major catabolite of histamine, are both selectively chemotactic for human eosinophils. These reagents cross-deactivated eosinophils. Kay (1977) observed the same situation using guinea pig eosinophils. Inhibition or enhancement of the chemotaxis induced by endotoxin-activated serum by the use of histamine H_2 and H_1 receptor antagonists, respectively, has also been reported (Clark *et al.*, 1975; Kay, 1977). The effects of using combinations of histamine and either of the ECF-A peptides can be either synergistic or inhibitory, emphasizing only the complexity of the situations (Clark *et al.*, 1977; Goetzl and Austen, 1977). It seems that sequential exposures resulted in no cross-deactivation, but, simultaneously, the combination of ECF-A and histamine deactivated eosinophils in regard to subsequent chemotaxis toward either one (Turnbull *et al.*, 1977). Litt (1976) has attributed the apparent eosinophilotactic activity of histamine to its acidity.

4.3. Neutrophil-Derived Factors

In a series of reports Czarnetzki, Konig, and Lichtenstein (Czarnetzki *et al.*, 1976; Konig *et al.*, 1976, 1977) have focused attention on the neutrophil as another cell which can be stimulated to yield an eosinophil chemotactic factor (ECF). Artificial stimulation of basophils, neutrophils, and even eosinophils themselves with a Ca^{2+} ionophore A23187 leads to the release of an ECF which preferentially attracts eosinophils and has an approximate molecular weight of 500–1000. Anti-IgE was shown to elicit ECF-A activity only from basophils, while neither anti-IgE nor the Ca^{2+} ionophore elicited any chemotactically active substances from exposed lymphocytes. The anti-IgE data indicate that this ECF is distinct from mast cell- or basophil-released ECF-A. Phagocytosis of zymosan, preferably complement-coated zymosan, by neutrophils also leads to the release of this ECF.

The total ECF activity obtainable on stimulation of neutrophils is not extractable from unstimulated neutrophils. This observation plus the kinetics of release of this ECF indicates that much of the released material is generated and released on stimulation. Thus the production, cell source, and stimulation mechanisms distinguish this ECF from ECF-A. A variety of inactivators of ECF, which appear to act on the ECF directly, have been described as being produced by human peripheral blood leukocytes. An immediately obvious functional setting which would involve neutrophil phagocytosis followed by rapid eosinophil accumulation is not apparent. However, the description of these phenomena opens up the possibilities of another setting for local tissue eosinophilia which must now be considered, and the occurrence of eosinophils at the periphery of acute inflammatory, neutrophil-rich abscesses is not without some precedent (Bass, 1975b).

4.4. Lymphocyte-Derived Factors

4.4.1. Eosinophil Chemotactic Factor-Precursor (ECF_p)

A soluble link between the antigen activation of sensitized lymphocytes and attraction of eosinophils has been provided by the work of Cohen and Ward (1971) and Torisu *et al.* (1973). In these studies in the guinea pig, it was shown that on appropriate stimulation lymphocytes produced and released a soluble substance (lymphokine) which reacted with homologous immune complexes (the antibody being of the IgG_2 class) in the absence of complement. As produced, the lymphokine possessed the antigenic nature of the stimulating antigen because it could be adsorbed by specific-antibody-affinity chromatography. After the interaction of this lymphokine precursor-like substance (ECF_p) with specific immune complexes, the complexes could be removed, and the fluid phase contained chemotactic activity for eosinophils which was active both *in vitro* and *in vivo* in the dermis.

4.4.2. Eosinophil Stimulation Promoter (ESP) and Chemotactic Factor

Another product of activated lymphocytes which affects eosinophils has been described in the mouse (Colley, 1973, 1976; Greene and Colley, 1974, 1976; James and Colley, 1975; Pelley *et al.*, 1976; Lewis *et al.*, 1977) and man (Kazura *et al.*, 1975; Warren *et al.*, 1976). In the mouse, this activity is synthesized *de novo* by antigen-stimulated, sensitized T lymphocytes and has been assayed by its ability to stimulate increased migration of eosinophils out of an agarose droplet. The moiety responsible for this activity is a heat-stable (60°C/30 min) protein which has a molecular weight in the range of 25,000–50,000. By these criteria, ESP activity was inseparable from that of an eosinophil chemotactic factor produced by lymphocytes (ECF-L) under identical culture conditions (Lewis *et al.*, 1977). It seems quite plausible that one moiety could be responsible for both activities.

The eosinophil chemotactic nature and eosinophil-influencing abilities of lymphokines are compatible with the sometimes-described presence of eosinophils within the strong cell-mediated immune reactions sites (Arnason and Waksman, 1963; Parish, 1970; Speirs *et al.*, 1974; Hirashima and Hayashi, 1976; Hirashima *et al.*, 1976).

4.5. Other Chemotactic Substances

4.5.1. Substances Derived from Tumors

Wasserman *et al.* (1974) have isolated an ECF-A-like material from a large-cell anaplastic carcinoma of the lung from a patient with tumor-associated and peripheral blood eosinophilia. The material is less acidic than ECF-A and has tentatively been termed "ECF-Ca" (Goetzl and Austen, 1977). It is thought that this situation resembles the ectopic production of certain hormones by tumors.

Culture supernatant fluids obtained from cultures of lymph node cells from patients with Hodgkin's disease had more preferential chemotactic activity for eosinophils (as opposed to neutrophils) than similar fluids produced by the nodes of lymphocytic lymphoma patients or reactive hyperplasia patients (Kay *et al.*, 1975). Chemotactic activity was associated with molecular-sieve fractions with estimated molecular weights of 500, 2000, 6000, and 30,000. It is possible that the production of such materials could account for the often-observed lymph node eosinophilia noted in Hodgkin's disease (Stuart, 1970; Parmley and Spicer, 1974).

4.5.2. Substances Generated by Platelet Activity

Turner *et al.* (1975) described the generation of chemotactic activity for eosinophils and neutrophils by the action of platelet lipoxygenase on arachidonic acid. This activity is distinct from the prostaglandin-associated activities produced by the platelet cyclooxygenase system. Goetzl *et al.* (1977) have extended the studies of one of these products, and it appears to influence eosinophils more than neutrophils.

4.5.3. Substances Obtained from Tissues or Sera

Extracts of skin lesion sites undergoing immediate and delayed reactions have yielded chemotactic activities which were active on eosinophil-rich cell populations (Hirashima and Hayashi, 1976). Early skin reactivity was associated with an ECF-A-like, low molecular weight moiety, and delayed skin test sites provided more of a thermolabile factor with an approximate molecular weight of 70,000.

Heat-inactivated (37°C/1 hr and 56°C/1 hr) sera from patients with a wide variety of inflammatory diseases have been seen to contain higher concentrations of eosinophil chemotactic activity than sera from normal subjects (Robinson and Miller, 1975). Sera from patients with bronchial asthma did not contain this eosinophil chemotactic activity.

5. Functional Roles of Eosinophils and Clinical Relationships

5.1. Atopic Allergies

5.1.1. Mechanisms of Interaction

Immunoglobulin E-mediated hypersensitivity states such as anaphylaxis, asthma, allergic rhinitis, and some drug allergies have long been associated with either local or systemic eosinophilia, and elevated IgE levels in either secretions or serum have often been correlated with the occurrence of eosinophilia. However, there are a number of examples with eosinophilia in patients with either normal IgE levels or an absence of circulating IgE, and patients with IgE myelomas do not necessarily have eosinophilia (Beeson and Bass, 1977). Therefore, the presence of IgE itself may not be sufficient to induce eosinophilia, and not all eosinophilias require IgE elevation. Rather, the relationship between atopic allergies and eosinophils would seem to be predicated on more than a mere concomitancy or association. These cells become intimately involved in the actual anaphylactic and IgE-mediated hypersensitivity reaction process.

The most popular role cast for eosinophils within such reactions is that of a modulator, or homeostatic regulator, whose presence would help ameliorate some of the potentially detrimental effects of the reaction in local tissues (Austen *et al.*, 1976; Kay, 1977; Hubscher, 1977). The localization of eosinophils within such reaction sites can be explained on the basis of the chemotactic and deactivating properties of either or both ECF-A and histamine (Kay *et al.*, 1971; Goetzl and Austen, 1977; Clark *et al.*, 1975, 1977) due to IgE-mediated mast cell degranulation. On their arrival, there are several components of eosinophils which may interact with the pharmacological mediators released by mast cells and basophils (see Section 2.3). An antihistaminic capability has been ascribed to the histaminase which is released by human eosinophils as a consequence of phagocytosis or interaction with the Ca^{2+} ionophore A23187 (Zeiger *et al.*, 1976; Zeiger and Colten, 1977). The effects of released histaminase could play a role in dampening the effects of histamine released from mast cells or basophils. Furthermore, the eosinophil-derived inhibitor (EDI) reported by Hubscher (1975a,b) could lead to an inhibition of histamine release. The components of EDI are indistinguishable from prostaglandins E_1 and E_2 and appear to inhibit the release of histamine by increasing intracellular levels of cyclic AMP in the degranulating target cells.

Parmley and Spicer (1974) have demonstrated arylsulfatase within eosinophils, and Wasserman *et al.* (1975) have shown that this enzyme from human eosinophils can inactivate another mast-cell-derived mediator, SRS-A. Arylsulfatase B from a variety of sources has been shown to have this activity. Phospholipase D is an additional eosinophil-associated enzyme which may exert a modulatory role by its ability to inactivate platelet-activating factor (PAF) (Kater *et al.*, 1976). PAF is released from basophils by anaphylactic triggering and can cause additional mediator release (histamine and serotonin) via the aggregation of platelets (Benveniste *et al.*, 1972). The major basic protein (MBP) of eosinophils, isolated by Gleich and colleagues (Gleich *et al.*, 1973, 1974; Gleich, 1977), can inactivate SRS-A and heparin. Experimental results reported by Jones and Kay (1976) have implicated the eosinophil in a negative control mechanism regulating the replenishment of granular contents (histamine) after cutaneous anaphylaxis. In these studies, histamine stores within skin test sites on guinea pigs depleted of eosinophils returned to normal levels much more rapidly than those on guinea pigs with a normal complement of eosinophils.

It is important to emphasize that the complexity of effects attributed to some of the modulators noted, the amounts of some of the substances possibly made available via eosinophils, and the inherent differences in some of the species models studied require that some caution be exercised in model building based on current information. However, the potential for eosinophils to play a major role in modulating overzealous IgE-mediated reactions is now the focus of much well-deserved attention. Further attempts to analyze the microenvironmental conditions during such interactions should provide additional insights into the relative importance of the interactions reported.

5.1.2. Atopic Clinical Conditions and Eosinophilia

a. Bronchial Asthma. Uncomplicated asthma is only rarely accompanied by pulmonary eosinophilia. However, moderate peripheral blood eosinophilia frequently occurs, and nasal secretions from patients with asthma often contain eosinophils (Lowell, 1967). In asthmatic patients, Gupta *et al*. (1975) noted a correlation between elevated peripheral blood eosinophil levels, a decrease in the number of circulating T lymphocytes, and an increase in serum IgE levels. Most cases exhibiting pulmonary eosinophil infiltrates and asthma involve extrinsic etiological agents such as *Aspergillus*, and are dependent on both IgE-mediated and immune complex-mediated reactions (Pepys and Simon, 1973).

b. Bronchial Asthma Preceding Polyarteritis Nodosa. It has been reported that bronchial asthma can progress to polyarteritis and that when this occurs the condition is associated with very high peripheral blood eosinophilia (Wilson and Alexander, 1945). This syndrome occurs more often in adults and usually has a rapid progression. It was proposed that in this situation the underlying asthma was more likely to be "intrinsic" in origin, by which was meant nonatopic rather than IgE mediated.

c. Seasonal Rhinitis. The development of seasonal rhinitis has been shown to be associated with moderate blood and nasal eosinophilias (Lowell, 1967; Stickney and Heck, 1944). Elevated levels of antiragweed IgE antibodies have also been observed in nasal secretions from ragweed-allergic rhinitis patients (Tse *et al*., 1970). Mild systemic exposure to an appropriate allergen has been seen to result in a twofold increase in circulating eosinophil levels in rhinitis patients 24 hr after injection (Lowell, 1967).

d. Drug-Related Elevated IgE and Eosinophilia. Eosinophilia is commonly associated with atopic responsiveness to a wide variety of drugs. Zolov and Levine (1969) demonstrated a good correlation between levels of circulating reaginic antibody (but not IgG or IgM) against penicillin and the development of eosinophilia during penicillin therapy. Davis and Hughes (1974) have reported that the majority of patients who develop dermal eruptions during gold therapy have elevated IgE and circulating eosinophil levels. Although these patients were receiving the gold therapy as treatment for rheumatoid arthritis, which can also be associated with eosinophilia (see Section 5.2.2c), it seemed clear that in this study the eosinophilia was a drug-induced phenomenon probably mediated via an IgE mechanism.

e. Atopic Dermatitis. Atopic dermatitis is usually associated with local eosinophilia which reaches a peak by 24 hr (Eidinger *et al*., 1964; Felarca and Lowell, 1971) and can be associated with elevated eosinophil levels in the peripheral blood (Öhman and Johansson, 1974) or in nasal secretions of children (Crawford, 1960). Dermal eosinophilic responses to insect bites, particularly those to which sensitization may have occurred, are commonly observed, and either can be seen within a few hours to 1 or 2 days (Goldman *et al.*, 1952) or take the form of "dermal eosinophilic granulomas" persisting for months or years (Allen, 1948).

5.2. Immune-Complex-Mediated Disorders

5.2.1. Mechanisms of Interaction

The previously noted chemotactic activities of the products of complement activation provide a mode of involving eosinophils in reactions in which complement-fixing antigen-antibody complexes participate. Furthermore, aggregated non-complement-fixing immunoglobulins could be related, as could a variety of other agents, either through the activation of the alternate complement pathway or by being phagocytosed by neutrophils with the subsequent release of neutrophil-derived ECF.

However, as summarized by Beeson and Bass (1977), it is difficult to envision why an accumulation of eosinophils would be advantageous at the sites of such reactions. Eosinophils can phagocytize immune complexes. However, they may do so preferentially for those involving non-complement-fixing IgE (Ishikawa *et al.*, 1974; Greco *et al.*, 1973). Their relative differences in numbers and abilities lead to doubts concerning any possible advantages they may have in removing such complexes. In fact, eosinophils are not commonly associated with clinical situations known for immune complex involvement. However, they are occasionally associated with certain disease entities which are at least in part due to immune complexes. The question of why is essentially unanswered.

5.2.2. Clinical Conditions Associated with Eosinophilia

a. Bullous Pemphigoid. Person and Rogers (1977) noted that eosinophils were prominent in the cellular infiltrate in the blister fluids of patients with bullous pemphigoid. The lesions also contained immunoglobulins of the IgG, IgA, and IgM classes and components of the complement sequences, but did not contain IgE. The possibility that the IgE was selectively removed by the eosinophils seems unlikely.

b. Allergic Alveolitis. Allergic alveolitis, induced by a variety of extrinsic agents and typified by bronchopulmonary aspergillosis, has been demonstrated to involve at least IgE- and IgG-mediated immune mechanisms (Pepys and Simon, 1973). It is not known whether the eosinophilia associated with this syndrome (see above) depends on either or both of these phenomena. Katzenstein *et al.* (1975) have described a related syndrome, bronchocentric granulomatosis, which involves eosinophil-rich granulomas in the bronchi as well as peripheral eosinophilia and which may be related to circulating precipitins and other reactivities against fungal agents.

c. Rheumatoid Arthritis. Peripheral blood eosinophilia has been noted in some patients with rheumatoid arthritis (Panush *et al.*, 1971; reviewed in Beeson and Bass, 1977; and Gupta, 1977). A paradoxical situation appears to exist in that eosinophilia has not been generally observed in the synovial fluids in rheumatoid arthritis. Four of the five patients studied by Panush *et al.* (1971) did exhibit synovial eosinophilia: this aspect may be resolved by more data regarding the eosinophil levels in synovial fluids of specific patients exhibiting concomitant peripheral blood eosinophilia.

d. Ulcerative Colitis. In a study by Marcussen (1974), 78% of ulcerative colitis patients who exhibited circulating anticolon antibodies also had eosinophilia of the colonic exudate. Riis and Anthonisen (1964) noted that in their series of nonspecific proctocolitis 28% of 67 patients had peripheral blood eosinophilia and 80% of 74 patients demonstrated eosinophilia in the inflammatory colonic exudate.

5.3. Syndromes of Varied or Unknown Etiologies

A wide variety of apparently unrelated clinical situations may be associated with either localized or systemic eosinophilia of varying intensities. Beeson and Bass (1977) have admirably cited, described, and summarized an enormous literature concerning these syndromes, and Lukens (1972) and Gupta (1977) have condensed much of this information into lists of eosinophilia-related disease states. A few of these conditions will be considered below, accompanied by only minimal literature citations. The reviews by Beeson and Bass (1977), Gupta (1977), Ottesen (1976), and Lukens (1972) are recommended for more examples and further detail concerning these entities.

5.3.1. Loffler's Syndrome

Loffler's syndrome is a usually transient pulmonary and peripheral eosinophilia induced by various etiologies ranging from drug-induced allergies to migrating tissue parasites. Often the syndrome is of idiopathic origin.

5.3.2. Hypereosinophilic Syndrome

The term "hypereosinophilic syndrome" is used to include a spectrum of states (Hardy and Anderson, 1968; Chusid *et al.*, 1975) which usually involve high counts of circulating, mature eosinophils ($> 1500/mm^3$) of chronic duration, accompanied by some organ involvement. The heart is the organ most commonly and severely affected. Loffler's eosinophilic endomyocarditis is a prolonged hypereosinophilic state associated with progressive, dense endocardial thickening and mural thrombus formation, which leads to heart failure (Roberts *et al.*, 1969). Spry and Tai (1976) have reported that not only were eosinophil levels elevated in this condition but also the cells themselves were altered. They were observed to express more Fc receptors for IgG, to exhibit more active phagocytosis mediated via C3b receptors, and to be more vacuolated, with altered granules (see Section 2.4). Hepatosplenomegaly and neurological manifestations of a variety of central nervous system dysfunctions are often observed in patients with hypereosinophilic syndrome.

5.3.3. Immunodeficiency Diseases

Several primary immunodeficiency diseases present with eosinophilia. These include a variety of agammaglobulinemias, dysgammaglobulinemias, and Wiskott–Aldrich syndrome. A possible correlation has been described between the susceptibility of most of these patients to infection with *Pneumocystis carinii* and their eosinophilia (Jose *et al.*, 1971). Jeunet and Good (1968) have reported examples of the other extreme in regard to eosinophils and immunodeficiency. They have observed profound peripheral blood and bone marrow eosinopenia or a total absence of eosinophils associated with a unique, spindle cell thymoma with hypogammaglobulinemia. The total absence of eosinophils is a very rare finding.

5.3.4. Estrus-Related Uterine Eosinophilia

Rytömma (1960) has provided a detailed account of the tissue distribution of eosinophils in the rat. One of the most striking aspects of this study was that the number of eosinophils in the uterus of mature rats was controlled by the estrous cycle. Immature or late-stage pregnant rats had zero eosinophils per 0.1 mm^2 of uterine tissue. During estrus this number was 105. Tchernitchin and co-workers have demonstrated an estrogen receptor on the surface of rat uterine (Tchernitchin *et al.*, 1974) and human endometrial (Tchernitchin *et al.*, 1971) eosinophils. They have hypothesized that these cells, which accumulate in large numbers in the uterus of immature rats as soon as 5 min after estrogen administration, are responsible for early uterine changes such as increased vascular permeability and water imbibition. Ross and Klebanoff (1966) have shown that eosinophils which emigrate to the rat uterus come from the bloodstream and that these cells undergo lysis in association with the profound uterine changes which occur during the estrous cycle. As noted by Beeson and Bass (1977), it is totally unknown whether the overwhelming preponderance of eosinophilia-related disorders in males, as opposed to females, could have any relationship to this estrogen receptor or the role of the eosinophil in the uterine setting.

5.4. Neoplasias

5.4.1. Eosinophilic Leukemia

The diagnosis of true eosinophilic leukemia rather than a leukemoid state, i.e., an eosinophilia due to a nonneoplastic, often idiopathic etiology, has proven to be difficult (Hardy and Anderson, 1968; Rickles and Miller, 1972; Spitzer and Garson, 1973; Chusid *et al.*, 1975). Documented cases of eosinophilic leukemia do exist, but their differential diagnosis remains difficult in the face of other hyper-eosinophilias and even pseudoeosinophilias (Yam *et al.*, 1972).

5.4.2. Carcinomas and Sarcomas

Eosinophilia has been reported in occasional patients with malignancies. Isaacson and Rapoport (1964) demonstrated that the occurrence of eosinophilia does not depend on the type of tumor involved, as emphasized by the observation that the incidence of eosinophilia in each specific type of tumor in their review series corresponded well to the relative frequency of occurrence of that type of tumor. As cited above (Wasserman *et al.*, 1974; Goetzl and Austen, 1977), evidence has been presented that ectopic production of a peptide eosinophilotactic factor

(ECF-Ca) by the tumor may account for the eosinophilia associated with some neoplasias.

5.4.3. Hodgkin's Disease

Eosinophil infiltration of the nodes during Hodgkin's disease is often given as one aspect of the histological description of this condition (Stuart, 1970). Parmley and Spicer (1974) have noted some structural differences in the eosinophils present. The observed increase in the "small granules" is thought to be related to the increased maturity of the eosinophils. The majority of patients with Hodgkin's disease do not have high peripheral blood eosinophil counts. Kay *et al*. (1975) have cultured lymph node cells from Hodgkin's disease patients and described several chemotactic factors for eosinophils in these preparations (see Section 4.5.1). These findings could possibly account for the accumulation of eosinophils in these nodes.

5.4.4. Radiation-Related Eosinophilia

Ghossein *et al*. (1975); Ghossein and Stacey (1973) have reported a condition which they have termed radiation-related eosinophilia. In this situation an eosinophilia occurs in approximately 40% of the patients who have received high-voltage irradiation as therapy for malignant tumors located below the diaphragm. The relationship to the type of tumor, if any, is unexplained. Ghossein and colleagues have correlated the occurrence of this phenomenon with a good prognosis and indicate that its prognostic significance is equal to analyzing the patient's ability to respond to DNCB by a cell-mediated response. Patients with both radiation-related eosinophilia and a positive DNCB response had the best prognosis.

5.5. Infectious Diseases

5.5.1. Viral, Bacterial, Fungal, and Protozoal Infections

Dramatic eosinopenia is observed during most acute infections. Beeson and Bass (1977) have reviewed the literature concerning infections by widely diverse acute and chronic etiological agents and concluded by emphasizing a correlation between the ability of an organism to induce an acute inflammatory reaction and its ability to bring about concomitant eosinopenia. Noninflammatory acute infections are negligible in their effects on eosinophil levels, and (see below) chronic inflammatory responses are often associated with eosinophilia. Thus eosinopenia is observed during the febrile or exanthematous stages of a variety of viral infections: measles, rubella, varicella, and dengue. Febrile bacterial infections of essentially all etiologies are characterized by eosinopenia. The major exception appears to be an eosinophilia which occurs during scarlet fever (Freidman and Holtz, 1935).

Bass (1975a,b) has demonstrated that the eosinopenia of acute infections (*E. coli* pyelonephritis, Coxsackie viral pancreatitis, pneumococcal abscess) occurs independently of the adrenal stimulation which might be suspected in stressful situations. On analysis, the rapid drop in circulating levels of eosinophils is followed by a rapid accumulation of these cells at the periphery of the inflammatory site and an inhibition of the "release mechanism" governing mature eosinophil egress from the marrow. If the process is prolonged, an inhibition of eosinophilopoiesis can occur. Eosinopenia could be produced in adrenalectomized mice with eosinophilia by administration of a material from an acute lesion exudate produced by a pneumococcal abscess (Bass, 1977; Beeson and Bass, 1977).

Most fungal infections do not cause eosinophilia. Coccidiodomycosis and allergic bronchopulmonary aspergillosis are exceptions to this statement. The situation with aspergillosis (see above) is perhaps typically complex in that both IgE-mediated and IgG-immune-complex-mediated hypersensitivity states contribute to this syndrome (Pepys and Simon, 1973).

Beeson and Bass (1977) acknowledge the difficulty of dealing with the protozoan disease literature due to the possibility that many such patients often also have concomitant infections with metazoan parasites, but their review and that of Conrad (1971) have led to the summation that eosinophilia can occur occasionally in some tissue-invasive protozoal infections but is not typical of most protozoan diseases. One exception to this general rule might be made for overt *Pneumocystis carinii* infections. With the close association of eosinophilia in this disease with its occurrence in immunodeficient patients (see above) (Jose *et al.*, 1971), some questions remain as to which factors are most central to the development of the observed eosinophilia.

5.5.2. Helminthic Infections

a. Eosinophilia. Infections with metazoan (nematode, cestode, and trematode) parasites are the most common conditions which exhibit eosinophilia. In the case of tissue-invasive or migratory metazoans, eosinophil levels are usually considerably elevated and stable (Conrad, 1971). These conditions generally include trichinosis, schistosomiasis, filariasis, visceral larvae migrans, strongyloidiasis, hydatid cyst disease, ascariasis (especially the pulmonary phase), fascioliasis, and paragonimiasis. This generalization does not apply universally to those parasites which neither enter the host tissues (remaining in the intestinal tract) nor induce substantial, persistent inflammatory responses. Helminthic infections less likely to be associated with eosinophilia are enterobiasis (pinworm), trichuris infection (whipworm), hookworm infections, and tapeworm (*Taenia*) infection.

Tropical eosinophilia is almost certainly due to a filarial infection (species uncertain) and provides an example of a Löffler's syndrome for which a probable etiology has been described (Donohugh, 1963). Patients with tropical eosinophilia have very high IgE levels and complement-fixation titers against dirofilarial antigens. These titers fall on treatment with the antifilarial drug diethylcarbamazine (Neva *et al.*, 1975). This serves as a reminder that most helminth infections are accompanied by strong, sustained IgE responses. It is clearly possible that some aspects of helminth-related eosinophilia are associated with the mechanisms by which atopic conditions can influence eosinophils (see Sections 4.2 and 5.1). It is also known that the T-lymphocyte–lymphokine relationships with eosinophils are operative in most helminthic infections. These interactions have been intensely studied in trichinosis (Basten *et al.*, 1970; Basten and Beeson, 1970; Boyer *et al.*, 1970; Warren *et al.*, 1976) and schistosomiasis (Colley, 1973, 1974, 1976; Kazura *et al.*, 1975; Pelley *et al.*, 1976; Phillips and Colley, 1978) (see Section 4.4).

b. Functional Roles Proposed for Eosinophils in Helminthic Infections. Trichinella infections: Grove *et al.* (1977) have recently used antieosinophil serum (AES) to deplete circulating, mature eosinophils during primary murine *Trichinella spiralis* infection. They observed that the number of muscle-stage larvae which developed in the absence of eosinophils was double that obtained in intact control mice. Interestingly, AES treatment did not affect the number of intestine-dwelling adult worms, which were eliminated at the normal time. Thus depletion of eosinophils during this infection resulted in the abrogation of a previously undetected protective, stage-specific immunity against the tissue-phase parasite, which developed during primary infection. Ruitenberg *et al.* (1977) have also reported elevated (fivefold) numbers of muscle-stage larvae in another setting, the athymic (nude) mouse. Peripheral blood eosinophilia did not occur in this model; its absence could explain the increased number of larvae and thus be in agreement with Grove *et al.* (1977). However, in the nude mouse, the adult worms were not eliminated. It is therefore unclear whether their continued productivity could account for the increase in muscle larvae, rather than it resulting from a lack of eosinophil participation.

Schistosoma infections: There are now two distinct roles proposed for eosinophils during schistosomiasis. Butterworth (1977) has reviewed the data pertinent to the eosinophil's role in protective immunity against invading larvae (schistosomula). The other function currently ascribed to the eosinophil involves the destruction of schistosome eggs and thus relates to the immunopathological aspects of the disease process (James and Colley, 1976; Phillips and Colley, 1978).

There are three main lines of evidence which implicate the eosinophil as an effector cell in the protective immune response against reinfection. (1) Butterworth *et al.* (1974, 1975, 1977a,b) have demonstrated that human eosinophils can damage radiolabeled schistosomula *in vitro*. Eosinophils from normal subjects accomplish this in conjunction with sera from schistosoma patients through an opsonizing, IgG-antibody-dependent, complement-independent reaction. (2) Hsu *et al.* (1974) and von Lichtenberg *et al.* (1976) have provided histopathological evidence that eosinophils are prominent in the dermal reactions against schistosomula. These reactions are thought to represent a major aspect of the protective response. (3) Mahmoud *et al.* (1973) have used antieosinophil serum (AES) to provide another type of evidence which implicates eosinophils in antischistosomal protection (Mahmoud *et al.*, 1975b). Administration of AES led to the depletion of circulating and tissue eosinophils and concomitantly abrogated the protective immunity induced by chronic infection. Depletion of other leukocytes by specific antisera did not affect the level of protection.

Although all the requisite conditions and ramifications for protection against schistosomiasis are not yet understood, these several types of evidence indicate that resistance may require dermal or perhaps pulmonary reactions focused on schistosomula involving antibody and eosinophils. High-level peripheral blood eosinophilia is not required, because passive transfer of immune serum into normal mice can convey protection (Sher *et al.*, 1975). Furthermore, eosinophils obtained from chronic schistosomiasis patients vary in their ability to induce ^{51}Cr release from schistosomula, perhaps indicating a blocking of the appropriate receptors necessary for eosinophil participation in this antibody-mediated cell (eosinophil)-dependent cytotoxicity (Butterworth *et al.*, 1977b).

In vivo and *in vitro* studies support a separate, distinct role for the eosinophil within egg-induced hepatic granulomas which provide the major immunopathogenic process of murine, and possibly human, schistosomiasis mansoni (Warren, 1972; Phillips and Colley, 1978). At certain times during granuloma formation, eosinophils compose approximately 50% of the cells within the lesions (Mahmoud *et al.*, 1975a). During the period when destruction of the central egg occurs (von Lichtenberg *et al.*, 1973), Bogitsh (1971) has described the degranulation of eosinophils on the surfaces of eggs within murine hepatic granulomas. James and Colley (1976, 1978a,b) have analyzed the schistosome egg-eosinophil interaction in an *in vitro* cocultivation system. Eosinophils obtained from *S. mansoni*-infected mice are capable of destroying *S. mansoni* eggs, while other cells are not. This reaction requires an antigenically intact egg. Normal eosinophils do not participate in this reaction. The eosinophil-mediated egg destruction can be abrogated by pretreatment of the eosinophils with trypsin and subsequently restored by sera containing high titers of antibody against eggs. This ability of the serum can be removed by a solid-phase antigen immunoadsorbent column. Furthermore, normal eosinophils can be activated either by immune serum or by incubation in a lymphokine- (ESP; ECF-L) containing culture supernatant fluid. The mechanism by which activated or antibody-armed eosinophils bring about the destruction of a shell-encased egg many times their own size is still unknown. Furthermore, while it is known that eggs, antiegg antibody, eosinophils, and ESP all exist within the granuloma, it is not known (Phillips and Colley, 1978) whether the *in vitro* system observed reflects the functional activities of these cells within the microenvironment of the granulomas.

6. Concluding Statement

There appears to have been a recent upsurge of interest in the eosinophil. We would submit that the resultant "advances" have been accomplished by the use of several new methodologies and approaches, and have been predicated on the long-suffering, unwavering enthusiasm of several staunch disciples of eosinophilology. Yet there is one epithet which is still most often used to refer to the eosinophil. The term applied is "an enigma." Functional roles are beginning to be hypothesized for these cells. More is now known about those factors and responses which influence them, and their distinctive nature is being unraveled. Still, the basis of the presumed essential functional uniqueness of eosinophils remains elusive. Therefore, instead of redefining our more enlightened state of ignorance by a recapitulation of this chapter, we would prefer to mention some of the areas of investigation that would seem to require initiation and/or continued emphasis.

Rather than testing the ability of the eosinophil to compete within systems designed to test the nature of other cells, studies should be designed to define the distinctive aspects of the eosinophil. Toward this end, perhaps more substrates could be derived from mast cell components, or parasite structures could be used to test the enzymatic capabilities of eosinophils. The work regarding the surface receptors on eosinophils points to the possibility of redefining a general eosinophilia into subpopulations based on maturity and functional capabilities, or even on undefined empirical differences. Likewise, antigenic differences, only now incipiently indicating differences in maturity, should be further exploited. The mechanisms which regulate the production of these cells ought to be extensively explored in relationship to both normal and accelerated conditions. Questions regarding functional roles for eosinophils will require the ability to discern the extent to which the plethora of interactions between eosinophils and their neighborhood affect the outcome of their activities. The dilemma is that *in vivo* systems are too complex to be understood, and *in vitro* models are too simplistic to be believed. Major efforts will be needed to define the functional capacities of the eosinophil within the actual or simulated microenvironments in which it is presumed that eosinophils express themselves.

Our current knowledge is provocative. Eosinophils now appear to be capable of both effector and regulator capacities. The challenge is to remove from the eosinophil the label "enigma" and to alter its "associated with" status to that of being referred to in its own right.

ACKNOWLEDGMENTS

The writing of this chapter and personal research cited were supported in part by the Research and Education Service of the Veterans Administration, the Edna McConnell Clark Foundation, and NIH Grant No. AI 11289. We are indebted to Mrs. Judith O'Connell for her excellent, dedicated secretarial assistance and to Dr. Stephen Kayes for his cogent comments regarding the manuscript.

7. References

Allen, A. C., 1948, Persistent "insect bites" (dermal eosinophilic granulomas) stimulating lymphoblastomas, histiocytoses, and squamous cell carcinomas, *Am. J. Pathol.* **24**:367–375.

Anwar, A. R. E., and Kay, A. B., 1977a, Membrane receptors for IgG and complement (C4, C3b, and C3d) on human eosinophils and neutrophils and their relation to eosinophilia, *J. Immunol.* **119**:976–982.

Anwar, A. R. E., and Kay, A. B., 1977b, The ECF-A tetrapeptides and histamine selectively enhanced human eosinophil complement receptors, *Nature (London)* **269**:522–524.

Archer, G. T., and Hirsch, J. G., 1963a, Motion picture studies on degranulation of horse eosinophils during phagocytosis, *J. Exp. Med.* **118**:287–294.

Archer, G. T., and Hirsch, G. F., 1963b, Isolation of granules from eosinophil leukocytes and study of their enzyme content, *J. Exp. Med.* **118**:277–292.

Archer, G. T., Air, G., Jackas, M., and Morell, D. B., 1965, Studies on rat eosinophil peroxidase, *Biochim. Biophys. Acta* **99**:96–101.

Archer, R. K., 1963, Factors affecting blood eosinophilia and eosinopenia, in: *The Eosinophil Leukocytes,* pp. 12–17, Davis, Philadelphia.

Archer, R. K., and Broome, J., 1963, Studies on the peroxidase reaction in living eosinophils and other leucocytes, *Acta Haematol.* **29**:147–156.

Arnason, B. G., and Waksman, B. H., 1963, The retest reaction in delayed hypersensitivity, *Lab. Invest.* **12**:737–747.

Austen, K. F., Wasserman, S. I., and Geotzl, E. J., 1976, Mast cell-derived mediators: Structural and functional diversity and regulation of expression, in: *Molecular and Biological Aspects of the Acute Allergic Reaction,* 33rd Nobel Symposium (S. G. O. Johansson, K. Strandberg, and B. Urnas, eds.), pp. 293–318, Plenum, New York.

Baehner, R. L., and Johnston, R. B., 1971, Metabolic and bactericidal activities of human eosinophils, *Br. J. Haematol.* **20:**277–285.

Bainton, D. F., and Farquhar, M. G., 1970, Segregation and packaging of granule enzymes in eosinophil leukocytes, *J. Cell Biol.* **45:**54–73.

Bass, D. A., 1975a, Behavior of eosinophil leukocytes in acute inflammation. I. Lack of dependence on adrenal function, *J. Clin. Invest.* **55:**1229–1236.

Bass, D. A., 1975b, Behavior of eosinophil leukocytes in acute inflammation. II. Eosinophil dynamics during acute inflammation, *J. Clin. Invest.* **56:**870–879.

Bass, D. A., 1977, Reproduction of the eosinopenia of acute infection by passive transfer of a material obtained from inflammatory exudate, *Infect. Immun.* **15:**410–416.

Basset, E. G., Baker, J. R., Baker, P. A., and Myers, D. B., 1976, Comparison of collagenase activity in eosinophil and neutrophil fractions from rat peritoneal exudates, *Aust. J. Exp. Biol. Med. Sci.* **54:**459–465.

Basten, A., and Beeson, P. B., 1970, Mechanism of eosinophilia. II. Role of the lymphocyte, *J. Exp. Med.* **131:**1288–1305.

Basten, A., Boyer, M. A., and Beeson, P. B., 1970, Mechanism of eosinophilia. I. Factors affecting the eosinophil response of rats to *Trichinella spiralis, J. Exp. Med.* **131:**1271–1287.

Beeson, P. B., and Bass, D. A., 1977, The eosinophil, in: *Major Problems in Internal Medicine,* Vol. XIV (L. H. Smith, Jr., ed.), Saunders, Philadelphia.

Benveniste, J., Hensen, P. M., and Cochrane, C. G., 1972, Leukocyte-dependent histamine release from rabbit platelets: The role of IgE, basophils, and a platelet-activating factor, *J. Exp. Med.* **136:**1356–1377.

Bogitsh, B. J., 1971, *Schistosoma mansoni:* Cytochemistry of eosinophils in egg-caused early hepatic granulomas in mice, *Exp. Parasitol.* **29:**493–500.

Boyer, M. H., Basten, A., and Beeson, P. B., 1970, Mechanism of eosinophilia. III. Suppression of eosinophilia by agents known to modify immune responses, *Blood* **36:**458–469.

Breton-Gorius, J., and Reyes, F., 1976, Ultrastructure of human bone marrow cell maturation, in: *International Review of Cytology* (G. H. Bourne and J. F. Danielli, eds.), pp. 251–321, Academic, New York.

Bujak, J. S., and Root, R. K., 1974, The role of peroxidase in the bactericidal activity of human blood eosinophils, *Blood* **43:**727–736.

Burns, C. P., and Hoak, J. C., 1975, Freeze-etch studies of the granules of human mast cells and eosinophils, *J. Ultrastruct. Res.* **50:**143–149.

Butterworth, A. E., 1977, The eosinophil and its role in immunity to helminth infection, *Cur. Top. Microbiol. Immunol.* **77:**127–168.

Butterworth, A. E., Sturrock, R. F., Houba, V., and Rees, P. H., 1974, Antibody-dependent cell-mediated damage to schistosolula *in vitro, Nature (London)* **252:**503–505.

Butterworth, A. E., Sturrock, R. F., Houba, V., Mahmoud, A. A. F., Sher, A., and Rees, P. H., 1975, Eosinophils as mediators of antibody-dependent damage to schistosomula, *Nature (London)* **256:**727–729.

Butterworth, A. E., Coombs, R. R. A., Gurner, B. W., and Wilson, A. B., 1976, Receptors for antibody-opsonic adherence on the eosinophils of guinea pigs, *Int. Arch. Allergy Appl. Immunol.* **51:**368–377.

Butterworth, A. E., David, J. R., Franks, D., Mahmoud, A. A. F., David, P. H., Sturrock, R. F., and Houba, V., 1977a, Antibody-dependent eosinophil-mediated damage to ^{51}Cr-labeled schistosomula of *Schistosoma mansoni:* Damage by purified eosinophils, *J. Exp. Med.* **145:**136–150.

Butterworth, A. E., Remold, H. G., Gouba, V., David, J. R., Franks, D., David, P. H., and Sturrock, R. F., 1977b, Antibody-dependent eosinophil-mediated damage to ^{51}Cr-labeled schistosomula of *Schistosoma mansoni:* Mediation by IgG, and inhibition by antigen-antibody complexes, *J. Immunol.* **118:**2230–2236.

Cao, A., Coppa, G., Marcucci, F., and Furbetta, M., 1973, Alkaline phosphatase and lactate dehydrogenase isoenzymes of human eosinophils, *Clin. Chim. Acta* **45:**101–102.

Chusid, M. J., Dale, D. C., West, B. C., and Wolff, S. M., 1975, The hypereosinophilic syndrome: Analysis of fourteen cases with review of the literature, *Medicine* **54:**1–27.

Clark, R. A. F., Gallin, J. I., and Kaplan, A. P., 1975, The selective eosinophil chemotactic activity of histamine, *J. Exp. Med.* **142:**1462–1476.

Clark, R. A. F., Sandler, J. A., Gallin, J. I., and Kaplan, A. R., 1977, Histamine modulation of eosinophil migration, *J. Immunol.* **118:**137–145.

Cline, M. J., 1972, Microbicidal activity of human eosinophils, *J. Reticuloendothel. Soc.* **12**:332–339.

Cohen, S., and Ward, P. A., 1971, *In vitro* and *in vivo* activity of a lymphocyte and immune complex-dependent chemotactic factor for eosinophils, *J. Exp. Med.* **133**:133–146.

Cohen, S. G., Sapp, T. M., Rizzo, A. P., and Kostage, S. T., 1964, Experimental eosinophilia. VII. Lymph node responses to altered gamma globulins, *J. Allergy* **35**:346–355.

Colley, D. G., 1973, Eosinophils and immune mechanisms. I. Eosinophil stimulation promoter (ESP): A lymphokine induced by specific antigen or phytohemagglutinin, *J. Immunol.* **110**:1419–1423.

Colley, D. G., 1974, Variations in peripheral blood eosinophil levels in normal and *Schistosoma mansoni*-infected mice, *J. Lab. Clin. Med.* **83**:871–876.

Colley, D. G., 1976, Eosinophils and immune mechanisms. IV. Culture conditions, antigen requirements, production kinetics and immunologic specificity of the lymphokine eosinophil stimulation promoter, *Cell. Immunol.* **24**:328–335.

Connell, J. T., 1969, Abnormal eosinophils, eosinophilia and basophilia in methimazole neutropenia, *Ann. Allergy* **27**:595–602.

Conrad, M. E., 1971, Hematologic manifestations of parasitic infections, *Sem. Hematol.* **8**:267–303.

Crawford, L. V., 1960, A study of the nasal cytology in infants with eczemoid dermatitis, *Ann. Allergy* **18**:59–64.

Czarnetzki, B. M., Konig, W., and Lichtenstein, L. M., 1976, Eosinophil chemotactic factor (ECF). I. Release from polymorphonuclear leukocytes by the calcium ionophore A 23187, *J. Immunol.* **117**:229–234.

Dale, D. C., Hubert, R. T., and Fauci, A., 1976, Eosinophil kinetics in hypereosinophilic syndrome, *J. Lab. Clin. Med.* **87**:487–495.

Davis, P., and Hughes, G. R. V., 1974, Significance of eosinophilia during gold therapy, *Arthritis Rheum.* **17**:964–968.

Desser, R. K., Himmelhoch, S. R., Evans, W. H., Januska, M., Mage, M., and Shelton, E., 1972, Guinea pig heterophil and eosinophil peroxidase, *Arch. Biochem. Biophys.* **148**:452–465.

Donohugh, D. L., 1963, Tropical eosinophilia: An etiologic inquiry, *N. Engl. J. Med.* **269**:1357–1364.

Ehrlich, P., 1879, Über die spezifischen Granulationen des Blutes, *Arch. Anat. Physiol.*, 571–599.

Eidinger, D., Wilkinson, R., and Rose, B., 1964, A study of cellular responses in immune reactions using the skin window technique. I. Immediate hypersensitivity reactions, *J. Allergy* **35**:77–85.

Felarca, A. B., and Lowell, F. C., 1971, The accumulation of eosinophils and basophils at skin sites as related to intensity of skin reactivity and symptoms in atopic disease, *J. Allergy Clin. Immunol.* **48**:125–133.

Fine, D. P., Buchanan, R. D., and Colley, D. G., 1973, *Schistosoma mansoni* infection in mice depleted of thymus-dependent lymphocytes. I. Eosinophilia and immunologic responses to a schistosomal egg preparation, *Am. J. Pathol.* **71**:193–206.

Foot, E. C., 1965, Eosinophil turnover in the normal rat, *Br. J. Haematol.* **11**:439–445.

Freidman, G., and Holtz, E., 1935, The behavior of eosinophiles in rheumatic fever, *J. Lab. Clin. Med.* **21**:225–233.

Ghidoni, J. J., and Goldberg, A. F., 1966, Light and electron microscopic localization of acid phosphatase activity in human eosinophils, *Am. J. Clin. Pathol.* **45**:402–405.

Ghossein, N. A., and Stacey, R., 1973, The prognostic significance of radiation-related eosinophilia, *Radiology* **107**:631–633.

Ghossein, N. A., Bosworth, J. L., Stacey, P., Muggia, F. M., and Krishnaswamy, V., 1975, Radiation-related eosinophilia: Correlation with delayed hypersensitivity, lymphocyte count, and survival in patients tested by curative radiotherapy, *Radiology* **117**:413–417.

Gilman, P. A., Jackson, D. P., and Guild H. G., 1970, Congenital agranalocytosis: Prolonged survival and terminal acute leukemia, *Blood* **36**:576–585.

Gleich, G. J., 1977, The eosinophil: New aspects of structure and function, *J. Allergy Clin. Immunol.* **60**:73–82.

Gleich, G. J., Loegering, D. A., and Maldonado, J. E., 1973, Identification of a major basic protein in guinea pig eosinophil granules, *J. Exp. Med.* **137**:1459–1471.

Gleich, G. J., Loegering, D. A., Kueppers, F., Bajaj, S. P., and Mann, K. G., 1974, Physicochemical and biological properties of the major basic protein from guinea pig eosinophil granules, *J. Exp. Med.* **140**:313–332.

Goetzl, E. J., and Austen, K. F., 1975, Purification and synthesis of eosinophilotactic tetrapeptides of human lung tissue: Identification as eosinophil chemotactic factor of anaphylaxis, *Proc. Natl. Acad. Sci. USA* **72**:4123–4127.

Goetzl, E. J., and Austen, K. F., 1976, Structural determinants of the eosinophil chemotactic activity of the acidic tetrapeptides of eosinophil chemotactic factor of anaphylaxis, *J. Exp. Med.* **144:**1424–1437.

Goetzl, E. J., and Austen, K. F., 1977, Eosinophil chemotactic factor of anaphylaxis (ECF-A): Cellular origin, structure and function, *Monogr. Allergy* **12:**189–197.

Goetzl, E. J., Woods, J. M., and Gorman, R. R., 1977, Stimulation of human eosinophil and neutrophil polymorphonuclear leukocyte chemotaxis and random migration by 12-L-hydroxy-5,8,10,14-eicosatetraenoic acid, *J. Clin. Envest.* **59:**179–183.

Goldman, L., Rockwell, E., and Richfield, D. F., 1952, Histopathological studies on cutaneous reactions to the bites of various arthropods, *Am. J. Trop. Med. Hyg.* **1:**514–525.

Greco, D. B., Fujita, Y., Ishikawa, T., and Arbesman, C. E., 1973, Antigen-antibody complexes in/on eosinophils in nasal secretions from patients allergic to ragweed, *J. Allergy Clin. Immunol.* **51:**124–125 (abstr.).

Greenberg, M. L., and Chikkappa, G., 1971, Eosinophil production and survival in a patient with eosinophilia (leukemia?), *Blood* **38:**826 (abstr.).

Greene, B. M., and Colley, D. G., 1974, Eosinophils and immune mechanisms. II. Partial characterization of the lymphokine eosinophil stimulation promoter, *J. Immunol.* **113:**910–917.

Greene, B. M., and Colley, D. G., 1976, Eosinophils and immune mechanisms. III. Production of the lymphokine eosinophil stimulation promoter by mouse T lymphocytes, *J. Immunol.* **116:**1078–1083.

Grove, D. I., Mahmoud, A. A. F., and Warren, K. S., 1977, Eosinophils and resistance to *Trichinella spiralis*, *J. Exp. Med.* **145:**755–759.

Gupta, S., 1977, Eozynofile: Ich budowa czynośći i znaczenie w klinice, *Pol. Arch. Med. Wewn.* **57:**435–445.

Gupta, S., Frenkel, R., Rosenstein, M., and Grieco, M. H., 1975, Lymphocyte subpopulations, serum IgE, and total eosinophil counts in patients with bronchial asthma, *Clin. Exp. Immunol.* **22:**438–445.

Gupta, S., Ross, G. D., Good, R. A., and Siegal, F. P., 1976, Surface markers of human eosinophils, *Blood* **48:**755–763.

Halberg, F., and Visscher, M. B., 1950, Regular diurnal physiological variation in eosinophil levels in five stocks of mice, *Proc. Soc. Exp. Biol. Med.* **75:**846–847.

Hardy, W. R., and Anderson, R. E., 1968, The hypereosinophilic syndromes, *Ann. Intern. Med.* **68:**1220–1229.

Herion, J. C., Glasser, R. M., Walker, R. I., and Palmer, J. G., 1970, Eosinophil kinetics in two patients with eosinophilia, *Blood* **36:**361–370.

Hirashima, M., and Hayashi, H., 1976, The mediation of tissue eosinophilia in hypersensitivity reaction. I. Isolation of two different chemotactic factors from DNP-*Ascaris* extract-induced skin lesion in guinea pig, *Immunology* **30:**203–212.

Hirashima, M., Honda, M., and Hayashi, H., 1976, The mediation of tissue eosinophilia in hypersensitivity reactions. II. Separation of a delayed eosinophil chemotactic factor from macrophage chemotactic factors, *Immunology* **31:**263–271.

Hsu, C. K., Hsu, S. H., Whitney, Jr., R. A., and Hansen, C. T., 1976, Immunology of schistosomiasis in athymic mice, *Nature (London)* **262:**397–399.

Hsu, S. Y. L., Hsu, H. F., Penick, G. D., Lust, G. L., and Osborne, J. W., 1974, Dermal hypersensitivity to schistosome cercariae in rhesus monkeys during immunization and challenge, *J. Allergy Clin. Immunol.* **54:**339–349.

Hubscher, T. T., 1975a, Role of the eosinophil in the allergic reactions. I. EDI—An eosinophil-derived inhibitor of histamine release, *J. Immunol.* **114:**1379–1388.

Hubscher, T. T., 1975b, Role of the eosinophil in the allergic reactions. II. Release of prostaglandins from human eosinophilic leukocytes, *J. Immunol.* **114:**1379–1393.

Hubscher, T. T., 1977, Immune and biochemical mechanisms in the allergic disease of the upper respiratory tract: Role of antibodies, target cells, mediators and eosinophils, *Ann. Allergy* **38:**83–90.

Hubscher, T. T., and Eisen, A. H., 1971, Allergen binding to human peripheral leukocytes, *Int. Arch. Allergy Appl. Immunol.* **41:**689–699.

Hudson, G., 1968, Quantitative study of the eosinophil granulocytes, *Sem. Hematol.* **5:**166–186.

Isaacson, N. H., and Rapoport, P., 1946, Eosinophilia in malignant tumors: Its significance, *Ann. Intern. Med.* **125:**893–902.

Ishikawa, T., Wicker, K., and Arbesman, C. E., 1974, *In vitro* and *in vivo* studies on uptake of antigen–antibody complexes by eosinophils, *Int. Arch. Allergy Appl. Immunol.* **46**:230–248.

Iverson, D., DeChatelet, L. R., Spitznagel, J. K., and Wang, P., 1977, Comparison of NADH and NADPH oxidase activities in granules isolated from human polymorphonuclear leukocytes with a fluorometric assay, *J. Clin. Invest.* **59**:282–290.

James, S. L., and Colley, D. G., 1975, Eosinophils and immune mechanisms: Production of the lymphokine eosinophil stimulation promoter (ESP) *in vitro* by isolated intact granulomas, *J. Reticuloendothel. Soc.* **18**:283–293.

James, S. L., and Colley, D. G., 1976, Eosinophil-mediated destruction of *Schistosoma mansoni* eggs, *J. Reticuloendothel. Soc.* **20**:359–374.

James, S. L., and Colley, D. G., 1978a, Eosinophil-mediated destruction of *Schistosoma mansoni* eggs *in vitro*. II. The role of cytophilic antibody, *Cell. Immunol.* **38**:35–47.

James, S. L., and Colley, D. G., 1978b, Eosinophil-mediated destruction of *Schistosoma mansoni* eggs. III. Lymphokine involvement in the induction of eosinophil functional abilities, *Cell. Immunol.* **38**:48–58.

Jenkins, V. K., Trentin, J. J., Speirs, R. S., and McGarry, M. P., 1972, Hemopoietic colony studies. VI. Increased eosinophil-containing colonies obtained by antigen pretreatment of irradiated mice reconstituted with bone marrow cells, *J. Cell. Physiol.* **79**:413–422.

Jeunet, F. S., and Good, R. A., 1968, Thymoma, immunologic deficiences and hematological abnormalities, in: *Immunologic Deficiency Disease in Man: Proceedings,* Vol. 4(1) (R. A. Good and D. Bergsma, eds.), pp. 192–206, National Foundation, New York.

Jones, D. G., and Kay, A. B., 1976, The effect of anti-eosinophil serum on skin histamine replenishment following passive cutaneous anaphylaxis in the guinea pig, *Immunology* **31**:333–336.

Jose, D. G., Gatti, R. A., and Good, R. A., 1971, Eosinophilia with *Pneumocystis carinii* pneumonia and immune deficiency syndromes, *J. Pediatr.* **79**:748–754.

Kashiwa, H. K., and Hungerford, G. F., 1958, Blood leucocyte response in rats fed a magnesium deficient diet, *Proc. Soc. Exp. Biol. Med.* **99**:441–443.

Kater, L. A., Goetzl, E. J., and Austen, K. F., 1976, Isolation of human eosinophil phospholipase D, *J. Clin. Invest.* **57**:1173–1180.

Katzenstein, A. L., Lievow, A. A., and Freidman, P. J., 1975, Bronchocentric granulomatosis, mucoid impaction, and hypersensitivity reactions to fungi, *Am. Rev. Resp. Dis.* **111**:497–537.

Kay, A. B., 1970a, Studies on eosinophil leucocyte migration. I. Eosinophil and neutrophil accumulations following antigen–antibody reactions in guinea pig skin, *Clin. Exp. Immunol.* **6**:75–86.

Kay, A. B., 1970b, Studies on eosinophil leucocyte migration. II. Factors specifically chemotactic for eosinophils and neutrophils generated from guinea pig serum by antigen–antibody complexes, *Clin. Exp. Immunol.* **7**:723–737.

Kay, A. B., 1977, Eosinophil leucocytes: Recruitment, localization and function in immediate-type hypersensitivity, *Monogr. Allergy* **12**:222–230.

Kay, A. B., Stechschulte, D. J., and Austen, K. F., 1971, An eosinophil leukocyte chemotactic factor of anaphylaxis, *J. Exp. Med.* **133**:602–619.

Kay, A. B., Shin, H. S., and Austen, K. F., 1973, Selective attraction of eosinophils and synergism between eosinophil chemotactic factor of anaphylaxis (ECF-A) and a fragment cleaved from the fifth component of complement (C5a), *Immunology* **24**:969–976.

Kay, A. B., McVie, J. G., Stuart, A. E., Krajewski, A., and Turnbull, L. W., 1975, Eosinophil chemotaxis of supernatants from cultured Hodgkin's lymph node cells, *J. Clin. Pathol.* **28**:502–505.

Kazura, J. W., Mahmoud, A. A. F., Karbs, K. S., and Warren, K. S., 1975, The lymphokine eosinophil stimulation promoter and human schistosomiasis mansoni, *J. Infect. Dis.* **132**:702–706.

Keller, H. U., and Sorkin, E., 1969, Studies on chemotaxis. XIII. Differences in the chemotactic response of neutrophil and eosinophil polymorphonuclear leucocytes, *Int. Arch. Allergy* **35**:279–287.

Klebanoff, S. J., 1968, Myeloperoxidase–halide–hydrogen peroxide antibacterial system, *J. Bacteriol.* **95**:2131–2138.

Konig, W., Czarnetzki, B. M., and Lichtenstein, L. M., 1976, Eosinophil chemotactic factor (ECF). II. Release from human polymorphonuclear leukocytes during phagocytosis, *J. Immunol.* **117**:235–241.

Konig, W., Czarnetzki, B. M., and Lichtenstein, L. M., 1977, Generation and release of eosinophil chemotactic factor from human polymorphonuclear leukocytes, *Monogr. Allergy* **12:**198–212.

Lachmann, P. J., Kay, A. B., and Thompson, R. A., 1970, The chemotactic activity for neutrophil and eosinophil leucocytes of the tri-molecular complex of the fifth, sixth and seventh components of human complement (C567) prepared in free solution by the "reactive lysis" procedure, *Immunology* **19:**895–899.

Lehrer, R. I., and Cline, M. J., 1969, Leukocyte myeloperoxidase deficiency and disseminated candidiasis: The role of myeloperoxidase in resistance to *Candida* infection, *J. Clin. Invest.* **48:**1478–1488.

Lewis, F. A., Carter, C. E., and Colley, D. G., 1977, Eosinophils and immune mechanisms. V. Demonstration of mouse spleen cell-derived chemotactic activities for eosinophils and mononuclear cells and comparisons with eosinophil stimulation promoter, *Cell. Immunol.* **32:**86–96.

Litt, M., 1964, Eosinophils and antigen–antibody reactions, *Ann. N.Y. Acad. Sci.* **116:**964–985.

Litt, M., 1976, Studies in experimental eosinophilia. XI. Dependence of eosinophilia, apparently induced by histamine, on acidity, *Int. Arch. Allergy App. Immunol.* **50:**473–487.

Lowell, F. C., 1967, Clinical aspects of eosinophilia in atopic disease, *J. Am. Med. Assoc.* **202:**875–878.

Lukens, J. N., 1972, Eosinophilia in children, *Pediatr. Clin. North Am.* **19:**969–981.

Mahmoud, A. A. F., and Warren, K. S., 1977, Anti-percursor eosinophil serum: Comparison with anti-mature eosinophil serum, *Clin. Res.* **25:**478A (abstr.).

Mahmoud, A. A. F., Warren, K. S., and Boros, D. L., 1973, Production of a rabbit anti-mouse eosinophil serum with no cross-reactivity to neutrophils, *J. Exp. Med.* **137:**1526–1531.

Mahmoud, A. A. F., Warren, K. S., and Graham, R. C., Jr., 1975a, Anti-eosinophil serum and the kinetics of eosinophilia in schistosomiasis mansoni, *J, Exp. Med.* **142:**560–674.

Mahmoud, A. A. F., Warren, K. S., and Peters, P. A., 1975b, A role for the eosinophil in acquired resistance to *Schistosoma mansoni* infection as determined by anti-eosinophil serum, *J. Exp. Med.* **142:**805–813.

Mahmoud, A. A. F., Stone, M. K., and Kellermeyer, R. W., 1977, Eosinophilopoietin: A circulating low molecular weight peptide-like substance which stimulates the production of eosinophil in mice, *J. Clin. Invest.* **60:**675–682.

Mann, P. R., and Cruickshank, C. N. D., 1975, An eosinophilotactic factor derived from rat mast cells, *J. Pathol.* **115:**91–96.

Marcussen, H., 1974, Fluorescent anti-colon antibodies and inflammatory eosinophilia in ulcerative colitis, *Scand. J. Gastroenterol.* **9:**575–577.

McGarry, M. P., and Miller, A. M., 1974, Evidence for the humoral stimulation of eosinophil granulocytopoiesis in *in vivo* diffusion chambers, *Exp. Hematol.* **2:**372–379.

McGarry, M. P., Speirs, R. S., Jenkins, V. K., and Trentin, J. J., 1971, Lymphoid cell dependence of eosinophil response to antigen, *J. Exp. Med.* **134:**801–814.

McGarry, M. P., Miller, A. M., and Colley, D. G., 1977, Humoral regulation of eosinophil granulocytopoiesis, in: *Experimental Hematology Today* (S. Baum and G. D. Ledney, eds.), pp. 63–70, Springer-Verlag, New York.

McRipley, R. J., and Sbarra, A. J., 1967, Role of the phagocyte in host-parasite interactions. XII. Hydrogen–peroxide–myloperoxidase bactericidal system in the phagocyte, *J. Bacteriol.* **94:**1425–1430.

Metcalf, D. D., Gadek, J. E., Raphael, G. D., Frank, M. M., Kaplan, A. P., and Kaliner, M., 1977, Human eosinophil adherence to serum-treated sepharose: Granule-associated enzyme release and requirement for activation of the alternative complement pathway, *J. Immunol.* **119:**1744–1750.

Mickenberg, I. D., Root, R. K., and Wolff, S. M., 1972, Bactericidal and metabolic properties of human eosinophils, *Blood* **39:**67–80.

Miller, A. M., and McGarry, M. P., 1976, A diffusible stimulator of eosinophilopoiesis produced by lymphoid cells as demonstrated with diffusion chambers, *Blood* **48:**293–300.

Miller, A. M., Colley, D. G., and McGarry, M. P., 1976, Spleen cells from *Schistosoma mansoni*-infected mice produce diffusible stimulator of eosinophilopoiesis *in vivo, Nature (London)* **161:**506–507.

Miller, F., DeHarven, E., and Palade, G. E., 1966, The structure of eosinophil leukocyte granules in rodents and in man, *J. Cell Biol.* **31:**349–362.

Nakatsui, T., Taketomi, Y., and Uchino, H., 1972, Ultrastructural localization of alkaline phosphatase in human granulocytes, lymphocytes and platelets of normals and of some hematological disorders, *Acta Haematol. Jpn.* **35**:47–68.

Neva, F. A., Kaplan, A. P., Pacheco, G., Gray, L., and Danaraj, T. J., 1975, Tropical eosinophilia: A human model of parasitic immunopathology, with observations on serum IgE levels before and after treatment, *J. Allergy Clin. Immunol.* **55**:422–429.

Nielsen, K., Fogh, L., and Andersen, S., 1974, Eosinophil response to migrating *Ascaris suum* larvae in normal and congenitally thymus-less mice, *Acta Pathol. Mocrobiol. Scand. B* **82**:919–920.

Öhman, S., and Johansson, S. G. O., 1974, Allergen-specific IgE in atopic dermatitis, *Acta Derm. Venereol.* **54**:283–290.

Ottesen, E. A., 1976, Eosinophilia and the lung, in: *Immunologic and Infectious Reactions in the Lung* (C. Kirkpatrick and H. Reynolds, eds.), pp. 289–332, Dekker, New York.

Ottesen, E. A., Stanley, A. M., Gelfand, J. A., Gadek, J. E., Frank, M. M., Nash, T. E., and Cheever, A. W., 1977, Immunoglobulin and complement receptors on human eosinophils and their role in cellular adherence to schistosomules, *Am. J. Trop. Med. Hyg.* **26**:134–141 (suppl.).

Panush, R. S., Franco, A. E., and Schur, P. H., 1971, Rheumatoid arthritis associated with eosinophilia, *Ann. Intern. Med.* **75**:199–205.

Parish, W. E., 1970, Investigations on eosinophilia. The influence of histamine, antigen–antibody complexes containing $\gamma 1$ or $\gamma 2$ globulins, foreign bodies (phagocytosis) and disrupted mast cells, *Br. J. Dermatol.* **82**:42–64.

Parish, W. E., 1972a, Eosinophilia, II. Cutaneous eosinophilia in guinea pigs mediated by passive anaphylaxis with IgG 1 or reagin, and antigen–antibody complexes; its relation to neutrophils and to mast cells, *Immunology* **23**:19–34.

Parish, W. E., 1972b, Eosinophilia. III. The anaphylactic release isolated human basophils of a substance that selectively attracts eosinophils, *Clin. Allergy* **2**:381–390.

Parmley, R. T., and Spicer, S. S., 1974, Cytochemical and ultrastructural identification of a small type granule in human late eosinophils, *Lab. Invest.* **30**:557–567.

Parwaresch, M. R., Walle, A. J., and Arndt, D., 1976, The peripheral kinetics of human radiolabelled eosinophils, *Virchows Arch. B.* **21**:57–66.

Pelley, R. P., Karp, R., Mahmoud, A. A. F., and Warren, K. S., 1976, Antigen dose response to specificity of production of the lymphokine eosinophil stimulation promoter, *J. Infect. Dis.* **134**:230–237.

Pepys, J., and Simon, G., 1973, Asthma, pulmonary eosinophilia, and allergic alveolitis, *Med. Clin. North Am.* **57**:573–591.

Person, J. R., and Rogers, R. S., III, 1977, Bullous and cicatricial pemphigoid. Clinical histopathologic and immunopathologic correlations, *Mayo Clin. Proc.* **52**:54–66.

Phillips, S. M., and Colley, D. G., 1978, Immunologic aspects of host responses to schistosomiasis: Resistance, immunopathology, and eosinophil involvement, *Prog. Allergy,* **24**:49–182.

Phillips, S. M., DiConza, J. J., Gold, J. A., and Reid, W. A., 1977, Schistosomiasis in the congenitally athymic (nude) mouse. I. Thymic dependency of eosinophilia, granuloma formation, and host morbidity, *J. Immunol.* **118**:594–599.

Polliack, A., and Douglas, S. D., 1975, Surface features of human eosinophils: A scanning and transmission electron microscopic study of a case of eosinophilia, *Br. J. Haematol.* **30**:65–70.

Ponzio, N. M., and Speirs, R. S., 1973, Lymphoid cell dependence of eosinophil response to antigen. III. Comparison of the rate of appearance of two types of memory cells in various lymphoid tissues at different times after priming, *J. Immunol.* **110**:1363–1370.

Ponzio, N. M., and Speirs, R. S., 1975, Lymphoid cell dependence of eosinophil response to antigen. VI. The effect of selective removal of T or B lymphocytes on the capacity of primed spleen cells to adoptively transferred immunity to tetanus toxoid, *Immunology* **28**:243–251.

Presentey, B., and Szapiro, L., 1969, Hereditary deficiency of peroxidase and phospholipids in eosinophilic granulocytes, *Acta Haematol.* **41**:359–362.

Rabellino, E. M., and Metcalf, D., 1975, Receptors for C3 and IgG on macrophage, neutrophil and eosinophil colony cells grown *in vitro, J. Immunol.* **115**:688–692.

Rickles, F. R., and Miller, D. R., 1972, Eosinophilic leukemoid reaction, *J. Pediatr.* **80**:418–428.

Riis, P., and Anthonisen, P., 1964, Eosinophilia in peripheral blood and inflammatory exudate in non-specific proctocolitis, *Acta Med. Scand.* **175**:85–89.

Roberts, W. C., Liegler, D. G., and Carbone, P. P., 1969, Endomyocardial disease and eosinophilia. A clinical and pathologic spectrum, *Am. J. Med.* **46**:28–42.

Robinson, L. D., Jr., and Miller, M. E., 1975, SECA, a new mediator of the human eosinophil response, *J. Allergy Clin. Immunol.* **56**:317–322.
Rogovine, V. V., Muravieff, R. A., Frolova, W. M., Geranina, N. G., and Piruzyan, L. A., 1875, Ultrastructural cytochemistry of peroxidase and acid phosphatase in mice maturing eosinophils, *Experientia* **31**:1031–1033.
Ross, R., and Klebanoff, S. J., 1966, The eosinophilic leukocyte. Fine structure studies of changes in the uterus during the estrous cycle, *J. Exp. Med.* **124**:653–659.
Ruitenberg, E. J., Elgersma, A., Kruizinga, W., and Leenstra, F., 1977, *Trichinella spiralis* infection in congenitally athymic (nude) mice. Parasitological, serological and haematological studies with observations in intestinal pathology, *Immunology* **33**:581–587.
Ruscetti, F. W., Cypess, R. H., and Chervenick, P. A., 1976, Specific release of neutrophilic- and eosinophilic- stimulating factors from sensitized lymphocytes, *Blood* **47**:757–765.
Rytömma, T., 1960., Organ distribution and histochemical properties of eosinophil granulocytes in the rat, *Acta Pathol. Microbiol. Scand. Suppl.* **140**:1–118.
Rytömma, T., and Teir, H., 1961, Relationship between tissue eosinophils and peroxidase activity, *Nature (London)* **192**:271–272.
Salmon, S. E., Cline, M. J., Schultz, J., and Lehrer, R. I., 1970, Myeloperoxidase deficiency: Immunologic study of a genetic leukocyte defect, *N. Engl. J. Med.* **282**:250–253.
Samter, M., 1965, Eosinophils, in: *Immunological Disease* (M. Samter and H. L. Alexander, eds.), pp. 242–245, Little, Brown, Boston.
Schriber, R. A., and Zucker-Franklin, D., 1975, Induction of bleed eosinophilia by pulmonary embolization of antigen-coated particles: The relationship to cell-mediated immunity, *J. Immunol.* **114**:1348–1353.
Seeman, P. M., and Palade, G. E., 1967, Acid phosphatase localization in rabbit eosinophils, *J. Cell Biol.* **34**:745–756.
Sher, R., and Glover, A., 1976, Isolation of human eosinophils and their lymphocyte-like rosetting properties, *Immunology* **31**:337–341.
Sher, A., Smithers, R. R., and Mackenzie, P., 1975, Passive transfer of acquired resistance to *Schistosoma mansoni* in laboratory mice, *Parasitology* **70**:347–357.
Speirs, R. S., and Meyer, R. K., 1949, The effects of stress, adrenal and adrenocorticotropic hormones on the circulating eosinophils of mice, *Endocrinology* **45**:403–429.
Speirs, R. S., Gallagher, M. T., Rauchwerger, J., Heim, L. R., and Trentin, J. J., 1973, Lymphoid cell dependence of eosinophil response to antigen. II. Location of memory cells and their dependence upon thymic influence, *Exp. Hematol.* **1**:150–158.
Speirs, R. S., Speirs, E. E., and Ponzio, N. M., 1974, Eosinophils in humoral and cell-mediated responses, in: *Developments in Lymphoid Cell Biology* (A. A. Gottlieb, ed.), pp. 51–73, CRC, Cleveland.
Spitzer, G., and Garson, O. M., 1973, Lymphoblastic leukemia with marked eosinophilia: A report of two cases, *Blood* **42**:377–384.
Spry, C. J. F., 1971a, Mechanism of eosinophilia. V. Kinetics of normal and accelerated eosinopoiesis, *Cell Tissue Kinet.* **4**:351–364.
Spry, C. J. F., 1971b, Mechanism of eosinophilia. VI. Eosinophil mobilization, *Cell Tissue Kinet.* **4**:365–374.
Spry, C. J. F., and Tai, P. C., 1976, Studies on blood eosinophils. II. Patients with Loffler's cardiomyophathy, *Clin. Exp. Immunol.* **24**:423–434.
Stickney, J. M., and Heck, F. J., 1944, Clinical occurrence of eosinophilia, *Med. Clin. North Am.* **28**:915–919.
Stryckmans, P. A., Cronkite, E. P., Greenberg, M. L., and Schiffer, L. M., 1968. Kinetics of eosinophil leukocyte proliferation in man, *Proc. 12th Congr. Int. Soc. Haematol*, New York, p. F19 (abstr.).
Stuart, A. E., 1970, Immunological aspects of reticulum cell neoplasia, *Br. Med. J.* **4**:423–424.
Tai, P. C., and Spry, C. J. F., 1976, Studies on blood eosinophils. I. Patients with a transient eosinophilia, *Clin. Exp. Immunol.* **24**:415–422.
Takenaka, T., Okuda, M., Kawabori, S., and Kubo, K., 1977, Extracellular release of peroxidase from eosinophils by interaction with immune complexes, *Clin. Exp. Immunol.* **28**:56–60.
Tanaka, Y., and Goodman, J. R., 1972, Eosinophils, in: *Electron Microscopy of Human Blood Cells*, pp. 138–146, Harper and Row, New York.

Tchernitchin, A., Hasbun, J., Peña, G., and Vega, S., 1971, Autoradiographic study of the *in vitro* uptake of estradiol by eosinophils in human endometrium, *Proc. Soc. Exp. Biol. Med.* **137:**108–110.

Tchernitchin, A., Roorijck, J., Tchernitchin, X., Vandenhende, J., and Galand, P., 1974, Dramatic early increase in uterine eosinophils after estrogen administration, *Nature (London)* **148:**142–143.

Torisu, M., Yoshida, T., Ward, P. A., and Cohen, S., 1973, Lymphocyte-derived eosinophil chemotactic factor. II. Studies on the mechanism of activation of the precursor substance by immune complexes, *J. Immunol.* **111:**1450–1458.

Tse, K. S., Wicher, K., and Arbesman, C. E., 1970, IgE antibodies in nasal secretions of ragweed-allergic subjects, *J. Alelrgy* **46:**352–358.

Turnbull, L. W., and Kay, A. B., 1976, Eosinophils and mediators of anaphylaxis. Histamine and imidazole acetic acid as chemotactic agents for human eosinophil leucocytes, *Immunology* **31:**797–802.

Turnbull, L. W., Evans, D. P., and Kay, A. B., 1977, Human eosinophils, acidic tetrapeptides (ECF-A) and histamine: Interactions *in vitro* and *in vivo, Immunology* **32:**57–63.

Turner, S. R., Tainer, J. A., and Lynn, W. S., 1975, Biogenesis of chemotactic molecules by the arachidonate lipoxygenase system of platelets, *Nature (London)* **257:**680–681.

von Lichtenberg, F., Erickson, D. G., and Sadun, E. H., 1973, Comparative histopathology of schistosome granulomas in the hamster, *Am. J. Pathol.* **72:**149–178.

vonLichtenberg, F., Sher, A., Gibbons N., and Doughty, B. L., 1976, Eosinophil-enriched inflammatory response to schistosomula in the skin of mice immune to *Schistosoma mansoni, Am. J. Pathol.* **84:**479–500.

Walls, R. S., 1976, Lymphocytes and specificity of eosinophilia, *S. Afr. Med. J.* **50:**1313–1318.

Walls, R. S., and Beeson, P. B., 1972, Mechanism of eosinophilia. VIII. Importance of local cellular reactions in stimulating eosinophil production, *Clin. Exp. Immunol.* **12:**111–119.

Walls, R. S., Basten, A., Leuchars, E., and Davies, A. J. S., 1971, Mechanisms for eosinophilic and neutrophilic leucocytoses, *Br. Med. J.* **3:**157–159.

Ward, P. A., 1969, Chemotaxis of human eosinophils, *Am. J. Pathol.* **54:**121–128.

Ward, P. A., Cochrane, C. G., and Müler-Eberhard, H. J., 1965, The role of serum complement in chemotaxis of leukocytes *in vitro, J. Exp. Med.* **122:**327–346.

Warren, K. S., 1972, The immunopathogenesis of schistosomiasis: A multidisciplinary approach, *Trans. R. Soc. Trop. Med. Hyg.* **66:**417–434.

Warren, K. S., Darp, R., Pelley, R. P., and Mahmoud, A. A. F., 1976, The eosinophil stimulation promoter test in murine and human *Trichinella spiralis* infection, *J. Infect. Dis.* **134:**277–280.

Wasserman, S. I., Goetzl, E. J., Ellman, L., and Austen, K. F., 1974, Tumor-associated eosinophilotactic factor, *N. Engl. J. Med.* **290:**420–424.

Wasserman, S. I., Goetzl, E. J., and Austen, K. F., 1975, Inactivation of slow reacting substance of anaphylaxis by human eosinophil arylsulfatase, *J. Immunol.* **114:**645–649.

West, B. C., Galb, N. A., and Rosenthal, A. S., 1975, Isolation and partial characterization of human eosinophil granules, *Am. J. Pathol.* **81:**575–588.

Wilson, K. S., and Alexander, H. L., 1945, The association of periarteritis nodosa, bronchial asthma and hypereosinophilia, *J. Lab. Clin. Med.* **30:**361–363 (abstr).

Yam, L. T., Li, C. Y., Necheles, T. F., and Katayama, I., 1972, Pseudoeosinophilia eosinophilic endocarditis, and eosinophilic leukemia, *Am. J. Med.* **53:**193–202.

Zeiger, R. S., and Colten, H. R., 1977, Histaminase release from human eosinophils, *J. Immunol.* **118:**540–543.

Zeiger, R. S., Twarog, F. J., and Colten, H. R., 1976, Histaminase release from human granulocytes, *J. Exp. Med.* **144:**1049–1061.

Zolov, D. M., and Levine, B. B., 1969, Correlation of blood eosinophilia with antibody classes. Studies with the penicillin hypersensitivity system, *Int. Arch. Allergy* **35:**179–193.

Zucker-Franklin, D., 1974, Eosinophil function and disorders, *Adv. Intern. Med.* **19:**1–25.

3

Lymphocyte Subpopulations and Functions in Hypersensitivity Disorders

SUDHIR GUPTA and ROBERT A. GOOD

1. Introduction

During the last 15 years, progress in understanding the structure and functions of lymphoid organs, cells, and molecules has provided us with a better understanding of their role in various immunological phenomena. This has brought us to a point of clinical application. Animal experiments and studies of experiments of nature in humans have led to the discovery of a two-component concept of immunity (Cooper *et al.*, 1965). Figure 1 depicts our current concept of this two-cell system of immunity. It is now clear that cells originating from the hemangioblasts of yolk sac develop into mature hematopoietic cells. It seems likely that cells of the yolk sac contain the precursors of all the major hematopoietic elements. During development, these pluripotent stem cells migrate to the fetal liver, where they not only can give rise to an additional population of stem cells but also may be induced to differentiate along several additional lines.

From yolk sac, fetal liver, and postnatal bone marrow, cells that can act as precursors of the lymphoid apparatus are derived. Lymphoid stem cells follow two different routes to differentiate into two major classes of lymphocytes, T and B lymphocytes. These cells can function as prethymic cells. They enter the thymus and interact with thymic epithelium and, possibly under the influence of a family of "thymic hormones," differentiate into relatively more mature postthymic T cells. These T cells, when stimulated by appropriate stimuli either *in vivo* or *in*

SUDHIR GUPTA and ROBERT A. GOOD • Memorial Sloan-Kettering Cancer Center, New York, New York 10021. This work was supported in part by grants from National Institutes of Health CA-19267, CA-08748, NS-11457, AI-11843, AG-00541, the Zelda R. Weintraub Cancer Fund.

vitro, respond by proliferation and/or the production of a variety of soluble mediators, the lymphokines. T lymphocytes tend to be distributed selectively in certain areas of peripheral lymphoid tissues. They occupy preferentially the deep cortical regions of lymph nodes and the parafollicular and perivascular accumulations in the Malpighian white matter of the spleen.

The T-cell population is a circulating and recirculating population and therefore represents a readily mobilizable pool of cells which can easily be depleted from the circulation either by thoracic duct drainage or by treatment with antilymphocyte serum. T lymphocytes are responsible for the expression of cell-mediated immunity, that is, delayed-type hypersensitivity, for solid-tissue allograft rejection reactions, for initiation of graft vs. host reactions, and for defense against many viruses, fungi, and facultative intracellular bacteria; they also provide a mechanism for detection and destruction of malignant cells.

By an alternative pathway, lymphoid stem cells are processed in fetal liver and adult bone marrow to differentiate into B lymphocytes, precursors of immunoglobulin-synthesizing and secreting plasma cells. B lymphocytes, when stimulated either *in vivo* or *in vitro*, differentiate into plasma cells to synthesize and secrete specific antibodies—the immunoglobulins M, G, A, D, and E. B lymphocytes and their immunoglobulin products represent a major bullwark against encapsulated high-grade pyogenic pathogens. B lymphocytes are concentrated in the far cortical areas of the lymph node. B cells and plasma cells make up the majority of cells in the medullary cords of the node. B cells and plasma cells of IgA and IgE classes are predominantly located in the subepithelial regions as, for example, the lamina propria of the gastrointestinal tract, in glands along the gastrointestinal tract, in Peyer's patches, and in the pharyngeal tonsils.

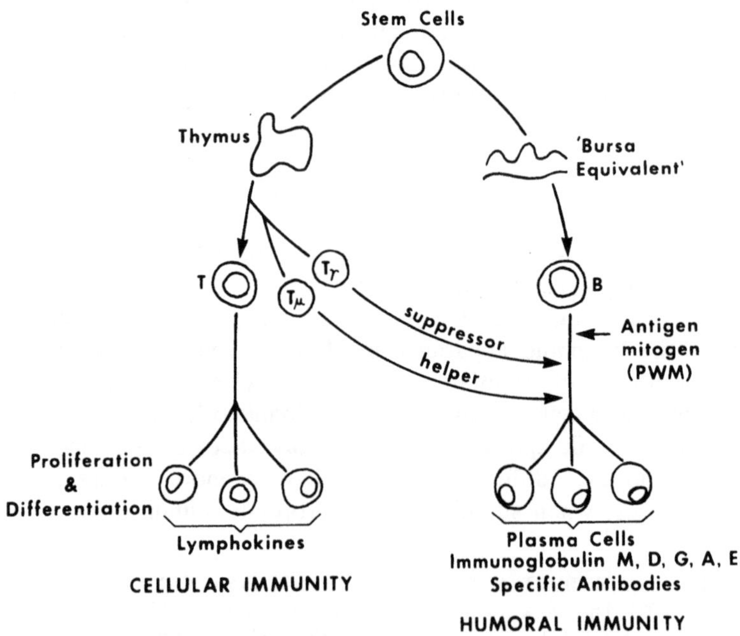

Figure 1. Cellular and humoral systems of immunity.

During the process of differentiation and maturation, lymphocytes develop into subpopulations having a variety of surface and intracellular markers, and they acquire distinct functions. In this chapter we will review the development of lymphoid cells and discuss the phenotypes and functions of the subpopulations. In addition, we will discuss perturbations of the lymphocytes and lymphocyte subpopulations in patients with hypersensitivity disorders.

2. Development of Thymus and T Lymphocytes

The thymus originates about 6 weeks of gestational age from the third and fourth pharyngeal pouches. It develops from an ectodermal–endodermal junction, and its epithelial components probably contain derivatives of both ecodermal and endodermal germ layers. Although the thymus is originally epithelial in nature, small lymphocytes are demonstrable histologically within this organ by the eighth to ninth week of gestation (Solomon, 1971; Papiernik, 1970). In man, the origin of these thymic lymphocytes is unknown; however, animal studies suggest that prethymic hematopoietic stem cells originating in yolk sac or fetal liver enter the thymus through its circulation and establish themselves as thymic stem cells in this organ. Here the cells undergo a rapid proliferation. The lymphoid tissue of the thymus becomes differentiated into cortex and medulla. Most lymphocytes spawned within the thymus seem never to leave the organ but die and are destroyed there by unknown mechanism(s). The proliferative process is most extensive in the cortical area, and the developing and proliferating cells seem to shift to the medullary region, from which they ultimately are discharged as T cells into the circulation and peripheral lymphoid tissue. A number of studies of lymphoid organs from fetuses (11–26 weeks' gestational age) have demonstrated the presence of up to 95% of cells forming spontaneous rosettes with sheep RBC (Wybran *et al.*, 1972, 1973; Hayward and Ezer, 1974) and 95–100% cells reacting with anti-fetal thymocyte antiserum (HTLA antigen) as shown by indirect immunofluorescence (Touraine *et al.*, 1974; Stites *et al.*, 1975). A small proportion of sheep erythrocytes (SRBC) forming cells are found in blood and splenic lymphocytes from fetuses of 12–20 weeks' gestational age.

Dwyer *et al.* (1972), employing [^{125}I]flagellin and autoradiography, have examined the appearance of antigen-binding cells in the thymuses from 22 human fetuses. The mean number of antigen-binding cells was highest in fetal thymuses (182/10^4 cells), compared to 60/10^4 cells in children's thymuses or 5/10^4 in the thymuses from young adults.

A number of investigators have studied the response of human fetal lymphocytes to phytohemagglutinin (PHA). Pegrum *et al.* (1968), employing a single dose of PHA and autoradiography, detected a fourfold increase in tritiated thymidine uptake in thymocytes from 22 fetal thymuses (16–24 weeks' gestational age). Fetal spleen cells responded less uniformly, and little or no response was obtained with bone marrow or liver cell cultures. However, Kay *et al.* (1970) could demonstrate response of fetal thymocytes to PHA as early as 14 weeks' gestation. A direct correlation was observed among the onset of thymic PHA responsiveness, the demarcation of thymus into cortex and medulla, and a rise in peripheral blood lymphocyte counts (Playfair *et al.*, 1963). Papiernik (1970) observed a progressive increase in the degree of lymphocyte transformation after stimulation with PHA until 18 weeks' gestational age. Thereafter, the responses decline to a level seen with adult thymus cells. Simultaneous morphological study suggests that thymic medulla is the probable source of PHA-responsive thymocytes. August *et al*. (1971) found that the PHA-responsive cells appeared in fetal spleen (14–16 weeks' gestation) approximately 2 weeks after the appearance of the same cell population in the thymus. Stites *et al*. (1976) in a time-dose kinetic study of the response of lymphocytes to PHA observed that PHA-responsive cells were present in thymus at 10 weeks and in the spleen and peripheral blood 3–4 weeks later. Bone marrow and fetal liver cells failed to respond to PHA. A tendency for an increase in PHA-induced DNA synthesis with increasing fetal age in all responsive organs was noted.

Pegrum *et al*. (1968) reported that fetal thymocytes, fetal liver lymphoid cells, and occasionally spleen cells are capable of responding to both normal adult and leukemic lymphocytes in a unidirectional mixed lymphocyte reaction (MLR). Carr *et al*. (1973) demonstrated the dissociation between the strong response of lymphoid cells from fetal liver to allogeneic lymphocytes and their failure to respond to PHA. MLR-responsive cells were also present in fetal spleen and thymuses. These studies suggest that MLR response is a more primitive response than is PHA reactivity. Stites *et al*. (1976) in a dose–response kinetic study found that MLR-responsive cells are present in fetal liver lymphoid cells as early as 7.5 weeks' gestational age. The real question about these very early responses is whether or not they are true immunological responses or whether they represent proliferative responses of hematopoietic cells to allogeneic stimuli that are not truely immunological in nature.

In addition to causing lymphocyte proliferation, phytohemagglutinin can induce *in vitro* nonspecific target cell destruction (Holm and Perlmann, 1967). Stites *et al*. (1972) examined PHA-induced cytotoxicity in a number of lymphoid tissues from fetuses ranging from 14 to 18 weeks' gestational age, using chicken RBC labeled with ^{51}Cr as target cell and measuring the release of ^{51}Cr as an index of lymphocyte-mediated cytotoxicity. Thymocytes failed to respond to PHA by expressing cytotoxicity. Lymphocytes from fetal bone marrow responded in an opposite manner, i.e., they produced cytotoxic cells after PHA stimulation; however, they failed to proliferate in response to PHA. Peripheral blood and splenic lymphocytes from the same fetuses responded to PHA both by proliferating and by destroying the xenogeneic target cells. Fetal liver cells failed to respond to PHA stimulation in either test.

Asantila *et al*. (1973) reported that the splenocytes from 13- to 23-week-old human fetuses were able to elicit graft-vs.-host reaction in rats (GVHR) and were more active than 18- to 23-week-old thymuses.

Touraine *et al*. (1977) studied *in vitro* expression of differentiation antigens on human T lymphocytes. T-cell precursors first expressed surface differentiation antigen (human T-lymphocyte antigen, HTLA) and then acquired the capacity to form rosettes with SRBC. The latter marker could not be induced when cells with HTLA had been eliminated. The proliferative responses to PHA, Con A, or allogeneic stimuli appeared to be characteristic of later stages in differentiation that also can be induced or amplified *in vitro* by incubation of bone marrow cells with thymopoietin or thymic extracts. When mitogen-responsive cells were eliminated by exposing them to 5-bromodeoxyuridine and light, the allogeneic response remained and even was enhanced. Understanding of the development of T-cell phenotypes and receptors *in vivo* has been provided by the study of a patient with DiGeorge's syndrome who underwent a thymus transplant in order to achieve immunological reconstitution. The same sequence of differentiation events observed *in vitro* also occurred *in vivo*. In the mouse, PHA-responsive spleen cells were first eliminated by treating with PHA and then with 5-bromodeoxyuridine and light. Such cells when injected into a lethally irradiated allogeneic recipient produced GVH. Inactivation of PHA-responsive cells did not result in decrease of the GVHR, indicating that the GVHR-inducing cells are distinct from the cells that respond to PHA. The scheme of sequential and bifurcational development of the human T cell is shown in Figure 2. Thymocytes in general lack receptors for both IgM ($T\mu$) and IgG ($T\gamma$) (Gupta and Good, 1978c). This indicates that receptors for μ and γ heavy chains develop on T cells after the appearance of receptors for SRBC. The temporal relationship among the expression of $T\mu$ and $T\gamma$ receptors, receptors for mitogens, and those responsible for allogeneic responses remains to be elucidated.

3. Development of B Lymphocytes

The most extensive studies of mammalian B-cell development have been carried out in mice. Small B cells with surface IgM are not detected by immunofluorescence in fetal liver until 16–17 days' gestation; however, large surface IgM-negative cells, positive for cytoplasmic IgM, may be found 4–5 days earlier (Raff *et al.*, 1976; Gelfand *et al.*, 1974; Nossal and Pike, 1973). Rosenberg and Parish (1977) observed a population of large lymphoid cells in 12-day fetal liver that adhere to carbonyl iron and bear small amounts of Ig, detected by formation of small rosettes with anti-Ig-coated RBC. These cells differ clearly from the small, nonadherent, surface-IgM-positive B lymphocytes which appear after the 16th day of embryonation. It seems that both these techniques detect the same precursor of B-lymphocyte lineage (pre-B cells). These pre-B cells have now been found also in rabbits and in human fetal liver. Pre-B cells lack stable surface IgM, since their development cannot be blocked by exposure to anti-μ antibodies either *in vivo* or *in vitro* (Raff *et al.*, 1976; Melchers *et al.*, 1977; Burrows *et al.*, 1977).

Gathings *et al.* (1977) investigated the ontogeny of B lymphocytes with regard to the presence of immunoglobulin. Pre-B cells are present in the human fetal liver

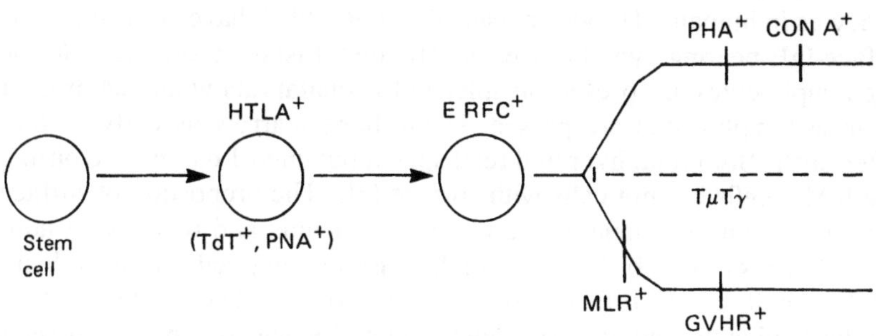

Figure 2. Scheme of differentiation of human T cells.

(7.5-week fetus), which lacks surface-IgM-bearing B lymphocytes. Based on morphological and kinetic criteria, pre-B cells can be broadly subdivided into two classes. One type is large in size ($\approx$ 17 μm), has a deeply indented or convoluted nucleus, and is rapidly dividing. The other is smaller in size ($\approx$ 8 μm). These also lack surface IgM, and only 1% are labeled by a 45-min pulse with [^{3}H]thymidine. In this way, they are similar to surface-IgM-bearing B cells. Evidence indicates that pre-B cells are progenitors of B lymphocytes: (1) large, actively proliferating pre-B cells are evidenced by kinetic studies; (2) pre-B cells are present in normal frequency in the bone marrow of boys with X-linked agammaglobulinemia in which both surface-Ig-positive B lymphocytes and plasma cells are virtually absent (Volger *et al.*, 1976); (3) in rabbits heterozygous for κ-chain allotypes (b4b5), pre-B cells express only one of the alternative alleles (Hayward *et al.*, 1977).

In the human, mouse, and rabbit, pre-B cells are found predominantly in the fetal liver and bone marrow but may be present in lower frequencies in fetal spleen, blood, and lymph nodes. Pre-B cells that are found in fetal spleen, blood, and lymph nodes are small, whereas both small and large pre-B cells are present in fetal liver and bone marrow. In fetuses older than 13 weeks, pre-B cells and surface-IgM-bearing B lymphocytes are present in approximately equal proportions in liver and bone marrow. B lymphocytes bearing only surface IgM develop earlier than do cells bearing other Ig classes (Vossen and Hijman, 1975; Gupta *et al.*, 1976c; Gathings *et al.*, 1976), and expression of surface IgD, surface IgG, and surface IgA occurs exclusively on immature B cells which also bear surface IgM. The ratio of lymphocytes bearing only IgM to those bearing both surface IgM and surface IgD probably serves as a good index of maturity of a given B-cell population.

The major fraction of B lymphocytes in fetuses older than 12 weeks' gestation bear both surface IgM and surface IgD; the great majority of lymphocytes with surface IgG or surface IgA also bear surface IgM. During fetal life (1) the proportion of B cells with surface IgM only, as opposed to those bearing both surface IgM and surface IgD, is much higher in fetal liver and bone marrow than in spleen, blood, and lymph nodes, and (2) surface IgG, surface IgA, and surface IgD appear independently on lymphocytes bearing IgM. Studies of the presence of the four surface Ig isotypes indicate that B cells from neonatal humans may simultaneously bear three or more surface Ig isotypes, whereas surface IgG+ and surface IgA+ B lymphocytes in adult peripheral blood usually express only the single isotype.

No studies are available regarding the ontogeny of surface-IgE-bearing B lymphocytes in humans. However, Ishizaka *et al.* (1978) have studied the ontogeny of surface-IgE-bearing lymphocytes in Hooded Listar strain rats. Surface-IgE-bearing lymphocytes are present in spleen of neonatal rats within 24 hr after birth. IgE-bearing lymphocytes are present in the bone marrow as early as the fourth day after birth. Both fetal liver and fetal spleen obtained 1 day before birth contain surface IgM+ cells but not cells with surface IgE. The proportion of surface IgE+ cells in the spleen and bone marrow rapidly expands and reaches an adult level within 3–4 weeks after birth. Most of the IgE-bearing cells from both newborn and adult animals carry surface IgM. Capping experiments have demonstrated that ϵ-chain determinants and μ-chain determinants belong to separate molecules. In newborn spleen the percentage of cells which have both surface IgE and IgM is higher than that of cells with surface IgG_{2a} at their surface. The following evidence indicates that cells with surface IgE+ are derived from cells that are IgM+: (1) IgM-bearing cells appear before the appearance of IgE-bearing lymphocytes, and (2) the treatment of newborn mice and rats with anti-IgM antibody suppresses the production of IgE (Manning *et al.*, 1976). However, Dwyer *et al.* (1976) reported that the anti-IgM treatment of newborn mice suppressed both IgM and IgG antibody responses to ovalbumin but failed to affect the IgE antibody response. It is possible that the suppression by anti-IgM is less effective on cells that have both IgE and IgM at their surface or that further differentiation of IgE+ and IgM+ double cells to IgE-bearing cells may continue in the mouse even after anti-IgM treatment.

The findings in rat, mouse, and now in human are in agreement with the view that precursors for each immunoglobulin class are B cells derived directly from separate cell lines that bear IgM. No longer do we need consider an obligatory IgM → IgG → IgA sequence, with successive switches in their development (Figure 3).

The Fc receptors and complement receptors on lymphocytes have also been studied in fetal liver and bone marrow (Gupta *et al.*, 1976c). Fc receptor-positive cells having lymphocyte morphology are found in frequencies comparable to those of B lymphocytes that have surface Ig; however, large pre-B cells (cIgM+ SIgM−) do not bear Fc receptors. Complement-receptor-bearing cells having lymphoid morphology are present in fetal liver in lower proportions than those with surface Ig and Fc receptor, and are absent during early gestational periods when the other two receptors are already present. No critical analysis of the temporal relationship of appearance of C3 receptors and surface immunoglobulins other than IgM have been published. A scheme of ontogeny of B-cell receptors is outlined in Figure 4.

Trinchieri *et al.* (1975) examined antibody-dependent cellular cytotoxicity

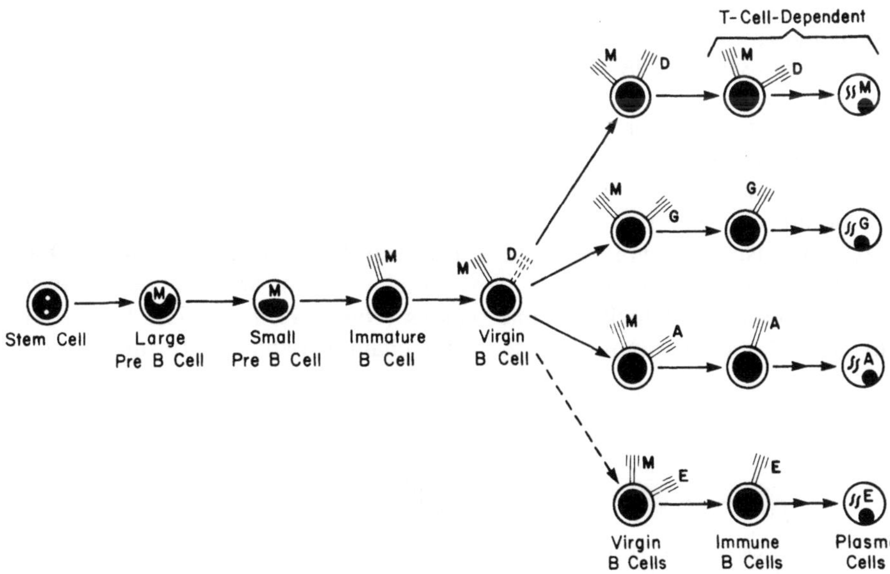

Figure 3. Ontogenic development and differentiation of B lymphocytes.

(ADCC) in cells from human fetuses 9–14 weeks old. ADCC could not be detected in liver, spleen, thymus, or bone marrow. Therefore, it can be concluded that functionally active ADCC effector cells appear late during ontogenetic development.

4. Lymphocyte Markers

During the process of differentiation and maturation, lymphoid cell subpopulations display a variety of markers. These distinct subpopulations are identified by the presence of surface markers, enzymatic markers, and metabolic markers (Table 1). Lymphocyte markers have recently been reviewed (Gupta, 1976, 1977; Siegal and Good, 1977; Gupta and Kapoor, 1979).

4.1. Surface Immunoglobulin

Readily demonstrable surface immunoglobulin, which is produced by the cell that is carrying the Ig on its surface, is a characteristic of B lymphocytes (a precursor of the plasma cell). Surface immunoglobulin can be shown to move over the cell surface while still attached to the membrane (Brown and Greaves, 1974). Approximately 10^5 antigen receptor molecules are present on a single B lymphocyte (Rabellino *et al.*, 1971). The surface immunoglobulin molecules are strictly oriented, with the combining sites oriented outward (Froland and Natvig, 1972a) and with the CH3 homology region closest to the membrane. Surface immunoglobulins may be detected by using fluorochrome-conjugated antiimmunoglobulin antisera directed against heavy- (μ, δ, α, γ, and ϵ) or light- (κ and λ) chain determinants. Approximately 10–14% of human lymphocytes in the peripheral blood express surface immunoglobulin, as identified by staining with a fluorescein isothiocyanate-conjugated $F(ab')_2$ antiimmunoglobulin antisera. Surface-IgM-bearing lymphocytes compose most of the circulating B lymphocytes, and only a minor population of B cells possess surface IgG, IgA, or IgE. Among IgG subclasses, IgG_2 appears to be the dominant IgG subclass on the surface of B lymphocytes (Froland and Natvig, 1972a). A restriction of Ig classes, IgG subclasses, and Gm antigens has been demonstrated on lymphocyte membrane (Froland and Natvig, 1972a, 1973). One exception to this restriction is that IgM and IgD can be demonstrated on the same cells by a double-staining technique (Fu *et al.*, 1974; Knapp *et al.*, 1973; Salsano *et al.*, 1974; Natvig *et al.*, 1975). Therefore, one cell may express two separate genes for the constant part of membrane-bound immunoglobulin heavy chains. However, by using idiotypic antisera it has been demonstrated that the IgD and IgM on the same cell have identical hypervariable regions and thus appear to use the same gene to code their variable regions (Natvig *et al.*, 1975). Forre *et al.* (1976) studied the distribution of Ig heavy-chain variable (VH) subgroups on

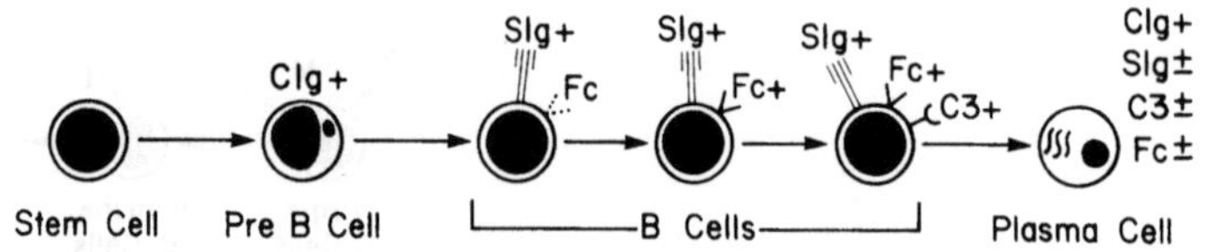

Figure 4. Sequential differentiation of B-cell receptors.

peripheral blood lymphocytes using antisera specific for the VH subgroup. Lymphocytes from healthy controls were stained with fluorescein isothiocyanate-conjugated $F(ab')_2$, anti-VHI, anti-VHII, and anti-VHIII subgroup antisera. The percentages of cells stained with antisera against VHI, VHII, and VHIII subgroups were 2.9%, 5.0%, and 5.5%, respectively. T lymphocytes and thymocytes did not stain with these antisera, suggesting that no VH antigens are present on these cells; however, the limitations of the sensitivity of immunofluorescence assay does not permit one to rule out absolutely the presence of a small amount of one or more of these heavy-chain antigens.

IgD-like molecules have been reported to be present on the surface of lymphocytes from man, mouse, rats, rabbits, monkeys, chicken, and tortoises. The surface IgD is quite susceptible to proteolysis. IgD may function as a supplementary antibody receptor, having a unique influence on the direction of differentiation to be taken by a B cell subsequent to stimulation by an immunogen.

The precise biological role of IgD still remains to be defined. It seems likely that IgD plays some role in "fine tuning" or modulation of the B-cell response, rather than having a more direct on-and-off signalling function. Bourgois *et al.* (1977) have suggested that IgD may play a regulatory role through the elicitation

TABLE 1. Markers of Lymphoid Cell Subpopulations

B-cell lineage	
Stem cell	?Alloantigen
Pre-B cells	Intracytoplasmic IgM
	?MRBC receptors
	?Terminal deoxynucleotidyltransferase (TdT)
B cells	Surface immunoglobulin
	MRBC receptors
	Epstein–Barr virus receptor
	IgG Fc receptors
	Complement component receptors
	IgM Fc receptors
	B-cell alloantigens ("Ia-like")
T-cell lineage	
Stem cell	?Alloantigen
Pre-T cells	Terminal deoxynucleotidyltransferase (TdT)
	HTLA
	Peanut agglutinin
T cells	HTLA
	SRBC receptors
	Acid α-naphthylacetic esterase
	IgG Fc receptors ($T\gamma$)
	IgM Fc receptors ($T\mu$)
	T_{H1}, T_{H2} antigen
	Histamine receptors
Third-population "unclassified" lymphoid cells	
	IgG Fc receptors
	Complement component receptors
	Receptors for EBV
	"Ia-like" antigen

of an antiidiotypic response. According to their suggestion, IgD, in whole or in part, is lost from the surface of B cells as a result of immunogenic presentation and an extreme sensitivity to proteolysis. The released IgD then is presumed to stimulate a specific regulatory antiidiotype antibody response which then functions by recognition of cell-surface Ig still remaining on the cell. IgM and IgD receptors display allelic exclusion on any individual cell; they come from the same chromosome (haplotype exclusion) and share the same variable region. These results suggest that there are separate V gene copies for each heavy chain and that individual lymphocytes become committed to one or the other heavy-chain complex early in their development. Immature B cells possess IgM receptors only. Mature B lymphocytes possess both IgM and IgD in varying proportions. After activation by antigen or mitogen, IgD is lost. Immature B cells are very susceptible to tolerance induction. The susceptibility of mature B cells to tolerance induction is increased by anti-δ antiserum, suggesting that IgD plays a role in preventing tolerance induction.

4.2. Receptors for IgG Fc

Receptors for IgG Fc are present on all B lymphocytes, third-population cells, and a minority of human T cells. Fc receptors on T cells are discussed in separate section in this chapter (see Section 14). Recent studies of murine and human lymphocytes have demonstrated that different subpopulations of cells have Fc receptors having different binding avidities for soluble antigen–antibody complexes. Arbeit *et al.* (1977) have shown that the Fc receptors of human B lymphocytes and the third-population cells can be clearly distinguished.

1. The Fc receptors of B lymphocytes have an appreciably lower avidity for complexed IgG than do the Fc receptors of third-population cells. The concentration of soluble immune complexes required to detect binding to the Fc receptors of third-population cells is 100 times less than that required for B-cell Fc receptors. This is the reason why third-population cells but not B cells will bind to Ripley EA (human O Rh^+ cells and anti-D RBC antibody complexes) (Froland *et al.*, 1974), whereas both subpopulations bind to OXRBC-IgG antibody complexes (Hallberg *et al.*, 1973) and homologous aggregated IgG (Dickler and Kunkel, 1972). This difference in the avidity of Fc receptors for immune complexes may reflect either the presence on these cells of different Fc receptors with different affinity or the presence of the same receptors with differences in density, distribution, or mobility of the receptors on the surface membrane.

2. Another distinguishing characteristic is the close association of Fc receptors on B cells with human "Ia-like" antigens. The $F(ab')_2$ fragments of antibodies against these alloantigens inhibit the binding of aggregated IgG to B cells but not to third-population cells. This may be due to lack of "Ia-like" antigens on third-population cells. Nelson *et al.* (1977) failed to detect B-cell alloantigens on third-population cells. Humphrey *et al.* (1976), using a different system, found a small proportion of third-population cells (10–20%) reacting with their antisera. These differences in Fc receptors on B and third-population cells may have functional relevance. Third-population cells are active in antibody-dependent cytotoxicity, whereas B cells do not mediate such cytotoxicity (Wisloff and Froland, 1973). B-cell Fc receptors, via their association with "Ia-like" antigens, may play a significant role in the regulation of immune responses.

An intact Fc portion of IgG seems to be essential for the induction of antibody-dependent cell-mediated cytotoxicity (Larsson and Perlmann, 1972). Inhibition studies of ADCC performed by Wisloff *et al.* (1974b) also confirmed that the reactive site is located on the Fc part of the molecule, since the Fc fragments prepared from pooled human immunoglobulin as well as from single IgG_1 and IgG_3 myeloma proteins effectively inhibited cytotoxicity while no or only weak inhibition was observed with the $F(ab')_2$ and Fab fragments. The Fc portion of IgG_2 inhibited ADCC poorly, and IgG_4 showed almost no inhibition. To be more precise as to which Fc portion of Ig is involved in the interaction with the effector cells, Wisloff *et al.* (1974a) used a PFc′ fragment, which roughly corresponds to the CH3 homology region. Since very little inhibition was found with this fragment, the authors concluded that the immunoglobulin structures reacting with the lymphocyte Fc receptor are situated in the CH2 region. Fc fragments from IgG_3 subclass protein, which contains an extension of the *N*-terminal part of the Fc piece, had significantly higher inhibitory capacity than the Fc fragment when the comparison was made on a molar basis. Since the extended *N*-terminal part of the Fc fragment is also included in the $F(ab')_2$ fragment, which does not inhibit ADCC, the importance of this part of the molecule is probably to stabilize the CH2 region for the expression of its biological activity. Therefore, it can be inferred that the site involved in binding to an effector cell is located within the CH2 region. However, it is possible that the importance of the CH2 region is to maintain the structural integrity of the entire Fc region.

Lymphocyte Fc receptors may also have biological functions such as the concentration and transport of antigen–antibody complexes (Brown *et al.*, 1970), and they may facilitate interaction between the receptor-bearing lymphocytes and lymphocytes with surface immunoglobulin (Schmidtke and Unanue, 1971). The biological significance of Fc receptors has been reviewed (Kerbel and Davies, 1974).

4.3. Complement Receptors

A relationship between cells of the immune system and components of the complement system has also been recognized in recent years. B lymphocytes express membrane receptors for C3b, C3d, C4b, C1q, and possibly factor B of alternative pathways of complement activation (Bianco *et al.*, 1970; Ross *et al.*, 1973; Bokish and Sobel, 1974; Sobel and Bokish, 1975; Halbwach *et al.*, 1975). Although many other tissue cells, notably macrophages, polymorphs, eosinophils, and platelets, have receptors for complement components, these receptors may not be identical to the C3b receptor on lymphocytes (Ross *et al.*, 1973; Gupta *et al.*, 1976b). C3 receptors are present on most but not all B lymphocytes. A small proportion of third-population cells (Gupta, unpublished observation), peripheral blood T cells (Chiao *et al.*, 1974), and fetal thymocytes also carry C3 receptors (Jondal *et al.*, 1973; Stein and Miller-Hormelink, 1977). Halbwach *et al.* (1975) detected an activity resembling factor B of the alternative pathway of complement activation by a functional assay involving incubation of lymphocytes with cobra venom factor and factor D. They concluded that lymphocytes either secrete or have on their surface "factor-B-like" activity. It has not yet been possible, however, to detect factor B serologically on the lymphocyte surface. The factor B is lacking from thymocytes and human erythrocytes. Although factor B in serum could be regarded as a fluid phase receptor for C3b, it seems unlikely that C3b receptor on lymphocytes is factor B. C3b receptors on lymphocytes are not blocked either by cobra venom factor in the fluid phase or by an antiserum to factor B. Erythrocytes do have C3b but lack factor-B-like activity. Therefore, it can be concluded that factor B is not the same molecule as the C3b receptor. It will be of considerable significance to elucidate the role of factor B in lymphocyte functions and cell interactions.

Sobel and Bokish (1975) reported that the C4b receptor is present on virtually all of the same cell types which have C3b receptors, with the exception of certain human lymphoblastoid cell lines that have receptors for C3b but lack those for C4b (Bokish and Sobel, 1974; Ross and Polley, 1974). The biological function of the C4b receptors appears to be similar to that of the C3b receptors. In contrast, the C1q receptors are present on both T and B lymphocytes. Approximately 3×10^5 molecules of C1q bind to each lymphocyte. C1q binding to the receptor on lymphocytes is markedly favored in medium of low ionic strength, whereas variations in the pH of the medium between 6.0 and 7.5 have no significant effect on C1q binding. The C1q receptor is trypsin sensitive but resistant to treatment with neuraminidase or DNase. The finding that C1q binds to T lymphocytes and Raji cells which lack membrane-bound Ig and to Daudi cells devoid of detectable amounts of β_2-microglobulin suggested that the C1q receptor is also distinct from these membrane markers. The biological significance of the C1q receptor is presently unknown. It is possible that the receptor mediates binding of immune complexes. It is proposed that the receptor binds an activated C1, which leads to activation of complement sequence and results in a change of cell activity.

Approximately 6000 C3 molecules are required for maximal binding to a lymphocyte. This receptor is trypsin sensitive. C3b and C3d receptors are serologically distinct and cap independently on the lymphocyte surface. Antibody production may be modulated by membrane disturbance due to the recognition of the antigen and also of C3 (Nussenzweig, 1974). Complement may participate in the initial events that take place on the lymphocyte surface during antigenic stimulation and that lead to antibody production. In addition, complement receptors may contribute to the follicular localization of antigen (Brown *et al.*, 1970) to certain areas in lymphoid organs, presumably for the induction of the immune response (Mitchell and Abbott, 1965; Nossal *et al.*, 1968).

C8 has been shown to be associated with lymphocytes and can be utilized by the cells in complement-mediated destruction of target cells carrying the C567 complex (McConnell and Lachmann, 1976), which can be inhibited by $F(ab')_2$ anti-C8 antiserum.

Apart from a putative C2 inhibitor (Bernard *et al.*, 1976), no other complement inhibitors have yet been demonstrated on the surface of lymphocytes.

4.4. Receptors for Mouse Erythrocytes

Mouse erythrocytes (MRBC) form spontaneous rosettes with a subpopulation of human B lymphocytes (Stathopoulos and Elliott, 1974; Gupta and Grieco, 1975; Gupta *et al.*, 1975b, 1976a, 1977). Approximately 7–8% of peripheral blood lymphocytes bind to MRBC. Double-labeling experiments have demonstrated that MRBC bind to most of the B cells with surface IgM (Gupta *et al.*, 1976a). The blocking experiments and study of primary and secondary immunodeficiency (Gupta *et al.*, 1976a, 1978a; Gupta and Good, 1976, 1977c; Koziner *et al.*, 1977) have clearly demonstrated that MRBC bind to the surface of B lymphocytes through a receptor that is independent of surface Ig and through receptors for IgG Fc and C3. Neuraminidase treatment of lymphocytes permits the binding of MRBC with B cells as well as with a subpopulation of third-population cells. The study of ontogeny of lymphocyte receptors in human fetal liver has demonstrated that the receptors for binding of MRBC appear as early as surface IgM (Gupta *et al.*, 1976c) and possibly at the pre-B-cell stage. The binding of MRBC can be partially blocked by anti-Ia antiserum (Gupta, unpublished data), suggesting either that the receptor for MRBC shares "Ia antigen" for its binding to B cells or that the two receptors are located very closely together. The binding of MRBC appears to correlate inversely with the sialic acid content of B-cell membrane. MRBC do not bind to monocytes, eosinophils, granulocytes, T lymphocytes, or thymocytes (Gupta *et al.*, 1976a). The nature of membrane receptors for MRBC remains to be elucidated.

4.5. Epstein–Barr Virus (EBV) Receptor

Epstein–Barr virus has an interesting relationship with human lymphocytes. The virus is clearly lymphotropic in man and in New World monkeys. Jondal and Klein (1973) demonstrated that EBV binds to the surface of some B blasts of long-term cultured lymphoid cell lines, but apparently no T cells were able to bind EBV. Greaves *et al.* (1975) demonstrated that virtually every B lymphocyte binds EBV, but there is no detectable binding to T cells. Recently, it has been shown that a proportion of third-population cells also carry receptors for EBV (E. Klein, personal communication). EBV does not bind to thymocytes or activated T cells. The closely linked disappearance and reappearance of EBV receptors and complement receptors in the P3HR-1 clone (originally isolated from the Burkitt lymphoma lines) strongly suggests that these two receptors are either identical or closely linked constituents of the cell membrane (Klein *et al.*, 1978). This apparent restriction of EBV-binding sites to B lymphocytes (and perhaps some epithelial cells as evidenced by the presence of the EBV genome in nasopharyngeal carcinoma) provides an adequate explanation of the B-cell origin of most long-term lymphoid cell lines (Greaves *et al.*, 1975; Jondal *et al.*, 1973; Thomas and Phillips, 1973). It implies that B lymphocytes are a target *in vivo* for transformation by EBV.

4.6. Receptors for Spontaneous Rosette Formation with *Macaca* Monkey RBC

Pelligrino *et al.* (1975) reported spontaneous rosette formation of *Macaca speciosa* monkey red blood cells with human B lymphocytes. *Macaca* monkey RBC rosette-forming cells were positive for surface immunoglobulin and C3d receptors. In contrast, no SRBC rosette-forming T cells bind to monkey RBC. Several lymphoblastoid cell lines with B-cell characteristics but not cell lines with T-cell characteristics formed spontaneous rosette formation with monkey RBC. Inhibition experiments showed that the structure on the lymphoid cell surfaces mediating the adherence of monkey RBC was independent of surface immunoglobulin as well as of the receptors for IgG Fc, C3b, and C3d. Approximately 25% of peripheral lymphocytes bind to monkey RBC, and, since only 10–14% of peripheral lymphocytes are B cells [as determined by $F(ab')_2$ antiimmunoglobulin antisera], it is apparent that monkey RBC also bind to a population other than B cells, possibly to the so-called third-population cells.

4.7. Human "Ia-like" Alloantigens

In addition to serologically defined HLA antigens (HLA-A,B,C), the HLA gene complex includes determinants which regulate the ability to stimulate mixed leukocyte cultures (MLC). The latter capacity, however, seems to be restricted to the B cells, third-population cells, and macrophages. This system has been designated "LD" (lymphocyte defined). In man, during studies on certain alloantisera that selectively inhibited MLC it was observed that antibodies were present with a striking specificity for alloantigens present on B but not on T lymphocytes; these were demonstrable by serological methods (Wernet *et al.*, 1975). These antigens are distinct from HLA determinants and are designated as B alloantigens or "Ia-like" antigens. At least two loci appear to be responsible for the synthesis of these polymorphic allotypic antigens. These antigens are detected by immunofluorescence staining, cytotoxicity, and radioimmunoassay serotyping. There appears to be complete divergence of Fc receptors and Ia determinants on cell line Daudi, which expresses both systems strongly, and cell line B 35M, which has Ia-like antigens but no detectable Fc receptors. Several analogies between the murine Ia system and human B-cell alloantigens have become apparent. If human "Ia-like" alloantigens are related to *Ir* gene products, the inhibition of immune responses *in vitro* by such antisera might be postulated. In an exclusive series of antigen-stimulation experiments to examine the effect of anti-"Ia-like" antibodies, Wernet (1976) reported that B-cell alloantibodies could inhibit secondary immune responses of human peripheral blood lymphocytes when the alloantibodies are reacted with the B cells prior to antigen exposure.

By adsorption studies and direct cytotoxic tests, as well as by indirect immunofluorescence, it became clear that human "Ia-like" antigens are not restricted to B lymphocytes. Recently, it has been shown that the "Ia-like" antigens are present on a subset of T cells which also have IgG Fc receptors (Samarut *et al.*, 1977). Some evidence suggests that other T-cell subpopulations [T cells with IgM receptors ($T\mu$) and T cells lacking both IgM and IgG receptors ($T\emptyset$)] might also have "Ia-like" antigens on their surface (Gupta, unpublished observations). The tissue distribution of human "Ia-like" alloantigens is shown in Table 2. Winchester *et al.* (1977, 1978) observed that by pretreating the bone marrow *in vitro* with anti-Ia-like antibodies and complement they could inhibit both myeloid and erythroid colony formation. These findings suggest that "Ia-like" determinants are expressed on progenitor cells of erythroid and granulocyte lineage.

4.8. Human Thymic Lymphocyte Antigens (HTLA)

Using heterologous anti-T-cell antiserum, a number of investigators have delineated the presence of human specific T-lymphocyte antigen (HTLA) (Yata *et al.*, 1973; Touraine *et al.*, 1974; Woody *et al.*, 1975; Ablin and Morris, 1973). This antiserum detects approximately 65% peripheral blood T cells and 97% thymocytes. There is a small population of T cells which bear HTLA but lack receptors for SRBC (Yata *et al.*, 1973). Woody *et al.* (1975) examined the effects of anti-HTLA antisera and complement on functions of lymphocytes. Treatment with anti-HTLA antiserum and complement exhibited marked inhibition of responsiveness to Con A but little decrease in PHA or PWM stimulations. MLC reaction was inhibited when responder cells were treated with the antiserum and complement. Cell-mediated lymphocytotoxicity and blastogenesis to antigens were also markedly inhibited, but only little effect on the release on MIF and lymphotoxin production was observed. These data suggest that subpopulations of T cells carry HTLA. The nature of HTLA has been partially characterized. Owen and Fanger (1976) characterized the antigen ($T\alpha_2$) as a protein of 86,000 daltons distinct from the antigen that binds SRBC. Anderson and Metzgar (1978) isolated an HTLA antigen of 150,000 daltons.

4.9. Receptor for Sheep Erythrocytes

Numerous studies have demonstrated that the binding of sheep erythrocytes to human lymphocytes is characteristic of T cells lacking surface immunoglobulins. The formation of rosettes between lymphocytes and sheep erythrocytes (E) is very susceptible to technical variations which influence both the proportion of rosette-forming lymphocytes and the strength of erythrocyte binding to lymphocytes. Depending on experimental conditions, the values of rosette-forming lymphocytes vary from 27% to 80%. Sheep erythrocytes form rosettes only with viable lymphocytes. Rosette formation can be inhibited by antilymphocyte serum, azathioprine, sodium cyanide, antimycin, iodoacetamide, trypsin, phospholipase A, ficin, and phytohemagglutinin (PHA). The inhibition by trypsin, phospholipase A, and ficin is reversible but can be blocked by sodium iodoacetate and not by cyclohexamide (reviewed in Gupta, 1977a). Neuraminidase has been reported to inhibit, to increase, or to produce no effect on rosette formation.

The biochemical nature of the receptor for sheep erythrocytes is not very well

TABLE 2. Distribution of "Ia-like" Alloantigens in man

Tissue	"Ia-like" antigens
B lymphocytes	+
T lymphocytes[a]	+
Third-population cells[a]	+
Macrophages	+
Epidermal cells (Langerhans' cells)	+
Endothelial cells (umbilical cord vein)	+
Spermatozoa	+
Fetal liver cells (14th week)	+
Progenitor cells (granulocytic and erythroid lineage)	+
Platelets	−
Fibroblasts	−
Erythrocytes	−
Liver	−
Brain	−

[a] Subpopulation.

understood. Inhibition of rosette formation by trypsin suggests that the receptor is trypsin sensitive and probably glycoprotein in nature. Owen and Fanger (1974, 1976), using an anti-human thymus antibody, reported the isolation of two antigens (Ts and Tα_2) from normal peripheral blood T lymphocytes. The Ts antigen appears to be the receptor for sheep erythrocytes as judged by its ability to block antithymocyte globulin-induced inhibition of spontaneous rosette formation with SRBC. This blocking activity was associated with two antigenically similar glycoproteins of molecular weights 65,000 (Ts_1) and 30,000 (Ts_2). Tα_2 is a protein with a molecular weight of 86,000.

4.10. Receptors for Rhesus Monkey Erythrocytes

Lohrmann and Novikovs (1974) reported spontaneous rosette formation of a large population of peripheral blood lymphocytes and thymocytes with rhesus monkey erythrocytes. From normal adults, a linear correlation existed between the percentages of rossette-forming cells with rhesus monkey RBC and with sheep erythrocytes. Less that 2% rhesus monkey erythrocyte rosette-forming cells were surface immunoglobulin positive. Therefore, these investigators concluded that rhesus monkey erythrocytes bind to human T cells. Rosette formation with monkey erythrocytes was more sensitive to trypsin treatment than SRBC rosette formation. ATG abolished SRBC rosette formation at high titers; however, no effect was observed on rosette formation with monkey RBC. Rosette inhibition with monkey RBC was more sensitive than with SRBC to EDTA. Sodium azide completely inhibited SRBC rosette formation but had only minimal effect on rosette formation with monkey RBC. These data suggest that rhesus monkey RBC bind to the same T cells to which SRBC bind; however, there appear to be two distinct receptors on T cells.

4.11. Receptors for *Helix promatia* Hemagglutinin

Helix promatia A hemagglutinin (HP) is a multivalent invertebrate agglutinin which has been obtained in a highly purified state. It has a molecular weight of 79,000 and consists of six identical or closely similar polypeptide chains of an approximate molecular weight of 13,000, each containing one carbohydrate binding site and one intrachain disulfide bridge. HP agglutinated human A RBC but not B or O RBC.

Hammerstrom *et al.* (1973) demonstrated that 70% of peripheral blood lymphocytes have receptors for HP. These receptors are present on most T cells and are easily detected by immunofluorescence when neuraminidase-treated lymphocytes are incubated with fluorochrome-labeled HP. Although the majority of the circulating B cells lack receptors for HP, studies have now clearly demonstrated that they are present in 15% of B cells from adult peripheral blood (Hellstrom *et al.*, 1976). These lymphocytes have on their surface IgM and/or IgD. This implies that approximately 1% of all peripheral blood HP-positive lymphocytes are B cells. In cord blood the total proportion of HP positive was not significantly different from that found in adult peripheral blood, but the percentage of B cells was higher and more than 80% of them had HP receptors. This means that approximately 20% of all HP-positive lymphocytes in cord blood are B cells. Recently, it has also been shown that B cells from patients with CLL also have receptors for HP (Hellstrom *et al.*, 1976). These two observations suggest that the receptor for HP on B cells is present on cells which are relatively immature. The relationship between HP and other receptors on the surface of B cells is not known at present. It is possible that, like receptors for MRBC, HP receptors could represent a differentiation marker. The binding property of the HP receptor on B cells appears to be different from that on the majority of T cells. This difference is well brought out by fractionation on HP-Sepharose. HP receptor on B cells binds more weakly with HP than do the bulk of the HP-positive T lymphocytes. This indicates either that B cells have, operationally, a lower concentration of HP receptors than the majority of the T cells or that their HP-binding structures differ from those on HP-positive T cells.

4.12. Receptors for Spontaneous Autorosette Formation

Baxley *et al.* (1973) demonstrated that human thymocytes, tonsils, and peripheral blood T cells bind spontaneously to autologous RBC. However, there was a difference in their binding to T cells in different compartments. Thymocytes bind to both untreated and neuraminidase-treated RBC, whereas T cells from tonsils and peripheral blood bind only to neuraminidase-treated human RBC. Rosette formation was inhibited by pretreatment of lymphocytes with sodium azide or proteolytic enzymes, 50°C for 7 min, or anti-T-cell (but not anti-B-cell) serum. A number of other investigators have since confirmed the observation of Baxley *et al.* (1973) that a subpopulation of human periperal blood T cells bind spontaneously to autologous erythrocytes (Sandilands *et al.*, 1974; Dewar *et al.*, 1974; Gluckman and Montambault, 1975). The functional properties of this subpopulation of T cells remains to be determined.

4.13. α-Naphthyl-acetate Esterase

The histochemical demonstration of nonspecific α-naphthyl-acetate esterase (ANAE) activity in monocytes is useful for the identification of these cells in mixed mononuclear cell suspensions. Recently, ANAE activity has been demonstrated to be present also in human peripheral blood T cells and certain mitogen-stimulated T lymphocytes (Ranki *et al.*, 1976; Totterman *et al.*, 1977). Knowles *et al.* (1978) examined ANAE activity in the peripheral blood and tissue lymphocytes using a modified method. They found that the percentages of SRBC rosette-forming T cells and ANAE-positive lymphocytes were nearly comparable in the peripheral blood. A distinctive staining pattern characterized the T lymphocytes, and this distribution could readily be distinguished from monocyte staining. Discrepancies have been observed in certain tissues such as spleen and thymus. Fewer thymocytes demonstrated ANAE activity (Knowles *et al.*, 1978; Kulenkampff *et al.*, 1976) when compared with SRBC rosette-forming cells. In spleen, ANAE activity was demonstrated in non-T cells. Grossi *et al.* (1978) reported ANAE activity to be present in $T\mu$ cells but lacking in $T\gamma$ cells. The histochemical demonstration of ANAE is simple and reproducible, and preparations may be counterstained to provide simultaneous cytomorphological detail. Such stained cells can be mounted as a permanent record.

4.14. Distribution of Lymphocyte Subpopulations in Peripheral Blood, Tissues, and Extravascular Fluids

Peripheral blood, spleen thymus, bone marrow, lymph nodes, tonsils, appendix, and a number of extravascular fluids have been examined for the proportions of lymphocytes subpopulations. These are summarized in Table 3, and only a few of them will be discussed in detail. Peripheral blood and lymph nodes appear to have similar distributions of T and B lymphocytes. Both tonsils and spleen are rich in B lymphocytes. Approximately 50% of lymphocytes are T cells and the other 50% are B cells. In tonsils, surface-IgA-bearing B cells are present in much higher proportions than in other compartments, except in human appendix (Mizumoto, 1976). Cerebrospinal fluid and aqueous humor from the eye contain predominantly T lymphocytes (Manconi *et al.*, 1976, 1978).

A number of recent publications have dealt with the cellular contents of human colostrum and milk. Ogra and Ogra (1978) and Diaz-Jouanen and Williams (1974) reported 40–50% T cells in human colostrum and milk, and Parmely *et al.* (1976) reported approximately 34% B lymphocytes. However, Manconi *et al.* (1978) reported that 80–100% of the lymphoid cells in colostrum are T cells and that no B lymphocytes are present in these secretions. The reason for these discrepancies remains to be elucidated. Interestingly, the last authors found as many Fc receptor-positive cells as T cells, suggesting that the majority of the T cells in human colostrum are T cells with IgGFc (Tγ) receptors. Parmely *et al.* (1976) studied *in vitro* functions of lymphocytes from human milk. Milk lymphocytes were found to be hyporesponsive to nonspecific mitogens and to respond less to histocompatibility antigens on allogeneic cells than do T lymphocytes of the blood. In most cases, the colostrum T lymphocytes did not respond to *Candida albicans* even though blood lymphocytes from the same patients responded vigorously to other antigens. By contrast, the Kl capsular antigen of *Escherichia coli* induced significant proliferation in lymphocytes from milk but failed to stimulate blood lymphocytes. This dichotomy of reactivity may reflect the accumulation of particular lymphocyte clones in the breast and is consonant with the

TABLE 3. Lymphocyte Subpopulations in Blood, Tissues, and Extravascular Fluids

	E(T) (%)	EA(Fc) (%)	EAC(C3) (%)	SIg (%)
Tonsils	58.7	37.8	43.5	42.4
Blood	84.7	20.3	9.7	12.5
Thymus	>99.0	1.0	1.0	<0.5
Lymph nodes	75.6	20.0	8.0	18.0
Spleen	40.0	30.0	44.0	24.0
Bone marrow	10.0	25.0	20.8	10.0
Appendix	38.2	ND	30.8	60.0
Colostrum	50.2	—	—	34.6
Aqueous humor (cataract)	88.3	—	—	—
Cerebrospinal fluid	93.0	—	2.0	—

concept that immunity of mammary tissue at the T lymphocyte level is a local immunity perhaps originating in the gut-associated lymphoid tissue (GALT) or bronchial-associated lymphoid tissue (BALT) and part of a mucosal-associated lymphoid tissue (MALT).

5. Functional Properties of Human T, B, and Third-Population Cells

The advances in technology of separating and purifying distinct lymphocyte subpopulations have contributed to our understanding regarding interactions of various lymphocyte subpopulations in immunological phenomena. By using these techniques, T, B, and third populations have been extensively studied for their functional characteristics. A list of these functions is summarized in Table 4.

6. Proliferative Responses to Mitogens, Antigens, and Allogeneic Cells

It is evident that PHA, Con A, and PWM are capable of inducing proliferation in T, B, and third-population cells (Chess *et al.*, 1974c). PWM does not stimulate purified B cells in complete absence of T cells. Chess *et al.* (1974a) have reported that purified B cells do respond to PHA and Con A. Receptors for Con A and PHA have been demonstrated on both T and B lymphocytes (Henkart and Fisher, 1975). Con A was found to bind to about twice as much labeled protein as PHA

TABLE 4. Functions of Human Lymphocyte Subpopulations

Properties	T cells	B cells	"Third-population" cells
Proliferative responses[a]			
Antigen	+	−	−
Allogeneic cells (R)	+	−	−
Allogeneic cells (S)	±	+	+
Cytotoxic responses			
Cell-mediated lympholysis	+	−	?
Antibody-dependent cytotoxicity	+ [b]	−	+
Natural killer activity	+ [b]	−	+
Mitogen-induced cytotoxicity	+	+	+
Lymphokine production			
Leukocyte migration inhibition factor	+	+	+
Macrophage migration inhibition factor	+	+	+
Blastogenic factor	+	+	+
Lymphotoxin (α)	+	+	+
Interferon	+	+	?
Receptors for Epstein–Barr virus	−	+	+
Antibody production	−	+	+
Miscellaneous			
Precursors of B cells	−	−	+
Precursors of T cells	−	−	+
Precursors of granulocytes	−	−	+
Precursors of erythrocytes	−	−	+

[a] R, Responder; S, stimulator.
[b] Subpopulation.

on whole peripheral blood lymphocytes. Although the degree of proliferative response is higher in T cells, the B cells also respond quite well. The proliferative response of third-population cells is comparable to that of B lymphocytes (MacDermott *et al.*, 1975).

Recently, Sakane and Green (1978) studied the proliferative response of lymphoid cell subpopulations when stimulated with protein A from *Staphylococcus aureus*. Both T and B but not third-population cells responded to protein A. Responses in the two populations were comparable. Interestingly, the response of unfractionated lymphocytes to protein A was consistently two- to three-fold higher than that of purified T lymphocytes or that of purified non-T lymphocytes. The addition of mitomycin-treated T cells greatly enhanced the non-T-lymphocyte proliferation to protein A. Similarly, mitomycin-treated non-T lymphocytes also promoted the protein A response of T lymphocytes. These findings suggest that the synergistic interaction of T- and non-T-lymphocyte populations in protein A responsiveness is required for the maximal response. Brochier *et al.* (1976) have reported that a water-soluble mitogen from *Nocardia* acts specifically to generate a T-independent B-cell response.

Only T cells appear to respond with proliferation to antigens from mumps, rubella, and SKSD (Chess *et al.*, 1974b). Both B and third-population cells fail to proliferate when stimulated with these antigens. In one-way mixed-leukocyte culture reactions, only T cells respond by proliferation, whereas B cells, third-population cells, and a subpopulation of T cells are capable of stimulating the responding T cells (Sondel *et al.*, 1975b; Gupta, unpublished observations).

Whereas rabbit B lymphocytes can be induced to proliferate and differentiate after treatment with antiimmunoglobulin antisera (Kishimoto and Ishizaka, 1975), antiimmunoglobulin specific for human M, G, or A did not stimulate synthesis of DNA by purified T cells, but purified B lymphocytes responded weakly. T- plus B-cell populations were more responsive. Cultures containing mitomycin-treated B cells plus purified T cells could also be stimulated to proliferate, thus indicating that T cells could be induced to proliferate by antiimmunoglobulin treatment of T- and B-cell mixtures.

7. Lymphocyte Mitogenic Factor (LMF)

Antigen-stimulated lymphocyte mitogenic factor (LMF) is produced only by T cells and not by B cells (Rocklin *et al.*, 1974a). This factor is antigen specific and causes a proliferative response in unseparated cells, T cells, and B cells. B cells do not produce antigen-stimulated LMF. However, Kasakura (1977) reported LMF production by both T and B lymphocytes. LMF produced by T cells differed in some respects from LMF produced by B lymphocytes: (1) The production of T-cell LMF was accelerated when the T lymphocytes were stimulated by allogeneic cells. In contrast, LMF activity from mixed cultures of B cells was not different from that produced by pure cells of B. LMF produced in unmixed B-cell cultures stimulated both B and T cells to proliferate, whereas LMF produced by cultures of T cells stimulated only B cells to proliferate. Blomgren (1976) reported LMF production by both T and B lymphocytes after stimulation with either PHA or PWM. Con A covalently bound to Sepharose-triggered B-cell preparations to higher MF release than either T cells or unfractionated lymphocyte suspensions.

8. Migration Inhibition Factor (MIF)

All three populations (T, B, and third population) produced migration inhibition factor (MIF) after stimulation with mumps, rubella, or SKSD antigen preparations (Chess *et al.*, 1974b; Rocklin *et al.*, 1974a). Despite the absence of antigen-induced proliferation of the B cells, MIF was produced only by B cells obtained from specifically sensitized individuals. B cells produce more MIF than do T cells. MIF produced by T or B cells was found to be identical when fractionated on Sephadex G-100. MIF is produced by B cells even in the presence of BuDR, antigen, and light.

Chess *et al.* (1975a) have examined T and B lymphocytes for their capacity to produce another mediator, leukocyte migration inhibitory factor (LIF). This material is distinct from MIF and inhibits migration of human PMN but not human monocytes. Both T and B cells from sensitized donors produced LIF when stimulated *in vitro* with PPD, candida, and SKSD. LIF production was antigen specific. T and B lymphocytes from donors lacking delayed hypersensitivity to PPD or monilia failed to elaborate LIF.

9. Interferon Production

Epstein *et al.* (1974), using purified T- and B-cell preparations isolated by fluorescence-activated cell sorter, demonstrated that both populations respond to PHA and PWM *in vitro* in the presence of macrophages by proliferation and the production of interferon. However, selective T-cell interferon production could be assessed at 3 days in culture; B-cell interferon production was delayed to 5 and 7 days. T cells or T-cell products were ineffective in inducing or accelerating B-cell interferon at 3 days. It must be emphasized that this lymphocyte-derived interferon is distinctly different and not nearly so well characterized as are the interferons produced by nonlymphoid cells.

10. Chemotactic Factors

Altman and Kirchner (1972) and Altman *et al.* (1975) examined the capacity of both T and B lymphocytes to produce chemotactic factors for neutrophils. T lymphocytes were stimulated with PHA and B lymphocytes were stimulated by erythrocytes sensitized with antibody and complement (EAC) which bind to their C3 receptors. Both T and B lymphocytes produced chemotactic factors with a molecular weight of approximately 12,500 having identical isoelectric points. Although chemotactic lymphokines produced by T and B cells are relatively homogeneous by gel filtration, they appear to contain two isoelectrically distinct species. One has a major peak with isoelectric point at pH 10.1 and a lesser peak with isoelectric point at pH 5.6. No chemotactic activity was found in the 12 more alkaline fractions which followed the chemotactic peak. These findings suggest that both T and B cells, although possessing different membrane receptors and requiring different mechanisms of activation to initiate lymphokine synthesis, produce physicochemically identical chemotactic factors.

11. Cell-Mediated Lympholysis (CML)

A number of investigators using murine and human lymphocytes have shown that cytotoxic cells can be generated during *in vitro* sensitization in a unidirectional mixed-lymphocyte culture reaction. The sensitization phase of this reaction appears to be dependent on the recognition of lymphocyte-defined (LD) antigens on the stimulating cells, whereas the cytotoxic cells generated kill only those cells bearing serologically defined (SD) antigens in common with those of the sensitizing cells. Only T cells are found to have cell-mediated cytotoxic potential, while isolated B and third-population cells are not cytotoxic in this assay (Sondel *et al.*, 1975a; MacDermott *et al.*, 1975). Moreover, B cells, when sensitized in the presence of T cells and isolated 6 days after *in vitro* sensitization, do not generate cytotoxic activity. However, B cells and third-population cells are at least as efficient as T cells in triggering T cells to proliferate in a one-way MLC and in generating killer T cells.

12. Antibody-Dependent and Spontaneous Cell-Mediated Cytotoxicity

Antibody-dependent cell-mediated cytotoxicity (ADCC) was thought to be a function of third-population cells (Perlmann and Perlmann, 1970; Wisloff *et al.*, 1974a). Recent studies have clearly demonstrated that both third-population cells and T cells mediate both ADCC and spontaneous lymphocyte-mediated cytotoxicity (SLMC) (West *et al.*, 1978; Gupta *et al.*, 1978b). Both Tγ and third-population cells appear to have similar cytotoxic potential in ADCC and SLMC (Gupta *et al.*, 1978b). In contrast, B cells lack both ADCC and SLMC properties. ADCC is an active energy-requiring phenomenon. The inhibition of both aerobic and anaerobic energy production in the effector cells (non-T, non-B cells) completely abolishes cytotoxicity (Trinchieri and de Marchi, 1975).

13. Precursor Cells among the So-Called Third Population of Lymphocytes

Recently, it has been demonstrated that third-population cells, under appropriate experimental conditions, can be differentiated into T cells, B cells, granulocytes, and erythrocytes; therefore, included among the cells of this population is a heterogeneous assortment of committed precursor cells (Richman *et al.*, 1978; Nathan *et al.*, 1978 Chess *et al.*, 1974c).

14. Human T-Cell Subpopulations

During the process of differentiation and maturation, human T lymphocytes develop receptors for Fc portions of immunoglobulins (Dickler *et al.*, 1974; Ferrarini *et al.*, 1975; Chiao *et al.*, 1975). This section will detail the properties of these T-cell subpopulations.

Human T lymphocytes are subclassified into at least three distinct subpopulations that may be identified by the presence or absence of surface receptors for the immunoglobulin molecule. Approximately 50–60% of peripheral blood T lymphocytes have receptors for IgM (Tμ cells) and about 10% of peripheral blood T lymphocytes have receptors for IgG (Tγ cells). Approximately 20–30% of peripheral blood T lymphocytes lack receptors for either IgM or IgG (TØ) cells. These three subpopulations of human T lymphocytes can be readily enumerated and precisely purified by a rosette assay using OXRBC-IgM (for Tμ) and OXRBC-IgG complexes (for Tγ). Using such an assay system, these populations, particularly Tμ and Tγ cells, have been extensively studied for their morphology and functions in various immunological phenomena and for perturbations of numbers and functions in a variety of primary and secondary immunodeficiency disorders (Gupta and Good, 1977a,b, 1978a; Gupta *et al.*, 1978a, 1979c; Moretta *et al.*, 1977). For detailed studies of these interesting T-cell subpopulations, readers are referred to recent reviews (Gupta and Good, 1978b; Moretta *et al.*, 1978; Gupta, 1978, 1979; Gupta and Kapoor, 1979).

14.1. Specificity of Immunoglobulin Receptors on T-Cell Subpopulations

The receptor for IgM on Tμ cells has specificity for the Fc portion of the IgM molecule (Ferrarini *et al.*, 1976; McConnell and Hurd, 1976; Moretta *et al.*, 1975). IgM appears to bind to the T-cell receptor by its CH4 domain (Conradie and Bubb, 1977). Preud'homme *et al.* (1977) have demonstrated that T-cell receptors can bind to monomeric 8 S human IgM. The apparent affinity of T-cell receptors for IgM is higher for monomeric than for pentameric IgM. This conclusion was reached by analysis of inhibition of rosette formation of T cells with pentameric IgM isolated from serum of patients with Waldenstrom's macroglobulinemia and 8 S native IgM purified from the serum of a pateint with macroglobulinemia having both 8 S and 19 S monoclonal IgM peaks. It appears that the intact intrachain disulfide bridges may be the requirement for IgM binding to the receptors on the surface of T cells. Recently, it has been shown that receptors for IgM are not confined to T cells but also can be demonstrated on certain normal B cells and B cells from certain patients with chronic lymphocytic leukemia (Ferrarini *et al.*, 1977; Pichler and Knapp, 1977, 1978).

Specificity of the IgG receptor on purified T cells has not yet been reported. It is possible that the Tγ cells may bind to the Fc portion of all subclasses of human IgG.

14.2. Histamine Receptors

Recently, T-cell subpopulations have been examined for the presence of histamine receptors (Rocklin *et al.*, 1979). Purified T lymphocytes from peripheral blood were passed over histamine-coated or noncoated Sepharose beads and then examined for the proportions of Tμ and Tγ cells. Approximately 50% of the Tγ cells were retained by histamine beads, while the remaining 50% passed through the column. This finding indicates that there exist at least two subpopulations of Tγ cells, those which are histamine receptor positive (H+) and those which are histamine receptor negative (H−). Functional analyses of these two subpopulations of Tγ cells are being carried out. Initial studies in certain *in vitro* systems suggest that H+ Tγ cells function as suppressor cells and H− Tγ cells participate in spontaneous and antibody-dependent cytotoxicity (Gupta *et al.*, unpublished observations).

14.3. Morphology of Tμ and Tγ Cells

Both light and electron microscopic and histochemical examination of purified Tμ and Tγ cells have revealed distinct morphological characteristics (Grossi *et al.*, 1978). By transmission electron microscopy, Tμ cells are smaller medium-sized lymphocytes. They have a rather smooth surface with relative paucity of cytoplasmic organelles and contain one or two large spots of ANAE. Tγ cells possess many long surface microvilli. Their cytoplasm is rich in mitochondria and has many single ribosomes, scattered strands of rough endoplasmic reticulum, and distinctive vesicles. The Golgi apparatus of the Tγ cells is also well developed, showing piles of microtubules and cisterns. Characteristic granules are seen in Tγ cells which comprise a dense matrix surrounded by a unit membrane. These granules are located between the Golgi apparatus and the overlying plasma membrane. The release of vesicular contents on short-term culture of Tγ cells is inhibited by cytochalasin B. Some of the Tγ cells were found to be capable of endocytosis of IgG antibody-coated erythrocytes.

14.4. Sensitivity of T-Cell Subpopulations

We have recently studied the effect of irradiation, corticosteroids, and thymopoietin on T-cell subpopulations. Purified T lymphocytes were irradiated (500 r, 1000 r, 2000 r, 3000 r) and treated with corticosteroids (2.5–200 μg/ml prednisolone) or thymopoietin (50–500 ng/ml) and examined for the proportions of Tμ and Tγ cells (Gupta and Good, 1977b). Tγ cells were found to be sensitive to low-dose irradiation (500 r and 1000 r), their number being greatly reduced by exposure to such relatively low dosages. However, at high doses of irradiation (2000 r and 3000 r), Tμ cells were also decreased. It appears that decrease in Tγ cells at low-dose irradiation is consequent to functional inhibition rather than direct cytotoxicity, since the viability of the irradiation-treated cell population continues to be more than 95%. At high doses the influence of irradiation was attributed to both functional inhibition and cell death (viability 70%). Corticosteroids at high concentrations (prednisolone 50 μg/ml or equivalent dose of hydrocortisone) *in vitro* resulted in a decrease of Tγ cells in a few subjects. Haynes and Fauci (1978) examined *in vivo* effects of a single dose of hydrocortisone on T-cell subpopulations 4 hr following intravenous injection. The proportions of Tμ cells were significantly decreased while the proportions of Tγ cells were increased. At 24 hr proportions of Tμ and Tγ returned to the initial level. This *in vivo* effect of hydrocortisone may be due to redistributions of T-cell subsets since Tμ cells are more mobile, and they might be readily driven out of circulation under the influence of hydrocortisone. Thymopoietin treatment of T-lymphocyte populations at a critical concentration of 100 ng/ml increased the proportion of Tγ cells. This observation indicates that the total peripheral blood T cells contain precursors for Tγ cells.

Mingari *et al.* (1978) investigated the effect of treatment of T cells with proteolytic enzymes on the expression of Tμ and Tγ receptors. IgM receptor is highly susceptible to both trypsin and pronase, whereas the IgG receptor is resistant to trypsin and sensitive only to high concentrations of pronase. After pronase treatment IgM receptors on T cells reappear within 2 hr, and resynthesis is completed in 6 hr. IgG receptors reappear in 4–6 hr after pronase treatment and the resynthesis is completed within 12 hr.

14.5. RNA Content of Tμ and Tγ Cells

Andreeff *et al.* (1978) studied the RNA and DNA content of human lymphocyte subpopulations by staining them with the metachromatic dye acridine orange and measuring the fluorescence of individual cells by flow cytofluorometry. Non-T cells have a unimodal distribution, with a sharp peak and an exponential distribution toward higher RNA values. T cells have a bimodal distribution with two separate peaks. When T cells are separated into Tμ and Tγ cells, each population displays a unimodal distribution. Tγ cells have the lowest content of RNA per cell; Tμ cells have twice as much RNA per cell as Tγ cells. These differences in the RNA content may represent yet another marker, a metabolic marker for T-cell subsets.

14.6. Compartmental Distribution of T-Cell Subsets

We have recently examined the distribution of Tμ and Tγ in lymphoid compartments (Gupta and Good, 1978c). Results are shown in Table 5. Tμ cells are present in comparable proportions among peripheral blood, cord blood, bone marrow, lymph nodes, and tonsils. The spleen contains very low proportions of Tμ cells. Tγ cells are present in comparable proportions among peripheral blood, bone marrow, and tonsils. Cord blood has significantly increased proportions of Tγ cells when compared with those in the peripheral blood of older children and adults. The spleen is very rich in Tγ cells. Normal lymph nodes lack Tγ cells almost completely. Thymuses, in general, have very low proportions of both Tμ and Tγ cells. However, occasional thymus from older subjects and thymic tissue from a patient with thymoma and hypogammaglobulinemia showed Tγ cells in proportions approaching those found in the normal peripheral blood. The significance of these observations remains to be elucidated. The data, however, suggest that Ig receptors are expressed on T lymphocytes only after the cells of this lineage have left the thymus. Does this finding mean that thymic hormones act on the

TABLE 5

Lymphoid compartment		Tμ (%) mean ± SD	Tγ (%) mean ± SD
Peripheral blood	(60)[a]	52.0 ± 10.8	10.3 ± 4.8
Cord blood	(20)	45.0 ± 10.3	14.5 ± 6.9
Lymph nodes	(3)	43.7 ± 15.8	0.3 ± 0.3
Thymus	(8)	2.1 ± 3.5	3.1 ± 3.2
Bone marrow	(4)	55.0 ± 23.8	8.5 ± 4.4
Tonsils	(5)	41.2 ± 15.4	7.0 ± 7.1
Spleen	(1)	10.0	45.0

[a] In parentheses, number of patients studied.

thymocytes to induce them to express Ig receptors only outside the thymus? Or, alternatively, is this expression of this level of differentiation antigen dependent? Studies of acute T-cell lymphoblastic leukemia have revealed that certain T-cell blasts possess both IgM and IgG receptors (Moretta *et al.*, 1977a; Beck *et al.*, 1978). This finding might be interpreted to indicate that the Tμ and Tγ cells develop from common thymocytes. It is not clear at the present time which of the receptors comes first in the differentiative expression. From studies of the ontogeny of surface Ig classes on B lymphocytes, it might be reasonable to propose that IgM receptors are expressed first on the surface of T cells followed by a later switching to receptors for IgG. Studies of ontogeny of T-cell subsets in human embryos should provide the answer to this question.

14.7. Response of T-Cell Subpopulations to Mitogens and Allogeneic Cells

Moretta *et al.* (1976) described the proliferative responses of Tμ and Tγ cells to phytohemagglutinin (PHA) and concanavalin A (Con A). Purified Tμ, Tγ, and Tγ-depleted T cells were cultured with PHA or Con A for 3 days and proliferative response was determined by [^{3}H]thymidine incorporation. In both the experiments with Con A, the kinetics of the proliferative response to varying concentrations of Con A was almost identical for Tμ and Tγ cells. However, Tγ cells from one of two donors tested had a much lower proliferative response that did the Tμ or the unfractionated T-cell population. Tμ and Tγ cells demonstrated distinct dose responses of the proliferative response to PHA. Isolated Tγ cells responded very poorly to any concentration of PHA, and isolated Tμ cells required much higher concentrations of PHA than was required by the unfractionated T-cell population to produce the same peak proliferative response. The poor proliferative response to Tγ cells may not be an intrinsic characteristic of Tγ cells; rather, subpopulations of Tγ cells might exist within the total population of Tγ cells, and one of these may be induced by PHA to become suppressor for another Tγ subpopulation. Such a relationship could account for the poor proliferative response of Tγ to PHA (autoregulation).

We have recently studied the proliferative responses of Tμ, Tγ and TØ cells (as responder cells) to allogeneic mononuclear cells, monocyte-depleted lymphoid cells, B cells, or third-population (TP) cells as stimulator cells. All three subpopulations responded similarly to one another and to unseparated T cells in mixed-leukocyte cultures. Similarly, in the mouse, MLC responsiveness has been shown for both IgG Fc+ and IgG Fc− subpopulations of T lymphocytes (Stout *et al.*, 1976).

14.8. Leukocyte Migration Inhibition Factor Production

Kapadia *et al.* (1978) examined T-cell subpopulations for their capacity to produce leukocyte migration inhibition factor (LMIF) when stimulated *in vitro* with PHA and Con A. Purified Tμ, Tγ, and TØ cells were cultured with or without Con A or PHA for 72 hr. Mitogen-stimulated (test) and mitogen-reconstituted (control) supernates were tested for LMIF activity on isolated normal neutrophils. Tμ and TØ cells produced LMIF in amounts comparable to that produced by unfractionated lymphocytes. However, Tγ either did not produce or produced less

LMIF than that produced by $T\mu$ cells. This study demonstrates yet another functional difference between $T\mu$ and $T\gamma$ cells.

14.9. Locomotor Properties of T-Cell Subpopulations

O'Neill and Parrott (1977) demonstrated that human T and non-T cells move toward either endotoxin-activated serum or casein. However, non-T cells respond less to casein. The different distribution of $T\mu$ and $T\gamma$ cells in various lymphoid compartments suggested that these subpopulations might have different locomotor properties. $T\mu$, $T\gamma$, and $T\emptyset$ cells from human peripheral blood and human tonsils were examined for their locomotor response toward the chemoattractant casein (Parrott *et al.*, 1978). $T\gamma$ cells from both human tonsils and peripheral blood do not move toward casein. $T\emptyset$ cells move well and $T\mu$ cells move even better toward casein. Prior incubation with AB serum blocked the movement of the T cells. Since AB serum blocks the receptor for IgM (on $T\mu$ cells), we proposed that the receptors for chemostimulant and for IgM Fc on $T\mu$ cells might be very closely associated or even overlap. However, in subsequent studies, purified human IgM failed to block the chemotactic or chemokinetic activity of $T\mu$ cells, at a time when IgM Fc receptors were completely blocked (Gupta, unpublished observations). This finding would suggest that the receptor(s) for chemoattractants is distinct from that of IgM Fc receptor.

14.10. Suppressor and Helper Functions of T-Cell Subsets

Recently, Moretta *et al.* (1977) studied the role of T-cell subpopulations in regulating the B-cell differentiation into plasma cells. Purified B cells were cocultured for 7 days with total T, $T\gamma$-depleted, and $T\gamma$-enriched cell fractions in the presence of PWM. At the end of 7 days, cultures were examined for the proliferative response and the number of plasma cells containing intracytoplasmic immunoglobulin. A $T\gamma$-depleted population provided a helper influence in a dose-dependent manner. Further separation of $T\gamma$-depleted fraction into $T\mu$ and $T\mu$-depleted demonstrated that $T\mu$ cells provide most of the helper effect. The observations established that $T\mu$ cells have helper activity for regulating B-cell differentiation. However, Hayward *et al.* (1978) have demonstrated that $T\mu$ cells, when activated *in vitro* with Con A, could suppress Ig production, suggesting that functionally distinct subpopulations exist within the $T\mu$-cell population. Gupta *et al.* (1979a), by treating purified $T\mu$ cells with 40 μg/ml of Con A, could demonstrate a switch in certain $T\mu$ cells to $T\gamma$ cells.

$T\gamma$ cells did not exert helper activity; therefore, this population was examined for their suppressor activity. $T\gamma$ cells have been shown to suppress the B-cell differentiation induced by $T\mu$ in the presence of PWM. This suppression by $T\gamma$ cells was found to be dose dependent. Irradiation (3000 r) of $T\gamma$ cells results in complete abrogation of suppressor activity. We have also shown that $T\gamma$ cells are radiosensitive (Gupta and Good, 1977b). Interaction with immune complexes is necessary for the $T\gamma$ cells to act to suppress B-cell differentiation. In contrast, Haynes and Fauci (1978) have demonstrated that the interaction of immune complexes with $T\gamma$ cells abrogates their capacity to suppress development of plaque-forming cells when $T\gamma$ cells are activated with Con A. Further suppression of B-cell differentiation requires that Tγ cells be present at the beginning of the cultures. Tγ cells will not suppress B-cell differentiation if B cells have been cocultured with Tμ cells in the presence of PWM for 1 or 2 days prior to the addition of Tγ cells (Moretta *et al.*, 1978). These studies suggest that Tγ cells do not suppress B cells by a direct cytotoxic mechanism, but rather by suppressing the influence of the helper T cells.

Shou *et al.* (1976) have shown that when human peripheral blood mononuclear cells are incubated with a high (supramitogenic) dose of concanavalin A for 18–48 hr, a suppressor activity for the proliferative response of cells to PHA, Con A, allogeneic cells, or antigens is generated. These Con-A-activated cells also act as suppressors for B-cell differentiation to immunoglobulin-synthesizing and -secreting plasma cells (Schwartz *et al.*, 1977). However, to understand the precise cellular basis of such an induced suppression, we studied the effect of Con A activation (in a dose response manner) on purified T cells in an 18-hr culture by assaying the proportions of Tμ and Tγ cells and *in vitro* functions for suppression of B-cell differentiation (Gupta *et al.*, 1978b). At the low concentrations (1–2.5 μg/ml), Con A increased the proportions of Tμ cells and enhanced the helper influence in the differentiation of B cells to plasma cells. At 40 μg/ml Con A, decreased proportion of Tμ and an increased proportion of Tγ cells were observed. Under these circumstances, marked suppression of B-cell responses was observed. Similar observations were found when Con A was used in cultures for 48 hr. These results indicate that the helper activity of low doses of Con-A-activated T cells is due to an increase in Tμ cells. Suppressor activity at higher doses of Con A appears to be attributable to a decrease in the proportion of Tμ cells and an increased proportion of Tγ cells. This analysis appears to be consonant with the view that precursors of both Tμ and Tγ cells exist in the TØ population in the peripheral blood. At a high concentration (40 μg/ml) of Con A, the inverse change in the proportions of Tμ and Tγ cells may have been a result of certain Tμ cells switching to Tγ cells (Gupta *et al.*, 1979a), which would support the observation of Hayward *et al.* (1978), who demonstrated that Tμ cells when activated with Con A could suppress immunoglobulin synthesis by B lymphocytes.

14.11. Antibody-Dependent (ADCC), Spontaneous (SLMC), and Mitogen-Induced (MICC) Cytotoxicity

We have recently investigated the subpopulations of T cells for their ADCC and SLMC activity (Gupta *et al.*, 1978b). Tγ cells have ADCC activity against chicken erythrocytes coated with IgG-anti-chicken RBC antibody as target cells and SLMC activity against cells of K562 cell line as target cells. Furthermore, we investigated the subpopulations of Tγ cells (i.e., histamine receptor H+ and histamine receptor H−) for ADCC and SLMC activity. By depleting the H+ T cells, we could enrich SLMC and ADCC activity of T cells, suggesting that SLMC and ADCC activities of Tγ cells are confined to H− Tγ cells (Gupta *et al.*, unpublished observations).

Cordier *et al.* (1978) examined Tγ and Tγ-depleted cells for their mitogen-induced capacity to kill the target chicken RBC. In this assay, effector cells (Tγ and Tγ-depleted cells) were cocultured with PHA and ^{51}Cr-labeled CRBC for a period of 24 hr and specific Cr release was measured. These authors reported that most of the mitogen-induced cellular cytotoxicity (MICC) resided in $T\gamma$ cells. However, Pichler *et al.* (1978), using almost similar system, reported MICC in both $T\mu$- and $T\gamma$-cell populations. The significance of MICC in relation to hypersensitivity disorders remains to be determined.

Recently, some preliminary studies of T-cell subsets have been carried out in patients with allergic disorders. Ong *et al.* (1979) have examined T-cell subpopulations in ten adult patients with allergic rhinitis who had intradermal tests positive for ragweed allergen. No significant differences in the proportions of $T\mu$ or $T\gamma$ cells were observed when compared with age-matched controls. However, when T cells were exposed to 50 μg antigen E/ml *in vitro,* ragweed-sensitive subjects responded by developing a significant increase in the proportions and numbers after overnight incubation of $T\mu$ cells and with no change in the proportion of $T\gamma$ cells. In contrast, in control subjects antigen E induced a significant increase in the proportions of $T\gamma$ cells and no change in $T\mu$ cells. The functional analysis of these two subsets in relation to allergen-specific antibody production in patients with allergic disorders remains to be determined.

Gupta *et al.* (1979b) have studied nine children with extrinsic bronchial asthma. Four of nine children were receiving aminophyllin for the bronchial spasm and remaining five were not receiving any medication at a time when studies of T-cell subsets were performed. The children in the latter group had in their circulation both $T\mu$ and $T\gamma$ cells in proportions comparable to those of age- and sex-matched controls. However, patients in the former groups had significantly lower proportion of $T\mu$ cells. To determine whether this low proportion of $T\mu$ cells was due to aminophyllin, T cells from normal healthy controls were incubated *in vitro* with aminophyllin, isoproterenol, and phenylphrine and examined for the proportions of $T\mu$ and $T\gamma$ cells. Both aminophyllin and isoproterenol (agents known to increase cyclic AMP) at a concentration of 10^{-3}–10^{-5} M produced significant reduction in the proportions of $T\mu$ cells and had no effect on $T\gamma$ cells. In contrast, phenylephrine (an agent known to increase cyclic GMP) at a concentration of 10^{-3} M produced a significant increase in the proportions of $T\mu$ cells. Therefore, it can be concluded that receptors for IgM on T cells ($T\mu$ cells) are very sensitive to modulatory effects of agents known to alter the levels of cyclic nucleotides, and receptors for IgG on T cells ($T\gamma$) are relatively resistant. Studies are in progress to analyze the effects of adrenergic agonists and antagonists on the functional activities of T-cell subsets.

The following section will review major lymphocyte subpopulations in certain hypersensitivity diseases.

15. Atopic Dermatitis

Atopic dermatitis or eczema has been defined as an allergic dermatosis characterized by erythema, intense itching, and vesiculation. Atopic dermatitis was first distinguished from other eczemas and prurigos about 1885 by the French dermatologists Besniere and Brocq. Over the years it was noted that the skin changes were often associated with certain allergic manifestations, especially hay fever and asthma. About 1930 it was hypothesized that these skin lesions are cutaneous analogues of asthma and hay fever, and the term "atopic dermatitis" was coined.

16. Cellular Immunity

Most of the studies of cell-mediated immunity in patients with atopic dermatitis and contact dermatitis have been reported during the last decade. One of the earliest descriptions of impaired cell-mediated immunity in patients with atopic dermatitis, using a patch test to common contact sensitizer, was made by Rostenberg and Sulzberger (1937).

16.1. T Lymphocytes

McGeady and Buckley (1975) studied 21 children ranging in age from 22 months to 17 years, who had eczema. These patients were not receiving systemic steroids at the time of study; however, many were using topical steroids. A significant diminution in the number of circulating T cells was found. It is not clear whether this reduction in circulating T cells was secondary to a systemic effect of topically administered corticosteroids, since topical application of corticosteroids on eczematous skin might be absorbed systemically. Carapeto *et al.* (1976) and Luckasen *et al.* (1974) also found low proportions of circulating T lymphocytes in patients with atopic dermatitis and contact dermatitis. Secher *et al.* (1977) studied 20 patients with contact dermatitis, 18 patients with atopic dermatitis, and two patients with mixed dermatitis and found no significant alterations in the proportions of circulating T lymphocytes. Similarly, Grove *et al.* (1975a) found no differences in absolute numbers of T lymphocytes in 35 patients with atopic eczema when compared with those of controls.

Strannegard *et al.* (1976) examined 113 patients with atopic eczema. These included 50 patients with atopic eczema alone and 63 with atopic eczema and asthma. The proportions of T lymphocytes were significantly reduced when compared with controls. No difference was observed between the group with eczema alone and the group with both eczema and asthma. Strannegard and Strannegard (1977) examined 215 patients with atopic eczema, rhinoconjuctivitis, asthma, or a combination of these presentations. The relative and absolute numbers of peripheral T cells were found to be significantly decreased.

Rachelefsky *et al.* (1976) studied 37 patients with atopic dermatitis and found a low percentage of T cells in 11 patients; when the mean value of T cells of the entire group was compared with that of the control group, no significant difference was observed. Clinical and laboratory evaluation of these 11 patients was not different from that of the remaining 26 patients. Dupree *et al.* (1975) found normal proportions of T lymphocytes in 13 patients with atopic diathesis (including eczema) from that of normal. However, they did not present their data separately for the group with atopic eczema.

As described in Chapter 5 of this book, by Ishizaka and Ishizaka, T lymphocytes regulate the production of IgE. Since patients with atopic eczema usually have higher levels of serum IgE, lymphocytes from these patients were evaluated for suppressor T cells. In a preliminary study a loss of suppressor T cells in certain patients with atopic eczema was reported (Baker and Gordon, 1977).

16.2. Lymphocyte Transformation

Lobitz *et al.* (1972) demonstrated diminished proliferative response to PHA of two patients with atopic dermatitis. McGeady and Buckley (1975) studied the proliferative response of lymphocytes from 21 children with atopic eczema to mitogens (PHA, Con A, and PWM) and antigens (*C. albicans* and tetanus toxoid). They found a significant impairment of the blastogenic response to Con A, PWM, and candida. Grove *et al.* (1975a), however, found no impairment of PHA responses in the 35 patients with atopic eczema that they studied. No correlation was made between the severity of disease and alterations in lymphocyte transformation.

Dupree *et al.* (1975) also found no abnormalities in PHA-induced lymphocyte transformation in 13 patients with atopic dermatitis. In contrast, Rachelefsky *et al.* (1976) found significantly depressed PHA response by lymphocytes from all 37 patients with atopic dermatitis. This abnormality was observed only when the concentrations of PHA used were 6.3 μg, 3.1 μg, and 1.6 μg; no significant depression was observed when PHA at concentrations of 12.5 μg, 25 μg, and 100 μg was used.

Strannegard *et al.* (1976) reported results of lymphocyte proliferation in response to PHA, Con A, and PWM from 91 patients with atopic eczema. Proliferative responses to PHA and, to a lesser degree, Con A were significantly depressed, whereas stimulation with PWM was unaffected. Strannegard and Strannegard (1977) examined the effect of sera from atopic and nonatopic children on mitogen and antigen responses. Sera from atopic children were not merely less stimulatory than normal for the proliferative responses of normal or atopic lymphocytes to Con A, PHA, PDD, but rather exercised a pronounced inhibitory effect in some cases. Inhibition by atopic serum appeared to be an early event in lymphocyte mitogenesis and not due to C-reactive protein, IgE, or factors binding to mitogens.

16.3. Delayed-Type Hypersensitivity

Rostenberg and Sulzberger (1937) described a low incidence of positive patch tests to common contact sensitizers in patients with atopic dermatitis. Similarly, Palacios *et al.* (1966) and Jones *et al.* (1973) found that patients with atopic eczema were less readily sensitized by 2,4-dinitrochlorobenzene and to *Rhus* extracts. Lobitz *et al.* (1972) reported two patients with atopic dermatitis who failed to respond at 48 hr to intradermal injections of a variety of ubiquitous bacterial and fungal agents. McGeady and Buckley (1975) divided their 21 children with atopic eczema into three groups based on the severity and distribution of their dermatitis. Intradermal skin tests with SK-SD and candida were evaluated. The children with most severe dermatitis (group I) exhibited marked depression of delayed cutaneous hypersensitivity; delayed unresponsiveness was also present in group II children (localized eczema). Patients in group III with nearly healed atopic dermatitis all had positive reactions to one or both antigens. Grove *et al.* (1975a) also found significant impairment of delayed skin reactivity to bacterial, viral, and mycotic antigens. These studies are at variance with the results of Palacios *et al.* (1966). These latter authors did not give any information regarding clinical status of their patients. However, if the data of Shick and Dick tests concerning toxins, which are uninterpretable, and mumps antigen are excluded from their results, only 19 of 32 patients had positive delayed hypersensitivity to other antigens tested. Dupree *et al.* (1975) found no abnormality in delayed cutaneous hypersensitivity to *C. albicans* and SK-SD in 13 patients with atopic dermatitis.

16.4. Humoral Immunity

Humoral immunity in atopic dermatitis has been evaluated much more extensively than the cellular immunity, and there is more agreement than disagreement regarding alterations in humoral immunity reported by various investigators.

16.5. B Lymphocytes

B lymphocytes in patients with atopic dermatitis have been reported to be normal or increased in proportions and/or absolute number. The disagreement among the authors appears to be largely due to the different techniques used to quantify B lymphocytes. Cormane *et al.* (1974) and Rachelefsky *et al.* (1976) reported increased numbers of total B cells as determined by surface Ig; the increase in B cells in the study of Cormane *et al.* (1974) was due to an increased number of IgA-bearing lymphocytes in contact dermatitis. Carapeto *et al.* (1976) also reported increases in surface-IgE- and IgA-bearing B lymphocytes. No correlation was observed between increases in B-cell numbers and clinical status of patients. Unfortunately, in the study of Rachelefsky *et al.* (1976) monospecific antiimmunoglobulin antisera were not used. Secher *et al.* (1977) found normal proportions of B lymphocytes in patients with atopic dermatitis and contact dermatitis; however, proportions of IgE-bearing lymphocytes were increased in atopic dermatitis when compared to controls. In their controls the mean value of IgE-bearing B cells was 3.2%, which makes us think that the purity and specificity of anti-IgE antiserum used might have been poor since we have found only occasional IgE-bearing B lymphocytes in the peripheral blood of healthy controls and patients with a wide number of diseases. McGeady and Buckley (1975) found normal numbers of Ig-bearing B lymphocytes in 21 patients with atopic dermatitis. No increase in the proportions of IgE-bearing lymphocytes was observed. However, they found an increased proportion of IgA-bearing B lymphocytes in the blood. These authors also reported an increase in B lymphocytes having complement receptors in the patients with atopic dermatitis. It is now well established that not all the B cells bear complement receptors and not all the complement-receptor-bearing lymphocytes are B cells; therefore, lymphocytes with complement receptors should not be considered synonymous with the B cells.

16.6. Serum Immunoglobulins

In the absence of extraordinary antigenic stimulation, the serum IgE level of an individual remains relatively constant. However, markedly elevated IgE levels occur in some, but not all, humans in association with a variety of helminth infestations. The level of IgE in serum is frequently elevated in individuals with allergic diseases. Orgel *et al.* (1974) studied serum immunoglobulins in American-born Filipino children and compared them with those of Caucasian children. Serum concentrations of IgG, IgM, and IgA were significantly higher in the healthy Filipino group than in the Caucasian control group. However, the differences between atopic and nonatopic subjects and between eczematous and noneczematous subjects were not significantly different for IgG, IgA, or IgM within a comparable racial group. Serum IgE levels were higher in atopic subjects of both racial groups when compared with the nonatopic group. Buckley *et al.* (1968) also reported comparable levels of serum IgM, IgG, IgA, and IgD in both atopic and nonatopic groups. McGeady and Buckley (1975) reported elevated levels of serum IgE in most of their patients with atopic eczema. Rachelefsky *et al.* (1976) reported elevated serum IgE levels in patients with atopic dermatitis; however, no significant difference was observed in serum IgE levels between a group of patients with low T-cell numbers and another group with normal T-cell numbers. Church *et al.* (1976) determined serum IgE concentrations and the presence of allergen-specific IgE in 23 patients with atopic dermatitis. Elevated serum IgE levels were observed in 83% of patients, and this elevation was independent of age and sex. A direct correlation was observed between the serum IgE levels and the clinical severity of disease. Similar correlation between the severity of the dermatitis and the concentration of IgE has been reported by Hoffman *et al.* (1975) and Johnson *et al.* (1974). Because the skin in atopic dermatitis is physiologically abnormal, the efficacy of skin testing for allergen identification has been questioned (Rosenberg and Solomon, 1971). The use of the RAST test has been reported to be helpful in defining both inhalant and food allergy (Church *et al.*, 1976; Hoffman *et al.*, 1975). The relationship among elevated serum IgE, impaired T-cell immunity, and pathogenesis of disease, however, still remains unclear. The elevated IgE levels could be due to defects in cell-mediated immunity, in particular the defect of suppressor T cells. The role of T cells in the regulation of IgE responses is discussed in great detail in Chapter 5.

17. Bronchial Asthma and Allergic Rhinitis

Immunological studies in patients with bronchial asthma and allergic rhinitis have demonstrated the involvement of both immediate (manifested by positive skin tests, anti-allergen-specific IgE antibody, and increased levels of serum IgE) and delayed-type hypersensitivity (manifested by depressed cell-mediated immunity). In this section, we will discuss the results of investigations of both humoral and cell-mediated immunity in patients with bronchial asthma and allergic rhinitis, and the effects of immunotherapy on lymphocyte populations.

17.1. Cell-Mediated Immunity: T Lymphocytes

Yocum *et al.* (1976) studied 17 patients with allergic rhinitis selected for markedly elevated levels of total serum IgE > 300 IU/ml. The proportions of T lymphocytes were comparable to those of control groups. Delayed cutaneous hypersensitivity to dermatophytin, mumps, tetanus-diphtheria toxoid, and streptokinase-streptodornase (SK-SD) demonstrated 76.3% positive test to SK-SD. Grove *et al.* (1975b) demonstrated high proportions of negative delayed cutaneous hypersensitivity reactions to ubiquitous antigens. Strannegard *et al.* (1976) reported lower proportions of T lymphocytes in 51 patients with allergic rhinitis when compared with controls. In one of the above studies, absolute numbers of T lymphocytes were reported, which is certainly critical in ultimate evaluations.

In patients with allergic bronchial asthma, numbers and percentages of circulating T lymphocytes have been reported to be normal or decreased. Gupta *et al.* (1975a), Strannegard *et al.* (1976), and Saraclar *et al.* (1977) reported significantly lower proportions of circulating T lymphocytes in patients with bronchial asthma when compared with age- and sex-matched controls. Gupta *et al.* (1975a) reported absolute T lymphopenia in 43% of patients with bronchial asthma, and Gottlieb and Hanifin (1974) reported T lymphopenia in 25% of their patients with asthma. Contrary to these studies, other investigators have reported normal proportions (Neiburger *et al.*, 1978; Thomson *et al.*, 1977) or absolute numbers (Thomson *et al.*, 1977; Saraclar *et al.*, 1977; Lang *et al.*, 1978) of T lymphocytes in patients with bronchial asthma. These discrepancies could be attributed to the differences in techniques and/or to an effect of drug therapy, because it has been shown that agents which *in vitro* increase intracellular cAMP inhibit rosette formation with SRBC (Galant and Remo, 1975). Lang *et al.* (1978) reported both normal proportions and normal absolute numbers of "active" T cells in patients with bronchial asthma. Thomson *et al.* (1977) found increased proportions and absolute numbers of "null" cells (defined as cells lacking surface Ig and receptors for SRBC and IgG Fc) and normal proportions and absolute numbers of K or third-population cells (non-T, non-B Fc receptor +).

Recently, Lang *et al.* (1978) examined the effects of sympathomimetic and cholinergic stimulation on T lymphocytes (for their rosette formation with SRBC) from patients with bronchial asthma. The β-adrenergic drug isoproterenol (10^{-3} M) inhibited formation of "active" E rosettes in asthmatics by only 18.0% as compared to 60.8% inhibition in the control group. Carbamylcholine (10^{-5} M), a cholinergic agonist, also showed a lower-than-normal response in asthmatics, 34.3% enhancement of "active" E rosetting compared to a 52.4% enhancement in the controls. The α-adrenergic agent phenylephrine (10^{-5} M) exhibited equally enhancing effects in both groups. Isoproterenol (10^{-3} M) had a minimal effect on inhibition of long-incubation "total" E rosettes in both control and asthmatic groups. This β-adrenergic abnormality further supported the β-blockade theory of asthma of Szentivanyi.

Verhaegen *et al.* (1977) studied the effect of histamine on the capacity of T lymphocytes to form rosettes with SRBC both in normals and in allergic subjects. Histamine had no effect on the capacity of T lymphocytes to form E rosettes in healthy subjects, but it significantly inhibited the rosette formation of T cells with SRBC in patients with allergies. This study suggests that increased sensitivity to the action of histamine characterizes T lymphocytes from allergic subjects.

17.2. Lymphocyte Transformation and Mediator Production in Response to Mitogens and Antigens

Studies on mitogen stimulation of lymphocytes from allergic patients have given divergent results. Pass *et al.* (1966) found a normal response to PHA, whereas Fjelde and Kopecka (1967) demonstrated depressed responses to PHA in asthmatic patients. Yocum *et al.* (1976) observed normal proliferative responses of lymphocytes from patients with allergic rhinitis when stimulated with PHA, Con A, and PWM. In another report, Strannegard *et al.* (1976) reported similar results in patients with allergic rhinitis; however, these authors demonstrated depressed responses to PHA and Con A and normal response to PWM in patients with bronchial asthma. Hanifen and Gottlieb (1974) suggested that serum IgE may inhibit mitogenic responses. However, in none of the above studies did any correlation exist between depressed proliferative response and levels of serum IgE. Strannegard and Strannegard (1977) examined the effect of sera from atopic and nonatopic children on the lymphocyte DNA synthesis induced by PHA, Con A, and PPD. Atopic sera were found to be inhibitory for mitogenic responses of lymphocytes to Con A. No significant inhibitory effect was observed on PHA- and PPD-induced lymphocyte proliferation. Sera from some of the servely ill atopic patients almost completely abolished mitogen-induced lymphocyte DNA synthesis. Inhibition by atopic serum appeared to be an early event in lymphocyte mitogenesis and not due to C-reactive protein, IgE, or factors binding to mitogens. Lymphocytes from atopic children were no more sensitive to suppressive influences of atopic serum factors than were lymphocytes from adult blood donors. These findings suggest that the T-cell defect in atopic patients may be partly caused by serum factors; however, these findings need further confirmation and documentation in a large series of studies.

In the limited number of published reports evaluating human lymphocyte responsiveness to pollen allergies, conflicting results were obtained (Zeitz *et al.*, 1966; Girard *et al.*, 1967; Richter and Naspitz, 1968; Maini *et al.*, 1971; Weisberg *et al.*, 1972; Rocklin *et al.*, 1974b; Evans *et al.*, 1976; Black *et al.*, 1976; Gatien *et al.*, 1975; Geha *et al.*, 1975). Most investigators reported a greater overall responsiveness by lymphocytes from atopic persons to allergens than by those from nonatopic controls (Zeitz *et al.*, 1966; Girard, *et al.*, 1967; Richter and Naspitz, 1968; Maini *et al.*, 1971; Rocklin *et al.*, 1974b; Evans *et al.*, 1976; Gatien *et al.*, 1975; Geha *et al.*, 1975); however, others have reported that lymphocytes from normal subjects also respond vigorously to pollen antigens (Weisberg *et al.*, 1972; Black *et al.*, 1976). Buckley *et al.* (1977) studied DNA synthetic responses of cultured lymphocytes from normal subjects, cord blood, atopic subjects, and patients with agammaglobulinemia to purified ragweed antigens E, K, and Ra3. Vigorous DNA synthetic responses to antigen E occurred with lymphocytes of patients from all groups. The mean day on which maximal responses occurred was 8.7. No significant intergroup difference in DNA synthetic response to pollen antigens was observed. The major reason for divergent results among published studies appears to be that, in most studies, cultures were harvested prior to the average time of peak lymphocyte responsiveness to pollen allergens *in vitro*. The proliferative responses of lymphocytes from nonatopic subjects to a variety of crude pollen extracts observed by Weisberg *et al.* (1972) led them to suggest that the apparent nonspecific stimulation was possibly artifactual and due to an interaction of heparin with the pollen extracts. However, Buckley *et al.* (1977) found that lymphocytes from normal nonatopic subjects respond equally well to purified ragweed antigen E whether cultured in a heparin-free, serum-supplemented medium or in a plasma-supplemented medium. The findings of proliferative responses to purified pollen allergens by lymphocytes from nonatopic normal, newborn, and agammaglobulinemic subjects suggest that purified ragweed pollen antigens are either ubiquitous and lead to cell-mediated responsiveness in all subjects with intact cell-mediated immunity or have mitogenic properties in addition to their known antigenic properties. As a matter of fact, the molecular weight of purified ragweed antigen E (37,800) is close to the molecular weights of the purified mitogens of concanavalin A (25,500) and pokeweed (22,000 to 32,000) (Lis and Sharon, 1973; Ling and Kay, 1975; Waxdal, 1975; King *et al.*, 1967).

Rocklin *et al.* (1974b) studied the lymphocytes from patients with ragweed hay fever and from controls for their capacity to produce mitogenic factor and migration inhibition factor when stimulated with ragweed antigen E (AgE). Cell-free supernates from AgE-stimulated and control cultures were assayed on autologous lymphocytes for increased tritiated thymidine incorporation 6 days later. Net mitogenic activity of supernates obtained from antigen-stimulated patient's lymphocytes was significantly greater that that obtained from control lymphocytes. Lymphocytes from 24/28 patients were found to produce significant quantities of mitogenic factor compared to lymphocytes from only 1/17 controls.

Supernates obtained from control cultures and lymphocytes stimulated by AgE and SK-SD were assayed for their inhibitory activity on the migration of guinea pig macrophages in capillary tubes. The mean percent migration inhibition for supernates obtained from patient's lymphocytes stimulated by 50 μg/ml of RAgE was significantly greater than that of supernates from control lymphocytes. The two groups produced similar amounts of MIF in response to SK-SD. These findings indicate that a majority of patients with ragweed hay fever make a broad immune response to one of the major antigenic determinant (RAgE) in ragweed extract.

17.3. Humoral Immunity: B Lymphocytes

The number of B lymphocytes in patients with allergic bronchial asthma and rhinitis is found to be within the range of normal controls (Thomson *et al.*, 1977; Gupta *et al.*, 1975a; Luckasen *et al.*, 1974). However, Yocum *et al.* (1976) reported significantly increased proportions of C3 (EAC) receptor-bearing cells in patients with allergic rhinitis. Their values for normal controls, however, were abnormally high (35%) as compared to those reported by several other investigators. It seems likely that these authors did not exclude monocytes (which form EAC rosettes) from their enumerations. Saraclar *et al.* (1977) also reported an increased number of EAC-positive lymphoid cells in patients with allergic rhinitis and/or bronchial asthma. These investigators depleted the phagocytic cells by carbonyl iron prior to assay for lymphocyte subpopulation. The procedure for depleting phagocytic cells, however, is known to produce alterations in the proportions of T and B cells. Neiburger *et al.* (1978) found increased proportions of surface-IgM-bearing B lymphocytes in patients with rhinitis and asthma. No significant difference was observed in the proportions of B cells with surface IgG, IgA, or IgE. Following (8 months) immunotherapy the proportions of IgM-bearing B lymphocytes returned to control values. No significant change in serum IgM level was observed. B cells with other surface immunoglobulins remained essentially unchanged. Saraclar *et al.* (1977) compared the lymphocyte subpopulations in patients without immunotherapy to those in patients on immunotherapy. They found no significant difference between the two groups. However, unlike Neiburger *et al.* (1978), they did not perform a sequential prospective study. The significance of these findings remains to be determined.

Becker and Buckley (1978) examined the biosynthesis of IgE by peripheral blood mononuclear cells from patients with asthma and/or eczema who had elevated levels of serum IgE and normal nonatopic controls with normal levels of serum IgE. Supernates from both unstimulated cells were assayed for IgE by double-antibody radioimmunoassay. Maximum IgE synthesis occurred on day 7 of cultures. IgE was present in supernates of unstimulated cultures from ten normal controls in a concentration of 165 pg/ml. In PWM-stimulated cultures, IgE could be detected in a concentration of 480 ± 358. In contrast, IgE concentrations in supernates from unstimulated mononuclear cell cultures from patients with asthma were 969 ± 437 pg/ml, and in PWM-stimulated cultures the concentrations of IgE were 869 ± 396 pg/ml. When cocultures of normal and patients with mononuclear cells were done, in unstimulated cultures, there was 87% inhibition of IgE biosynthesis. The findings were similar in PWM-stimulated cultures. This study indicates that peripheral B cells in patients with elevated IgE are already maximally stimulated and cannot be further stimulated by PWM. The suppression of IgE biosynthesis in coculture experiments reflects the presence of cells in normal mononuclear cell populations that inhibit IgE biosynthesis by the patient's cells. In contrast, no significant suppression of IgM or IgG was observed, suggesting that the suppression is specific for IgE. These studies imply that patients with elevated IgE levels may have a deficiency of suppressor cells that regulate IgE biosynthesis in normal individuals.

17.4. Serum Immunoglobulins

In 1968 Johansson reported elevated serum IgE levels in patients with allergic asthma. In these patients, the mean IgE concentrations were 6 times higher than in healthy subjects. However, patients with nonatopic asthma showed normal IgE levels. The maximum increase in serum IgE levels was observed in atopic eczema, less in allergic bronchial asthma, and least in with allergic rhinitis (Berg and Johansson, 1969). Increased levels of IgE in patients with allergic rhinitis and bronchial asthma have been reported by a number of investigators (Gupta *et al.*, 1975a; Yocum *et al.*, 1976; Dahlstrom *et al.*, 1973; Neiburger *et al.*, 1978; Orgel *et al.*, 1974).

17.5. Antibody-Dependent Cell-Mediated Cytotoxicity (ADCC)

As discussed earlier in this chapter, cells responsible for ADCC activity were first described as "K" cells and identified by the lack of receptors for SRBC or surface Ig but as cells having a receptor for IgG Fc. Thomson *et al.* (1977) found normal proportions and normal absolute numbers of K cells in patients with extrinsic bronchial asthma. They observed ADCC activity by asthmatic lymphocytes against IgG-sensitized Chang liver cells to be comparable to that of controls. Flaherty *et al.* (1977) also examined the mononuclear cells as well as granulocytes from controls, patients with allergic asthma, and patients with nonallergic (intrinsic) asthma for their ADCC activity against target chicken RBC sensitized with IgG.

Most patients with intrinsic bronchial asthma had a reduced ADCC capacity, but this function was normal in patients with extrinsic bronchial asthma. The abnormality did not correlate with the severity of asthma or with treatment. Polymorphonuclear granulocytes from both extrinsic and intrinsic asthma had ADCC comparable to that of controls. This study suggests that an effector cell abnormality as reflected in ADCC activity is inherent in the mononuclear cell population, perhaps in the third-population cells, in patients with intrinsic asthma.

17.6. Cyclic Nucleotides in Leukocytes of Atopic Subjects

Parker and Smith (1973) reported that lymphocytes are the main component of leukocyte subpopulations responsible for decreased cAMP production in asthma. Makino *et al.* (1977) compared the cAMP response of lymphocytes from normals and asthmatic subjects to norepinephrine (β_1-stimulator) and salbutamol (β_2-stimulator). The maximum cAMP production in lymphocytes after exposure to salbutamol (10^{-3} M) was significantly less in the asthmatic group than in normals (only one-third that of normals). No significant difference in maximum cAMP response to norepinephrine (10^{-3} M) was observed between the two groups. These findings further support the hypothesis that there exists a selective blockage of β_1-receptors in asthma. The abnormality of β_2-receptors in asthma may be attributable to a diminished number of receptors, diminished binding affinity for β_2-stimulants, diminished activity of the catalytic unit of adenylate cyclase, or increased activity of phosphodiesterase. Sokol and Beall (1975) found no difference in numbers or binding affinity of leukocyte epinephrine receptors of normal and asthmatic subjects. Diminished activity of adenylate cyclase also seems unlikely since Parker and Smith (1973) and Busse (1975) reported normal response to prostaglandin E_1. Mue *et al.* (1975) found phophodiesterase activity of leukocytes from asthmatics to be similar to that of normals. Parker *et al.* (1973) observed increased cAMP production in lymphocytes from asthmatic subjects after treatment with 100–200 mg/day of hydrocortisone. Logdon *et al.* (1972) also reported similar findings in asthmatic children. Makin *et al.* (1977) observed that asthmatic patients receiving corticosteroid treatment had decreased cAMP production in lymphocytes with salbutamol when compared with the patients who were not receiving corticosteroids. It is possible that these patients were receiving corticosteroids in amounts that were not sufficient to restore the activity of β-adrenergic receptors. Lee *et al.* (1977) found that β-adrenergic stimulation of cAMP and glycogenolysis was significantly reduced in the asthmatic subjects when compared with controls. Prostoglandin E produced less of a rise in cAMP in asthmatics than in normals, but the difference was not significant and glycogenolysis was normal. Cortisol potentiated the effect of isoproterenol and PGE_1 *in vitro*, but in the presence of cortisol the response of the asthmatic cells to isoproterenol was still lower than that of cells from normals.

17.7. Polymorphonuclear Leukocyte and Monocyte Chemotaxis in Atopic Disease

Recent investigations have brought forward an association among atopy, hyperimmunoglobulinemia E, recurrent infection, and defective polymorphonuclear (PMN) and monocyte chemotaxis (Clark *et al.*, 1973; Hill and Quie, 1974; Van Scoy *et al.*, 1975; Snyderman *et al.*, 1977; Rogge and Hanifin, 1976). Most of these patients were first identified because of undue susceptibility to infection. Furukawa and Altman (1978) examined PMN and MN chemotaxis in patients with atopic dermatitis and allergic rhinitis and asthma. Atopic patients without infection had a low prevalence of PMN chemotactic defect (4%). The presence or absence of this abnormality was not related to serum IgE levels. Snyderman *et al.* (1977) reported a much higher incidence (30%) of PMN chemotactic defect in patients with atopic eczema. Infection at the time of study could be one of the explanations for the discordance of the results of these two groups of investigators. Hill *et al.* (1976) have found that certain atopic individuals have PMN chemotactic defect only immediately prior to and during episodes of infection. Furukawa and Altman (1978) and Snyderman *et al.* (1977) reported that high proportions (39% and 57%) of patients with allergic asthma and/or eczema demonstrated depressed MN chemotaxis. Snyderman *et al.* (1977) found that sera from six of eight patients with atopic eczema inhibited the chemotaxis of normal MNs. However, Furukawa and Altman (1978) failed to find evidence of inhibitors for chemotaxis in sera from their patients. These discrepancies could be due to differences in methodology. Furukawa and Altman (1978) used C5a and bacterial chemotactic factors as chemoattractants, whereas Snyderman used lymphocyte-derived chemotactic factor. Monocytes and macrophages are essential for proper initiation and control of most immune response. Therefore, abnormal MN chemotaxis could play a role in the faulty regulation of humoral and/or cellular immunity that occurs in atopy.

18. Drug Hypersensitivity

Immunological aspects of drug allergy are discussed in detail in Chapter 10. This section will briefly review changes in lymphocyte populations in patients with well-documented histories of hypersensitivity to certain drugs.

Scheffer *et al.* (1975) examined peripheral blood lymphocytes from six asthmatic patients suspected of having acute (three cases) or subacute (three cases) adverse reactions to cromolyn inhalation. Patients with acute adverse reactions presented with anaphylaxis, oropharyngeal edema, or urticaria; subacute reactions were manifested by polymyositis, pericarditis, and pulmonary infiltrates or cutaneous eruptions. No correlation between the occurrence or nature of the reaction and the duration of cromolyn therapy or dose of cromolyn was found. Both acute and subacute adverse reactions to cromolyn were associated with alterations in the *in vitro* immunological parameters. Lymphocytes from patients with acute and subacute adverse reactions produced migration inhibitory factor (MIF) and incorporated increased amounts of [^{3}H]thymidine when challenged with cromolyn. Production of MIF in response to cromolyn was not observed with lymphocytes from patients who were cromolyn tolerant or of normal subjects. In contrast, lymphocyte transformation was seen in four or nine cromolyn-tolerant patients. Thus MIF production may differentiate patients with clinical evidence of reaction to cromolyn from cromolyn-tolerant patients. Two of the three patients with subacute reactions were distinguished from those with acute reactions by the presence of elevated serum binding of cromoglycate. This binding activity resided in the IgG fraction and subsided within 4 months following discontinuation of drugs. Lymphocyte transformation was also short lived, becoming negative in five of six patients at 6 weeks. MIF production was still demonstrable after 10 months in two of the three patients with subacute reactions. Immunological reactions to cromolyn appear to be heterogeneous and may include either cell-mediated immunity, antibody-mediated immunity, or both. Both T and B lymphocytes may thus be activated in adverse reactions to cromolyn. While proliferative response to specific antigen (cromolyn in this case) is a function of T cells, antibody production and MIF production probably require both cell types.

The presence of eosinophilia during the course of nitrofurantoin pneumonitis has been reported (Hailey *et al.*, 1969). Geller *et al.* (1977) studied peripheral blood mononuclear cells from five patients with acute nitrofurantoin pleuropulmonary reactions. All patients had profound lymphopenia, and four had eosinophilia. The two patients available for testing had decreased total numbers of both T cells and B cells (EAC rosettes). The authors entertained the possibility of change in lymphocyte traffic, with lymphocytes leaving the circulation to enter the pulmonary infiltration. Other possibilities that nitrofurantoin might also interfere with lymphocyte life-span or production were also entertained. All three patients tested had negative lymphocyte proliferative response to nitrofurantoin. Bone *et al.* (1976) also observed negative blastogenic response to nitrofurantoin in a patient with desquamative interstitial pneumonia following long-term treatment with nitrofurantoin. Rocklin and David (1971) reported similar results in a patient with nitrofurantoin syndrome. However, Goldstein and Janicki (1974) and Pearsall *et al.* (1974) reported positive lymphocyte transformation to nitrofurantoin during 2½ years after treatment in patients presenting with acute pulmonary reactions in nitrofurantoin. Lundgren *et al.* (1975) also observed positive lymphocyte transformation response to nitrofurantoin in two patients with chronic pulmonary lesions associated with nitrofurantoin. The reason(s) for these discrepancies in the results by various investigators remains to be determined. Thus the diagnosis of various nitrofurantoin hypersensitivity reactions relies on clinical data. The mechanisms of these reactions presently remain unclear.

Reidenberg and Caccese (1975) studied thymidine uptake by lymphocytes from 43 patients with suspected drug allergy, when stimulated *in vitro* with the specific drug to which they appeared to be allergic. These drugs included INH, furosemide, chlorapropamide, and phenobarbital. Only 12 of 43 patients had increased thymidine uptake by their drug-treated lymphocytes. Thymidine uptake decreased with time after the suspect drug was stopped, and all the tests eventually became negative. However, in this study many false-negative and false-positive results were observed.

Bassi *et al.* (1976) reported the presence of IgE antibody in sera from five of 20 patients who had episodes ascribable to rifampicin sensitization. These antibodies cross-react with rifampicin and with the chromophoric moiety of rifampicins, but not with the side chain of rifampicin. Significant histamine release was obtained *in vitro* when leukocytes were incubated with sera from these five patients together with rifampicin. The reasons for failure to detect specific IgE and specifically induced release of histamine by the sera from the remaining 15 patients are unclear. It is possible that levels of anti-rifampicin IgE are below the sensitivity of the assay employed. Perhaps more antigen is required for histamine release when lower amounts of IgE are bound per cell.

Webster and Thompson (1974) examined *in vivo* and *in vitro* reactivity to ampicillin polymer in patients with infections mononucleosis as well as other individuals with and without a history of having received ampicillin. *In vivo* skin testing proved largely inconclusive, as did investigations of specific penicilloyl antibodies. *In vitro* stimulation was produced by polymeric ampicillin but not by the purified monomeric form, and the reaction appeared to be independent of prior experience of the drug or of other penicillins. Ampicillin polymer stimulated "unsensitized" lymphocytes. The compound transformed lymphocytes in all the clinical groups and to roughly the same extent. The polymer also stimulated cells from newborn infants whose mothers had not received any penicillin during pregnancy, reinforcing the idea of the "nonspecific" nature of this effect. In conclusion, evidence for an operation of specific humoral or cellular immune mechanisms directed against ampicillin in those patients who develop a rash following therapy is minimal.

19. Summary

In this chapter we have reviewed the current status of lymphocyte subpopulations with regard to their surface markers and functions in various immunological phenomena. Evidence has been presented which causes doubt about the significance of immunoglobulin receptors on T-cell subpopulations as distinct cells with helper or suppressor activities. Immunological perturbations in atopic disorders are subtle; the most consistent abnormality in cell-mediated immunity, however, is observed only in severe atopic dermatitis. Critical and double-blind studies of various immunological functions in hypersensitivity disorders are required in order to clarify the contradictory results already reported in the literature.

ACKNOWLEDGMENT

The authors wish to thank Secretarial Service of Sloan-Kettering Institute for the preparation of the manuscript.

20. References

Ablin, R. J., and Morris, A. J., 1973, Thymus-specific antigens on human thymocytes and on thymus-derived lymphocytes, *Transplantation* **15:**415.

Altman, L. C., and Kirchner, H., 1972, The production of monocyte chemotactic factor by agammaglobulin chicken spleen cells, *J. Immunol.* **109:**1149–1151.

Altman, L. C., Chassy, B., and Mackler, B. F., 1975, Physiochemical characterization of chemotactic lymphokines produced by human T and B lymphocytes, *J. Immunol.* **115:**18–21.

Anderson, J. K.,and Metzgar, R. S., 1978, Detection and partial characterization of human T and B lymphocyte membrane antigens with antisera to HSB and SB cell lines, *J. Immunol.* **120:**262–271.

Andreeff, M., Beck, J. D., Darzynkiewicz, Z., Traganos, F., Gupta, S., Melamed, M., and Good, R. A., 1978, RNA content in human lymphocyte subpopulations, *Proc. Natl. Acad. Sci.* **75:**1938–1942.

Arbeit, R. D., Henkart, P. A., and Dickler, H. B., 1977, Differences between Fc receptors of two lymphocyte subpopulations of human peripheral blood, *Scand. J. Immunol.* **6:**873–878.

Asantila, T., Sorvari, T., Hirvonen, J. and Toiramen, P., 1973, Xenogeneic reactivity of human fetal lymphocytes, *J. Immunol.* **11:**984–989.

August, C. S., Berkel, A. E., Driscoll, S. and Merler, E., 1971, Ontogeny of lymphocyte function in the developing human fetus, *Pediatr. Res.* **5**:539.

Baker, G. P., and Gordon, B., 1977, Atopic dermatitis—A disease of suppressor T cell deficiency, and its treatment with the immunostimulant drug levamisole, *Am. Congr. Allery Immunol. Sci. Abstr. No. 77793.45*, 217.

Bassi, L., DiBerardinoh, and Silvestri, L. G., 1976, IgE antibodies in patients allergic to rifampicin. *Int. Arch. Allergy Appl. Immunol.* **51**:390–394.

Baxley, G., Bishop, G. B., Cooper, A. G., and Wortis, H. H., 1973, Rosetting of human red blood cells to thymocytes and thymus-derived cells, *Clin. Exp. Immunol.* **15**:385–392.

Beck, J. D., Mertelsman, R., Haghbin, M., Good, R. A., and Gupta, S., 1978, Characterization of T cell acute lymphocytic leukemia (ALL) by Fc receptors and multiple cell markers, *Proc. Am. Assoc. Cancer Res.* **19**:172.

Becker, W. G., and Buckley, R. H., 1978, *In vitro* studies of IgE biosynthesis, *J. Allergy Clin. Immunol.* **61**:177.

Berg, T., and Johansson, S. G. D., 1969, IgE concentrations in children with atopic diseases: A clinical study, *Int. Arch. Allergy* **36**:219–232.

Bernard, A., Boumsell, L., and Good, R. A., 1976, Complement inhibitors released from leukocytes. II. Evidence that lymphocytes release and produce an inhibitor of C_2 activation, *Cell Immunol.* **22**:351–357.

Bianco, C., Patrick, R., and Nussenzweig, V., 1978, A population of lymphocytes bearing a membrane receptor for antigen-antibody-complement complexes. I. Separation and characterization, *J. Exp. Med.* **132**:702–720.

Black, P. L., Marsh, D. G., Jarrett, E., Delespesse, G. J., and Bias, W. B., 1976, Family studies of association with HLA and specific immune responses to highly purified pollen antigens, *Immunogenetics* **3**:349–368.

Blomgren, H., 1976, Evidence for the release of mitogenic factors by both T and B lymphocytes in the human, *Scand. J. Immunol.* **5**:1173–1178.

Bokish, V. A., and Sobel, A. T., 1974, Receptor for the fourth component of complement on human B lymphocytes and cultured human lymphoblastoid cells, *J. Exp. Med.* **140**:1336–1347.

Bone, R. C., Wolfe, J., Sobonya, R. E., Kerby, G. R., Stechshulte, D., Ruth, W. E., and Welch, M., 1976, Desquamative interstitial pneumonia following long-term nitrofurantoin therapy, *Am. J. Med.* **60**:697–701.

Bourgois, A., Abney, E. R., and Parkhouse, R. M. E., 1977, Mouse immunoglobulin receptors on lymphocytes: Identification of IgM and IgD molecules by tryptic cleavage and a postulated role for cell surface IgD, *Eur. J. Immunol.* **7**:210–213.

Brochier, J., Bona, C., Ciorbaru, R., Revillard, J. P., and Chedid, L., 1976, A human T-independent B lymphocyte mitogen extracted from *Nocardia opaca, J. Immunol.* **117**:1434–1439.

Brown, G., and Greaves, M. F., 1974, Cell surface markers for human T and B lymphocytes, *Eur. J. Immunol.* **4**:302–310.

Brown, J. C., de Jusus, D. G., Holborow, E. J., and Harris, G., 1970, Lymphocyte mediated transport of aggregated human γ-globulin into germinal center areas of normal mouse spleen, *Nature (London)* **228**:367–369.

Buckley, R. H., Dees, S. C., and O'Fallon, W. M., 1968, Serum immunoglobulins. I. Levels in normal children and in uncomplicated childhood allergy, *Pediatrics* **41**:600–611.

Buckley, R. H., Seymour, F., Sonal, S. O., Ownby, D. R., and Becker, W. G., 1977, Lymphocyte responses to purified ragweed allergens *in vitro*. I. Proliferative responses in normal newborn agammaglobulinemia and atopic subjects, *J. Allergy Clin. Immunol.* **59**:70–78.

Burrows, P. D., Lawton, A. R., and Cooper, M. D., 1977, Effect of anti-μ suppression and cyclophosphamide on pre-B cells in mice, *Fed. Proc.* **36**:1302.

Busse, W. W., 1975, Impaired inhibition of lysosomal enzyme release from neutrophils in asthma, *Clin. Res.* **23**:502.

Carapeto, F. J., Winkelmann, R. K., and Jordan, R. G., 1976, T and B lymphocytes in contact and atopic dermatitis, *Arch. Dermatol.* **112**:1095–1100.

Carr, M. C., Stites, D. P., and Fudenberg, H. H., 1973, Dissociation of responses to phytohemagglutinin and adult allogeneic lymphocytes in human foetal lymphoid tissues, *Nature (London) New Biol.* **241**:279–281.

Chess, L., MacDermott, R. P., and Schlossman, S. F., 1974a, Immunologic functions of isolated human lymphocyte subpopulations. I. Quantitative isolation of human T and B cells and responses to mitogen, *J. Immunol.* **113:**1113–1121.

Chess, L., MacDermott, R. P., and Schlossman, S. F., 1974b, Immunolgic functions of isolated human lymphocyte subpopulations. II. Antigen triggering of T and B cells *in vitro, J. Immunol.* **113:**1123–1127.

Chess, L., MacDermott, R. P., Sondel, P. M., and Schlossman, S. F., 1974c, Cells involved in human cellular hypersensitivity, in: *Progress in Immunology II* (L. Brent and J. Holborow, eds.), p. 125, North-Holland, Amsterdam.

Chess, L., Rocklin, R. E., MacDermott, R. P., David, J. R., and Schlossman, S. F., 1975a, Leukocyte inhibitory factor (LIF): Production by purified human T and B lymphocytes, *J. Immunol.* **115:**315–317.

Chess, L., Levine, H., MacDermott, R. D., and Schlossman, S. F., 1975b, Immunologic functions of isolated human lymphocyte subpopulations. VI. Further characterization of surface Ig negative, E rosette negative (null cell) subsets, *J. Immunol.* **115:**1438–1487.

Chiao, J. W., Pantic, V. S., and Good, R. A., 1974, Human peripheral lymphocytes bearing both B-cell complement receptors and T-cell characteristics for sheep erythrocytes detected by a mixed rosette method, *Clin. Exp. Immunol.* **18:**483–490.

Chiao, J. W., Pantic, V. S., and Good, R. A., 1975, Human lymphocytes bearing receptor for complement components and SRBC, *Clin. Immunol. Immunopathol.* **4:**545–555.

Church, J. A., Kleban, D. G., and Bellanti, J. A., 1976, Serum immunoglobulin E concentrations and radioallergosorbant test in children with atopic dermatitis, *Pediatr. Res.* **10:**97–99.

Clark, R. A., Root, R. K., Kimball, H. R., and Kirkpatrick, C. M. 1973, Defective neutrophil chemotaxis and cellular immunity in a child with recurrent infections, *Ann. Intern. Med.* **78:**515.

Conradie, J. D.,and Budd, M. D., 1977, CH_4 domain of IgM has cytophilic activity for human lymphocytes, *Nature (London)* **265:**160–162.

Cooper, M. D., Peterson, R. D. A., and Good, R. A., 1965, Delineation of the thymic and bursal lymphoid systems in the chicken, *Nature (London)* **205:**143–146.

Cordier, G., Samarut, C., and Revillard, J. P., 1978, Contribution of lymphocytes bearing Fcγ receptors to PHA-induced cytotoxicity, *Immunology* **35:**49–56.

Cormane, R. H., Husz, S., and Hammerlinck, F., 1974, Immunoglobulin and complement-bearing lymphocytes in allergic contact dermatitis and atopic dermatitis, *Br. J. Dermatol.* **90:**597–605.

Dahlstrom, G., Johansson, G., and Kiviloog, 1973, Immunoglobulin IgE concentrations in an adult clinical material with chronic obstructive pulmonary disease, *Scand. J. Resp. Dis.* **54:**73–77.

Dewar, A. E., Stuart, A. E., Parker, A. C., and Wilson, C., 1974, Rosetting cells in autoimmune hemolytic anemia, *Lancet* **2:**519.

Diaz-Jouanen, and Williams, R. C., 1974, T and B lymphocytes in human colostrum, *Clin. Immunol. Immunopathol.* **3:**248–255.

Dickler, H. B., and Kunkel, H. G., 1972, Interaction of aggreated γ-globulin with B lymphocytes, *J. Exp. Med.* **136:**191–196.

Dickler, H. B., Adkinson, M. F., and Terry, W. D., 1974, Evidence for individual human peripheral blood lymphocytes bearing both B and T cell markers, *Nature (London)* **247:**213–245.

Dupree, E., Friedman, J. M., Lard, R. W., and Goldman, A. S., 1975, Cell-mediated immunity in atopic dermatitis, *J. Allergy Clin. Immunol.* **55:**102.

Dwyer, J. M., Rosenbaum, J. T., and Lewis, S., 1976, The effect of antigen suppression of γM and γG on the production of γE, *J. Exp. Med.* **143:**781–790.

Dwyer, J. M., Warner, N. L., and McKay, I. R., 1972, Specificity and nature of the antigen-combining sites on fetal and mature thymus lymphocytes, *J. Immunol.* **108:**1439–1946.

Epstein, L. B., Kreth, H. W., and Herzenberg, L. A., 1974, Fluorescence activated cell sorting of human T and B lymphocytes. II. Identification of the cell type responsible for interferon production and cell proliferation in response to mitogens, *Cell. Immunol.* **12:**407–421.

Evans, R., Rocklin, R. E., Pence, H. E., and Kaplan, H. M., 1976, The effect of immunotherapy on humoral and cellular responses in ragweed hay fever, *J. Clin. Invest.* **57:**1378–1385.

Ferrarini, M., Moretta, L., Abrile, R., and Durante, M. L., 1975, Receptors for IgG molecules on human lymphocytes forming spontaneous rosettes with sheep red cells, *Eur. J. Immunol.* **5:**70–72.

Ferrarini, M., Moretta, L., Mingari, M. C., Tonda, P., and Pernis, B., 1976, Human T cell receptor for IgM specificity for the pentameric Fc fragment, *Eur. J. Immunol.* **6:**520–521.

Ferrarini, M., Hoffman, T., Fu, S. M., Winchester, R. J., and Kunkel, H. G., 1977, Receptors for IgM on certain human B lymphocytes, *J. Immunol.* **119:**1525–1529.

Fjelde, A., and Kopecka, B., 1967, Cell transformation and mitogenic effects in blood leukocyte cultures of atopic dermatitis patients, *Acta Derus-Vener.(Stockholm)* **47:**168.

Flaherty, K. D., Martin, J. M., Strom, W. W., Kriz, R. J., Surfus, M. T., and Reed, C. E., 1977, Antibody-dependent cellular cytotoxicity in asthmatics, *J. Allergy Clin. Immunol.* **58:**48–53.

Forre, O., Natvig, J. B., Froland, S. S., and Johnson, P. M., 1976, Distribution of heavy-chain variable-region (VH) subgroups on human lymphocytes, *Scand. J. Immunol.* **5:**1221–1228.

Froland, S. S., and Natvig, J. B., 1972, Surface bound immunoglobulins on lymphocytes from normal and immunodeficient humans, *Scand. J. Immunol.* **1:**1–12.

Froland, S. S., and Natvig, J. B., 1972b, Class, subclass and allelic exclusion of membrane bound Ig of human B lymphocytes, *J. Exp. Med.* **136:**409–414.

Froland, S. S., and Natvig, J. B., 1973, Identifications of three different human lymphocyte populations by surface markers in T and B lymphocytes in humans, *Transplant. Rev.* **16:**114–162.

Froland, S. S., Wisloff, F., and Michaelson, T. E., 1974, Human lymphocytes with receptors for IgG: A population of cells distinct from T- and B-lymphocytes, *Int. Arch. Allergy* **47:**124–138.

Fu, S. M., Winchester, R. J., and Kunkel, H. G., 1974, Occurrence of surface IgM, IgD and free light chains on human lymphocytes, *J. Exp. Med.* **139:**451–456.

Furukawa, C. T., and Altman, L. C., 1978, Defective monocyte and polymorphonuclear leukocyte chemotaxis in atopic disease, *J. Allergy Clin. Immunol.* **61:**288–293.

Galant, S. P., and Remo, R. A., 1975, β-Adrenergic inhibition of human T lymphocyte rosettes, *J. Immunol.* **114:**512–513.

Gathings, W. E., Cooper, M. D., Lawton, A. R., and Alford, C. A., 1976, B cell ontogeny in humans, *Fed. Proc.* **35:**393.

Gathings, W. E., Lawton, A. R., and Cooper, M. D., 1977, Immunofluorescent studies of the development of pre-B cells, B lymphocyte and immunoglobulin isotype diversity in humans, *Euro. J. Immunol.* **7:**804–810.

Gatien, J. G., Merler, E., and Cotten, H. R., 1975, Allergy to ragweed antigen E: Effect of specific immunotherapy on the reactivity of human T lymphocytes *in vitro, Clin. Immunol. Immunopathol.* **4:**32–37.

Gausset, P., Delespesse, G., Hubert, G., Kennes, B., and Govairts, A., 1976, *In vitro* response of subpopulations of human lymphocytes. II. DNA synthesis induced by anti-immunoglobulin antibodies, *J. Immunol.* **116:**446–453.

Geha, R. S., Cotten, H. R., Schneeberger, E., and Merler, E., 1975, Cooperation between human thymus derived and bone marrow-derived lymphocytes in antibody response to ragweed antigen E *in vitro, J. Clin. Invest.* **56:**386–390.

Gelfand, M. C., Elfenbein, G. J., Frank, M. M., and Paul, W. E., 1974, Ontogeny of B lymphocytes. II. Relative rates of appearance of lymphocytes bearing surface immunoglobulin and complement receptors, *J. Exp. Med.* **139:**1125–1141.

Geller, M., Flaherty, D. K., Dickie, H. A., and Reed, C. E., 1977, Lymphoma in acute nitrofurantoin pleuropulmonary reactions, *J. Allergy Clin. Immunol.* **59:**445–448.

Girard, J. P., Rose, N. R., Kunz, M. L., Kobayashi, S., and Arbesman, C. E., 1967, *In vitro* lymphocyte transformation in atopic patients: Induced by antigens, *J. Allergy* **39:**65–81.

Gluckman, J. C., and Montambault, P., 1975, Spontaneous autorosette-forming cells in man: A marker for a subset population of T lymphocytes, *Clin. Exp. Immunol.* **22:**302–310.

Goldstein, R. A., and Janicki, B. W., 1974, Immunologic studies in nitrofurantoin-induced pulmonary diseases, *Med. Ann. D.C.* **43:**115.

Gottlieb, B. R., and Hanifin, J. M., 1974, Circulating T cell deficiency in atopic dermatitis, *Clin. Res.* **22:**159A (abstr.).

Greaves, M. F., Brown, G., and Rickinson, A., 1975, Receptors for Epstein–Barr virus on human B lymphocytes, *Clin. Immunol. Immunopathol.* **3:**514–524.

Grossi, C. E., Webb, S. R., Zicca, A., Lydyard, P. M., Moretta, L., Mingari, M. C., and Cooper, M. D., 1978, Morphological and histochemical analyses of two human T-cell subpopulations bearing receptor for IgM or IgG, *J. Exp. Med.* **147:**1405–1417.

Grove, D. I., Reid, J. G., and Forbes, I. F., 1975a, Humoral and cellular immunity in atopic eczema, *Br. J. Dermatol.* **92:**611–618.

Grove, D. I., Burston, T. O., Wellby, M. L., Ford, R. M., and Forbes, I. J., 1975b, Humoral and cellular immunity in asthma, *J. Allergy Clin. Immunol.* **55:**152–163.

Gupta, S., 1976, Surface markers of human T and B lymphocytes: Their profile in primary immunodeficiency, N.Y. State Med. J. **76**:24–30.

Gupta, S., 1977, Znaczniki powierzchniowe subpopulacji limfocyton ludzkich, ich znaczenie biologiczne oraz badania w niedoborach immunologicznych 1 rozrostach ukladu lemfoidalnego, *Pol. Arch. Med. Wewn.* **57**:149–172.

Gupta, S., 1978, Functionally distinct subpopulations of human T lymphocytes: A review, *Clin. Bull.* **8**:100–107.

Gupta, S., 1979, T cell subpopulations: Structure, functions and profile in normals and patients with primary immunodeficiency, lymphoproliferative and autoimmune disorders, *Pol. Arch. Wein. Med.* **61**:161–165 (Pol).

Gupta, S., and Good, R. A., 1976, Mouse erythrocyte rosette-forming immunocytes in primary immunodeficiency, *Cell. Immunol.* **27**:147–148.

Gupta, S., and Good, R. A., 1977a, Subpopulations of human T lymphocytes. I. Studies in immunodeficient patients, *Clin. Exp. Immunol.* **30**:222–228.

Gupta, S., and Good, R. A., 1977b, Subpopulations of human T lymphocytes. II. Effect of thymopoietin, corticosteroids, and irradiation, *Cell. Immunol.* **34**:10–18.

Gupta, S., and Good, R. A., 1977c, Rosette-formation with mouse erythrocytes. V. Relationship of mouse erythrocyte rosette-forming cells to cells with surface immunoglobulin and receptors for C_3 and IgG Fc in primary immunodeficiency disorders, *Clin. Immunol. Immunopathol.* **8**:520–529.

Gupta, S., and Good, R. A., 1978a, Subpopulations of human T lymphocytes. V. T lymphocytes with receptors for immunoglobulin M and G in patients with primary immunodeficiency disorders, *Clin. Immunol. Immunopathol.* **11**:292–302.

Gupta, S., and Good, R. A., 1978b, Human T cell subsets in health and disease, in: *Human Lymphocyte Differentiation: Its Application to Cancer* (B. Serrou and C. Rosenfeld, eds.), pp. 367–374, Elsevier/North-Holland Biomed Press, Amsterdam.

Gupta, S., and Good, R. A., 1978c, Subpopulations of human T lymphocytes. III. Quantitation and distribution in peripheral blood, cord blood, tonsils, bone marrow, thymus, lymph nodes and spleen, *Cell Immunol.* **36**:263–270.

Gupta, S., and Grieco, M. H., 1975, Rosette formation with mouse erythrocytes. I. A probable marker for human B lymphocytes, *Int. Arch. Allergy Appl. Immunol.* **49**:734–742.

Gupta, S., and Kapoor, N., 1979, Lymphocyte subpopulations: Surface intracellular, enzymatic markers and functions, in: *Infections Complicating the Abnormal Host* (M. H. Grieco, ed.), Yorke Medical Book, New York.

Gupta, S., Frenkel, R., Rosenstein, M., and Grieco, M. H., 1975a, Lymphocyte subpopulations, serum IgE and total eosinophil counts in patients with bronchial asthma, *Clin. Exp. Immunol.* **22**:438–445.

Gupta, S., Good, R. A., and Siegal, F. P., 1975b, Spontaneous mouse erythrocyte rosette formation with human "B" lymphocytes, *Clin. Res.* **23**:411A.

Gupta, S., Good, R. A., and Siegal, F. P., 1976a, Rosette-formation with mouse erythrocytes. III. Studies in primary immunodeficiency and lymphoproliferative disorders, *Clin. Exp. Immunol.* **26**:204–213.

Gupta, S., Ross, G. D., Good, R. A., and Siegal, F. P., 1976b, Surface markers of human eosinophils. *Blood* **48**:755–763.

Gupta, S., Pahwa, R., O'Reilly, R., Good, R. A., and Siegal, F. P., 1976c, Ontogeny of lymphocyte subpopulations in human fetal liver, *Proc. Natl. Acad. Sci. USA* **73**:919–922.

Gupta, S., Pahwa, R., Siegal, F. P., and Good, R. A., 1977, Rosette-formation with mouse erythrocytes. IV. T, B and third population cells in human tonsils, *Clin. Exp. Immunol.* **28**:347–351.

Gupta, S., Safai, B., and Good, R. A., 1978a, Subpopulations of human T lymphocytes. IV. Distribution and quantitation in patients with mycosis fungoides and Sezary syndrome, *Cell. Immunol.* **39**:18–26.

Gupta, S., Fernandes, G., Nair, M., and Good, R. A., 1978b, Spontaneous and antibody-dependent cell-mediated cytotoxicity by human T cell subpopulations, *Proc. Natl. Acad. Sci. USA* **75**:5137–5141.

Gupta, S., Schwartz, S. A., and Good, R. A., 1978c, Effect of Con A on human T cell subpopulations, *J. Allergy Clin. Immunol.* **16**:144.

Gupta, S., Safai, B., and Good, R. A., 1978d, Rosette-formation with mouse erythrocytes. VI. T, B and third population cells in mycosis fungoides and effect of leukophoresis, *Am. J. Hematol.* **4**:133–140.

Gupta, S., Schwartz, S. A., and Good, R. A., 1979a, Subpopulations of human T lymphocytes. VIII. Cellular basis of Con A induced T cell-mediated suppression of immunoglobulin production by B cells from normal humans, *Cell. Immunol.* **43**:242–251.

Gupta, S., Fikrig, S., and Good, R. A., 1979b, Effects of agents modifying cyclic nucleotide levels on T cell subsets and locomotion of T cells, *J. Allergy Clin. Immunol.* **63**:143.

Gupta, S., Kapadia, A., Kapoor, N., and Good, R. A., 1979c, Immunoregulatory T lymphocytes in patients with primary immunodeficiency disorders, *Ind. J. Med. Res.* **69**:645–650.

Hailey, F. J., Glascock, H. W., and Hewitt, W. F., 1969, Pleuropneumonic reactions to nitrofurantoin, *N. Engl. J. Med.* **281**:1087–1090.

Halbwach, L., McConnell, I., and Lachmann, P. J., 1975, The demonstration of lymphocytes of an activity resembling factor B of the alternative pathway of complement activation, in: *Membrane Receptors of Lymphocytes* (M. Seligmann, J. L. Preud'homme, and F. M. Kourilsky, eds.), pp. 141–150, American Elsevier, New York.

Hallberg, T., Gurner, B. W., and Coombs, R. R. A., 1973, Opsonic adherence of sensitized ox red cells to human lymphocytes as measured by rosette-formation, *Int. Arch. Allergy* **44**:500–513.

Hammerstrom, S., Hellstrom, U., Perlmann, P., and Dillner, M. L., 1973, A new surface marker on T-lymphocytes of human peripheral blood, *J. Exp. Med.* **138**:1270–1275.

Hanifin, J. M., and Gottlieb, B. R., 1974, IgE inhibits T-cell rosette formation, *Clin. Res.* **22**:328A.

Haynes, B. F., and Fauci, A. S., 1978, The differential effect of *in vivo* hydrocortisone on the kinetics of subpopulations of human peripheral blood thymus-derived lymphocytes, *J. Clin. Immunol.* **61**:703–707.

Hayward, A. R., and Ezer, G., 1974, Development of lymphocyte populations in the human foetal thymus and spleen, *Clin. Exp. Immunol.* **17**:169–178.

Hayward, A. R., Simons, M., Lawton, A. R., Cooper, M. D., and Mage, R. G., 1977, Pre-B and B cells in rabbits, *Fed. Proc.* **36**:1295.

Hayward, A. R., Layward, L., Lydyard, P. M., Moretta, L., Dagg, M., and Lawton, A. R., 1978, Fc receptor heterogeneity of human suppressor T cells, *J. Immunol.* **121**:1–5.

Hellstrom, U., Mellstedt, H., Perlmann, P., Holm, G., and Petterson, D., 1976, Receptors for *Helix promatia* A hemagglutinin on leukemic lymphocytes from patients with chronic lymphocytic leukemia (CLL), *Clin. Exp. Immunol.* **26**:196–203.

Hellstrom, U., Perlmann, P., Robertson, E. S., and Hammerstrom, S., 1978, Receptors for *Helix promatia* A hemagglutinin (HP) on a subpopulation of human B cells, *Scand. J. Immunol.* **7**:191–197.

Henkart, P. A., and Fisher, R. I., 1975, Characterization of the lymphocyte surface receptors for Con A and PHA, *J. Immunol.* **114**:710–714.

Hill, H. R., and Quie, P. G., 1974, Raised serum IgE level and defective neutrophil chemotaxis in three children with eczema and recurrent bacterial infections, *Lancet* **1**:183.

Hill, H. R., Williams, P. B., Krueger, G. G., and Janis, B., 1976, Recurrent staphylococcal abscesses associated with defective neutrophil chemotaxis and allergic rhinitis, *Ann. Intern. Med.* **85**:39–43.

Hoffman, D. R., 1975, Specific IgE antibodies in atopic eczema, *J. Allergy Clin. Immunol.* **55**:256.

Hoffman, D. R., Yamamoto, F. Y., Geller, B., and Haddad, Z., 1975, Specific IgE antibodies in atopic eczema, *J. Allergy Clin. Immunol.* **55**:256–267.

Holm, G., and Perlmann, P., 1967, Cytotoxic potential of stimulated human lymphocytes, *J. Exp. Med.* **125**:721–736.

Humphrey, R. E., McCune, J. M., Chess, L., Herman, H. C., Malenka, D. J., Mann, D. L., Parham, P., Schlossman, S. F., and Strominger, J., 1976, Isolation and immunologic characterization of a human B lymphocyte-specific cell surface antigens, *J. Exp. Med.* **144**:98–112.

Ishizaka, K., Ishizaka, T., Okudaira, H., and Bazin, H., 1978, Ontogeny of IgE bearing lymphocytes in the rat, *J. Immunol.* **120**:655–660.

Johansson, S. G., 1968, Raised levels of a new immunoglobulin class (IgND) in asthma, *Lancet* **2**:951–953.

Johnson, E. E., Irons, J. S., Patterson, R., and Roberts, M., 1974, Serum IgE concentration in atopic dermatitis, *J. Allergy Clin. Immunol.* **54**:95.

Jondal, M., and Klein, G., 1973, Surface markers of human T and B lymphocytes. II. Presence of Epstein-Barr virus receptors on B lymphocytes, *J. Exp. Med.* **138**:1365–1378.

Jondal, M., Wigzell, H., and Aiuti, F., 1973, Human lymphocyte subpopulations: Classification according to surface markers and/or functional characteristics, *Transplant. Rev.* **16:**163–195.

Jones, H. E., Lewis, C. W., and McMarlin, S. L., 1973, Allergic contact sensitivity in atopic dermatitis, *Arch. Dermatol.* **107:**217–222.

Kapadia, A., O'Reilly, R. J., Good, R. A., and Gupta, S., 1978, Leukocyte migration inhibition factor (LMIF) production by human T cell subpopulation, *Fed. Proc.* **37:**1365.

Kasakura, S., 1977, Blastogenic factors—Production of T and B lymphocytes, *Immunology* **33:** 23–29.

Kay, H. E. M., Doe, J., and Hockley, A., 1970, Response of human foetal thymocytes to phytohemagglutinins, *Immunology* **18:**393–396.

Kerbel, R. S., and Davies, A. J. S., 1974, The possible biological significance of Fc receptors on mammalian lymphocytes and tumor cells, *Cell* **3:**105–112.

King, T. P., Normal, P. S., and Lichtenstein, L. M., 1967, Studies on ragweed pollen allergens. V, *Ann. Allergy* **25:**541–553.

Kiskimoto, T., and Ishizaka, K., 1975, Regulation of antibody response *in vitro*. IX. Induction of secondary anti-hapten IgG antibody response by anti-immunoglobulin and enhancing factor, *J. Immunol.* **114:**585–591.

Klein, G., Yejenov, E., Falk, F., and Westman, A., 1978, Relationship between Epstein-Barr virus (EBV)-production and the loss of the EBV receptor/complement receptor complex in a series of sublines derived from the same original Burkitt's lymphoma, *Int. J. Cancer* **21:**552–560.

Knapp, W., Bolhuis, R. L. H., Radl, J., and Hijman, W., 1973, Independent movement of IgD and IgM molecules on the surface of individual lymphocytes, *J. Immunol.* **11:**1295–1298.

Knowles, D. M., Hoffman, T., Ferrarini, M., and Kunkel, H. G., 1978, The demonstration of acid α-naphthyl acetate esterase activity in human lymphocytes: Usefulness as T-cell marker, *Cell Immunol.* **35:**112–123.

Koziner, B., Fillipa, D., Mertelsmann, R., Gupta, S., Clarkson, B., Good, R. A., and Siegal, F. P., 1977, Characterization of malignant lymphomas in leukemic phase by multiple differentiation markers of mononuclear cells: Correlation with clinical features and conventional morphology, *Am. J. Med.* **64:**556–567.

Kulenkampff, J., Janossy, G., and Greaves, M. F., 1976, Acid esterase in human lymphoid cells and leukemic blasts: A marker for T lymphocytes, *Br. J. Hematol.* **36:**231–240.

Lang, P., Goel, Z., and Grieco, M. H., 1978, Subsensitivity of T lymphocytes to sympathomimetic and cholinergic stimulation in bronchial asthma, *J. Allergy Clin. Immunol.* **61:**248–254.

Larsson, A., and Perlmann, P., 1972, Study of Fab and $f(ab')_2$ from rabbit IgG for capacity to induce lymphocyte-mediated target cell destruction *in vitro, Int. Arch. Allergy* **43:**80–88.

Lee, T. P., Busse, W. W., and Reed, C. E., 1977, Effect of beta adrenergic against prostaglandins and cortisol in lymphocyte levels of cyclic adenosine monophosphate and glycogen, *J. Allergy Clin. Immunol.* **59:**408–413.

Ling, N. R., and Kay, J. E., 1975, *Lymphocyte Stimulation*, American Elsevier, New York.

Lis, H., and Sharon, N., 1973, Plant lectins, *Annu. Rev. Biochem.* **42:**541–574.

Lobitz, W. C., Jr., Honeyman, J. F., and Winkler, W. W., 1972, Suppressed cell-mediated immunity in two adults with atopic dermatitis, *Br. J. Dermatol.* **86:**317–328.

Logdon, P. J., Middleton, E., Jr., and Coffey, R. G., 1972, Stimulation of leukocyte adenyl cyclase by hydrocortisone and isoproterenol in asthmatic and nonasthmatic subjects, *J. Allergy Clin. Immunol.* **50:**45–56.

Lohrmann, H. P., and Novikovs, L., 1974, Rosette formation between human T-lymphocytes and unsensitized rhesus monkey erythrocytes, *Clin. Immunol. Immunopathol.* **3:**99–111.

Luckasen, J. R., Sabatt, A., Goltz, R. W., and Kersey, J. H., 1974, T and B lymphocytes in atopic eczema, *Arch. Dermatol.* **110:**375–377.

Lundgren, R., Böck, O., and Wiman, L. G., 1975, Pulmonary lesions and autoimmune reactions after long-term nitrofurantoin treatment, *Scand. J. Resp. Dis.* **56:**208.

MacDermott, R. P., Chess, L., and Schlossman, S. F., 1975, Immunolgic functions of isolated human lymphocyte subpopulations. V. Isolation and functional analysis of a surface negative, E rosette-negative subset, *Clin. Immunol. Immunopathol.* **4:**415–424.

Maini, R. N., Dumonde, D. C., Faux, J. A., Hargreave, F. E., and Pepys, J., 1971, The production of lymphocyte mitogenic factor and migration-inhibition factor by antigen-stimulated lymphocytes of subjects with grass-pollen allergy, *Clin. Exp. Immunol.* **9:**449–465.

Makino, S., Ikemorik, Kashima, T., and Fukada, T., 1977, Comparison of cyclic adenosine monophosphate response of lymphocytes in normal and asthmatic subjects to epinephrine and salbutanol, *J. Allergy Clin. Immunol.* **59:**348–352.

Manconi, P. A., Zaccheo, D., Bugiani, O., *et al.*, 1976, T and B lymphocytes in normal cerebrospinal fluid, *N. Engl. J. Med.* **294:**49.

Manconi, P. A., Fadda, M. F., Cadoni, A., Cornaglia, P., Zaccheo, D., and Grifoni, V., 1978, Subpopulations of T lymphocytes in human extravascular fluids, *Intl. Arch. Allergy Appl. Immunol.* **56:**385–390.

Manning, D. D., Manning, J. K., and Reed, N. K., 1976, Suppression of reaginic antibody (IgE) formation in mice by treatment with anti-μ antiserum, *J. Exp. Med.* **144:**288–292.

McConnell, I., and Hurd, C. M., 1976, Lymphocyte receptors for rabbit IgM on human T lymphocytes, *Immunology* **30:**835–840.

McConnell, I., and Lachmann, P. J., 1976, Complement and cell membranes, *Transplant. Rev.* **32:**72–92.

McGeady, S. J., and Buckley, R. H., 1975, Depression of cell-mediated immunity in atopic eczema, *J. Allergy Clin. Immunol.* **56:**393–406.

Melchers, F., Andersson, J., and Phillips, R. A., 1977, Ontogeny of murine B lymphocytes: Development of Ig synthesis and of reactivities to mitogens and to anti-Ig antibodies, *Cold Spring Harbor Symp. Quant. Biol.* **41:**147–158.

Mingari, M. C., Moretta, L., Moretta, A., Moretta, M., Ferrarini, M., and Preud'homme, J. L., 1978, Fc receptors for IgG and IgM immunoglobulins on human T lymphocytes: Mode of re-expression after proteolysis or interaction with immune complexes, *J. Immunol.* **121:**767–770.

Mitchell, J., and Abbott, A., 1965, Ultrastructure of the antigen-retaining reticulum of lymph node follicles as shown by high-resolution autoradiography, *Nature (London)* **208:**500–502.

Mizumoto, T., 1976, B and T cells in the lymphoid tissues of human appendix, *Intl. Arch. Allergy Appl. Immunol.* **51:**80.

Moretta, L., Ferrarini, M., Durante, M. L., and Mingari, M. C., 1975, Expression of a receptor for IgM by human T cells *in vitro, Eur. J. Immunol.* **5:**565–568.

Moretta, L., Ferrarini, M., Mingari, M. C., Moretta, A., and Webb, S. R., 1976, Subpopulations of human T cells identified by receptors for immunoglobulins and mitogen responsiveness, *J. Immunol.* **17:**2171–2174.

Moretta, L., Mingari, M. C., Moretta, A., and Lydyard, P. M., 1977a, Receptors for IgM are expressed on acute lymphoblastic leukemic cells having T cell characteristics, *Clin. Immunol. Immunopathol.* **7:**405–409.

Moretta, L., Webb, S. R., Grossi, C. E., Lydyard, P. M., and Cooper, M. D., 1977b, Functional analysis of two human T cell subpopulations. Help and suppression of B cell responses by T cell bearing receptors for IgM (TM) or IgG (TG), *J. Exp. Med.* **146:**184–200.

Moretta, L., Ferrarini, M., and Cooper, M. D., 1978, Characterization of human T cell subpopulations as defined by specific receptors for immunoglobulins, *Contemp. Top. Immunobiol. 8:19–53.*

Mue, S., Ise, T., Ono, T., and Takishima, T., 1975, The leukocyte phosphodiesterase activity of human bronchial asthma, *Jpn. J. Allergy* **24:**490.

Nathan, D. G., Chess, L., Hillman, D. G., Clarke, B., Breard, J., Merler, E., and Housman, D. E., 1978, Human erythroid burst-forming unit: T cell requirement for proliferation *in vitro, J. Exp. Med.* **147:**324–339.

Natvig, J. B., Salsano, F., Froland, S. S., and Seavem, P., 1975, Membrane IgD and IgM on single cells carry same idiotype, in: *Membrane Receptors of Lymphocytes* (M. Seligmann, J. L. Preud'homme, and F. M. Kourilsky, eds.), pp. 13–24, American Elsevier, New York.

Neiburger, R. G., Neiburger, J. B., and Dockhorn, R. J., 1978. Distribution of peripheral blood T and B lymphocyte markers in atopic children and changes during immunotherapy, *J. Allergy Clin. Immunol.* **61:**88–92.

Nelson, D. L., Strober, W., and Abelson, L. D., 1977, Distribution of alloantigens on human Fc receptor bearing lymphocyte: The presence of alloantigens on sIg positive (B cells) but not sIg negative lymphocytes, *J. Immunol.* **118:**943–946.

Nossal, G. J. V., and Pike, B. L., 1973, Studies on the differentiation of B lymphocytes in the mouse, *Immunology* **25:**33–45.

Nossal, G. J. V., Abbot, A., Mitchell, J., and Lummuz, Z., 1968, Antigenic immunity. XV. Ultrastructural features of antigen capture in primary and secondary lymphoid follicles, *J. Exp. Med.* **127:**277.

Nussenzweig, V., 1974, Receptors for immune complexes on lymphocytes, *Adv. Immunol.* **19:**67–216.

Ogra, S. S., and Ogra, P. L., 1978, Immunologic aspects of human colostrum and milk, *J. Pediatr.* **92**:550–555.

O'Neill, G. J., and Parrott, D. M. V., 1977, Locomotion of human lymphoid cells. I. Effect of culture and con A on T and non-T lymphocytes, *Cell Immunol.* **33**:256–267.

Ong, K. S., Grieco, M. H., and Goel, Z., 1979, Differing responses of thymus-derived lymphocytes to *in vitro* challenge by antigen E in ragweed-sensitive and ragweed-non-sensitive subjects, submitted.

Orgel, H. S., Lenoir, M. A., and Bazaral, M., 1974, Serum IgG, IgA, IgM and IgE levels and allergy in Filipino children in United States, *J. Allergy Clin. Immunol.* **53**:213–222.

Owen, F. L., and Fanger, M. W., 1974, Studies on the human T-lymphocyte population. II. The use of a T cell specific antibody in the partial isolation and characterization of the human lymphocyte receptor for sheep red blood cells, *J. Immunol.* **113**:1138–1144.

Owen, F. L., and Fanger, M. W., 1976, Studies on the human T-lymphocyte population. IV. The isolation of T-lymphocyte antigens from peripheral lymphocytes, *Immunochemistry* **13**:121–127.

Palacios, J., Fuller, E. W., and Blaylock, W. K., 1966, Immunological capabilities of patients with atopic dermatitis, *J. Invest. Dermatol.* **47**:484–492.

Papiernik, M., 1970, Correlation of lymphocyte transformation and morphology in the human fetal thymus, *Blood* **36**:470–479.

Palacios, J., Fuller, E. W., and Blaylock, W. K., 1966, Immunological capabilities of patients with atopic dermatitis, *J. Invest. Dermatol.* **47**:484.

Papiernik, M., 1970, Correlation of lymphocyte transformation and morphology in the human fetal thymus, *Blood* **36**:470.

Parker, C. W., and Smith, J. W., 1973, Alterations in cyclic adenosine monophosphate metabolism in human bronchial asthma. I. Leukocyte responsiveness to B-adrenergic agents, *J. Clin. Invest.* **52**:48–59.

Parker, C. W., Huber, M. G., and Baumann, M. L., 1973, Alterations in cyclic AMP metabolism in human bronchial asthma. III. Leukocyte and lymphocyte response to steroids, *J. Clin. Invest.* **52**:1342–1354.

Parmely, M. J., Beer, A. E., and Billingham, R. E., 1976, *In vitro* studies on the T lymphocyte population of human milk, *J. Exp. Med.* **144**:358.

Parrott, D. M. V., Good, R. A., O'Neill, G. J., and Gupta, S., 1978, Heterogeneity of locomotion of human T cell subsets, *Proc. Natl. Acad. Sci. USA* **75**:2392–2395.

Pass, F., Larsen, W. G., and Lobitz, W. C., 1966, The cultured lymphocytes of atopic patients, *Ann. Allergy* **24**:426–429.

Pearsall, H. R., Ewatt, J., Tsoi, M. S., Sumida, A., Backus, D., Winterbauer, R. H., Webb, D. R., and Jones, H., 1974, Nitrofurantoin lung sensitivity report of a case with prolonged nitrofurantoin lymphocyte sensitivity and interaction of nitrofurantoin-stimulated lymphocytes with alveolar cells, *J. Lab. Clin. Med.* **83**:728–737.

Pegrum, G. D., Ready, D., and Thompson, E., 1968, The effect of phytohemagglutinin on human foetal cells grown in culture, *Br. J. Hematol.* **15**:371.

Pelligrino, M. A., Ferrone, S., and Theofilopoulos, A. N., 1975, Rosette formation of human lymphoid cells with monkey red blood cells, *J. Immunol.* **115**:1065–1071.

Perlmann, P., and Perlmann, H., 1970, Contectual lysis of antibody-coated chicken erythrocytes by purified lymphocytes, *Cell. Immunol.* **1**:300–315.

Pichler, W. J., and Knapp, W., 1977, Receptors for IgM coated erythrocytes on chronic lymphatic leukemia cells, *J. Immunol.* **118**:1010–1015.

Pichler, W. J., and Knapp, W., 1978, Receptors for IgM on human B lymphocytes, *Scand. J. Immunol.* **7**:105–109.

Pichler, W. J., Broder, S., Gendelman, F. W., and Nelson, J. L., 1978, Cytotoxic ability of purified human B, L, Tμ and Tγ lymphocytes, *Fed. Proc.* **37**:1272.

Playfair, J. H. L., Wolfendale, M. R., and Kay, H. E. M., 1963, The leukocytes of peripheral blood in human foetus, *Br. J. Hematol.* **9**:336–344.

Preud'homme, J. L., Gonnot, M., Tspais, A., Bruet, J. C., and Minaesco, C., 1977, Human T lymphocyte receptors for IgM: Reactivity with monomeric 8 S subunits, *J. Immunol.* **119**:2206–2208.

Rabellino, E., Colon, S., Grey, H. M., and Unanue, E. R., 1971, Immunoglobulins on the surface of lymphocytes. l. Distribution and quantitation, *J. Exp. Med.* **133**:156–167.

Rachelefsky, G. S., Opelz, G., Mickey, M. R., Kinchi, M., Terasaki, P. I., Siegal, S. C., and Steihm,

E. R., 1976, Defective T cell functions in atopic dermatitis, *J. Allergy Clin. Immunol.* **57**:569–575.

Raff, M. C., Megson, M., Owen, J. J. T., and Cooper, M. D., 1976, Early production of intracellular IgM by B lymphocyte precursors in mouse, *Nature (London)* **259**:224–226.

Ranki, A., Totterman, T. H., and Hayry, P., 1976, Identification of resting human T and B lymphocytes by acid α-naphtyl-acetate esterase staining combined with rosette-formation with *Staphylococcus aureus* Strain Cowan I, *Scand. J. Immunol.* **5**:1129–1138.

Reidenberg, M. M., and Caccese, R. W., 1975, Lymphocyte transformation tests and suspected drug allergy, *J. Lab. Clin. Med.* **86**:997–1002.

Richman, C. M., Chess, L., and Yankee, R. A., 1978, Purification and characterization of granulocyte progenitor cells (CFU-c) from human peripheral blood using immunologic surface markers, *Blood* **51**:1–8.

Richter, M., and Naspitz, C. K., 1968, The *in vitro* blastogenic response of lymphocytes of ragweed sensitive individuals, *J. Allergy* **41**:140–151.

Rocklin, R. E., and David, J. R., 1971, Detection *in vitro* of cellular hypersensitivity to drugs, *J. Allergy Clin. Immunol.* **48**:276–282.

Rocklin, R. E., MacDermott, R. P., Chess, L., Schlossman, S. F., and David, J. R., 1974a, Studies on mediator production by highly purified human T and B lymphocytes, *J. Exp. Med.* **140**:1303–1316.

Rocklin, R. E., Pence, H. E., Kaplan, H., and Evans, R., 1974b, Cell-mediated immune response of ragweed-sensitive patients to ragweed antigen E. *In vitro* lymphocyte tr ansformation and eloboration of lymphocyte mediators, *J. Clin. Invest.* **53**:735–744.

Rocklin, R. E., Breard, J., Gupta, S., Good, R. A., and Melmon, K. L., 1979, Characterization of the human blood lymphocytes that produce a histamine-induced suppressor factor (HSF), submitted.

Rogge, J. L., and Hanifin, J. M., 1976, Immunodeficiencies in severe atopic dermatitis, *Arch. Dermatol.* **112**:1391–1396.

Ross, G. D., and Polley, M. J., 1974, Human lymphocytes and granulocyte receptors for the fourth component of complement (C_4) and the role of granulocyte receptors in phagocytosis, *Fed. Proc.* **33**:759.

Rosenberg, A., and Solomon, J. M., 1971, Dermatitis and infantile eczema, in: *Immunological Diseases* (M. Samter, ed.), pp. 920–933, Little, Brown, Boston.

Rosenberg, Y. J., and Parish, C. R., 1977, Ontogeny of the antibody-forming cell line in mice. IV. Appearance of cell bearing Fc receptors, complement receptors, and surface immunoglobulin, *J. Immunol.* **118**:612–617.

Ross, G. D., Polley, M. J., Rabellino, E., and Grey, H. M., 1973, Two different-complement-receptors on human lymphocytes. One specific for C_3b and one specific for C_3b inactivator-cleaved C_3b, *J. Exp. Med.* **138**:798–811.

Rostenberg, A., and Sulzberger, M. B., 1937, Some results of patch tests, *Arch. Dermatol. Syphilol.* **35**:433.

Sakane, T., and Green, I., 1978, Protein A from *Staphylococcus aureus*—a mitogen for human T lymphocytes and B lymphocytes but not L lymphocytes, *J. Immunol.* **120**:302–311.

Salsano, F., Froland, S. S., Natvig, J. B., and Michaelson, T. E., 1974, Same idiotype of B lymphocyte membrane IgD and IgM: Formal evidence for monoclonality of chronic lymphocytic leukemia cells, *Scand. J. Immunol.* **3**:841–846.

Samarut, C., Gebuhrer, L., Brochier, J., Betnel, H., and Revillard, J. P., 1977, Presence of "Ia-like" antigens on human T lymphocytes bearing receptors for IgG, *Eur. J. Immunol.* **7**:908–910.

Sandilands, G., Gray, K., Cooney, A., Browning, J. D., and Anderson, J. R., 1974, Autorosette-formation by human thymocytes and lymphocytes, *Lancet* **1**:27.

Saraclar, Y., McGeady, S. J., and Mansmann, H. C., 1977, Lymphocyte subpopulations of atopic children and the effect of therapy upon them, *J. Allergy Clin. Immunol.* **60**:301–305.

Scheffer, A. L., Rocklin, R. E., and Goetzl, E. J., 1975, Immunologic components of hypersensitivity reactions to cromolyn sodium; *N. Engl. J. Med.* **293**:1220–1224.

Schmidtke, J., and Unanue, E. R., 1971, Interaction of macrophages and lymphocytes with surface immunoglobulin, *Nature (London) New Biol.* **223**:84–86.

Schwartz, S. A., Shou, L., Good, R. A., and Choi, Y. S., 1977, Suppression of immunoglobulin synthesis and secretion by peripheral blood lymphocytes from normal donors, *Proc. Natl. Acad. Sci. USA* **74**:2099–2103.

Secher, L., Svejgaard, E., and Hansen, G. S., 1977, T and B lymphocytes in contact and atopic dermatitis, *Br. J. Dermatol.* **97**:537–541.

Shou, L., Schwartz, S. A., and Good, R. A., 1976, Suppressor cell activity after Con A treatment of lymphocytes from normal donors, *J. Exp. Med.* **143**:1100–1110.

Siegal, F. P., and Good, R. A., 1977, Human lymphocyte differentiation markers and their application to immune deficiency and lymphoproliferative disease, *Clin. Hematol.* **6**:355–422.

Snyderman, R., Rogers, E., and Buckley, R. H., 1977, Abnormalities of leukotaxis in atopic dermatitis, *J. Allergy Clin. Immunol.* **60**:121–126.

Sobel, A. T., and Bokish, V. A., 1975, Receptors for C_4b and C_{1q} on human peripheral lymphocytes and lymphoblastoid cells, in: *Membrane Receptors of Lymphocytes* (M. Seligmann, J. L. Preud'homme, and F. M. Kourilsky, eds), pp. 151–160, American Elsevier, New York.

Sokol, W. N., and Beall, G. N., 1975, Leukocyte epinephrine receptors of normal and asthmatic individuals, *J. Allergy Clin. Immunol.* **55**:310–324.

Solomon, J. B., 1971, *Fetal and Neonatal Immunology,* American Elsevier, New York.

Sondel, P. M., Chess, L., MacDermott, R. P., and Schlossman, S. F., 1975a, Immunologic functions of isolated human lymphocyte subpopulations. III. Specific allogeneic lympholysis mediated by human T cells alone, *J. Immunol.* **114**:982–987.

Sondel, P. M., Chess, L., and Schlossman, S. F., 1975b, Immunologic functions of isolated human lymphocyte subpopulations. IV. Stimulation of MLC and CML by human T cells, *Cell Immunol.* **18**:351–359.

Stathopoulos, A., and Elliott, E. V., 1974, Formation of mouse or sheep red blood cell rosettes by lymphocytes from normal and leukemic individuals, *Lancet* **1**:600–602.

Stein, H., and Miller-Hormelink, H. K., 1977, Simultaneous presence of receptors for complement and sheep red blood cells on human fetal thymocytes, *Br. J. Hematol.* **36**:225–230.

Stites, D. P., Carr, M. C., and Fudenberg, H. H., 1972, Development of cellular immunity in the human fetus: Dichotomy of proliferative and cytotoxic responses of lymphoid cell to phytohemagglutinin, *Proc. Natl. Acad. Sci. USA* **69**:1440–1444.

Stites, D. P., Caldwell, J. P., Carr, M. C., and Fudenberg, H. H., 1975, Ontogeny of immunity in humans, *Clin. Immunol. Immunopathol.* **4**:519–527.

Stites, D. P., Carr, M. C., and Fudenberg, H. H., 1976, Ontogeny of cellular immunity in human fetus: Development of responses to phytohemagglutinin and to allogeneic cells, *Cell. Immunol.* **11**:257–271.

Stout, R. D., Waksal, S. D., and Herzenberg, L. A., 1976, The Fc receptor on thymus derived lymphocytes. III. Mixed lymphocyte reactivity and cell-mediated lymphocytic activity of Fc^- and Fc^+ T lymphocytes, *J. Exp. Med.* **144**:54–68.

Strannegard, I. L., and Strannegard, O., 1977, Influence of serum from atopic children on T lymphocytes, *Int. Arch. Allergy Appl. Immunol.* **55**:217–227.

Strannegard, I. L., Lindholm, and Strannegard, O., 1976, T lymphocytes in atopic children. *Intl. Arch. Allergy Appl. Immunol.* **56**:684–692.

Thomas, D. B., and Phillips, B., 1973, Membrane antigens specific for human lymphoid cells in the dividing phase, *J. Exp. Med.* **138**:64–70.

Thomson, N. C., Sandilands, G. P., Gray, K., and Reid, F., 1977, Increase in peripheral blood "null" cells in extrinsic bronchial asthma, *Clin. Exp. Immunol.* **30**:429–433.

Totterman, T. H., Ranki, A., and Hayry, P., 1977, Expression of the acid α-naphthyl-acetate esterase marker by activated and secondary T lymphocytes in man, *Scand. J. Immunol.* **6**:305–310.

Touraine, J. L., Touraine, F., Kiszkiss, D. F., Choi, Y. S., and Good, R. A., 1974, Heterologous specific antiserum for identification of human T lymphocytes, *Clin. Exp. Immunol.* **16**:502–520.

Touraine, J. L., Hadden, J. W., and Good, R. A., 1977, Sequential stages of human T lymphocyte differentiation, *Proc. Natl. Acad. Sci. USA* **74**:3414–3418.

Trinchieri, G., and de Marchi, M., 1975, Antibody-dependent cell-mediated cytotoxicity in humans. II. Energy requirement. *J. Immunol.* **115**:256–260.

Trinchieri, G., Bauman, P., de Marchi, M., and Tokes, Z., 1975, Antibody-dependent-cell-mediated cytotoxicity in humans. I. Characterization of the effector cell, *J. Immunol.* **115**:249–255.

Van Scoy, R. E., Hill, H. R., Ritts, R. E., Jr., and Quie, P. G., 1975, Familial neutrophil chemotaxis defect, recurrent bacterial infections, mucocutaneous candidiasis and hyperimmunoglobulinemia E, *Ann. Intern. Med.* **82**:766–777.

Verhaegen, H., DeCock, W., and DeCree, J., 1977, Histamine receptor-bearing peripheral T lymphocytes in patients with allergies, *J. Allergy Clin. Immunol.* **59**:266–268.

Vogler, L. B., Pearl, E. R., Gathings, W. E., Lawton, A. R., and Cooper, M. D., 1976, B lymphocyte precursors in bone marrow in immunoglobulin deficiency diseases, *Lancet* **2**:376.

Vossen, J. M., and Hijman, S. W., 1975, Membrane associated immunoglobulin determinants on bone marrow and blood lymphocytes in the pediatric age group and in fetal tissues, *Ann. N.Y. Acad. Sci.* **254**:262–279.

Waxdal, M. J., 1975, Differential stimulation of murine T and B cell populations by purified mitogens from pokeweed, in: *Immune Recognition* (A. S. Rosenthal, ed.), Academic Press, New York.

Webster, A. W., and Thompson, R. A., 1974, The ampicillin rash lymphocyte transformation by ampicillin polymer, *Clin. Exp. Immunol.* **18**:553–564.

Weisberg, S. C., Pan, P. M., and Mathews, K. P., 1972, The effects of pollen extracts on *in vitro* ^{3}H thymidine uptake of lymphocytes from normal individuals, *J. Allergy Clin. Immunol.* **49**:125 (abstr).

Wernet, P., 1976, Human Ia-type alloantigens: Methods of detection, aspects of chemistry and biology. Markers for disease states, *Transplant. Rev.* **30**:271–295.

Wernet, P., Winchester, R., and Kunkel, H. G., 1975, Serological detection and partial characterization of human MLC determinants with special reference to B-cell specificity, *Transplant. Proc. Suppl.* **1(7)**:193–200.

West, W., Boozer, R. B., and Herberman, R. B., 1978, Low affinity E rosette formation by the human K cells, *J. Immunol.* **120**:90–95.

Winchester, R. J., Ross, G. D., Jarowski, C. I., and Broxmeyer, H. E., 1977, Expression of Ia-like antigen molecules on human granulocytes during early phases of differentiation, *Proc. Natl. Acad. Sci. USA* **74**:4012–4016.

Winchester, R. J., Meyers, P. A., Broxmeyer, H. E., Wang, C. Y., Moore, M. A. S., and Kunkel, H. G., 1978, Inhibition of human erythropoietic colony formation in culture by treatment with Ia antisera, *J. Exp. Med.* **148**:613–618.

Wisloff, F., and Froland, S. S., 1973, Antibody-dependent lymphocyte-mediated cytotoxicity in man: No requirement for lymphocytes with membrane-bound immunoglobulins, *Scand. J. Immunol.* **2**:151–157.

Wisloff, F., Froland, S. S., and Michaelson, T. E., 1974a, Antibody-dependent cytotoxicity mediated by human Fc receptor bearing cells lacking markers for B and T lymphocytes, *Int. Arch. Allergy Appl. Immunol.* **47**:139–154.

Wisloff, F., Michaelson, T. E., and Froland, S. S., 1974b, Inhibition of antibody-dependent human lymphocyte-mediated cytotoxicity in immunoglobulin classes, IgG subclasses, and IgG fragments, *Scand. J. Immunol.* **3**:29–38.

Woody, J. N., Ahmed, A., Knudsen, R. C., Strong, D. M., and Sell, K. W., 1975, Human T-cell heterogeneity as delineated with a specific human thymus lymphocyte antiserum. *In vitro* effects on mitogen response, mixed leukocyte culture, cell-mediated lymphocytotoxicity and lymphokine production, *J. Clin. Invest.* **55**:956–966.

Wybran, J., Carr, M. C., and Fudenberg, H. H., 1972, The human rosette-forming cell as a marker of a population of thymus-derived cells, *J. Clin. Invest.* **51**:2537–2543.

Wybran, J., Carr, M. C., and Fudenberg, H. H., 1973, Effect of serum on human rosette forming cells in fetuses and adult blood, *Clin. Immunol. Immunopathol.* **1**:408–413.

Yata, J., Tsukimoto, I., and Tachibana, T., 1973, Human lymphocyte subpopulations: Human thymus-lymphoid tissue (HTL) antigen-positive lymphocytes forming rosettes with sheep erythrocytes and HTL antigen-negative lymphocytes interacting with antigen-antibody-complement complexes, *Clin. Exp. Immunol.* **14**:319–326.

Yocum, M. W., Strong, D. M., and Lakin, J. D., 1976, Competent cellular immunity in allergic rhinitis patients with elevated IgE, *J. Allergy Clin. Immunol.* **57**:384–388.

Zeitz, S. J., Van Arsdel, P. P., Jr., and McClure, D. K., 1966, Specific response of human lymphocytes to pollen antigens in tissue culture, *J. Allergy* **38**:321–329.

4

Molecular Properties of Allergens

T. P. KING

1. Allergens or Antigens

A wide variety of natural or synthetic substances which are foreign to the host can act as antigens or immunogens to induce immunological responses in man and animals. Most immunological responses are beneficial for the host, but some are not. The immunological responses harmful to the host are called "hypersensitivity" or "allergy." Allergic responses are classified into two types, immediate and delayed, on the basis of the lag in their appearance following challenge with allergen. The immediate type is mediated by specific antibodies of different immunoglobulin classes, while the delayed type is mediated by specifically activated T lymphocytes. The immediate type is further divided into those mediated by antibodies of the IgE class and those mediated by antibodies of Ig classes other than IgE; the IgE-mediated allergy is also known as "atopy." The chemical nature of the cellular component of T lymphocytes responsible for delayed-type allergy is as yet unknown.

Antigens which can induce any of the above forms of allergic responses are termed "allergens." Allergens involved in the IgE-mediated hypersensitivity are called "atopic allergens." Frequently, the term "allergen" is used to designate solely atopic allergen. In this chapter the broader definition of "allergen" is used.

The known antigens or allergens are usually proteins or polysaccharides, and, less commonly, polypeptides, nucleic acids, or low-molecular-weight chemicals which can form conjugates with body proteins. These portions of the antigen molecule which react with the specific antigen-binding receptor molecules of lymphocytes are termed "antigenic determinants." The antigenic determinants generated on reaction of low-molecular-weight chemicals with macromolecules are designated haptens.

T. P. KING • The Rockefeller University, New York, New York 10021.

The purpose of this chapter is to review some of the known findings of antigenic determinants of different antigens. These findings show that antigens which induce allergic responses are not different from those which do not. Induction of allergic responses does not depend on any specific chemical nature of antigens, but it does depend on the genetic control of the immunized individual and the mode of presentation of the antigen to the individual.

2. Types of Antigenic Determinants

Humoral antibody responses on antigen stimulation are known to require the collaboration of T and B lymphocytes. This has been shown for IgA, IgE, and IgG antibody responses (Katz and Benacerraf, 1972; Ishizaka, 1976; Tada, 1975). B cells are the precursors of antibody-secreting plasma cells. There are different subclasses of B cells specific for each Ig class of antibodies. T cells, in addition to their roles in delayed hypersensitivity and in cellular cytotoxicity (Dennert, 1976), possess helper (Claman and Chaperon, 1969) and suppressor (Gershon, 1974) functions for the regulation of antibody production by T and B cells. Studies of cell surface antigen markers have established that helper and suppressor cells are distinct subclasses of T cells (Cantor and Boyse, 1977).

The antigen receptor molecules of B lymphocytes are known to be conventional antibodies of different immunoglobulin classes. The antigen receptors of T lymphocytes have not yet been characterized biochemically. Analysis with antiidiotypic antibodies suggests that there is a close similarity between the specificities of T- and B-cell antigen-binding receptors (Binz and Wigzell, 1977; Rajewsky and Eichman, 1977). The close similarity of T- and B-cell antigen receptors suggests that their receptors can recognize and combine with the same antigenic determinants. However, this does not exclude the possibility that some antigenic determinants may have specificity or differential affinities for T and B cells of different subclasses.

As outlined earlier, both T and B lymphocytes are involved in allergy of the immediate type, while only T lymphocytes are involved in allergy of the delayed type. Therefore, an understanding of the antigenic determinants relevant to allergy of the immediate type will include the antigenic determinants for specific T and B cells which are active in antibody synthesis and in regulation of antibody synthesis, while an understanding of the antigenic determinants relevant to allergy of the delayed type will include the antigenic determinants for specific T cells which are active in cellular immunity and in its regulation.

3. B-Cell-Specific Antigenic Determinants

Most of our knowledge of B-cell-specific antigenic determinants is derived from studying the interactions of antigens with their specific IgG antibodies. At present, we have only limited or indirect data on the antigenic determinants reacting with antibodies of the other classes of immunoglobulins.

3.1. Experimental Approaches

All naturally occurring antigens contain several antigenic determinants. For example, the globular proteins sperm whale myoglobin and chicken egg white lysozyme, with molecular weights of 18,400 and 13,930, respectively, both contain at least five determinants reacting with IgG antibodies (Atassi, 1977; Atassi and Habeeb, 1977). The general approach for studying the determinants of a multivalent antigen involves selective cleavages at several different regions of the antigen molecules so that a series of overlapping fragments can be isolated and tested for their antigenic activities with specific IgG antibodies. To establish the minimal size and the key amino acid residues required for antigenic activity, further degradations of the active fragment, or, alternatively, of synthetic analogues of the active fragment, are made and studied.

The activities of the fragments in combining with the antigen-specific antibodies are measured either directly or indirectly. The direct method involves the use of radiolabeled fragments to follow the fragment–antibody interaction. The indirect method involves the inhibition of the antigen–antibody interaction by the fragment as measured by the decrease of the amount of immune precipitate formed or by the decrease of the amount of complement fixed. Most reported studies were made with whole-animal antisera. These findings may be taken to represent those of IgG-specific determinants, since the major antibody component of all hyperimmune animal antiprotein sera is of the IgG class.

A quantitative measure of the antigenic activity of a determinant is defined by its affinity constant for the specific antibody. The data from antigenically active peptides isolated from chicken egg white lysozyme indicate that the affinity constant of determinant–antibody interaction is in the range of 10^4–10^6 M^{-1} (Pecht *et al.*, 1971; Ha *et al.*, 1975). The affinity constant of a determinant in the interact protein can be several orders higher than that of the same determinant studied as an isolated small peptide because of possible conformational changes of the peptide segment on its separation from the remainder of the protein molecule (see below).

Detection of antigenic determinants with affinity constants less than 10^3 M^{-1} is difficult by the direct procedure described above. For example, in the direct-binding test, with antibody and test fragment concentrations both at 10^{-5} M, less than 1% of the fragment will be bound when the affinity constant is 10^3 M^{-1}. An antibody concentration of 10^{-5} M corresponds to that of a good antiserum with 1.6 mg/ml of antibody. In the inhibition of antigen–antibody precipitin reaction, where the concentration of test fragment is increased to 10^{-2} M (1000 times larger than that of antigen), it is possible to detect determinants with affinity constants of about 10^2 M^{-1}. However, the problem of contamination becomes serious when such large excesses of test fragments are used relative to the antigen.

The above procedures cannot be used for measuring antigenic determinant–IgE antibody interactions because serum total IgE levels for man and experimental animals are only in the range of μg/ml or less (Ishizaka, 1973). The specific IgE antibody levels must be less than μg/ml, corresponding to a molar concentration of less than 6 nM. The low serum concentration of IgE antibody means that it will be more difficult to detect determinants with weak affinity constants unless one can work with IgE-enriched fractions, which in practice are difficult to obtain. The low IgE antibody concentration requires specialized techniques for its detection. The most commonly used *in vitro* procedures for measuring human IgE antibodies are histamine-release assays from sensitive leukocytes and radioallergosorbent tests (RAST) (Adkinson and Lichtenstein, 1976; Johansson *et al.*, 1972).

Histamine-release assay is selective for IgE antibodies because only IgE molecules are bound to basophilic leukocytes and mast cells, while IgG molecules are not. Histamine release takes place in a dose-dependent fashion from IgE-sensitized leukocytes on challenge with appropriate antigen. Reaction of univalent antigenic fragment with cell-bound antibody does not lead to histamine release. Univalent antigenic fragments can be detected by their inhibition of histamine release on challenge with antigen.

In RAST, a solid adsorbent containing antigen is incubated with immune sera to adsorb antibodies of all classes, and the amount of IgE antibodies adsorbed is quantitated by a second adsorption with radiolabeled specific anti-IgE antibody. RAST is said to be sensitive in the range of picogram quantities of IgE antibody. For assaying antigens or their fragments, the procedure can be modified as an inhibition assay, that is, in the initial step of RAST, soluble antigen or fragment competes with insoluble antigen for antibodies (Foucard *et al.*, 1972).

3.2. Antigenic Determinants Reacting with IgG Antibodies: Size, Structure, and Conformation

Using the experimental approach described above, the antigenic determinants of several globulin protein antigens have been determined. These studies have been summarized in detail in several review articles (Arnon, 1974; Atassi, 1977; Benjamini *et al.*, 1972; Crumpton, 1974; Goodman, 1975; Sachs, 1974). The salient features from these studies will be given below.

The minimal size of a peptide antigenic determinant appears to be in the range of four to eight amino acid residues. This conclusion is indicated not only for the data of globular proteins but also for those of synthetic polypeptides of known repeating sequences and polypeptidyl–protein conjugates (Sage *et al.*, 1964; Arnon *et al.*, 1965; Schechter *et al.*, 1970). Antigenic determinants of polysaccharides and nucleic acids are approximately of the same size as those of proteins, and they contain about five monosaccharides or mononucleotides (Kabat, 1966).

Studies on the minimal size of peptide determinants are complicated by conformational differences in the intact and the degraded molecules. In all globular proteins, the long polypeptide chain is folded into a unique conformation. This conformation is stabilized by cooperative noncovalent interactions of the spatially or sequentially adjacent amino acid residues such as hydrogen bonds, ionic bonds, and hydrophobic bonds. When a peptide fragment is excised from the protein molecule, some of the stabilizing noncovalent interactions may be lost, and the flexible peptide can take on a wide spectrum of conformations. In assays for antigen activity, only the fraction of the peptide molecules having a conformation identical to that in the native antigen will interact with the antigen-specific antibody, and this will be reflected as a decreased affinity constant (Sachs, 1974).

To avoid the complication of conformation, Schechter *et al.* (1970) approached the problem of minimal size of antigenic determinants by the use of different protein immunogens to which peptides of defined structures (D-Ala)$_n$-Gly (n = 1–4) were attached. These short alanyl peptides were chosen because they are unlikely to assume ordered conformations. Cross-precipitation and inhibition tests were made with such antisera, using peptides of the general structure (D-Ala)$_n$ = 1–4) and (D-Ala)$_n$-Gly-ϵ-aminocaproic acid (n = 1–3) as inhibitors. The results showed that in all instances the determinant was a tetraalanine and that the lysyl residue of the protein carrier participated in the determinant only when the conjugated hapten was smaller than a tetrapeptide.

The antigenic determinants of proteins can be composed of amino acid residue sequentially adjacent to each other in the primary structure of the molecule or spatially adjacent but distant in the primary structure. Both types are known to be present in globular proteins, and they have been designated as "sequential" and "conformational" determinants (Sela, 1972). These two terms are convenient for the purpose of distinguishing the two types of determinants, but it is important to note that, as described earlier, the sequential determinants are dependent on the conformation of the molecule, just as the conformational determinants are.

In Table 1 are listed the IgG-specific antigenic determinants of two globular proteins, sperm whale myoglobin and chicken egg white lysozyme. Because of their known exact three-dimensional structures, the antigenic determinants of these two proteins were intensively studied in several laboratories (Arnon, 1974; Atassi, 1977; Crumptom, 1974; Ha *et al.*, 1975). The indicated antigenic determinants of myoglobin are all of the sequential type while those of lysozyme are of the conformational type. With both proteins, an admixture of their respective peptides indicated in Table 1 was found to inhibit better than 80% of the precipitin reaction of the native protein with its specific antisera. Essentially the same findings were obtained with several goat or rabbit antisera. However, there is some variation in the extent of contribution of each peptide to the overall specificity of each individual serum.

The antigenic determinants listed in Table 1 are about equally rich in polar and nonpolar amino acid residues. For the polar residues, they appear to contain more basic amino acid residues than acidic residues. This preponderance of basic amino acid residues is probably not of general significance because there are major antigenic determinants of other proteins, e.g., tobacco mosaic virus protein (Benjamini *et al.*, 1972), which are free of basic amino acid residues.

TABLE 1. Known Antigenic Determinants of Two Globular Proteins[a]

A.	Sperm whale myoglobin
	16 21
Site 1	Lys • Val • Glu • Ala • Asp • Val
	56 62
Site 2	Lys • Ala • Ser • Glu • Asp • Leu • Lys
	94 99
Site 3	Ala • Thr • Lys • His • Lys • Ile
	113 119
Site 4	His • Val • Leu • His • Ser • Arg • His
	145 151
Site 5	Lys • Tyr • Lys • Glu • Leu • Gly • Tyr
B.	Chicken egg white lysozyme
	6 7 13 14 125 126 128
Site 1	Cys • Glu • • • Lys • Arg • • • Arg • Gly • • • Arg
	62 87 89 93 96 97
Site 2	Trp • • • Asp • • • Thr • • • Asn • • • Lys • Lys
	33 34 113 114 116
Site 3	Lys • Phe • • • Asn • Arg • • • Lys •

[a] From Atassi (1977) and Atassi and Habeeb (1977).

The antigenic determinants in Table 1 also do not reveal any apparent distinguishing amino acid sequence or spatial arrangement of these residues, as compared to other portions of protein molecules which are immunologically inactive. A notable common feature of these determinants is their location in the known three-dimensional structure of the molecule. They are located at or near the corners of the folded polypeptide chain, and these corners usually represent the more exposed surface areas of the molecule. Similar findings were also made with another protein antigen of known tertiary structure, staphylococcal nuclease (Sachs, 1974).

It is noted that, while a peptide antigenic determinant is composed of four to eight amino acid residues, these residues do not necessarily contribute equally to the overall specificity (binding) of the determinant for the antibody-combining region. That is, one of these residues, because of its accessibility, makes a major contribution to the specificity of the determinant, and such a determinant is termed "immunodominant" (Lüderitz *et al.*, 1966). For example, haptenic groups which form part of the antigenic determinants of a protein are immunodominant because the binding energy of the determinant for the specific antibodies is determined primarily by the hapten portion of the molecule.

The general conclusion from the preceding paragraphs is that a globular protein contains a finite number of antigenic determinants of well-defined structures and sizes which react with IgG antibodies. These determinants are dependent on the conformation of the molecule, and they are located on the more exposed surface areas of the molecule. The determinants are recognized by all the animals tested, but their immunopotencies are not the same in individual animals.

3.3. Antigenic Determinants Reacting with IgM Antibodies

Most studies on antigenic determinants have been made with whole animal antisera. Because IgG antibodies are known to be the major components, the results are taken to indicate the specificity of the determinants reacting with the IgG class of antibodies. In one reported instance where separated IgG and IgM antibodies [from rabbit antisera specific for a protein conjugate with D-$(\mathrm{Ala})_n$ peptide] were used, antibody-combining sites of identical specificity and size were observed. Therefore, an antigenic determinant can have common specificity for an IgG and IgM antigen-binding site.

3.4. Antigenic Determinants Reacting with IgE Antibodies

No detailed characterization of IgE-specific antigenic determinants has yet been carried out even though many proteins, and, less frequently, polysaccharides, can induce both IgE and IgG responses in man and in experimental animals (*cf.* King, 1976). This lack is probably in part related to the following two experimental problems: the very low serum IgE antibody level relative to the IgG antibody levels, and the difficulty of inducing sustained IgE antibody responses in appropriate animal models. The second problem has been overcome with the findings that IgE antibody response is much more sensitive than IgG antibody response to the effects of adjuvant, dose of antigen, route of immunization, and genetic makeup of the host (Levine and Vaz, 1970).

Many of the atopic allergens are well-characterized proteins (*cf.* King, 1976). They are free of any unusual chemical groups, and they do not possess any special biochemical function. The only apparent structural requirement of an atopic allergen is the same as that of an antigen, namely, that it is foreign to the immunized host. Atopic allergy in man is believed to be under genetic control, because there is association of a person's sensitivity to a particular antigen with his major histocompatibility antigen (Marsh, 1975; Marsh *et al.*, 1977). The capability of several atopic allergens to react with IgE antibodies, as well as with IgG antibodies, is readily decreased by greater then a thousandfold on denaturation, chemical modification of its side chains, or proteolysis, as has been shown for the major allergens of ragweed and rye grass pollen, codfish, and bee venom. These results show that atopic allergens are like other globular protein antigens in that they give similar changes on such treatments. They also show that the majority of IgE-specific determinants or proteins are like the IgG-specific determinants. That is, they consist of only amino acid residues which are arranged in specific spatial arrays.

At present, we still lack data on the exact structure and size of an antigenic determinant of a protein allergen reacting with IgE antibodies. However, it is likely that antigenic determinants of a protein which react with IgE and IgG antibodies are the same, although the same determinant may have different affinities for IgE and IgG antibodies. This suggestion is based on the following considerations: First, the properties of IgE- and IgG-specific antigenic determinants of proteins are similar, as described above. Second, hapten–protein conjugates, e.g., penicilloyl proteins (Levine, 1972), are known to induce, in experimental animals and in man, the same hapten-specific IgE, IgG, and IgM antibodies. Third, the structural similarity of IgE and IgG molecules (Johansson *et al.*, 1972) suggests that both molecules may have the same kind of specificity.

4. T-Cell-Specific Antigenic Determinants

4.1. Experimental Approaches

T-cell antigen receptors have yet to be characterized and studied fully in solution. Therefore, it is not possible to determine directly the interaction of T-cell determinants with their specific receptors. Instead, recourse is made to study the interaction of determinants and their receptors at the functional level of cellular immune responses *in vitro* or *in vivo*.

There are three widely used techniques for studying cell-mediated immune responses (Morley *et al.*, 1973; Bloom and Glade, 1971). One is the delayed-type hypersensitivity following skin testing of the sensitized animal with the antigen or its fragments. The skin reaction is due to release of inflammatory mediator factor(s) following combination of antigen with its specific cellular antigen receptor. The second technique is the *in vitro* transformation of lymphocytes from sensitized donors. Lymphocyte transformation into blast cells takes place because of the release of mitogenic factor(s) on combination of antigen with its specific cellular receptor. The transformation is followed by the incorporation of thymidine into DNA of dividing cells. The third technique is the inhibition of macrophage migration from capillary tubes (MIF). Migration is inhibited because of release of mediator factors on combination of antigen with its specific cellular receptor; usually peritoneal exudate cells from sensitized donors, containing a mixture of lymphocytes and macrophages, are used.

It is not known whether a single subclass or different subclasses of T cells are involved in the above tests. Also, the role of antigenic valency in the above tests is not clear. There is agreement that a univalent antigen is active in skin tests and in inhibition of macrophage migration. But there is disagreement that a univalent antigen is active in lymphocyte transformation (Goodman *et al.*, 1974; Levy *et al.*, 1972; Spitler *et al.*, 1972).

While T-helper and T-suppressor cells can be differentiated by their cell surface alloantigens, T-helper cells and T cells mediating delayed-type hypersensitivity T-(DTH) cannot be so differentiated (Cantor and Boyse, 1977). Are T-helper and T-DTH cells the same? Do T-helper, T-suppressor, and T-DTH cells release the same mediator factors on reaction with antigens? Answers to these questions are not yet available. Therefore, it is not clear that the three techniques described above for studying cell-mediated immunity (delayed-type hypersensitivity) also measure the interaction of antigenic determinants with specific T-helper or T-suppressor cells. At present, there is no reported simple *in vitro* test for studying the interaction of determinants with specific T-helper or T-suppressor cells.

4.2. Size, Structure, and Conformation

T-DTH-cell determinants of protein antigens, like their B-cell determinants, are located on the surface of the molecules. This is illustrated by the studies on lysozyme (Miyagawa *et al.*, 1975a,b); the same set of lysozyme peptides, which contain residues located on the surface of the molecule, are dominant both in their binding with antilysozyme antibodies and in cell-mediated immunity.

The size of T-DTH-cell determinants for protein antigens appears to be in the range of tetra- to octapeptides, as is illustrated by studies of peptides from bovine encephalitogenic protein (Spitler *et al.*, 1972; Bergstrand and Källen, 1973), oxidized ferrodoxin (Levy *et al.*, 1972), and tobacco mosaic virus protein (Benjamini, 1977). Another observation in support of this conclusion is that guinea pigs responsive to polylysine develop cellular immunity when immunized with peptides larger than hexalysine (Schlossman *et al.*, 1969). For certain other chemicals which can serve as T-DTH cell determinants, their size can be even smaller than that of a tetrapeptide. This is illustrated by the report that L-tyrosine-*p*-azobenzenearsonate (molecular weight 409), and some of its derivatives can induce cellular immunity in guinea pigs (Leskowitz *et al.*, 1966; Alkan *et al.*, 1972).

Several protein antigens are known to contain some, if not all, antigenic determinants which have common specificity for humoral and cellular immunities. This was shown for lysozyme (Miyagawa *et al.*, 1975a,b), tobacco mosaic virus protein (Benjamini, 1977), and oxidized ferrodoxin (Levy *et al.*, 1972). On the other hand, studies with glucagon (a 29-residue peptide) showed that the antigenic determinants specific for humoral and cellular immunities were concentrated mainly in the amino-terminal 17 residues and the carboxyl-terminal 12 residues, respectively. However, when glucagon was used as an immunogen in the form of a conjugate with albumin, both halves of the glucagon molecule were equally important as determinants for antibody response (Senyk *et al.*, 1972). In addition to these examples of protein antigens, several haptens were shown to elicit both humoral and cellular immune responses in man and in experimental animals, for example, the penicilloyl group (Redmond and Levine, 1968) and the 2,4-dinitrophenyl group (Janeway, 1976). These findings taken together indicate that an antigenic determinant can have common specificity for both T- and B-cell antigen receptors and that such a determinant can bind T and B receptors with different affinities under different conditions.

Studies have also suggested the common specificity of B-cell and T-helper-cell determinants, since the capacity of heterologous albumins to serve as hapten carriers in determining secondary antihapten responses correlated well with their cross-reactivity at the antibody level (Rajewsky and Eichman, 1977).

A distinguished feature of T-cell determinants for protein antigens is the apparent lack of conformational dependence, which is in sharp contrast to the B-cell determinants. This is indicated by the cross-reactivity of native and denatured proteins in cellular immunity (Gell and Benacerraf, 1961). A recent example is the cross-reactivity of lysozyme and its fully reduced and carboxymethylated derivative in cell-mediated immunity (Thompson *et al.*, 1972).

The cross-reactivity of native and denatured proteins may also be present at the level of T-helper and/or T-suppressor cells, as suggested by the following findings: Antigen E, the major allergen of ragweed pollen, can be denatured on treatment with urea. The denatured antigen lacks the B-cell-specific determinants, as it did not react with anti-antigen E antibodies. Nor did the denatured antigen induce in mice or rabbits production of antibodies specific for the native antigen. The denatured antigen apparently retains the T-cell-specific determinants of the native antigen since pretreatment of mice with the denatured antigen primed the animals for both IgE and IgG antibody responses to the native antigen E (Ishizaka *et al.*, 1975). Also, repeated treatments of antigen-E-sensitized mice with the denatured antigen suppressed the ongoing IgE and IgG antibody responses to the native antigen (Takatsu *et al.*, 1975).

The lack of conformational dependence of protein antigens in cell-mediated immunity does not necessarily indicate that B- and T-cell determinants are structurally different. It may possibly be a consequence of differences in the affinities of T- and B-cell antigen receptors for their determinants. That is, the high affinity of a T-cell receptor for its specific determinant can compensate for the unfavorable equilibrium of ordered and disordered conformations.

5. Concluding Remarks

In all mammalian species studied, the ability of an individual to mount an immune response on challenge with specific antigens is known to be under genetic control; the genes involved reside in the chromosomal region known as the major histocompatibility gene complex (Benacerraf and McDevitt, 1972). As postulated in the clonal selection theory (Burnet, 1959), each individual possesses a set of lymphocyte antigen receptors of defined specificities. These specificities are determined by the genetic makeup of the individual. Only when the individual is challenged with an antigen meeting the specificities of the lymphocyte receptors will there be evoked a humoral or cellular immune response. Therefore, the specificity of an immune response rests on the individual under immunization as well as on the antigenic determinants present in the immunogen.

In this chapter, the emphasis is on the specificity of antigenic determinants. We can ask the following two questions: First, are there special structural requirements for antigenic determinants? Second, are these requirements different for the determinants specific for T or B lymphocytes and their subclasses?

The fact that chemicals as diverse as proteins, polysaccharides, and nucleic acids can be immunogenic indicates that there is no restriction as to the class of chemical compounds which can serve as antigens. Again, comparison of the structural data of peptide antigenic determinants with those of immunologically inactive peptides does not reveal any apparent unique features. The only apparent common features of peptide antigenic determinants which have been examined are (1) their size in the range of four to eight amino acid residues; (2) their accessibility, being located on the surface of the protein molecule; and (3) their dependence on the conformation of the native molecule for B-cell determinants, and an apparent lack of this conformational dependence for T-cell determinants.

The answer to our second question posed earlier, on the different structural requirements for determinants specific for T or B lymphocytes and their subclasses, also appears to be negative. With several proteins and hapten–protein conjugates, it has been shown that the same antigenic determinant is specific for both T and B cells. The apparent lack of conformational dependence of T-cell antigenic determinants can be taken to indicate that T-and B-cell determinants are structurally different since B-cell determinants depend on the conformation of the determinant. But there can be an alternative interpretation of this observation, namely, the affinity of T-cell antigen receptor is much higher than that of B-cell antigen receptor, so that it effectively compensates for the unfavorable equilibrium of the ordered and the disordered forms of antigenic determinant.

Finally, it is known that the type of immune response which is induced depends on the dose, the antigenic valency, and the physicochemical state of the antigen. The importance of the dose of antigen is illustrated by the findings that the optimal amounts of an antigen required to induce or suppress an IgE antibody response in a responder animal are significantly lower than those required for IgG antibody responses (Levine and Vaz, 1970). The importance of antigenic valency is indicated by the following two examples: (1) aggregated bovine γ-globulin, in contrast to its monomer, is ineffective in the induction of tolerance at the antibody level (Chiller and Weigle, 1972), and (2) chemically modified bacterial flagellins are more effective than the native protein in the induction of delayed hypersensitivity (Parish, 1974). The importance of the physicochemical state of the antigen is given by the example of induction of cell-mediated immunity for the hapten 2,4-dinitrophenyl group (DNP). Hapten-specific cellular immunity was not obtained in guinea pigs when DNP-albumin was used as the immunogen. However, such immunity was obtained when DNP-albumin was used in the presence of complete Freund's adjuvant or, alternatively, when DNP-dodecanoylated albumin was used (Dailey and Hunter, 1974).

These changes in the dose, the antigenic valency, and the physicochemical state of the antigens do not change the chemical nature of the antigenic determinants of the molecule, yet they can alter the type of immune response induced.

These facts argue strongly against the possibility that the determinants for different subclasses of T and B cells are structurally different, and they support the notion that an antigenic determinant can bind to different subclasses of T and B cells with varying affinities under different conditions. However, it is known that some antigens selectively elicit formation of antibodies belonging to specific subgroups of IgG (*cf.* Schur, 1972). As examples, IgG antibodies to dextrans were selectively found in the IgG_2 subgroups (Yount *et al.*, 1968), and IgG antibodies to clotting factor VIII (Anderson and Terry, 1968) and to grass pollen antigens (Van der Giessen *et al.*, 1976) were found in the IgG_4 subgroup. Thus we cannot exclude the possibility that there can be antigenic determinants specific for T or B cells, just as those shown for subgroups of IgG.

6. References

Adkinson, N. F., Jr., and Lichtenstein, L. M., 1976, Assessment of allergic states: IgE methodology and the measurement of allergen specific IgG antibody, in: *Clinical Immunobiology* (F. H. Bach and R. A. Good, eds.), pp. 305–344, Academic Press, New York.

Alkan, S. S., Williams, E. B., Nitecki, D. E., and Goodman, J. W., 1972, Antigen recognition and the immune response: Humoral and cellular immune responses to small mono- and bifunctional antigen molecules, *J. Exp. Med.* **135:**1228–1246.

Anderson, B. R., and Terry, W. D., 1968, Gamma G4-globulin antibody causing inhibition of clotting factor VIII, *Nature (London)* **217:**174–175.

Arnon, R., 1974, Conformation and physico-chemical factors influencing antigenicity, in: *Progress in Immunology II,* Vol. 2 (L. Brent and J. Holborow, eds.), pp. 5–15, North-Holland, Amsterdam.

Arnon, R., Sela, M., Yaron, A., and Sober, H. A., 1965, Polylysine-specific antibodies and their reaction with oligolysine, *Biochemistry* **4:**948–953.

Atassi, M. Z., 1977, The complete antigenic structure of myoglobin: Approaches and conclusions for antigenic structures of proteins, in: *Immunochemistry of Proteins,* Vol. 2 (M. Z. Atassi, ed.), pp. 77–176, Plenum, New York.

Atassi, M. Z., and Habeeb, A. F. S. A., 1977, The antigenic structure of hen egg-white lysozyme: A model for disulfide-containing proteins, in: *Immunochemistry of Proteins,* Vol. 2 (M. Z. Atassi, ed.), pp. 177–264, Plenum, New York.

Benacerraf, B., and McDevitt, H. O., 1972, Histocompatibility-linked immune response genes, *Science* **175:**273–279.

Benjamini, E., 1977, Immunochemistry of the tobacco mosaic virus, in: *Immunochemistry of Proteins,* Vol. 2 (M. Z. Atassi, ed.), pp. 265–310, Plenum, New York.

Benjamini, E., Michaeli, D., and Young, J. D., 1972, Antigenic determinants of proteins of defined sequence, *Curr. Top. Microbiol. Immunol.* **58:**85–134.

Bergstrand, H., and Källen, B., 1973, Antigenic determinants on bovine encephalitogenic protein: Localization of regions that induce transformation of lymph node cells from immunized rabbits, *Eur. J. Immunol.* **3:**287–292.

Binz, H., and Wigzell, H., 1977, Antigen binding, idiotopic T-lymphocyte receptors, *Contemp. Top. Immunobiol.* **7:**113–177.

Bloom, B. R., and Glade, P. R., 1971, *In Vitro Methods in Cell-Mediated Immunity,* Academic Press, New York.

Burnet, F. M., 1959, *The Clonal Selection Theory of Acquired Immunity,* Cambridge University Press, New York.

Cantor, H., and Boyse, E., 1977, Regulation of the immune response by T-cell subclasses, *Contemp. Top. Immunobiol.* **7:**47–67.

Chiller, J. M., and Weigle, W. O., 1972, Cellular basis of immunological unresponsiveness, *Contemp. Top. Immunobiol.* **1:**119–142.

Claman, H. N., and Chaperon, E. A., 1969, Immunologic complementation between thymus and marrow cells—A model for the two-cell theory of immunocompetence, *Transplant. Rev.* **1:**92–113.

Crumpton, M. J., 1974, Protein antigens: The molecular basis of antigenicity and immunogenicity, in: *The Antigens,* Vol. 2 (M. Sela, ed.), pp. 1–78, Academic Press, New York.

Dailey, M. O., and Hunter, R. L., 1974, The role of lipid in the induction of hapten-specific delayed hypersensitivity and contact sensitivity, *J. Immunol.* **112:**1526–1534.

Dennert, G., 1976, Thymus derived killer cells: Specificity of function and antigenic recognition, *Transplant. Rev.* **29:**59–88.

Foucard, T., Johansson, S. G. O., Bennich, H., and Berg, T., 1972, *In vitro* estimation of allergens by a radioimmune antiglobulin technique using human IgE antibodies, *Int. Arch. Allergy Appl. Immunol.* **43:**360–370.

Gell, P. G. H., and Benacerraf, B., 1961, Delayed hypersensitivity to simple protein antigens, *Adv. Immunol.* **1:**319–343.

Gershon, R. K., 1974, T cell control of antibody production, *Comtemp. Top. Immunobiol.* **3:**1–40.

Goodman, J. W., 1975, Antigenic determinants and antibody combining site, in: *The Antigens,* Vol. 3 (M. Sela, ed.), pp. 127–187, Academic Press, New York.

Goodman, J. W., Bellone, C. J., Hanes, D., and Nitecki, D. E., 1974, Antigen structural requirements for lymphocyte triggering and cell cooperation, in: *Progress in Immunology II,* Vol. 2 (L. Brent and J. Holborow, eds.) pp. 27–37, North-Holland, Amsterdam.

Ha, Y. M., Fujio, H., Sakato, N., and Amano, T., 1975, Further studies on the specificity of the *N*- and *C*-terminal antigenic determinant of hen egg white lysozyme, *Biken J.* **18:**47–60.

Ishizaka, K., 1973, Chemistry and biology of immunoglobulin E, in: *The Antigens,* Vol. 1 (M. Sela, ed.), pp. 479–528, Academic Press, New York.

Ishizaka, K., 1976, Cellular events in the IgE antibody response, *Adv. Immunol.* **23:**1–75.

Ishizaka, K., Okudaira, H., and King, T. P., 1975, Immunogenic properties of modified antigen E. II. Ability of urea-denatured antigen and 2-polypeptide chain to prime T cells specific for antigen E, *J. Immunol.* **114:**110–115.

Janeway, C. A., Jr., 1976, The specificity of T lymphocyte responses to chemically defined antigens, *Transplant. Rev.* **29:**164–188.

Johansson, S. G. O., Bennich, H. H., and Berg, T., 1972, The clinical significance of IgE, in: *Progress in Clinical Immunology,* Vol. 1 (R. S. Schwartz, ed.), pp. 157–181, Grune and Stratton, New York.

Kabat, E. A., 1966, The nature of an antigenic determinant, *J. Immunol.* **97:**1–11.

Katz, D. H., and Benacerraf, B., 1972, The regulatory influence of activated T cells and B cell responses to antigen, *Adv. Immunol.* **15:**1–94.

King, T. P., 1976, Chemical and biological properties of some atopic allergens, *Adv. Immunol.* **23:**77–105.

Leskowitz, S., Jones, V., and Zak, S., 1966, Immunochemical study of antigenic specificity in delayed hypersensitivity. V. Immunization with monovalent low molecular weight conjugates, *J. Exp. Med.* **123:**229–237.

Levine, B. B., 1972, Skin rashes with penicillin therapy: Current management, *New Engl. J. Med.* **286:**42–43.

Levine, B. B., and Vaz, N. M., 1970, Effect of combinations of inbred strain, antigen, and antigen dose on immune responsiveness and reagin production in the mouse: A potential mouse model for immune aspects of human atopic allergy, *Int. Arch. Allergy Appl. Immunol.* **39:**156–171.

Levy, J. G., Hull, D., Kelly, B., Kilburn, D. G., and Teather, R. M., 1972, The cellular immune response to synthetic peptides containing sequences known to be haptenic in performic acid-oxidized ferredoxin from *Clostridium pasteurianum, Cell. Immunol.* **5:**87–97.

Lüderitz, O., Staub, A. M., and Westphal, O., 1966, Immunochemistry of O and R antigens of *Salmonella* and related anterobactericeae, *Bacteriol. Rev.* **30:**192–255.

Marsh, D. G., 1975, Allergen and the genetics of allergy, in: *The Antigens,* Vol. 3 (M. Sela, ed.), pp. 271–359, Academic Press, New York.

Marsh, D. G., Goodfriend, L., and Bias, W. B., 1977, Basal serum IgE levels and HLA antigen frequencies in allergic subject. I. Studies with ragweed allergen Ra3, *Immunogenetics* **5:**217–233.

Miyagawa, N., Ashizawa, T., Kashiba, S., Miyagawa, S., Fujio, H., Ha, Y. M., and Amano, T., 1975a, Antigenic determinants of hen egg-white lysozyme in delayed hypersensitivity. I. Macrophage migration inhibition activities of lysozyme fragments, *Biken J.* **18:**215–228.

Miyagawa, N., Ashizawa, T., Kashiba, S., Miyagawa, S., Fujio, H., Ha, Y. M., and Amano, T., 1975b, Antigenic determinants of hen egg white lysozyme in delayed hypersensitivity. II. Antigenicity and immunogenicity of the *N*- and *C*-terminal peptide. *Biken J.* **18:**229–247.

Morley, J., Wolstencroft, R. A., and Dumonde, D. C., 1973, The measurement of lymphokines, in: *Handbook of Experimental Immunology,* Vol. 2 (D. M. Weir, ed.), pp. 28.1–28.23, Blackwell, Oxford.
Parish, C. R., 1974, Functional aspects of antigen structure in terms of tolerance and immunity, in: *Progress in Immunology II,* Vol. 2 (L. Brent and J. Holborow, eds.), pp. 39–55, North-Holland, Amsterdam.
Pecht, I., Maron, E., Arnon, R., and Sela, M., 1971, Specific excitation energy transfer from antibodies to dansyl-labeled antigen: Studies with the loop peptide of hen egg-white lysozyme, *Eur. J. Biochem.* **19:**368–371.
Rajewsky, K., and Eichman, K., 1977, Antigen receptors of T helper cells, *Contemp. Top. Immunobiol.* **7:**69–112.
Redmond, A. P., and Levine, B. B., 1968, Delayed skin reactions to benzylpenicillin in man, *Int. Arch. Allergy Appl. Immunol.* **33:**193–206.
Sachs, D. H., 1974, Proteins as antigens, in: *Current Topics in Biochemistry 1973* (C. B. Anfinsen and A. N. Schechter, eds.), pp. 73–107, Academic Press, New York.
Sachs, H. J., Deutsch, G. F., Fasman, G. D., and Levine, L., 1964, The serological specificity of the poly-alanine immune system, *Immunochemistry* **1:**133–144.
Schechter, B., Schechter, I., and Sela, M., 1970, Antibody combing sites to a series of peptide determinants of increasing size and defined structure, *J. Biol. Chem.* **245:**1438–1447.
Schlossman, S. F., Herman, J., and Yaron, A., 1969, Antigen recognition: *In vitro* studies on the specificity of the cellular immune response, *J. Exp. Med.* **130:**1031–1045.
Schur, P. H., 1972, Human gamma-G subclasses, in: *Progress in Clinical Immunology,* Vol. 1 (R. S. Schwartz, ed.), pp. 71–104, Grune and Stratton, New York.
Sela, M., 1972, Antigen design and immune response, *Harvey Lect.* **67:**213–246.
Senyk, G., Nitecki, D. E., Spitler, L., and Goodman, J. W., 1972, The immune response to glucagon in conjugated form, *Immunochemistry* **9:**97–110.
Spitler, L. E., von Muller, C. M., Fudenberg, H. H., and Eylar, E. H., 1972, Experimental allergic encephalitis: Dissociation of cellular immunity to brain protein and disease production, *J. Exp. Med.* **136:**156–174.
Tada, T., 1975, Regulation of reaginic antibody formation in animals, *Prog. Allergy* **19:**122–194.
Takatsu, K., Ishizaka, K., and King, T. P., 1975, Immunogenic properties of modified antigen E. II. Effect of repeated injections of modified antigen on immunocompetent cells specific for native antigen, *J. Immunol.* **115:**1469–1476.
Thompson, K., Harris, M., Benjamini, E., Mitchell, G., and Noble, M., 1972, Cellular and humoral immunity: A distinction in antigenic recognition, *Nature (London) New Biol.* **238:**20–21.
Van der Giessen, M., Haman, W. L., Van Kernebeek, G., Aalbesse, R. C., and Dieges, P. H., 1976, Subclass typing of IgG antibodies formed by grass pollen-allergic patients during immunotherapy, *Int. Arch. Allergy Appl. Immunol.* **50:**625–640.
Yount, W. J., Dorner, M. M., Kunkel, H. G., and Kabat, E. A., 1968, Studies on human antibodies. VI. Selective variations in subgroup composition and genetic markers, *J. Exp. Med.* **127:**633–646.

5

Immunoglobulin E: Biosynthesis and Immunological Mechanisms of IgE-Mediated Hypersensitivity

KIMISHIGE ISHIZAKA and TERUKO ISHIZAKA

1. Introduction

The presence of reaginic antibody in the serum of allergic patients was first demonstrated by Prausnitz and Küstner in 1921. The nature of the antibodies, however, remained unknown for 40 years until IgE was found in the serum of hay fever patients and identified as a carrier of reaginic antibody activity (K. Ishizaka *et al.*, 1966a,b; K. Ishizaka and T. Ishizaka, 1967). Indeed, an injection of purified IgE preparation from ragweed-sensitive individuals into normal skin resulted in the sensitization of the skin site for the Prausnitz–Küstner (P-K) reaction, and the removal of IgE antibody from the sera of atopic patients by anti-IgE was accompanied by loss of sensitizing activity. Subsequent studies have shown that association of reaginic activity with IgE is found not only in the ragweed system but also in the other allergen-reagin systems. Antigenic analysis of the immunoglobulin (K. Ishizaka *et al.*, 1967d) and identification of a unique myeloma protein ND as an E myeloma protein (Johansson and Bennich, 1967; Bennich *et al.*, 1969) established that IgE represents a unique immunoglobulin class.

KIMISHIGE ISHIZAKA and TERUKO ISHIZAKA • Department of Medicine and Microbiology, The Johns Hopkins University School of Medicine, Baltimore, Maryland 21239. The research was supported by research grants from U.S. Public Health Service, AI-10060, AI-11202, from the National Science Foundation, PCM-74-00857, and from the John A. Hartford Foundation. This is publication No. 313 from O'Neill Laboratories at The Good Samaritan Hospital.

Discovery of E myeloma protein established the physiochemical properties of this protein. IgE is an γ_1-glycoprotein with a sedimentation coefficient of 8.0 S and a molecular weight of 190,000 (Bennich and Johansson, 1968). The IgE molecules are composed of two heavy (ϵ) and two light chains, and the antigenic determinants, specific for the immunoglobulin class, are present in the carboxyl-terminal half (Fc portion) of the heavy chains. The knowledge about IgE provided immunochemical approaches to study mechanisms of reaginic hypersensitivity reactions, and these studies led to investigations of the regulation of IgE antibody formation. In this chapter, basic information obtained in these studies will be summarized for future application to clinical research.

2. Mechanisms of IgE-Mediated Hypersensitivity

2.1. Immunological Properties of IgE Antibody

The most important biological property of IgE antibody is the ability to sensitize homologous tissues for allergic reactions. The minimum concentration of IgE antibody required for sensitizing normal human skin for a positive P-K reaction is on the order of 0.2–0.3 ng/ml (K. Ishizaka *et al.*, 1967b). Sensitization of human skin by IgE but not by the other immunoglobulins is supported by so-called reversed-type P-K reactions (K. Ishizaka and T. Ishizaka, 1968a). Intracutaneous injection of a minute dose (10^{-4} μg) of the antibody specific for IgE into normal individuals resulted in induction of an erythema-wheal reaction, whereas even a thousand fold more of the antibodies specific for the other immunoglobulin classes, i.e., IgG, IgM, IgA and IgD, failed to do so. Since normal individuals have IgE which has affinity for target cells involved in P-K reactions, mechanisms of the skin reaction by anti-IgE are considered to result from combination of antibody with cell-bound normal IgE.

IgE antibodies are responsible for PCA reactions in the monkey with sera from atopic patients (K. Ishizaka *et al.*, 1967a). When *Macaca irus* was employed, about 30 times as much IgE antibody was required to sensitize monkey skin as required for P-K reactions in humans. It was also found that injection of anti-human IgE into monkey skin induced reversed-type PCA reactions (K. Ishizaka and T. Ishizaka, 1968a). The reaction is due to cross-reactivity of monkey IgE with antibodies against human IgE. On the other hand, human IgE antibody did not give PCA reaction in the guinea pig. This finding was supported by the fact that an intracutaneous injection of even 600 μg/ml of E myeloma protein followed by challenge of the guinea pig with anti-human IgE failed to induce reversed PCA reactions (T. Ishizaka *et al.*, 1970).

The IgE antibodies can sensitize not only skin but also other tissues such as lung. When monkey lung tissues were incubated *in vitro* with human reaginic serum containing anti-ragweed IgE antibody and the sensitized tissues were exposed to ragweed allergen, tissues released both histamine and slow-reacting substance of anaphylaxis (SRS-A), which contract bronchial smooth muscle. The sensitizing activity in the reaginic serum was removed by the adsorption of the serum with anti-IgE immunosorbent. The concentrations of IgG, IgM, and IgA in the supernatant after the adsorption were comparable to those in the original serum, but IgE concentration diminished to 0.1% after the adsorption. Failure of the supernatant to sensitize monkey lung tissues therefore indicates that IgE antibody is responsible for sensitization (T. Ishizaka *et al.*, 1970). Orange *et al.* (1971) reproduced similar experiments using human lung fragments and demonstrated that IgE antibody sensitized human tissues for the release of both histamine and SRS-A. Subsequently, Kay and Austen (1971) have shown that the allergen-IgE antibody reaction in human lung fragments resulted in a release of another chemical mediator which is chemotactic for eosinophils. The fact that IgE mediates the release of three functionally distinct chemical mediators which increase secretions, contract bronchial smooth muscle, and are chemotactic for eosinophils supports the idea that IgE is involved in respiratory allergy.

Sensitization of homologous species with IgE antibodies can be observed at the cellular level as well. Many years ago, Lichtenstein and Osler (1964) observed histamine release from isolated leukocytes of atopic patients on exposure to allergen, and Levy and Osler (1966) showed passive sensitization of normal human leukocytes with reaginic serum for antigen-induced histamine release. If the reaction of allergen with reaginic antibodies is actually responsible for the histamine release, one can suspect that IgE is bound to some leukocytes. Indeed, anti-IgE released histamine from leukocytes of atopic patients and of some normal individuals (T. Ishizaka *et al.*, 1969a). Furthermore, fixation of IgE to leukocytes on passive sensitization was demonstrated. As shown in Figure 1, incubation of leukocytes from a normal individual with an IgE-rich serum increased the sensitivity of the leukocytes to anti-IgE. Passive sensitization of leukocytes for reversed-type histamine release was accomplished with E myeloma protein as well; the sensitizing activity of the myeloma protein was comparable to that of IgE present in the reaginic serum. In the experiment shown in Figure 1, aliquots of normal

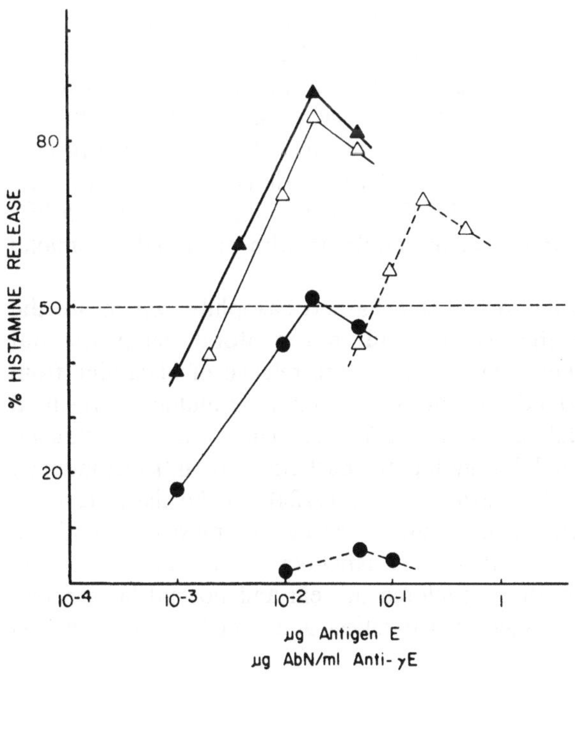

Figure 1. Histamine release from human leukocytes by anti-IgE or antigen E. Normal leukocytes released histamine by anti-IgE (△- - -△) but not by ragweed antigen E (●- - -●). After sensitization of the leukocytes with serum from a ragweed-sensitive individual, the leukocytes released histamine on exposure to antigen E (●——●). The sensitivity of the leukocytes to anti-IgE increased after the sensitization with serum (△——△) or with 3 µg/ml of E myeloma protein (▲——▲).

leukocytes were passively sensitized with a dilution of reaginic serum containing 3 μg/ml of IgE or with 3 μg/ml of purified E myeloma protein, and the sensitized cells were challenged with varying concentrations of anti-IgE. Dose–response curves of histamine release from the sensitized cells were superimposable. These results indicate that IgE combines with leukocytes on passive sensitization and that IgE antibody is responsible for antigen-induced histamine release from leukocytes.

2.2. Mechanisms of Sensitization

2.2.1. Target Cells for IgE

A question to be asked was the reason why IgE but none of the other immunoglobulins is able to mediate reaginic hypersensitivity reactions. As the allergic manifestations are induced by antigen–antibody reactions in the tissues, it is reasonable to speculate that IgE has a high affinity for tissues and cells. Reversed-type histamine release from human leukocytes and successful sensitization of monkey lung fragments *in vitro* with E myeloma protein provided an approach to demonstrate target cells for IgE. Incubation of human leukocytes with ^{125}I-labeled anti-IgE in the presence of EDTA, which prevented histamine release, followed by autoradiography of the leukocytes, clearly showed that almost all basophil granulocytes combined ^{125}I-labeled anti-IgE, while neutrophils, eosinophils, small lymphocytes, and monocytes did not (K. Ishizaka *et al.*, 1970b). The binding of anti-IgE with basophils was specific. If the same leukocytes were treated with ^{125}I-labeled anti-IgG, most of the neutrophils and monocytes were labeled, whereas basophils were not labeled. Furthermore, binding of IgE with basophils was demonstrated by incubating the leukocytes with ^{125}I-labeled E myeloma protein. Again, none of the leukocytes except basophil granulocytes combined radiolabeled IgE. Subsequently, Sullivan *et al.* (1971) demonstrated the presence of IgE molecules on basophil granulocytes by electron microscopy. All of these findings established that basophil granulocytes are target cells sensitized with IgE. The cells sensitized with IgE were studied in tissues as well. E myeloma protein injected into monkeys was detected on mast cells in various tissues such as the skin, omentum, small intestine, and bronchi. Treatment of these tissues with ^{125}I-labeled anti-IgE resulted in the binding of the antibody with mast cells (Tomioka and Ishizaka, 1971).

The presence of IgE molecules on mast cells and basophils, which are the major source of histamine in the tissues and in the blood, suggests that antigen–antibody reactions on these cells result in the release of histamine from the cells. Indeed, the antigen–antibody reactions on basophil granulocytes resulted in degranulation of the cells (T. Ishizaka *et al.*, 1971). Evidence was also obtained that no leukocyte other than basophil granulocytes participate in anti-IgE-induced histamine release from the cells (T. Ishizaka *et al.*, 1972a). At the tissue level, it was established that IgE–anti-IgE reactions on the surface of mast cells initiated the release of both histamine and SRS-A (T. Ishizaka *et al.*, 1972b). In the experiments shown in Table 1, both E myeloma protein and normal human IgG were injected into monkeys for passive sensitization and a cell suspension was prepared from their lungs. When the cell suspension was treated with either ^{125}I-labeled anti-IgE or anti-IgG and examined by autoradiography, anti-IgE labeled mast cells but not the other cells. Anti-IgG combined with macrophages and neutrophils but not with mast cells. Incubation of the cell suspension with anti-IgE at 37°C resulted in the release of both histamine and SRS-A, whereas anti-IgG failed to release either mediator. It is therefore clear that the IgE–anti-IgE reaction on mast cells initiates the release of both chemical mediators, whereas the IgG–anti-IgG reaction on macrophages does not. Since almost all histamine in the lung cell suspensions was associated with mast cells, it is apparent that the antigen–antibody reaction on mast cells initiates a sequence of enzymatic reactions in the cells leading to the release of histamine. The source of SRS-A is not settled. Bach and Brashler (1974) have shown that mast-cell-depleted rat peritoneal cells released SRS-A on exposure to calcium ionophores and suggested the possibility that the source of SRS-A is not necessarily mast cells. More recently, however, Jakschik *et al.* (1977) reported that purified rat mast cells released SRS-A on exposure to anti-IgE. A question still remains as to whether SRS-A released from mast cells may account for all SRS-A released *in vivo*.

2.2.2. Structures in IgE Molecules Essential for Sensitization

The sensitization of basophil granulocytes and mast cells by IgE but not by immunoglobulin of the other classes is due to the presence of unique structures in the IgE molecules. Accumulated evidence showed that structures essential for the binding with basophils and mast cells are present in the carboxyl-terminal half (Fc portion) of ϵ chains (*cf.* Figure 2). Among the fragments obtained by either papain or pepsin digestion, only the Fc fragments can block passive sensitization with IgE antibody (Stanworth *et al.*, 1968; K. Ishizaka *et al.*, 1970a). The ^{125}I-labeled Fc fragment but not the Fab fragment binds with human basophil granulocytes (K. Ishizaka *et al.*, 1970b). It was also found that monkey lung tissues sensitized with the Fc fragment released both histamine and SRS-A on exposure to anti-IgE (K. Ishizaka *et al.*, 1970a). Since anti-IgE did not induce histamine release from unsensitized tissues in this experiment, it appears that the Fc fragments actually bind with mast cells and sensitize them for histamine release. All of these findings

TABLE 1. Histamine and SRS-A Release from Lung Cell Suspension

Challenge	Antibody added (μg AbN/ml)	Histamine released (μg)	SRS-A released (unit)
Anti-IgE[a]	0.1	0.258	100
	0.02	0.312	120
	0.004	0.198	60
Anti-IgG	0.5	0.054	<10
	0.1	0.012	0
Buffer	0	0.006	0

[a] Since the donor of the lung cell suspension received both E myeloma protein and normal human IgG, anti-ϵ_0 antibody rather than anti-IgE was used for challenge.

indicate that IgE molecules combine with target cells through the Fc portion of the molecules.

It is well known that reaginic antibody is inactivated by heating at 56°C. Analysis of heated IgE antibody showed that antigen-binding activity of IgE antibodies is maintained after the heat treatment; however, the antibodies lose the ability to sensitize mast cells (K. Ishizaka *et al.*, 1967c). Experiments by Bennich and Dorrington (1972) revealed that heat inactivation of IgE antibody is due to structural changes in the Fc portion of the molecules. It is also known that reaginic antibody is susceptible to reduction-alkylation treatment. Susceptibility of each disulfide bond in IgE molecules to reducing reagents has been investigated and correlated with the biological activity of reduced-alkylated protein (Takatsu *et al.*, 1975a). The results of such experiments showed that cleavage of the inter-heavy-light chain bond, which is most susceptible to reducing reagents, did not affect the affinity of IgE molecules for target cells. After two additional disulfide bonds were cleaved by reduction in 2 mM dithiothreitol followed by alkylation, the protein could combine with target cells, but their affinity was significantly lower than that of native protein. Partial hydrolysis of the reduced alkylated protein as well as results of structural studies by Bennich and von Bahr-Lindström (1974) indicates that these disulfide bonds are intra-ϵ-chain bonds located between Fd and the hinge portion of the molecule (*cf.* Figure 2). These findings appear to be in conflict with the fact that the Fc portion is responsible for the binding of IgE molecules to target cells; however, later studies suggested the mechanisms involved. It was found that the Fc fragment obtained from the reduced-alkylated protein had affinity for basophils comparable to those of the Fc fragment obtained from the native protein. Indeed, the fragment had higher affinity than the reduced alkylated protein from which the fragment was obtained. These findings suggest strongly that a certain conformation in the Fc portion of the molecules is required for a high affinity and that such a conformational structure is affected by cleavage of disulfide bonds in the Fd portion. The affinity of IgE for the target cells was completely lost after cleavage of the fifth disulfide bond, which is an inter-ϵ-chain bond located at the carboxyl-terminal end of the $F(ab')_2$ (*cf.* Figure 2) (Stanworth *et al.*, 1970; Takatsu *et al.*, 1975a). These findings also support the concept that conformational structures in the Fc portion of the IgE molecules are involved in the binding with target cells.

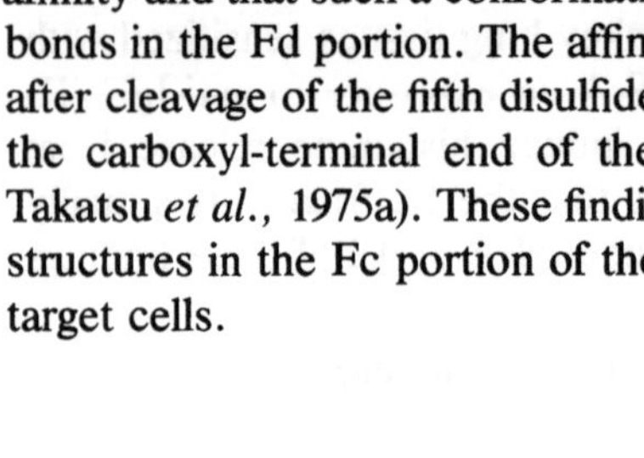

Figure 2. Structure of IgE. One of the two class-specific antigenic determinants (ϵ_1) is present in the Fc′ portion of ϵ-chains, and another determinant (ϵ_2) is present in the carboxyl-terminal portion of ϵ-chains. From Bennich and von Bahr-Lindström (1974).

The demonstration of IgE on human basophils and mast cells raised the question of how many IgE molecules are present on the cells and whether the binding of IgE with receptors is reversible. Since pure IgE was available only in humans at that time, we tried to determine the number of IgE molecules on human basophil granulocytes. Difficulties in the experiment were that basophils are only a minor component of human peripheral blood leukocytes and isolation of the cells in a relatively pure form is almost impossible. Thus we enumerated the number of IgE molecules on basophils by the C1a-fixation transfer technique using a basophil-rich fraction (T. Ishizaka *et al.*, 1973). The results of the experiment indicated that human basophils of normal and atopic individuals possess 10,000–40,000 IgE molecules per cell. After saturation of receptors with IgE with E myeloma protein, the number of IgE molecules per cell increased to 40,000–90,000, which represented the total number of receptor sites per cell (Table 2).

The binding of IgE with receptors is reversible. Cell-bound IgE rapidly dissociates when the cells are exposed to a pH lower than 4 (T. Ishizaka and K. Ishizaka, 1974). The results strongly suggest that covalent bonding is not involved in the binding. However, the affinity of IgE for basophils is quite high at the physiological condition. Determination of the proportion of receptors occupied by IgE at certain concentrations of serum IgE revealed that the equilibrium constant of the binding between IgE and receptor is on the order of 10^9 M^{-1} (T. Ishizaka *et al.*, 1973) (Table 2). Subsequently, Kulczycki and Metzger (1974) studied the binding between rat IgE and rat basophilic leukemia (RBL) cells. An advantage of this system is that a large quantity of pure RBL cells can be obtained by *in vitro* culture; thus the binding of ^{125}I-labeled rat IgE to the cells can be measured quantitatively. Their experiments indicated that an average number of receptor sites per leukemia cell was 500,000–1,000,000, and that the average equilibrium constant of the reaction was 9×10^9 M^{-1}. Similarly, Conrad *et al.* (1975) enumerated receptor sites on normal rat mast cells and reported that the number of IgE receptors is on the order of 300,000 per cell. An equilibrium constant of the binding reaction was estimated to be $1–2 \times 10^9$ M^{-1} (Table 2). Summarizing the data available in both human and rat systems, it is clear that IgE has high affinity for receptors on target cells. This explains why a minute dose of IgE antibody can sensitize the cells and why sensitization with IgE antibody is persistent.

TABLE 2. Receptors for IgE on Basophils and Mast Cells

Target cells	Receptors/cells ($\times 10^3$)	Equilibrium constant ($\times 10^9$)
Human basophils[a]	40–100	0.5–1.3
Rat basophilic leukemia cells	1000[b]	9.0[b]
	600[c]	1–2[c]
Rat peritoneal mast cells	300[c]	1–1.5[c]

[a] T. Ishizaka *et al.* (1973).
[b] Kulczycki and Metzger (1974).
[c] Conrad *et al.* (1975).

2.2.4. IgE-Receptors on Mast Cells

Attempts were made to characterize receptors for IgE using rat mast cells and basophilic leukemia cells. Bach and Brashler (1973) incubated rat reaginic serum with cell ghosts of normal peritoneal mast cells and found that the antibody could be adsorbed. Subsequently, König and Ishizaka (1976) have disrupted normal rat mast cells by sonication and recovered reagin-binding activity in the supernatant. Gel filtration of the fraction through a Sepharose 6B column showed that void volume fraction contained active components which combined both reaginic antibody and ^{125}I-labeled IgE. Availability of a large number of RBL cells by *in vitro* culture facilitated chemical identification of receptors. Conrad and Froese (1976) surface-labeled rat mast cells and RBL cells with ^{125}I and incubated the cells with rat E myeloma protein to saturate the receptors. Cells were then treated with a nonionic detergent, Nonidet P-40, and IgE–receptor complexes in the eluate were precipitated with anti-IgE. Analysis of the precipitates, dissolved in sodium dodecylsulfate (SDS) and urea, on SDS-polyacrylamide gel electrophoresis showed a major radioactive band which corresponded to a molecular weight of 62,000. Because the radioactive component was derived from plasma membrane and was coprecipitated with IgE–anti-IgE complexes, the component must be a receptor or its fragment. Subsequently, Kulczycki *et al.* (1976) have shown that the 62,000 component described by Conrad and Froese is a glycoprotein. They also found that the component has an atypical electrophoretic behavior often associated with glycoprotein. In 10–12% gel the mobility of the component corresponded to 45,000–50,000 daltons, and in 5.9% gel to 60,000–70,000 daltons. The component exposed to SDS, however, failed to combine with IgE. So far, active receptors have not been isolated. Nevertheless, the size of intact receptor molecules in NP-40 extract of RBL cells was estimated to be 130,000–150,000 by density gradient ultracentrifugation (Newman *et al.*, 1977; Conrad and Froese, 1978). Based on the molecular weight of free receptors, IgE, and IgE-receptor complex, Newman *et al.* (1977) concluded that the solubilized receptor molecule is monovalent with respect to binding with IgE.

Receptor molecules are insoluble in the absence of detergent. Hydrophobic properties of solubilized receptors suggest that a large part of the molecule is incorporated into membrane. Conrad and Froese (1976) have shown that radioiodination of receptors on RBL cells by the lactoperoxidase method was prevented if the receptors had been saturated with IgE. This finding suggests that only a small portion of a receptor molecule is exposed to the cell surface and that this area is almost completely covered by a single IgE molecule.

2.3. Immunological Mechanisms of IgE-Mediated Reactions

2.3.1. Bridging Hypothesis

It is well known that monovalent hapten induce neither anaphylaxis nor reaginic hypersensitivity reactions. For example, an intracutaneous injection of monovalent hapten failed to induce erythema-wheal reactions in patients sensitive to penicillin, while divalent and trivalent haptens did (Levine and Redmond, 1968). Since IgE-mediated hypersensitivity reactions can be induced either by the antigen or by anti-IgE, we have employed the latter reagent to study the mechanisms of the reactions. It was found that the $F(ab')_2$ fragments of anti-IgE induced erythema-wheal skin reactions in both normal and atopic individuals, released histamine from human leukocytes (K. Ishizaka and T. Ishizaka, 1968a), and released both histamine and SRS-A from monkey lung tissues which had been sensitized with IgE (T. Ishizaka *et al.*, 1970). Quantitatively, the ability of the $F(ab')_2$ fragments to induce the reaction was comparable to that of undigested antibody. In marked contrast, monovalent Fab′ monomer fragments failed to give any of these reactions. Induction of reversed-type allergy by $F(ab')_2$ but not by Fab′ monomer of anti-IgE suggested that bridging of two IgE molecules on target cells by a divalent ligand is the initial step of the reactions. Subsequently, Siraganian *et al.* (1975) studied antigen-induced histamine release from rabbit leukocytes and platelets mediated by antihapten IgE antibody. Rabbits were immunized with either benzyl penicilloyl derivatives of ovalbumin (BPO-OA) or dinitrophenyl derivatives of bovine γ-globulin (DNP-BGG), or both antigens, and their leukocytes were challenged by monovalent haptens, divalent haptens, or mixed divalent haptens containing both the DNP group and the BPO group in a molecule. Their results confirmed that bivalent, but not monovalent, haptens induced histamine release. More importantly, a mixed BPO-DNP divalent hapten failed to release histamine from the leukocytes of either BPO-primed or DNP-primed animals, but the same hapten released histamine if donors of leukocytes were immunized with both DNP-BGG and BPO-OA. A mixture of monovalent BPO-hapten and DNP-hapten did not induce histamine release. These findings are further evidence to indicate that the activation of basophils is due to dimer formation of two cell-bound IgE molecules.

Further evidence for the bridging hypothesis was obtained by studies of antigen–antibody complexes. When ragweed antigen E was added to IgE, IgG, or IgA antibody preparation from a ragweed-sensitive serum and antigen–antibody complexes thus formed were injected into normal human skin, only the complexes of IgE antibody with allergen provoked erythema-wheal reactions. Analysis of the allergen–antibody complexes indicated that the complex composed of one IgE antibody and two antigen molecules does not have skin reactivity, whereas the complexes containing two or more antibody molecules do (K. Ishizaka and T. Ishizaka, 1968b). These findings suggested the possibility that the antibody molecules brought into close proximity by antigen may interact with each other, and the antibody–antibody interaction may be involved in the induction of biological activity. The hypothesis was supported by the fact that nonspecifically aggregated IgE have the same activities as antigen–IgE antibody complexes. Intracutaneous injections of aggregated IgE or aggregated Fc fragments of IgE induced erythema-wheal reactions, and incubation of these materials with human leukocytes resulted in histamine release (K. Ishizaka *et al.*, 1970a; T. Ishizaka *et al.*, 1970). As expected, neither monomeric IgE or Fc fragments nor aggregated $F(ab')_2$ fragments induced such reactions. These findings suggested the possibility that interaction between the Fc portion of IgE molecules may be involved in the activation of enzyme sequences leading to the release of chemical mediators.

2.3.2. Role of IgE Receptors in Triggering

Requirement of the cross-linkage of cell-bound IgE molecules for triggering may be interpreted by an entirely different mechanism. It has been shown that IgE molecules are firmly bound to receptors even after the antigen (or anti-IgE) reacts with the molecules (T. Ishizaka and K. Ishizaka, 1975). Thus bridging of cell-bound IgE molecules by divalent antigen or anti-IgE probably brings two receptor molecules into close proximity. It is conceivable that such a local change or disturbance of membrane structures and/or possible interaction between adjacent receptor molecules may activate membrane-associated enzymes. If this is the case, one can expect that direct bridging of receptor molecules may induce histamine release without participation of cell-bound IgE. Thus we tested the hypothesis by using antibodies against receptor molecules (T. Ishizaka *et al.*, 1977). The IgE–receptor complexes were prepared based on the previous finding of Conrad and Froese (1976). RBL cells were saturated with rat IgE and the cells were extracted with 0.5% Nonidet P-40 (NP-40). The IgE-receptor complexes in the extract were precipitated with rabbit anti-rat IgE and a rabbit was immunized with the precipitates included in complete Freund's adjuvant. Antibodies against membrane components on RBL cells were purified by using RBL cells as an immunosorbent, and the purified antibodies were rendered specific for mast cells by adsorption with mast cell-depleted normal rat peritoneal cells. The final antibody preparation (anti-RBL) inhibited the binding of IgE with both mast cells and solubilized receptors, indicating that the preparation contained antireceptor antibodies.

Subsequent experiments showed that most of the antibodies in the anti-RBL preparation were actually antireceptor antibodies (Conrad *et al.*, 1978). RBL cells were surface labeled with ^{125}I, and an NP-40 extract of the cells was incubated with anti-RBL. Analysis of the antigen–antibody complexes by SDS gel electrophoresis showed that the major cell surface component, which binds with the antibody, had a molecular weight of 45,000 and corresponded to the receptor. More importantly, the binding of anti-RBL with the component was inhibited if the cells had been saturated with IgE before extraction with NP-40.

As expected, anti-RBL induced skin reactions in normal rats and noncytotoxic histamine release from normal mast cells (T. Ishizaka *et al.*, 1977). More importantly, skin reactions and histamine release by anti-RBL were inhibited if the receptors on mast cells had been saturated by IgE (Figure 3). The findings are in agreement with the fact that the binding of anti-RBL with receptor molecules was inhibited by saturation of receptors by IgE and indicated that antireceptor antibodies were responsible for triggering histamine release.

It was also found that the F(ab')$_2$ fragments of anti-RBL induced both skin reactions in normal rats and histamine release from mast cells, while the Fab' monomer fragments of the antibody failed to do so (T. Ishizaka and K. Ishizaka, 1978). Failure of the Fab' fragment to trigger the cells is not due to lack of binding. The Fab' fragments inhibited the binding of [^{125}I]-IgE with RBL cells *in vitro,* and an intracutaneous injection of the fragment into normal rats blocked passive sensitization of the skin sites with IgE antibodies. Therefore, it appears that direct bridging of receptor molecules by divalent antireceptor antibody causes histamine release but the binding of the monovalent antibody with the receptor is not

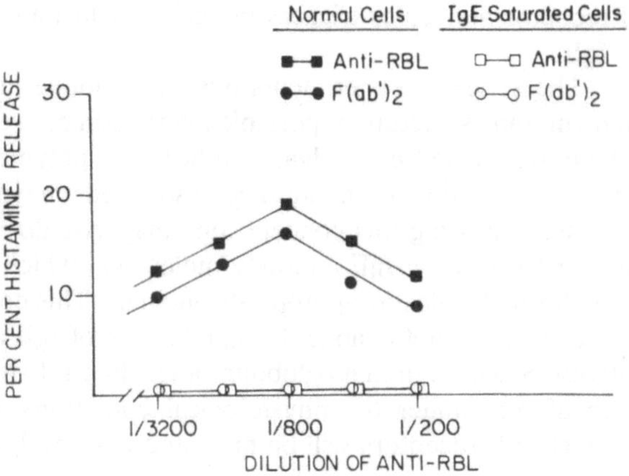

Figure 3. Inhibition of anti-RBL-induced histamine release by IgE. A portion of peritoneal cells were saturated with IgE. Both IgE-saturated cells and untreated cells were incubated with serial dilutions of either undigested anti-RBL or $F(ab')_2$ fragments of the antibody in the presence of phosphatidyl serine. From T. Ishizaka and K. Ishizaka (1978).

sufficient for the histamine release (Figure 4a–c). An interesting observation was that the Fab′ monomer fragment of anti-RBL can sensitize mast cells for reversed-type passive cutaneous anaphylaxis (PCA) reactions. When the Fab′ fragment of anti-RBL was injected intracutaneously into normal rats and the animals were challenged by the antibodies against rabbit IgG 2 hr later, skin sites which received the fragment of anti-RBL showed cutaneous anaphylaxis. The Fab′ monomer fragments and $F(ab')_2$ fragments of anti-RBL were comparable on a weight basis with respect to their ability to sensitize rats skin for the reversed PCA reactions. It appears that the reactions of the receptor-bound Fab′ fragments with anti-RGG (anti-Fab) induce skin reactions (Figure 4d). It should be noted that the mechanism of this reaction is similar to anti-IgE-induced histamine release in which receptor-bound IgE molecules are bridged by divalent anti-IgE (Figure 4e). Taken collectively, the results obtained with antireceptor antibodies clearly show that bridging

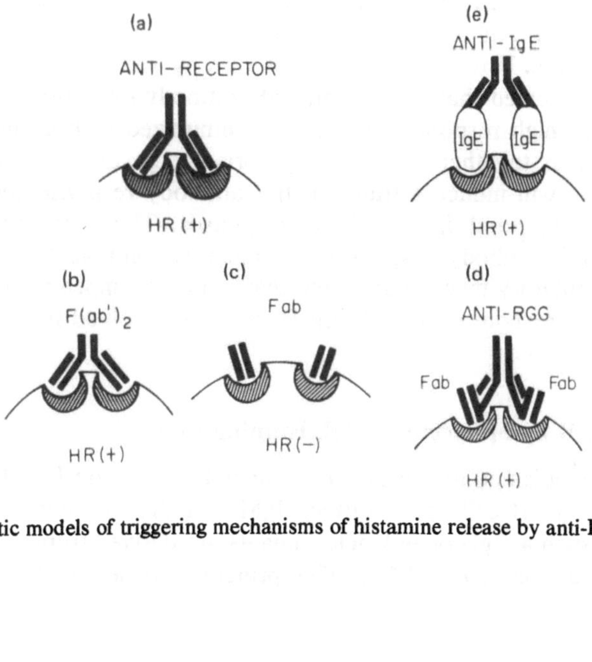

Figure 4. Schematic models of triggering mechanisms of histamine release by anti-RBL and anti-IgE.

of receptor molecules triggers the cells for histamine release without participation of IgE.

The series of experiments described above indicate that some local changes in membrane structure or possible interaction between adjacent receptor molecules, which are caused by bridging, rather than polymerization of IgE are responsible for the activation of membrane-associated enzymes, which leads to histamine release. Following this concept, one may visualize that IgE receptors serve as an anchor for specific IgE antibody molecules, which in turn mediate the bridging of receptor molecules by appropriate antigens. This concept of triggering mechanisms, however, does not change the significance of IgE antibodies in reaginic hypersensitivity. Since no immunoglobulin other than IgE will bind with IgE receptors with high affinity under the physiological conditions, triggering of histamine release through IgE receptors will be mediated only by IgE antibodies.

3. IgE Antibody Response and Regulation

A crucial role of IgE antibody in reaginic hypersensitivity and atopic diseases suggests strongly that prevention or suppression of IgE antibody formation is beneficial for atopic patients. Fortunately, the scope of our knowledge on the mechanisms of antibody responses has considerably broadened in the past decade. It is firmly established that collaboration of two distinct types of lymphocytes, i.e., bone marrow-derived precursors of antibody-forming cells (B cells) and thymus-derived lymphocytes (T cells), is essential for the induction of antibody responses to most protein antigens (reviewed by Katz and Benacerraf, 1972). This principle obtained with IgM and IgG antibody responses has been proven to be the case also with IgE antibody formation. No IgE antibody response was obtained in athymic nude mice (Michael and Bernstein, 1973), and T-independent antigens failed to raise IgE antibody response in experimental animals. From the immunological viewpoint, however, IgE antibody responses in experimental animals have certain characteristic features that are not easily demonstrated in IgG antibody response. In spite of the fact that the IgE antibody level in the serum of hay fever patients is persistent, it is rather difficult to obtain a persistent IgE antibody formation in rodents. However, extensive studies by Vaz *et al.* (1971) using inbred strains of mice revealed that a persistent IgE antibody formation is obtained only when genetically high responder strains are immunized with a minute dose of a potent immunogen together with an appropriate adjuvant. An increase of the immunizing dose will induce a transient IgE antibody response and cause dissociation between IgE and IgG antibody responses. These observations suggest strongly that IgE antibody responses are more susceptible than IgG antibody responses to regulatory mechanisms, and that immunocompetent cells involved in the IgE antibody response are different from those involved in the IgG antibody response.

3.1. Precursor B Lymphocytes of IgE-Forming Cells

Extensive studies on the surface immunoglobulin (Ig) on B cells in the mouse showed that virgin B cells bear surface IgM and that the lymphocytes bearing other isotypes such as IgG or IgA determinants are derived from the virgin B cells (reviewed by Lawton *et al.*, 1975). This principle applies to the IgE system as well. Ontogenetic development of IgE-bearing B lymphocytes in the rat showed that IgE-bearing B cells appear in the spleen within 24–48 hr after birth. These cells are detected in the bone marrow as well and bear both IgE and IgM determinants (K. Ishizaka *et al.*, 1978). Accumulated evidence indicates that the cells bearing both IgE and IgM are derived directly from IgM-bearing virgin B cells, and that neither antigen nor T cells are involved in the differentiation. It has been shown that IgE-bearing lymphocytes increase in all lymphoid tissues except the thymus following infection of rats with the nematode *Nippostrongylus brasiliensis* (Nb) (T. Ishizaka *et al.*, 1976). This response was observed even in neonatally thymectomized rats, which failed to form antibodies against hapten–protein conjugate (Urban *et al.*, 1977a). More recently, we have observed that the conversion of IgM-bearing cells to IgE-IgM double-bearing cells can be achieved by a soluble factor derived from mesenteric lymph node cells of the parasite-infected rats (Urban *et al.*, 1977b). Addition of cell-free culture supernatants of the mesenteric lymph node cells to normal bone marrow cell culture induces a significant increase of IgE-bearing cells. The increase in IgE-bearing cells is not due to the passive binding of IgE or its fragments to lymphocytes. Effect of the factor is specific; the factor does not increase either IgM-bearing cells or IgG-bearing cells in the bone marrow cultures. It was also found that essentially all IgE-bearing cells appearing in the bone marrow culture have both surface IgE and IgM (Urban and Ishizaka,1978). Separate experiments showed that this factor is derived from B cells rather than from T cells (Urban *et al.*, 1978). It is apparent that IgM-bearing virgin B cells can differentiate to IgM-IgE double-bearing cells by B-cell factor(s) without participation of T cells.

Evidence was obtained that the cells bearing both IgE and IgM are actually precursors of IgE-forming cells. If normal mesenteric lymph node cells, which contain the IgE-bearing B cells, are cultured with pokeweed mitogen (PWM), both IgM- and IgE-forming plasma cells develop in the culture within 5 days. Removal of IgE-bearing cells before stimulation with PWM diminishes the number of IgE-forming plasma cells without affecting the development of IgM-forming cells (Table 3). Since a large proportion of IgE-bearing cells also bear IgM, removal of IgM-bearing cells was accompanied by a marked decrease of IgE-bearing cells, and the

TABLE 3. Effect of Depletion of IgE-B Cells or IgM-B Cells on the Development of Ig-Forming Cells

	Ig-bearing cells		Ig-forming cells[b]	
Fractionation[a]	IgE (%)	IgM (%)	IgE	IgM
Unfractionated	3.5	14.3	50	190
IgE-B cell depletion	0.9	9.7	12	160
IgM-B cell depletion	1.0	1.4	20	60

[a] A mesenteric lymph node cell suspension was treated with either rabbit anti-IgE or anti-IgM antibody, and cell suspensions were placed on tissue culture dishes coated with anti-rabbit IgG. Nonadherent cells were cultured in microplates (2×10^5 cells per well).
[b] The number of Ig-forming cells per ten wells in which 2×10^6 nucleated cells were cultured.

number of both IgM- and IgE-forming plasma cells in the culture was diminished (*cf.* Table 3). The results indicated that cells bearing both IgE and IgM are already committed for IgE synthesis.

To get some idea on the nature of B memory cells committed for IgE synthesis, either IgM-bearing cells or IgE-bearing cells were depleted from the mesenteric lymph node cells of Nb-infected rats and the rest of the cells were cultured with Nb antigen. As expected, depletion of IgE-bearing cells resulted in a marked decrease of IgE-forming plasma cells without a significant effect on the development of IgM- and IgG_{2a}-forming plasma cells. Removal of 80% of the IgM-bearing cells significantly diminished all of the IgE-, IgG_{2a}-, and IgM-forming plasma cells. However, depletion of IgM-bearing cells was less effective than depletion of IgE-bearing cells to diminish IgE-forming plasma cells. The results suggested that B memory cells committed for IgE are composed of IgE-bearing cells and IgE-IgM double-bearing cells.

Previous studies on the *in vitro* secondary IgE antibody response of rabbit mesenteric lymph node cells, however, strongly suggested that the majority of IgE-B memory cells do not carry μ-chain determinants (Kishimoto and Ishizaka, 1972). Some years ago, we established an *in vitro* system in which secondary IgE antihapten antibody response can be determined (K. Ishizaka and Kishimoto, 1972). Mesenteric lymph node cells from rabbits immunized with alum-adsorbed DNP derivatives of ragweed antigen (DNP-Rag) or ascaris extract (DNP-Asc) produced not only IgM and IgG but also IgE antihapten antibodies *in vitro* on stimulation with homologous antigen. In order to deplete a certain population of B cells, mesenteric lymph node cells from DNP-Asc-primed rabbits were passed through a Sepharose immunosorbent coated with anti-μ, anti-γ, or anti-Fab (light-chain) antibody, and effluent cells were stimulated with DNP-Asc for 24 hr. The cells were cultured for 6 days in the absence of antigen, and antihapten antibodies in the culture supernatant were determined. The results of the experiment indicated that the anti-μ-chain column and the anti-γ-chain column removed immunocompetent cells required for IgM and IgG antibody responses, but the IgE antibody response was not affected. As expected, the anti-Fab column removed Ig-bearing cells and reduced all of the IgM, IgG, and IgE antibody responses. The results suggested that B memory cells committed for IgE antibody response are distinct from those for IgG and IgM antibodies, and do not bear μ- or γ-chain determinants.

Discrepancies between rabbit and rat systems may be due to differences in immunization regimen for priming B memory cells and/or species difference. Rat mesenteric lymph node cells were obtained 4–5 weeks after infection with Nb, while rabbits were immunized with alum-adsorbed DNP-Asc two or three times with 4-week intervals, and lymph node cells were obtained 10–12 days after a booster immunization. The proportion of IgM-IgE double-bearing cells and IgE-bearing cells in a B memory cell population might change depending on the period after priming. Nevertheless, findings obtained in both the rat and rabbit systems indicate that B memory cells committed for IgE synthesis and secretion bear ϵ-chain determinants on their surface.

3.2. Requirement of T-Helper Cells in IgE Response

The differentiation of IgE-bearing B cells to IgE-forming plasma cells requires T cells. If one cultures the B-cell-rich fraction from Nb-infected rats with T cells from either infected rats or normal rats in the presence of Nb antigen, IgE-forming plasma cells develop only in the presence of T cells from infected animals. T cells from normal rats fail to collaborate with IgE-bearing B cells for their differentiation. The results clearly show that antigen-primed T cells are required for the development of IgE-forming cells from B memory cells. The same principle is applied to the polyclonal response of IgE-bearing B cells to PWM. B cells from normal rat mesenteric lymph nodes do not differentiate to IgE-forming plasma cells in the absence of T cells.

Accumulated evidence indicates that helper T cells are involved in at least two stages of B-cell differentiation. One is the last stage of differentiation in which IgE-B memory cells differentiate to antibody-forming cells for secondary IgE antibody response. The conclusion was obtained in both the adoptive secondary antibody response in irradiated mice (Hamaoka *et al.*, 1973a) and in the *in vitro* IgE antibody response of antigen-primed rabbit mesenteric lymph node cells (Kishimoto and Ishizaka, 1973). A representative result of adoptive transfer experiments is shown in Figure 5. If one transfers spleen cells from DNP-KLH-primed mice into irradiated syngeneic mice and challenges the recipients with DNP-heterologous carrier conjuate such as DNP-OA, no anti-DNP IgE antibody is formed in the recipients. If OA-primed spleen cells are cotransferred together with DNP-KLH-primed cells and the recipients are challenged with DNP-OA, a marked IgE antihapten antibody response is observed. OA-specific helper cells are removed by treatment of the spleen cells with anti-θ antiserum and C, indicating that helper cells belong to T cells.

Similar studies using an *in vitro* IgE antibody response of rabbit mesenteric lymph node cells provided interesting facts on the dissociation between the helper function for IgE and IgG antibody responses. Mesenteric lymph node cells of a rabbit immunized with alum-precipitated dinitrophenyl derivatives of ascaris extract (DNP-Asc) produced both IgE and IgG antihapten antibodies *in vitro* on stimulation with homologous antigen but failed to form antibodies on stimulation with DNP derivatives of heterologous carrier such as ragweed antigen (DNP-Rag). If a supplemental immunization of alum-adsorbed Rag was given to DNP-Asc-primed animals, their lymph node cells formed both IgE and IgG antihapten antibodies on stimulation with either DNP-Asc or DNP-Rag (Table 4). The results

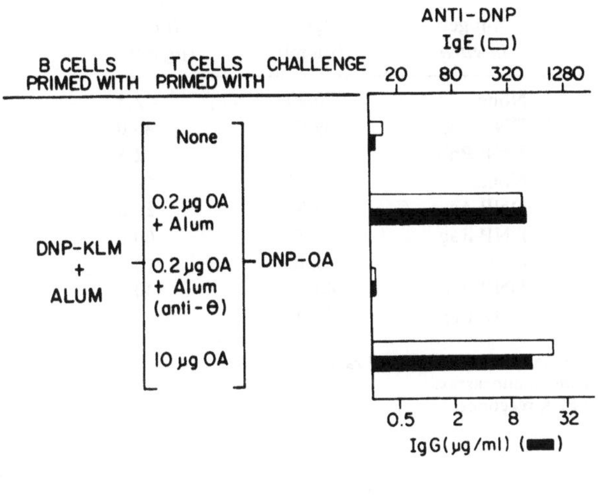

Figure 5. Adoptive secondary antibody responses in irradiated mice. Sources of B cells were primed with DNP-KLH in alum. Their spleen cells were transferred into irradiated syngeneic mice with or without spleen cells from ovalbumin-primed mice and the recipients were challenged by DNP-OA without adjuvant. Antihapten IgE antibody titer at day 10 and IgG antibody titer at day 21 are shown.

are similar to those obtained in adoptive transfer experiments in irradiated mice. When DNP-Asc-primed rabbits received a supplemental immunization of the same Rag antigen included in complete Freund's adjuvant, stimulation of their lymphocytes with DNP-Rag induced IgG but no IgE antihapten antibody response (Table 4). Stimulation of the same cell suspension with DNP-Asc gave both IgE and IgG antibody responses, indicating that hapten-primed IgE-B memory cells were present in the cell suspension. The results suggested that T-helper cells collaborating with IgE-B cells are distinct from those collaborating with IgG-B cells (Kishimoto and Ishizaka, 1973). Similar experiments in high-responder mice using adoptive transfer technique, however, failed to confirm the results (Hamaoka *et al.*, 1973b). However, Kimoto *et al.* (1977) succeeded in demonstrating the *in vitro* secondary IgE antibody response of spleen cells of Balb/c mice and studied the effect of adjuvant on priming of helper cells. These investigators immunized mice with Asc included in either alum or CFA and mixed their spleen cells with DNP-OA-primed spleen cells. The cell suspensions were stimulated with DNP-Asc *in vitro* and then cultured for the formation of antibodies. The results showed that T cells obtained by alum priming had helper activities for both IgG_1 and IgE antibody responses, whereas those obtained by CFA priming enhanced only IgG_1 antibody response. These findings collectively suggest that T-helper cells collaborating with IgE-B memory cells are different from those collaborating with IgG-B memory cells. As suggested by Katz *et al.* (1974), however, dissociation between IgE and IgG antibody responses could be due to different sensitivity of IgE-B cells vs. IgG-B cells to the same T-cell population. Since the differentiation of B memory cells is controlled by both helper and suppressor T cells (see below), dissociation between the two isotypes can be explained by different sensitivity of B cells. The third possibility to be considered is that two different subpopulations of T cells, i.e., "antigen-specific helper cells" and "isotype-specific helper cells," may be involved. The presence of allotype-specific helper and suppressor T cells (Herzenberg *et al.*, 1975) may support this possibility.

Another role of helper T cells in the IgE antibody response is that these cells

TABLE 4. Helper Function of Carrier-Specific Cells against Primary and Secondary Carriers for IgG and IgE Antibody Responses

		Anti-DNP	
Supplemental immunization[a]	Antigen *in vitro*	IgG[b] (μg/ml)	IgE[c] (μg/ml)
None	None	0.29	<2.5
	DNP-Asc	39.0	40.0
	DNP-Rab	0.35	<2.5
Ragweed Ag	None	0.32	<2.5
	DNP-Asc	18.5	20.0
	DNP-Rag	23.5	60.0
Ragweed Ag	None	0.40	<2.5
	DNP-Asc	40.0	40.0
	DNP-Rag	30.0	<2.5

[a] Supplemental immunization was given to DNP-Asc-primed rabbits.
[b] IgG antibody was measured by radioimmunoassay.
[c] IgE antibody was determined by PCA reactions.

participate in the development of B memory cells from their precursors. In the experiments shown in Figure 6, two groups of high-responder mice were immunized with alum-precipitated urea-denatured antigen, or the same antigen without adjuvant. The reason for using urea-denatured ovalbumin (UD-OA) in this experiment was that the modified antigen can prime T cells specific for native OA but do not prime B cells specific for the major antigenic determinants in native OA molecules (Takatsu and Ishizaka, 1975). These primed mice as well as control mice were then immunized with DNP-OA without adjuvant. Under the conditions employed, control mice failed to produce IgE antibody. However, mice primed with alum-adsorbed UD-OA formed antihapten IgE antibody. After 4 weeks, these mice were sacrificed, and hapten-specific B memory cells in their spleens were assessed the the adoptive transfer technique. The results showed that hapten-specific B memory cells for IgE antibody developed in the mice primed with alum-adsorbed UD-OA but not in the others. It appears that priming with alum-precipitated carrier enhanced the development of B memory cells committed for IgE. Indeed, the transfer of splenic T cells from the carrier-primed mice also enhanced the development of IgE-B memory cells.

3.3. Regulation of IgE Antibody Response by Suppressor T Cells

Both the development of IgE-B memory cells and the differentiation of B memory cells to IgE-forming plasma cells are regulated by antigen-specific sup-

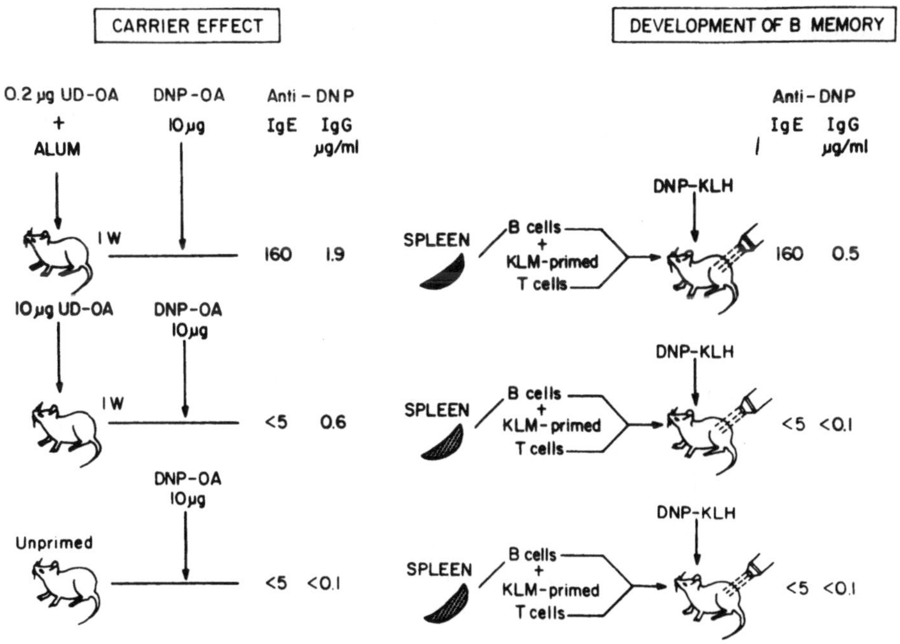

Figure 6. Role of carrier-primed T cells on the development of B memory cells. Mice were primed with urea-denatured ovalbumin (UD-OA) with or without adjuvant. One week later, they were immunized with 10 μg of DNP-OA without adjuvant. Four weeks after the immunization, hapten-primed B memory cells in their spleens were assessed by the adoptive transfer technique in irradiated mice.

pressor T cells. In previous studies on IgG and IgM antibody responses, most of the antigen-specific suppressor T cells are raised in low-responder mice; however, these cells can be generated even in high-responder strains. For example, (C57BL/6 × DBA/2) F_1 (BDF1) mice are one of the highest responders to OA, and they produce a high and persistent IgE antibody response when immunized with alum-adsorbed OA. However, repeated intravenous injections of OA or UD-OA into OA-primed mice induced the generation of OA-specific suppressor T cells. The splenic T cells from urea-denatured antigen-treated mice suppressed primary IgE antibody response of the recipient to alum-adsorbed DNP-OA (Takatsu and Ishizaka, 1976a). Suppression of IgE antibody response was specific for carrier; the splenic T cells from the UD-OA-treated mice failed to suppress anti-DNP antibody response to DNP-KLH.

Antigen-specific suppressor T cells depressed ongoing IgE antibody formation as well (Takatsu and Ishizaka, 1976b). In the experiment shown in Figure 7, BDF1 mice were immunized with a minute dose of OA included in alum. After IgE antibody titer reached maximum, 20 million splenic T cells of UD-OA-treated mice were transferred to the animals. Control mice received normal T cells. It is evident that IgE antibody titer declined after the transfer of suppressor T cells. Repeated transfer of suppressor T cells further diminished IgE antibody titer. Effect of suppressor T cells on the ongoing IgE formation suggests an important role of suppressor T cells on the regulation of IgE antibody response.

Throughout the studies described above, it was frequently observed that IgE antibody response was more susceptible to antigen-specific suppressor T cells than IgG antibody response. These findings suggest the possibility that suppressor T cells are involved in dissociation between IgE and IgG antibody responses. As described, a persistent IgE antibody response was obtained in high-responder BDF1 mice only when they were immunized with a minute dose (0.05 μg) of alum-adsorbed OA or DNP-OA. An increase of antigen dose for immunization resulted

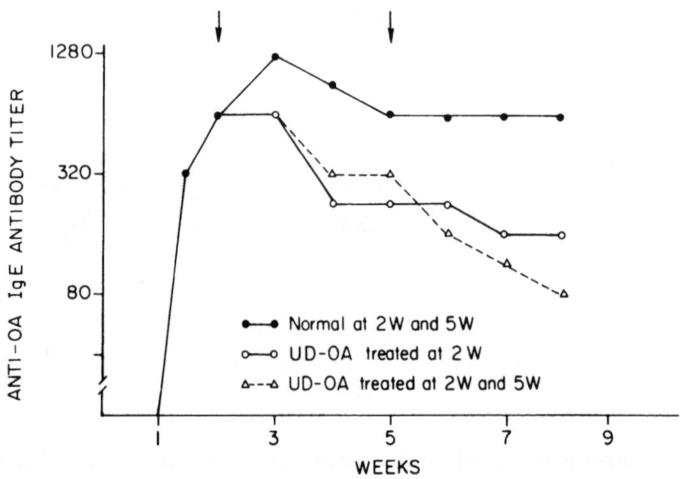

Figure 7. Depression of ongoing IgE antibody formation by suppressor T cells. All animals were immunized with alum-adsorbed OA. At 2 weeks, 2 × 10^7 splenic T cells from normal mice (•—•) or UD-OA treated mice (○—○, △—△). From Takatsu and Ishizaka (1976b).

in a transient IgE antibody response, although the magnitude of IgG antibody response rather increased (Figure 8). Determination of helper T cells and IgE-B memory cells developed in the groups of mice by adoptive transfer techniques indicated that spleen cells from the three groups of mice were comparable with respect to the helper activity of T cells and the size of IgE-B memory cell population. A difference between the high-dose group and the low-dose group was the presence of antigen-specific suppressor T cells in the former group. Thus suppressor T cells were demonstrated in splenic T cells of mice immunized with 10 μg OA but not in the animals primed with 0.05 μg OA (Tamura and Ishizaka, 1978). As discussed, transfer of suppressor T cells depressed ongoing IgE antibody response and frequently caused dissociation between IgG and IgE antibody responses. In the experiments shown in Figure 7, for example, IgE antibody diminished to ⅛ after the transfer of suppressor T cells, but IgG antibody titer of the same recipients was more than 50% of control mice. Taken collectively, a transient IgE antibody response by high-dose immunization is probably due to generation of suppressor T cells.

The possibility may be considered that antigen-specific suppressor T cells for IgE are distinct from those for IgG antibody response. As suggested by Katz *et al.* (1974), dissociation between IgE and IgG antibody responses could be due to different sensitivity of IgE-B cells vs. IgG-B cells to the same helper and suppressor T cells. Indeed, our findings on both the antigen E system and OA system can be explained by either of these hypotheses. In this context, observations by Kishimoto *et al.* (1976) suggest more strongly that suppressor T cells for IgE are distinct from those for IgG. These investigators found that preimmunization of Balb/c mice with DNP derivatives of tubercle bacilli (DNP-Tbc) suppressed IgE antibody response

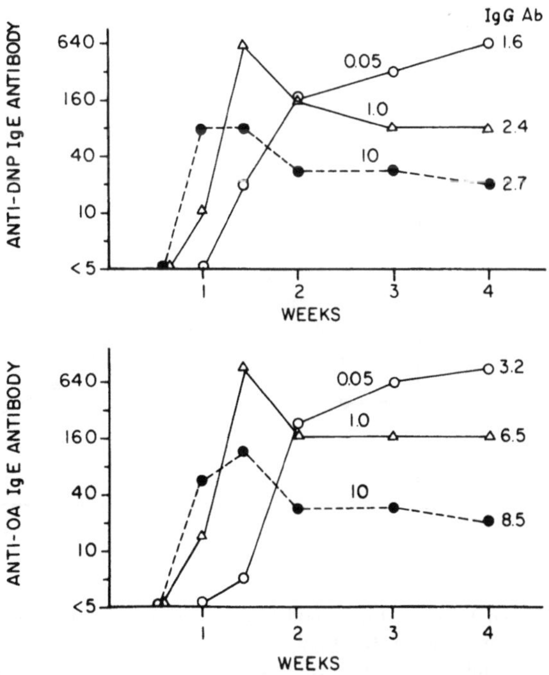

Figure 8. Effect of antigen dose on the kinetics of IgE antibody response. BDF1 mice were immunized with 0.05 μg (○—○), 1.0 μg (△—△), or 10 μg (●—●) of DNP-OA in 0.5 mg alum. Anti-DNP (upper) and anti-OA (lower) antibody responses were determined. IgG antibody titer at week 4 in terms of antigen-binding activity (μg/ml) is included in the figure. From Tamura and Ishizaka (1978).

of the animals to DNP-OA but enhanced IgG antibody responses. Furthermore, transfer of splenic T cells from DNP-Tbc-immunized mice into normal syngeneic mice suppressed primary IgE antibody response of the recipients to DNP-OA without affecting IgG antibody response. More recently, Suemura *et al.* (1977) reported that DNP-specific suppressor cells obtained by DNP-Tbc immunization actually suppressed *in vitro* IgE antibody response without affecting IgG antibody response. Combining these findings with previous observations on the dissociation of helper function for IgE and IgG antibody responses, they speculated that antigen-specific suppressor T cells for IgE may recognize and control helper T cells from the same immunoglobulin class and ultimately affect the differentiation of IgE-B cells. Weakness of the hypothesis is the lack of information for the mechanisms through which helper and/or suppressor T cells for a certain isotype will recognize B cells of the homologous isotype. Further studies on the cellular events are required to exclude one or the other hypothesis.

3.4. Experimental Model of Immunotherapy

It is well known that IgE antibody titer in the serum of ragweed-sensitive hay fever patients is persistent. In untreated patients, the IgE as well as IgG antibody titer significantly increases after each ragweed season. Quantitative measurements of IgE and IgG antibodies showed that an immunological effect of "hyposensitization treatment" or immunotherapy was dissociation between IgG and IgE antibodies (K. Ishizaka and T. Ishizaka, 1973) (Figure 9). Thus IgG antibody

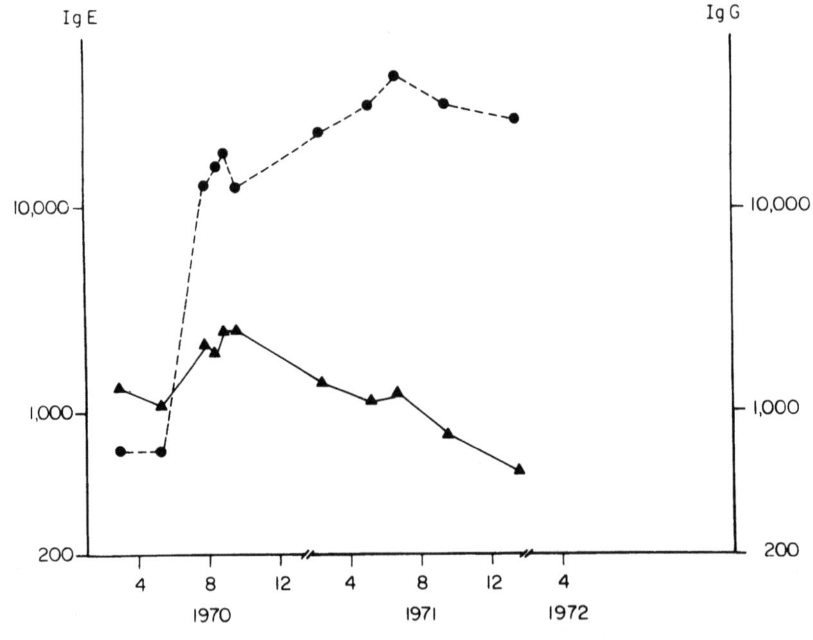

Figure 9. Effect of immunotherapy on IgE and IgG antibody titer in the serum of a ragweed-sensitive hay fever patient. Ragweed antigen was injected continuously for 2 years. IgE antibody (▲—▲) and IgG antibody (●---●) titers were measured by radioimmunoassay. From K. Ishizaka and T. Ishizaka (1973).

against ragweed antigen increased thirty- to fortyfold within 1–2 months after the initiation of the treatment. The IgE antibody titer usually increased significantly during this period, but the titer gradually declined thereafter. After 2 years of treatment, the IgE antibody level became significantly lower than the pretreatment level in more than 50% of the treated patients. The most significant effect of the treatment was suppression of secondary IgE antibody response. After a long-term treatment, most of the patients failed to show the secondary IgE antibody response after the ragweed season.

Because the T-cell population has the regulatory role in antibody response, we speculated that the effect of immunotherapy on the IgE antibody response may be due to some changes in the T-cell population and set up an animal model to analyze immunological effects of the treatment. In the course of our studies on antibody response to ragweed antigen E, we realized that urea-denatured antigen E and α-polypeptide chains isolated from the antigen molecules (King *et al.*, 1974) do not react with antibodies against the native allergen but stimulate antigen-primed T cells (K. Ishizaka *et al.*, 1974). It was also found that these modified antigens can prime T cells specific for the native antigen (K. Ishizaka *et al.*, 1975). Thus we studied the effect of repeated injections of modified antigens on the IgE antibody response. A/J strain mice were immunized with alum-adsorbed antigen E for a persistent IgE antibody response and 10 μg of UD-antigen or α-chain was injected once every week. As shown in Figure 10, the treatment diminished IgE antibody titer to native antigen E and suppressed IgE antibody response to a booster injection of native antigen. This treatment, however, did not affect the IgG antibody titer. If the same dose of native antigen E was injected every week to antigen-E-primed mice, IgG antibody titer increased. In these animals, IgE antibody titer was not significantly affected, but the treatment suppressed the secondary IgE antibody response to the antigen. It appears that the effect of repeated injections of modified antigen into antigen-E-primed mice is similar to that observed in treated patients.

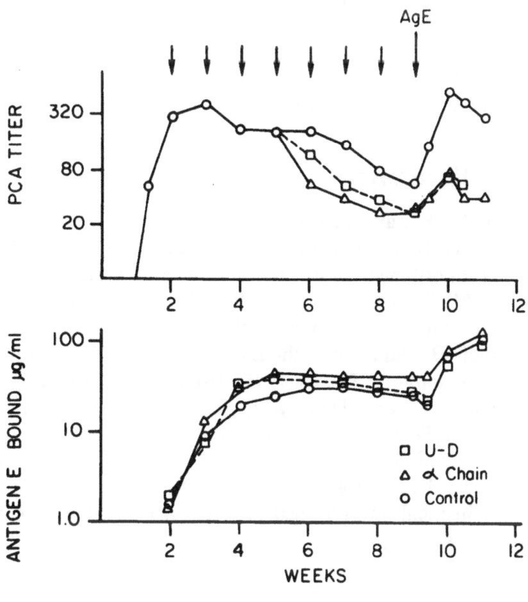

Figure 10. Effect of weekly injections of UD-antigen E or α-chain on the ongoing antibody formation to antigen E (AgE). All animals were immunized with 1 μg antigen E plus 1 mg alum and boosted with 10 μg antigen E in saline at week 9. Either 10 μg UD antigen or α-chain was injected once a week beginning from week 2. From K. Ishizaka *et al.* (1974).

In order to analyze the immunological effects of repeated antigen injections, helper activity and B memory cells in the treated animals were determined by adoptive transfer technique (Takatsu *et al.*, 1975b). The results showed that repeated injections of either native antigen or modified antigen diminished helper activity for both IgE and IgG antibody responses. The treatment with native antigen E increased both IgE-B memory cells and IgG-B memory cells for the antigen, while the activity of the B memory cells in the modified antigen-treated mice was less than that in untreated mice. Different effects of native and modified antigen on B-cell development probably explain why modified antigen was more effective than native antigen to depress the ongoing IgE antibody formation. In any event, the primary effect of the treatment appears to be depression of helper activity, which accounts for the suppression of secondary IgE antibody response. As already discussed, antigen-specific suppressor T cells are induced by repeated injections of antigen and regulate the ongoing IgE antibody formation. It appears, therefore, that depressed helper activity by repeated injections of antigen is due to the generation of suppressor T cells.

One may notice that modified antigens such as urea-denatured antigen E have an advantage for the generation of suppressor T cells. Since these antigens do not contain the major antigenic determinants in the native antigen molecules, a relatively high dose of modified antigens can be injected into atopic patients without causing side effects. As discussed above, high-dose antigen is favorable for the induction of antigen-specific suppressor T cells.

It should be noted that urea denaturation is not only the method for modification of allergens. Lee and Sehon (1978) recently reported that ragweed antigens or ovalbumin conjugated with polyethylene glycols has much lower allergenicity than the native antigen and that the administration of the conjugate suppressed both the primary and secondary IgE antibody response to the native antigen. Since the suppression of IgE antibody response by the modified antigen is carrier specific, the mechanism of suppression is probably due to generation of antigen-specific suppressor T cells. Considering the mechanisms involved in the regulation of IgE antibody formation through antigen-specific suppressor T cells, modification of allergen to tolerogen and an enhancement of suppressor T cells by changing the schedules of treatment would be one of the reasonable approaches to improve the effect of immunotherapy.

4. References

Bach, M. K., and Brashler, J. R., 1973, On the nature of the presumed receptor for IgE on mast cells. II. Demonstration of the specific binding of IgE to cell-free particulate preparations from rat peritoneal mast cells, *J. Immunol.* **111**:324.

Bach, M. K., and Brashler, J. R., 1974, *In vivo* and *in vitro* production of slow reacting substance in the rat upon treatment with calcium ionophores, *J. Immunol.* **113**:2040.

Bennich H., and von Bahr-Lindström, H., 1974, Structure of immunoglobulin E, in: *Progress in Immunology II*, Vol. 1 (L. Brent and J. Holborrow, eds.), p. 49, North-Holland, Amsterdam.

Bennich, H., and Dorrington, K., 1972, Structure and conformation of immunoglobulin E, in: *Biological Role of the Immunoglobulin E System* (K. Ishizaka and D. H. Dayton, eds.), p. 19, National Institute of Child Health and Human Development, Washington, D.C.

Bennich, H., and Johansson, S. G. O., 1968, Studies on a new class of human immunoglobulins. II. Chemical and physical properties, in: *Killander Gamma Globulin*, p. 199, Interscience, New York.

Bennich, H., Ishizaka, K., Ishizaka, T., and Johansson, S. G. O., 1969, Immunoglobulin E. A comparative study of γE globulin and myeloma IgND, *J. Immunol.* **102:**826.
Conrad, D. H., and Froese, A., 1976, Characterization of the target cell receptor for IgE. II. Polyacrylamide gel analysis of the surface IgE receptor from normal rat mast cells and from rat basophilic leukemia cells, *J. Immunol.* **116:**319.
Conrad, D. H., and Froese, A., 1978. Characterization of the target cell receptor for IgE. III. Properties of the receptor isolated from rat basophilic leukemia cells by affinity chromatography. *J. Immunol.* **120:**429.
Conrad, D. H., Bazin, H., Sehon, A. H., and Froese, A., 1975, Binding parameters of the interaction between rat IgE and rat mast cell receptors, *J. Immunol.* **114:**1688.
Conrad, D. H., Froese, A., Ishizaka, T., and Ishizaka, K., 1978, Evidence for antibody activity against the receptor for IgE in a rabbit antiserum prepared against IgE–receptor complexes, *J. Immunol.* **120:**507.
Hamaoka, T., Katz, D. H., and Benacerraf, B., 1973a, Hapten-specific IgE antibody responses in mice. II. Cooperative interactions between adoptively transferred T and B lymphocytes in the development of IgE response, *J. Exp. Med.* **138:**538.
Hamaoka, T., Katz, D. H., and Benacerraf, B., 1973b, Hapten-specific IgE antibody responses in mice. III. Establishment of parameters for generation of helper T cell function regulating the primary and secondary responses of IgE and IgG B lymphocytes, *J. Immunol.* **113:**958.
Herzenberg, L. A., Okumura, K., and Metzler, D. M., 1975, Regulation of immunoglobulin and antibody production by allotype suppressor T cell in mice, *Transplant. Rev.* **27:**57.
Ishizaka, K., and Ishizaka, T., 1967, Identification of γE antibodies as a carrier of reaginic activity, *J. Immunol.* **99:**1187.
Ishizaka, K., and Ishizaka, T., 1968a, Reversed type allergic skin reaction by anti-γE globulin antibodies in humans and monkeys, *J. Immunol.* **100:**554.
Ishizaka, K., and Ishizaka, T., 1968b, Induction of erythema wheal reactions by soluble antigen–IgE antibody complexes in humans, *J. Immunol.* **101:**68.
Ishizaka, K., and Ishizaka, T., 1968c, Human reaginic antibodies and immunoglobulin E, *J. Allergy* **42:**300.
Ishizaka, K., and Ishizaka, T., 1969, Immune mechanisms of reversed type reaginic hypersensitivity, *J. Immunol.* **103:**588.
Ishizaka, K., and Ishizaka, T., 1973, Role of IgE and IgG antibodies in reaginic hypersensitivity in the respiratory tract, in: *Asthma: Physiology, Immunopharmacology and Treatment* (K. F. Austen and L. M. Lichtenstein, eds.), pp. 55–70, Academic, New York.
Ishizaka, K., and Kishimoto, T., 1972, Regulation of antibody response *in vitro*. II. Formation of rabbit reaginic antibody, *J. Immunol.* **109:**65.
Ishizaka, K., Ishizaka, T., and Hornbrook, M. M., 1966a, Physicochemical properties of human reaginic antibody. IV. Presence of a unique immunoglobulin as a carrier of reaginic activity, *J. Immunol.* **97:**75.
Ishizaka, K., Ishizaka, T., and Hornbrook, M. M., 1966b, Physicochemical properties of human reaginic antibody. V. Correlation of reaginic activity with γE globulin antibody, *J. Immunol.* **97:**844.
Ishizaka, K., Ishizaka, T., and Arbesman, C. E., 1967a, Induction of passive cutaneous anaphylaxis in monkeys by human γE antibody, *J. Allergy* **39:**254.
Ishizaka, K., Ishizaka, T., and Hornbrook, M. M., 1967b, Allergen-binding activity of γE, γG, and γA antibodies in sera from atopic patients: *In vitro* measurements of reaginic antibody, *J. Immunol.* **98:**490.
Ishizaka, K., Ishizaka, T., and Menzel, A. E. O., 1967c, Physicochemical properties of reaginic antibody. VI. Effect of heat on γE, γG and γA antibodies in the sera of ragweed sensitive patients, *J. Immunol.* **99:**610.
Ishizaka, K., Ishizaka, T., and Terry, W. D., 1967d, Antigenic structure of γE globulin and reaginic antibody, *J. Immunol.* **99:**849.
Ishizaka, K., Ishizaka, T., and Lee, E. H., 1970a, Biologic function of the Fc fragments of E myeloma protein, *Immunochemistry* **7:**687.
Ishizaka, K., Tomioka, H., and Ishizaka, T., 1970b, Mechanisms of passive sensitization. I. Presence of IgE and IgG molecules on human leukocytes, *J. Immunol.* **105:**1459.
Ishizaka, K., Kishimoto, T., Delespesse, G., and King, T. P., 1974, Immunogenic properties of

modified antigen E. I. Presence of specific determinants for T cells in denatured antigen and polypepetide chains, *J. Immunol.* **113**:70.

Ishizaka, K., Okudaira, H., and King, T. P., 1975, Immunogenic properties of modified antigen E. II. Ability of urea-denatured antigen and α polypeptide chain to prime T cells specific for antigen E, *J. Immunol.* **114**:110.

Ishizaka, K., Ishizaka, T., Okudaira, H., and Bazin, H., 1978, Ontogeny of IgE bearing lymphocytes in the rat, *J. Immunol.* **120**:655.

Ishizaka, T., and Ishizaka, K., 1974, Mechanisms of passive sensitization. IV. Dissociation of IgE molecules from basophil receptors at acid pH, *J. Immunol.* **112**:1781.

Ishizaka, T., and Ishizaka, K., 1975, Biology of immunoglobulin E: Molecular basis of reaginic hypersensitivity, *Progr. Allergy* **19**:60.

Ishizaka, T., and Ishizaka, K., 1978, Triggering of histamine release from rat mast cells by divalent antibodies against IgE receptors, *J. Immunol.* **120**:800.

Ishizaka, T., Ishizaka, K., Johansson, S. G. O., and Bennich, H., 1969a, Histamine release from human leukocytes by anti-γE antibodies, *J. Immunol.* **102**:884.

Ishizaka, T., Ishizaka, K., Bennich, H., and Johansson, S. G. O., 1969b, Biologic activities of aggregated immunoglobulin E, *J. Immunol.* **104**:854.

Ishizaka, T., Ishizaka, K., Orange, R. P., and Austen, K. F., 1970, The capacity of human IgE to mediate the release of histamine and slow-reacting substance of anaphylaxis (SRS-A) from monkey lung, *J. Immunol.* **104**:335.

Ishizaka, T., Tomioka, H., and Ishizaka, K., 1971, Degranulation of human basophil leukocytes by anti-γE antibody, *J. Immunol.* **106**:705.

Ishizaka, T., DeBernardo, R., Tomioka, H., Lichenstein, L. M., and Ishizaka, K., 1972a, Identification of basophil granulocytes as a site of allergic histamine release, *J. Immunol.* **108**:1000.

Ishizaka, T., Tomioka, H., and Ishizaka, K., 1972b, Release of histamine and slow reacting substance of anaphylaxis (SRS-A) by IgE–anti-IgE reactions on monkey mast cells, *J. Immunol.* **108**:513.

Ishizaka, T., Soto, C., and Ishizaka, K., 1973, Mechanisms of passive sensitization. III. Number of IgE molecules and its receptor sites on human basophil granulocytes, *J. Immunol.* **111**:500.

Ishizaka, T., Urban, J. F., Jr., and Ishizaka, K., 1976, IgE formation in the rat following infection with *Nippostrongylus brasiliensis*. I. Proliferation and differentiation of IgE-bearing cells. *Cell. Immunol.* **22**:248.

Ishizaka, T., Chang, T. H., Taggart, M., and Ishizaka, K., 1977, Histamine release from rat mast cells by antibodies against rat basophilic leukemia cell membrane, *J. Immunol.* **119**:1589.

Jakschik, B., Sullivan, T. J., Kulczycki, A., Jr., and Parker, C. W., 1977, Release of slow reacting substances from rat mast cells, *Fed. Proc.* **36**:1328.

Johansson, S. G. O., and Bennich, H., 1967, Immunological studies of an atypical myeloma immunoblobulin, *Immunology* **73**:381.

Katz, D. H., and Benacerraf, B., 1972, The regulatory influence of activated T cells on B cell responses to antigen, *Adv. Immunol.* **15**:2.

Katz, D. H., Hamaoka, T., Newburger, P. E., and Benacerraf, B., 1974, Hapten-specific IgE antibody responses in mice. IV. Evidence for distinctive sensitivities of IgE and IgG B lymphocytes to the regulatory influence of T cells, *J. Immunol.* **113**:974.

Kay, A. B., and Austen, K. F., 1971, The IgE-mediated release of an eosinophil leukocyte chemotactic factor from human lung, *J. Immunol.* **107**:899.

Kimoto, M., Kishimoto, T., Noguchi, S., Watanabe, T., and Yamamura, Y., 1977, Regulation of antibody response in different immunoglobulin classes. II. Induction of *in vitro* IgE antibody response in murine spleen cells and demonstration of a possible involvement of distinct T helper cells in IgE and IgG antibody responses, *J. Immunol.* **118**:840.

King, T. P., Norman, P. S., and Tao, N., 1974, Chemical modification of the major allergen of ragweed pollen antigen E, *Immunochemistry* **11**:83.

Kishimoto, T., and Ishizaka, K., 1972, Regulation of antibody response *in vitro*. IV. Heavy chain antigenic determinants on hapten-specific memory cells, *J. Immunol.* **109**:1163.

Kishimoto, T., and Ishizaka, K., 1973, Regulation of antibody responses *in vitro*. VI. Carrier-specific helper cells for IgE and IgG antibody response, *J. Immunol.* **111**:720.

Kishimoto, T., Hirai, Y., Suemura, M., and Yamamura, Y., 1976, Regulation of antibody response in different immunoglobulin classes. I. Selective suppression of anti-DNP IgE antibody response by preadministration of DNP-coupled mycobacterium, *J. Immunol.* **117**:396.

König, W., and Ishizaka, K., 1976, Binding of rat IgE with the subcellular components of normal rat mast cells, *Immunochemistry* **13**:345.

Kulczycki, A., Jr., and Metzger, H., 1974, The interaction of IgE with rat basophilic leukemia cells. II. Quantitative aspects of the binding reaction, *J. Exp. Med.* **140**:1676.

Kulczycki, A., Jr., McNearney, T. A., and Parker, C. S., 1976, The rat basophilic leukemia cell receptor for IgE I. Characterization as a glycoprotein, *J. Immunol.* **117**:661.

Lawton, A. R., Kincade, P. W., and Cooper, M. D., 1975, Sequential expression of germ line genes in development of immunoglobulin class diversity, *Fed. Proc.* **34**:33.

Lee, W. Y., and Sehon, A. H., 1978, Suppression of reaginic antibodies with modified allergens. II. Abrogation of reaginic antibodies with allergens conjugated to polyethylene glycol, *Int. Arch. Allergy* **56**:193.

Levine, B. B., and Redmond, A. P., 1968, The nature of the antigen antibody complexes initiating the specific wheal-and-flare reaction in sensitized man, *J. Clin. Invest.* **47**:556.

Levy, D. A., and Osler, A. G., 1966, Studies on the mechanisms of hypersensitivity phenomena. XIV. Passive sensitization *in vitro* of human leukocytes to ragweed pollen antigen, *J. Immunol.* **97**:203.

Lichtenstein, L. M., and Osler, A. G., 1964, Studies on the mechanisms of hypersensitivity phenomena. IX. Histamine release from human leukocytes by ragweed pollen antigen, *J. Exp. Med.* **120**:507.

Michael, J. G., and Bernstein, I. L., 1973, Thymus dependence of reaginic antibody formation in mice, *J. Immunol.* **111**:1600.

Newman, S. A., Rossi, G., and Metzger, H., 1977, Molecular weight and valence of the cell surface receptor for immunoglobulin E, *Proc. Natl. Acad. Sci. USA* **14**:869.

Orange, R. P., Austen, W. G., and Sasten, K. F., 1971, Immunological release of histamine and SRS-A from human lung. I. Modulation by agents influencing cellular levels of cyclic 3′, 5′ adenosine monophosphate, *J. Exp. Med.* **134**:136S.

Siraganian, R. P., Hook, W. A., and Levine, B. B., 1975, Specific *in vitro* histamine release from basophils by bivalent haptens: Evidence for activation by simple bridging of membrane-bound antibody, *Immunochemistry* **12**:149.

Stanworth, D. R., Humphrey, J. H., Bennich, H., and Johansson, S. G. O., 1968, Inhibition of Prausnitz-Küstner reaction by proteolytic-cleavage fragments of a human myeloma protein of immunoglobulin class E, *Lancet* **2**:17.

Stanworth, D. R., Housley, J., Bennich, H., and Johansson, S. G. O., 1970, Effect of reduction upon the PCA-blocking activity of immunoglobulin E, *Immunochemistry* **7**:321.

Suemura, M., Kishimoto, T., Hirai, Y., and Yamamura, Y., 1977, Regulation of antibody responses in different immunoglobulin class. III. *In vitro* demonstration of IgE-class-specific suppressor function of DNP microbacterium-primed T cells and soluble factor released from these cells, *J. Immunol.* **119**:149.

Sullivan, A. L., Grimley, P. M., and Metzger, H., 1971, Electron microscopic localization of immunoglobulin E on the surface of human basophils, *J. Exp. Med.* **134**:1403.

Takatsu, K., and Ishizaka, K., 1975, Reaginic antibody formation in the mouse. VI. Suppression of IgE and IgG antibody response to ovalbumin following the administration of high dose urea-denatured antigen, *Cell. Immunol.* **20**:276.

Takatsu, K., and Ishizaka, K., 1976a, Reaginic antibody formation in the mouse. VII. Induction of suppressor T cells for IgE and IgG antibody responses, *J. Immunol.* **116**:1257.

Takatsu, K., and Ishizaka, K., 1976b, Reaginic antibody formation in the mouse. VIII. Depression of the on-going IgE antibody formation by suppressor T cells, *J. Immunol.* **117**:1211.

Takatsu, K., and Ishizaka, K., 1977, Reaginic antibody formation in the mouse. IX. Enhancement of suppressor and helper cell activities of primed spleen cells, *J. Immunol.* **118**:151.

Takatsu, K., Ishizaka, T., and Ishizaka, K., 1975a, Biological significance of disulfide bonds in human IgE molecules, *J. Immunol.* **114**:1838.

Takatsu, K., Ishizaka, K., and King, T. P., 1975b, Immunogenic properties of modified antigen E. III. Effect of repeated injections of modified antigen on immunocompetent cells specific for native antigen, *J. Immunol.* **115**:1469.

Tamura, S., and Ishizaka, K., 1978, Reaginic antibody formation in the mouse. X. Possible role of suppressor T cells in transient IgE antibody response, *J. Immunol.* **120**:837.

Tomioka, H., and Ishizaka, K., 1971, Mechanisms of passive sensitization. II. Presence of receptors for IgE on monkey mast cells, *J. Immunol.* **107**:971.

Urban, J. F., Jr., and Ishizaka, K., 1978, IgE-B cell generating factor from lymph node cells of rats infected with *Nippostrongylus brasiliensis*. II. Effector mechanisms of IgE-B cell generating factor, *J. Immunol.* **121**:199.

Urban, J. F., Jr., Ishizaka, T., and Ishizaka, K., 1977a, IgE formation in the rat following infection with *Nippostrongylus brasiliensis*. II. Proliferation of IgE-bearing cells in neonatally thymectomized animals, *J. Immunol.* **118**:1982.

Urban, J. F., Jr., Ishizaka, T., and Ishizaka, K., 1977b, IgE formation in the rat following infection with *Nippostrongylus brasiliensis*. III. Soluble factor for the generation of IgE-bearing lymphocytes, *J. Immunol.* **119**:583.

Urban, J. F., Jr., Ishizaka, T., and Ishizaka, K., 1978, IgE-B cell generating factor from lymph node cells of rats infected with *Nippostrongylus brasiliensis*. I. Source of IgE-B cell generating factor, *J. Immunol.* **121**:192.

Vaz, E. M., Vaz, N. M., and Levine, B. B., 1971, Persistent formation of reagins in mice injected with low doses of ovalbumin, *Immunology* **21**:11.

6

Mediators of Immediate Hypersensitivity

PHILIP C. HO, ROBERT A. LEWIS, K. FRANK AUSTEN, and ROBERT P. ORANGE

1. Introduction

The clinical manifestations of allergic disorders are related to the biological effects of immunologically released mediators of immediate hypersensitivity. The physicochemical characteristics, mechanisms of generation and release, and experimentally observed pathophysiological effects of these biological activities, including interactions with other effector pathways, provide a molecular and cellular basis for understanding the allergic disorders. The mediators of immediate hypersensitivity are pharmacologically active principles that act as local messengers between a primary target cell population and populations of secondary effector cells or tissues. The primary target cells release preformed and stored mediators and participate in the generation of those mediators which are newly formed subsequent to immunological challenge. Effector cells such as eosinophils, neutrophils, platelets, T lymphocytes, and monocytes are modulated by the action of the mediators and, in turn, amplify or regulate the inflammatory host response. The granule-associated preformed mediators of immediate hypersensitivity are released from mast cells and basophils subsequent to immunological challenge by a noncytotoxic process (Hastie, 1971; Austen and Becker, 1966). The process of degranulation necessitates cell membrane changes (Lagunoff, 1973), activation of membrane-

---

PHILIP C. HO and ROBERT P. ORANGE • Department of Immunology, The Hospital for Sick Children, University of Toronto, Toronto, Ontario M5G 1X8 Canada. ROBERT A. LEWIS and K. FRANK AUSTEN • Departments of Medicine, Robert B. Brigham Hospital and Harvard Medical School, Boston, Massachusetts 02120. R. A. L. is the recipient of a Young Investigator Research Grant of the National Heart, Lung, and Blood Institute, NIH (HL-21089).

On October 10, 1977, during the preparation of this chapter, Dr. Robert P. Orange suddenly passed away. We dedicate this chapter to him as an acknowledgment of his many contributions toward the characterization of SRS-A and the understanding of mast cell activation.

bound enzymes, metabolic energy, and ionic calcium flux, and is modulated by cellular levels of cyclic nucleotides and cytoskeletal binding agents; therefore, it resembles secretory processes in other cell types (Becker and Henson, 1973). This is confirmed by recent studies which have established release of mediators by granule secretion, using morphological (Lawson *et al.*, 1977) and chemical (Yurt and Austen, 1978) criteria.

Human lung (Schild *et al.*, 1951; Brocklehurst, 1960) and nasal polyp fragments (Kaliner *et al.*, 1973) obtained from allergic subjects release histamine, slow-reacting substance of anaphylaxis (SRS-A), and, at least as demonstrated in the latter tissue, eosinophil chemotactic factor of anaphylaxis (ECF-A) subsequent to challenge by specific antigen. These same chemical mediators, as well as a platelet-activating factor (PAF) (Bogart and Stechschulte, 1974), are obtained from human lung fragments (Orange *et al.*, 1971a; Kay and Austen, 1971) after passive sensitization by atopic serum, followed by challenge with specific antigen. Similarly, these same four factors are released from basophil-rich leukocyte suspensions (Grant and Lichtenstein, 1974; Lewis *et al.*, 1975). More recently, high-molecular-weight neutrophil chemotactic factor (NCF) has been shown to be released into the venous effluent in patients with cold urticaria following cold-induced angioedema (S. I. Wasserman *et al.*, 1977). Further, serotonin (Benditt *et al.*, 1955), chymase (Lagunoff and Benditt, 1963; Yurt and Austen, 1977), intermediate-molecular-weight eosinophil chemotactic factors (Boswell *et al.*, 1978), and heparin proteoglycan (Yurt *et al.*, 1977b) have been well defined as additional granule-associated activities released from the rat peritoneal mast cell; the two latter activities have been defined in the human lung as well (Boswell *et al.*, 1978; Metcalfe *et al.*, 1978). The prostaglandins and other metabolic products of arachidonic acid are formed secondary to membrane perturbation (Vane, 1976). The list of preformed and newly generated mediators (Table 1) includes both those mediators known to be released by immunologically mediated activation-secretion and those presumed to be released under the same circumstances by virtue of their subcellular localization (Lagunoff and Pritzl, 1976).

2. Physicochemical Characteristics, Metabolism, and Pharmacological Actions of Mediators

2.1. Preformed Mediators

2.1.1. Histamine

Histamine, or β-imidazolethylamine, is formed from L-histidine by the action of a specific enzyme, L-histidine decarboxylase, which requires pyridoxal-5-phosphate as a cofactor. The enzyme in rat mast cells appears to be located in the extragranular cytoplasm and is inhibited by brocresine (NSD 1055 or 4-bromo-3-hydroxybenzyloxyamine phosphate) (Slorach and Uvnäs, 1968). Under normal conditions, rat mast cell histamine is metabolized slowly, with an intracellular half-life of about 50 days (Schayer, 1952). In mast cells (Lloyd *et al.*, 1967), basophils (Orenstein *et al.*, 1977), and platelets (Åborg and Uvnäs, 1971), the membrane-bound granules which store histamine are composed largely of proteoglycan and

TABLE 1. Mediators of Immediate Hypersensitivity

Mediator	Physicochemical characteristics	Assays	Effects	Inhibitors and antagonists	Inactivation
		A. Preformed mediators			
Histamine	β-Imidazolyl-ethylamine, mol. wt. 111	Guinea pig ileum bioassay; fluorometric and radioenzymatic	Contraction of smooth muscles; increase of vascular permeability; stimulation of suppressor T lymphocytes; enhancement (H-1) or inhibition (H-2) of granulocyte chemotaxis	H-1, e.g., mepyramine H-2, e.g., cimetidine	Histaminase Histamine *N*-methyltransferase + monoamine oxidase
Serotonin	5-Hydroxytryptamine, mol. wt. 176	Estrous rat uterus bioassay; fluorometric and radioenzymatic	Increase of vascular permeability and anaphylaxis in the rat	Cyproheptadine Methylsergide	Monoamine oxidase
ECF-A	Val/Ala-Gly-Ser-Glu, mol. wt. 360–390	Chemotactic attraction of eosinophils in a modified Boyden chamber	Chemotactic attraction of eosinophils and neutrophils; eosinophil and neutrophil deactivation	*N*- and *C*-terminal tripeptides; high-dose histamine	Subtilisin Pronase Aminopeptidase-M Carboxypeptidase A
Intermediate-molecular-weight ECF peptides	Peptides, mol. wt. 1200–2500	As in ECF-A	As in ECF-A	Unknown	Carboxypeptidase A
NCF	Protein, mol. wt. >750,000	Chemotactic attraction of neutrophils in a modified Boyden chamber	Chemotactic attraction of neutrophils and eosinophils; neutrophil and eosinophil deactivation	Unknown	Unknown

(continued)

TABLE 1. Mediators of Immediate Hypersensitivity *(Continued)*

Mediator	Physicochemical characteristics	Assays	Effects	Inhibitors and antagonists	Inactivation
		A. Preformed mediators			
Heparin	Proteoglycan, mol. wt. 750,000 (rat mast cell)	Metachromasia by azure A; uronic acid content; anticoagulant activity	Anticoagulation; inhibition of complement activation	Protamine	Heparinase
Chymase	Protein, mol. wt. 29,000	Hydrolysis of *N*-benzoyltyrosine ethyl ester Hydrolysis of [^{125}I]casein	Proteolysis with chymotryptic specificity	Serotonin Heparin Chymotrypsin inhibitors	Unknown
N-Acetyl-β-D-glucosaminidase	Protein, mol. wt. 150,000	Hydrolysis of *p*-nitrophenyl-*N*-acetyl-β-D-glucosaminide	Cleavage of glucosamine residues	Product inhibitable	Unknown
Basophil (and lung) kallikrein of anaphylaxis	Protein	Generation of bradykinin	Via bradykinin	Trypsin inhibitors	Unknown
Arylsulfatase	Protein, mol. wt. 116,000 (A)	Hydrolysis of *p*-nitrocatechol sulfate	Inactivation of SRS-A	Phosphate Sulfate Product and substrate inhibitable	Unknown

		B. Newly generated mediators			
SRS-A	Acidic unsaturated sulfur-containing lipid, mol. wt. 300–500	Contraction of guinea pig ileum in the presence of atropine and mepyramine	Contraction of pulmonary smooth muscle; increase of vascular permeability	FPL55712	Arylsulfatases A and B
PAFs	Phospholipidlike, mol. wt. 700 (rat)	Release of [^{14}C]serotonin from platelets	Platelet aggregation; platelet degranulation	Unknown	Phospholipases A, C, and D
Prostaglandins and thromboxanes	C_{20} unsaturated carboxylated acids	Bioassay on rat stomach strip, rabbit aorta, guinea pig ileum, rat colon, and chick rectum in the presence of antagonists of other mediators GC-mass spectrometry	Bronchial muscle contraction (PGD_2, $PGF_{2\alpha}$, TXA_2), or relaxation (PGE_2) Platelet aggregation (TXA_2), or inhibition thereof (PGI_2, PGD_2) Vasodilatation, pyrogenesis, nociogenesis	Arachidonic acid metabolites with opposing effects as noted	Specific dehydrogenases
Lipid chemotactic factors	C_{20} unsaturated carboxylic acid (HETE) C_{17} unsaturated carboxylic acid (HHT) Uncharacterized lipids (from rat peritoneal exudate)	Chemotactic attraction of neutrophils and eosinophils in a modified Boyden chamber	Chemotaxis and chemokinesis of neutrophils (HHT, HETE, and rat lipid factor) and eosinophils (HETE, HHT)	Unknown	Unknown

protein. Membrane-free granules isolated from rat mast cells take up exogenous histamine avidly by a cationic exchange mechanism (Uvnäs, 1971). Within 1 min of the intravenous injection of [^{14}C]histamine into humans, over 95% of the radioactivity is converted to histamine metabolites (Beall and VanArsdel, 1960). Most of the histamine is methylated by histamine methyltransferase to form 1-methyl-4-(β-aminoethyl)imidazole (methylhistamine) and is then deaminated by monoamine oxidase (MAO) to form 1-methylimidazole-4-acetic acid. A second route involves the oxidation of histamine by a diamine oxidase (histaminase) to imidazole-4-acetic acid, which is then largely conjugated and excreted in the urine as 1-ribosyl-imidazole-4-acetic acid. Attempts to block one pathway result in accelerated catabolism by the alternate route.

Histamine may be quantitated by bioassay, using the cat or guinea pig terminal ileum in organ bath (Austen, 1976), by a fluorometric method (Shore, 1976), or by a sensitive radioenzymatic assay (Snyder and Taylor, 1976).

Since the introduction of a new class of histamine antagonists by Black *et al.*, (1972), the two types of histamine receptors postulated by Ash and Schild (1966) have been functionally further characterized. The receptors involved in the histamine-induced contraction of intestinal and bronchial smooth muscle are sensitive to the classical H-1 antihistamines. Histamine stimulation of gastric acid secretion and of chronotropic and inotropic cardiac effects is blocked by H-2 antagonists such as burimamide, metiamide, and cimetidine. Histamine suppresses IgE-mediated histamine release from basophils (Bourne *et al.*, 1971), lysosomal enzyme release from neutrophils (Zurier *et al.*, 1974), and allogeneic cell killing by T lymphocytes (Plaut *et al.*, 1973) via H-2 receptors. Histamine appears to mediate the H-2 effects by elevating the level of intracellular cyclic 3′,5′-adenosine monophosphate (cyclic AMP) (Douglas, 1975a). The urticarial lesions elicited by intracutaneous histamine require the combination of H-1 and H-2 antagonists for inhibition (Beaven, 1976). Similarly, the chemokinetic action of histamine on neutrophilic and eosinophilic polymorphonuclear leukocytes (Clark *et al.*, 1975) is abolished only by a combination of H-1 and H-2 antagonists (Clark *et al.*, 1977). Activation of the H-1 receptor enhances and that of H-2 inhibits the chemotactic response of these granulocytes to a cell-specific factor (Goetzl and Austen, 1976b). In general, H-1 actions are proinflammatory and H-2 actions are antiinflammatory.

Histamine enhances venular permeability *in vivo* by a direct contractile response of the endothelial cells lining the postcapillary venules; interendothelial gaps then allow free passage of plasma proteins and platelets from vessel lumen to tissue spaces (Majno *et al.*, 1969). This transient venular response allows transudation in early phases of the inflammatory response but is limited by tachyphylaxis to a second wave of histamine (Wilhelm, 1973). The effects of intravenous histamine on central and peripheral airways in the unanesthetized guinea pig (Drazen and Austen, 1975) and the medicated dog (Gold *et al.*, 1976; LaPierre *et al.*, 1976) are mediated in part by irritant receptors and reflex vagal stimulation. Atropine abolishes the increases in pulmonary resistance more readily than the decrease in compliance, suggesting that the latter occurs by both direct and reflex mechanisms. In the human, intravenous histamine raises pulmonary resistance in asthmatic airways but not in those of normal subjects (Newball, 1976), indicating that this may not be the critical pathway for histamine action on pulmonary mechanics. Both histamine (Weiss *et al.*, 1932) and an endogenous histamine liberator (Lecomte, 1957), when given intravenously to normal humans, elicit vasodilatation, urticaria, and angioedema, especially of the head and neck, hypertension, vomiting, tenesmus, and hyper- or hypoventilation, but no bronchospasm. These effects may relate to the pathophysiology of acute systemic anaphylaxis, where massive amounts of histamine are liberated into the systemic circulation. Indeed, more recently, venom-induced experimental anaphylaxis in the human has been shown to be associated with increased levels of serum histamine (Kaplan *et al.*, 1977). Elevated plasma histamine levels have also been observed in resting patients with basophilic leukemia (Beaven, 1976), in patients with exercise-induced asthma (McFadden and Soter, 1977), and transiently in patients with cold urticaria (Soter *et al.*, 1976; Kaplan *et al.*, 1975) following appropriate physical stimuli.

2.1.2. Serotonin

In the rat mast cell, serotonin (5-hydroxytryptamine) is a product of a relatively nonspecific decarboxylase acting on 5-hydroxytryptophan (Slorach and Uvnäs, 1968). Because the enzyme responsible for hydroxylating tryptophan to the precursor 5-hydroxytryptophan is absent, hydroxylation of tryptophan is the rate-limiting step. Serotonin is stored in rat mast cell granules, possibly bound to a chymotryptic enzyme termed chymase (Yurt and Austen, 1977, 1978). In humans and most other species, serotonin is found in the central nervous system, in the enterochromaffin cells of the gastrointestinal tract, and in platelet granules but not in mast cells (Sjoerdsma *et al.*, 1957). It is catabolized rapidly by monoamine oxidase of the pulmonary endothelial cells (Vane, 1969) and is excreted in the urine as 5-hydroxyindoleacetic acid.

Serotonin can be measured by bioassay on the estrous rat uterus or by a fluorometric assay (Spector, 1976). Specific antagonists include methylsergide (1-methyl-*d*-lysergic acid butanolamide) and cyproheptadine (Periactin) (reviewed by Douglas, 1975a). The *in vitro* effects of serotonin exhibit considerable species variation, and many tissue preparations demonstrate tachyphylaxis to repeated doses. *In vitro* preparations of isolated human bronchial tissue are not constricted by serotonin (Brocklehurst, 1958). *In vivo,* a role for serotonin in immediate hypersensitivity is established only for passive pulmonary anaphylaxis in the rat (Farmer *et al.*, 1975) and for systemic and cutaneous anaphylaxis in rat (Sanyal and West, 1958) and mouse (Gershon and Ross, 1962). In the rat, local application of serotonin to venular endothelium causes intercellular gaps similar to those produced by histamine (Wilhelm, 1973). Inhalation of serotonin aerosol by normal humans elicits no bronchoconstrictive effects (Herxheimer, 1955). Elevations in blood serotonin have been noted with attacks of flushing and diarrhea in the carcinoid syndrome (Sjoerdsma *et al.*, 1956) and in experimental angioedema in a patient with cholinergic urticaria (Kaplan *et al.*, 1975).

2.1.3. Eosinophil Chemotactic Factor of Anaphylaxis, Intermediate-Molecular-Weight Eosinophil Chemotactic Factors, and High-Molecular-Weight Neutrophil Chemotactic Factor

The immunological release of a selective chemoattractive factor for eosinophils was initially demonstrated in guinea pig (Kay *et al.*, 1971) and human (Kay and Austen, 1971) lung fragments. This factor, designated "eosinophil chemotactic factor of anaphylaxis" (ECF-A), was subsequently described in human nasal polyps (Kaliner *et al.*, 1973), human leukemic basophils (Lewis *et al.*, 1975), sera from patients with idiopathic acquired cold urticaria subjected to cold challenge (Soter *et al.*, 1976), and the bullous fluid from patients with bullous pemphigoid (Wintroub *et al.*, 1978). ECF-A is preformed in rat peritoneal mast cell granules (Wasserman *et al.*, 1974a) and in dispersed human lung mast cells (Paterson *et al.*, 1976b). The structural identity of the low-molecular-weight eosinophil chemotactic factors released immunologically from human, rat, and guinea pig has not been established.

Purification of the low-molecular-weight eosinophil chemotactic activity extracted from human lung by sequential chromatography over Sephadex G-25, Dowex-1, Sephadex G-10, and paper yielded two acidic tetrapeptides of 300–400 daltons. These were identified as Ala-Gly-Ser-Glu and Val-Gly-Ser-Glu and then synthesized (Goetzl and Austen, 1975). The synthetic tetrapeptides and purified low-molecular-weight eosinophil chemotactic factors, extracted or released as ECF-A, exhibited the same dose-response profile, with a peak chemotactic activity preferential for human eosinophils in the concentration range of 5×10^{-8} to 1×10^{-6} M, as assayed in modified Boyden chambers (Kay and Austen, 1971). Synthetic tetrapeptides and their analogues and tripeptide substituent fragments have been functionally characterized by assessing both their relative potencies as chemotactic factors and their abilities to inhibit directed migration of eosinophils toward a chemotactic stimulus (Goetzl and Austen, 1976a). Of four synthetic tetrapeptides (Ala/Val/Leu/Phe-Gly-Ser-Glu) with differing *N*-terminals, the leucyl tetrapeptide was most potent, and the phenylalanyl analogue the least. Mixtures of alanyl and valyl tetrapeptides tested in varying ratios had an action equal to that of each alone at a concentration equal to their sum, suggesting a common receptor. While reversal of the internal glycine and serine residues had no significant effect, deletion of the glycine residue led to a distinct reduction in chemotactic potency, indicating that the internal dipeptide has mainly a spacer function. Neither the *N*-terminal nor *C*-terminal tripeptides were chemotactically active. Preincubation of eosinophils with one-hundredth of the minimal chemotactic dose of either alanyl or valyl tetrapeptides impaired their subsequent response to the latter, demonstrating a uniquely low threshold of eosinophils to such deactivation. Each tetrapeptide cross-deactivated to a chemotactic C5 fragment of somewhat higher doses. Although neither the *N*- nor *C*-terminal tripeptides have significant chemotactic activity, the former demonstrates reversible stimulus-specific competitive inhibition and the latter demonstrates irreversible cell-directed inhibition. These observations imply that the eosinophil receptor for the acidic tetrapeptides binds the *N*-terminal region by a hydrophobic domain and is activated and deactivated by the *C*-terminal glutamic acid via an ionic domain (Goetzl and Austen, 1976a; Boswell *et al.*, 1976). The tetrapeptides of ECF-A also elicit directed migration of human neutrophils at tenfold higher concentrations in an interaction inhibited in the expected fashion by *N*- and *C*- terminal tripeptides (Goetzl and Austen, 1976b). Notably, however, ECF-A has no effect on monocytes (Goetzl and Austen, 1975). Histamine blocks the chemotactic response of human eosinophils to the tetrapeptides by an H-2 action and enhances the directed migratory response by an H-1 effect. The action of tetrapeptides in uncovering additional eosinophil C3b receptor activity (Anwar and Kay, 1977) may facilitate the host defense benefits derived from their chemotactic activation and deactivation. Eosinophilotactic activity of ECF-A tetrapeptides has also been observed when they are injected into marmoset or human skin (L. W. Turnbull *et al.*, 1977).

Other cells are also capable of releasing low-molecular-weight eosinophil chemotactic factors (ECF), albeit by other than IgE-dependent mechanisms. Low-molecular-weight ECFs obtained from extracts of human bronchogenic carcinomas (Wasserman *et al.*, 1974b), supernatants of tumor cell cultures, and urine from tumor-bearing patients (Goetzl *et al.*, 1978) are less acidic than the tetrapeptides of ECF-A. Neutrophils, when stimulated by phagocytosis or with the calcium ionophore A23187, release a low-molecular-weight ECF which is not preformed (Czarnetski *et al.*, 1976; König *et al.*, 1976) and is completely uncharacterized.

Eosinophilotactic peptides of 1200–2500 molecular weight (intermediate-molecular-weight ECF) with preferential chemotactic activity for eosinophils and secondary specificity for neutrophils are released anaphylactically with low-molecular-weight eosinophilotactic activity from rat mast cells. Three factors of different charge and hydrophobicity constitute the intermediate-molecular-weight ECF of the rat mast cell. These factors are chemotactic and not chemokinetic for eosinophils. A similar activity by size has been extracted from human lung, but has not been further characterized (Boswell *et al.*, 1978).

The peak of chemotactic activity appearing in the exclusion volume of Sephadex G-25 gel filtration of human lung or rat peritoneal extracts is preferentially chemotactic for neutrophils, but has not been physicochemically characterized (S. I. Wasserman *et al.*, 1977). Such a high-molecular-weight activity was first described in extracts of human leukemic basophils (Lewis *et al.*, 1975), but in no instance has its immunological release been documented. A high-molecular-weight NCF is released into the venous effluents of a cold-challenge extremity of patients with cold urticaria (S. I. Wasserman *et al.*, 1977). Purified high-molecular-weight NCF is greater than 750,000 and has a neutral isoelectric point. It is believed to be released from human mast cells because the time course of its appearance and disappearance in the monitored venous effluent corresponds to that of histamine and ECF-A (S. I. Wasserman *et al.*, 1977). It has a primary specificity for neutrophils, a secondary action on eosinophils, and no effect on monocytes.

The presumed effect of the chemotactic principles *in vivo* is to attract eosinophilic and neutrophilic granulocytes to the site of an immediate hypersensitivity reaction by a complex gradient of factors differing in size, charge, hydrophobicity, and relative chemotactic and chemokinetic activity, and to hold them by deactivation. The function of the responding eosinophil is considered later.

2.1.4. Heparin Proteoglycan

Heparin, a highly sulfated proteoglycan with anticoagulant properties, has been identified in rat peritoneal mast cells (Yurt *et al.*, 1977a) and is discharged subsequent to IgE-dependent degranulation (Yurt *et al.*, 1977b). Enzymatic degradation of commercial heparin with heparinase has revealed hexa- or octasaccharide repeating units that are composed of tri- and disulfated disaccharides linked alternately in a proportion of 3:1, respectively (Silva and Dietrich, 1975). Biosynthesis of mouse mastocytoma heparin occurs by the stepwise alternating transfer of uronic acid and *N*-acetylhexosamine monosaccharide units from the appropriate nucleotide sugars to the nonreducing termini of the growing glycosaminoglycan chains; sulfation occurs subsequent to polymerization and requires the presence of 3′-phosphoadenylyl sulfate (reviewed by Lindahl *et al.*, 1973). Heparin from mouse mast cell tumor is catabolized by tissue heparinase (Ögren and Lindahl, 1975, 1976). Commercial and mouse tumor heparin are present as degraded glycosaminoglycan side chains. Rat mast cell heparin is a protease-resistant material of 750,000 daltons. Since rat mast cell heparin incorporates [^{3}H]serine as well as [^{35}S]sulfate and undergoes cleavage by dilute base, a characteristic of extracellular proteoglycans with a xylosyl-seryl linkage, it is held to be an unusual proteoglycan (Yurt *et al.*, 1977a). Endogenous human heparin has been recognized in human lung (Engleberg, 1963) and both 60,000-dalton proteoglycan and 20,000-dalton glycosaminoglycan side chains have been isolated from dispersed, concentrated human lung mast cells (Metcalfe *et al.*, 1978). The smaller size of human heparin proteoglycan relative to that of the rat may reflect a greater susceptibility to cleavage of the polypeptide backbone and the effects of the human cell dispersion and isolation procedure.

Release of heparin from rat mast cells has been achieved by compound 48/80 (Fillion *et al.*, 1970), polymyxin B sulfate (Lagunoff, 1972), calcium ionophore A23187, and reverse anaphylaxis (Yurt *et al.*, 1977b). In these studies, the net percentage of heparin released after solubilization of the discharged granules correlated in a linear fashion with net percentage histamine release, and the released heparin was of comparable size to the residual heparin proteoglycan.

Heparin is quantitated by assays for metachromasia, uronic acid content, functional anticoagulant activity in whole plasma, and antithrombin III cofactor activity. On the basis of uronic acid content, both residual and immunologically released rat mast cell heparin exhibits about 10–20% of the anticoagulant and antithrombin cofactor activity of the low-molecular-weight commercial heparin glycosaminoglycans. Its anticomplementary activity against the alternative pathway protein involved in formation of the amplification C3 convertase (C3bBb) is equal to that of commercial heparin (Weiler *et al.*, 1978). Heparin appears to play an antiinflammatory role as a regulatory negative feedback factor (Austen, 1979).

2.1.5. Mast Cell Granule-Associated Enzymes

At least one proteolytic enzyme is released immunologically along with histamine and heparin from guinea pig lung (Ungar and Damgaard, 1955) and rat mast cells (Lagunoff and Pritzl, 1976). Rat mast cell granules contain a chymotrypsinlike enzyme which represents a major granule protein with a specific activity comparable to that of crystallized bovine pancreatic α-chymotrypsin (Lagunoff and Pritzl, 1976). The mechanism for granule solubilization to release full chymase and heparin activity is not known but could involve oxidative (Yurt and Austen, 1977) or enzymatic degradation of the heparin proteoglycan. The cationic chymase is composed of a single polypeptide chain of 29,000 molecular weight (Yurt and Austen, 1977) and is inhibited by serotonin, which presumably is stored at the active site (Yurt and Austen, 1977, 1978). Although chymotrypsin has been shown to degranulate rat mesenteric mast cells (Uvnäs and Antonsson, 1963), and neutrophil chymotryptic activity generates several putative extracellular functions (Venge and Olsson, 1975; Odeberg and Olsson, 1975; Hällgren and Venge, 1976a, b; Malemud and Janoff, 1975), a role for mast cell chymase in either eliciting further mast cell degranulation or in generating active peptides from plasma proteins has not been studied.

N-Acetyl-β-D-glucosaminidase is of about 150,000 molecular weight, accounts for about 1% of the total rat mast cell granule protein (Lagunoff and Pritzl, 1976), and degrades polysaccharides (Lagunoff *et al.*, 1970). Proteolytic activity that releases kinin activity from crude kininogen has been observed on treatment of rat mast cells with L-epinephrine and rat serum (Rothschild *et al.*, 1974) and with antigen challenge of sensitized (IgG_1) guinea pig lung (Brocklehurst and Lahiri, 1962; Jonasson and Becker, 1966). In the human, antigen challenge of IgE-sensitized lung fragments (Webster *et al.*, 1974) and peripheral leukocytes (Newball *et al.*, 1975a) results in the release of an activity capable of hydrolyzing the synthetic substrate tosyl-L-arginine methyl ester (TAMe). Human leukocyte suspensions also release a kallikrein activity for crude kininogen (Newball *et al.*, 1975b) that comigrates with the TAMe esterase on Sephadex G-200 (Lichtenstein, 1976). One additional enzyme, arylsulfatase A, is released in a linear relationship to histamine during coupled activation–secretion of the rat mast cell. It is thus presumed to reside in the secretory granule of that cell (MacDonald-Lynch *et al.*, 1978).

The contribution of such enzymes as chymase, glucosaminidase, and arylsulfatase A, and the chemotactic factor, high-molecular-weight NCF, to the total granule protein is unclear. The approximate molar ratio of heparin proteoglycan–chymase–serotonin–histamine of the granule is roughly 1:40:40:1200 (Yurt and Austen, 1977, 1978). The estimated 20 glycosaminoglycan side chains per heparin proteoglycan would bind two cationic chymases per anionic helical glycosaminoglycan chain. Serotonin would be positioned in the active chymase site, while histamine would have an ionic linkage to carboxyl groups of the sugars in the glycosaminoglycan disaccharide units or in the protein component of the granule (Austen, 1979).

2.2. Newly Generated Mediators

2.2.1. Slow-Reacting Substance of Anaphylaxis (SRS-A)

SRS-A is a low-molecular-weight unsaturated acidic sulfur-containing lipid with smooth muscle constricting and vasodilating effects *in vivo*. It is newly generated from a number of mast-cell-rich mammalian tissues subsequent to IgE-dependent or homocytotropic IgG-dependent histamine release as well as by nonimmunological stimuli in some other cells. Its precise chemical structure is as yet unidentified, and it is not clear whether SRS-As from different species and tissues are identical or are a family of structurally related compounds. It is presently defined by its physicochemical characteristics, its susceptibility to inactivation by arylsulfatases of several sources, its ability to contract the atropinized, antihistamine-treated guinea pig ileum, and its inhibition by a semispecific antagonist, FPL55712.

SRS-A adsorbs to proteins and to phospholipids such as lecithin (Brocklehurst, 1962; Orange *et al.*, 1973) so as to cochromatograph with the binding principle. In a chloroform-methanol-water biphasic system, SRS-A partitions into the theoretical upper phase as is characteristic of polar lipids (Orange *et al.*, 1973). The observation that SRS-A could be recovered from biological fluids in a stable form, free of protein, by ethanol extraction (Brocklehurst, 1962; Orange and Austen, 1969) permitted the accumulation of sufficient amounts of biological active SRS-A for preparative functional purification. Removal of contaminating phospholipids by base hydrolysis is followed by a desalting step on nonionic Emberlite XAD chromatography. DEAE chromatography (Rouser *et al.*, 1961) separates SRS-A from gangliosides, phosphatides, and neutral hexoses, and silicic acid chromatography (Orange *et al.*, 1973) eliminates contaminating hydrocarbons, steroids, and hydroxy acids. These procedures followed by Sephadex LH-20 gel filtration result in a greater than 100,000-fold purification of SRS-A on a function-to-weight basis, with recoveries of biological activity ranging from 15% to 35% of the starting material. From the LH-20 gel filtration, using polyethylene glycol as a marker, the molecular mass of SRS-A is estimated to be between 350 and 450 daltons. Estimates of the functional activity of purified preparations of SRS-A indicate that 1 unit of activity is equivalent to between 0.1 and 1.0 ng by weight (Orange *et al.*, 1973; Strandberg and Uvnäs, 1971).

The characteristic slow, protracted contraction produced by SRS-A on the atropinized, antihistamine-treated guinea pig ileum occurs without tachyphylaxis to further doses. One unit of SRS-A is defined as the concentration required to give a contraction of the ileum of equal amplitude to that produced by 5 ng of histamine/ml (in the absence of mepyramine). While other pharmacological principles such as neutral peptide (Wintroub *et al.*, 1974), kinins, and some prostaglandins (Orange and Austen, 1976) produce a similar slow contraction pattern, only the effect of SRS-A on this assay is inhibited by FPL55712 in less than μg/ml concentrations, with 50% inhibition occurring at a concentration of 25 ng/ml (Augstein *et al.*, 1973). The action of SRS-A on guinea pig ileum and airway smooth muscle is lost in a parallel dose-response fashion by treating the agonist with arylsulfatase or the smooth muscle preparation with FPL55712 (Orange *et al.*, 1974; Drazen *et al.*, 1978).

SRS-A activity is not susceptible to inactivation by a wide variety of enzymes, including trypsin, chymotrypsin, leucine aminopeptidase, pronase, phospholipases A, B, C, and D, neuraminidase, and 15-hydroxyprostaglandin dehydrogenase (reviewed by Orange and Austen, 1969; Orange *et al.*, 1973; Strandberg and Uvnäs, 1971). A sulfur moiety in active SRS-A samples was revealed by spark source mass spectrometry (Orange *et al.*, 1974), but the charge characteristics of SRS-A were against the presence of a sulfate group. The initial observation of an enzyme, arylsulfatase, that inactivates SRS-A (Orange *et al.*, 1974) was confirmed by similar observations on partially purified arylsulfatase B from human eosinophils (Wasserman *et al.*, 1975), arylsulfatase A or B from human lung (Wasserman and Austen, 1976) and crude arylsulfatase from guinea pig tissue (Kay *et al.*, 1976). Finally, arylsulfatases capable of inactivating SRS-A have been demonstrated in rat mast cells (Orange and Moore, 1976a) and in purified form from rat leukemic basophils (Wasserman and Austen, 1977). The cleavage of *p*-nitrocatechol sulfate (*p*NCS) by highly purified arylsulfatase A or B from human lung (Wasserman and Austen, 1976) or rat leukemic basophils (Wasserman and Austen, 1977) was competitively inhibited by SRS-A, indicating a common active site for both enzymatic cleavage of *p*NCS and inactivation of SRS-A.

Because only mast cells and basophils normally have surface receptors for IgE, the release of SRS-A from human lung (Kay and Austen, 1971), skin (Greaves *et al.*, 1972), nasal polyps (Kaliner *et al.*, 1973), and peripheral leukocytes (Grant and Lichtenstein, 1974) by IgE-dependent mechanisms is presumably dependent on coupled activation–secretion by these cells. Several lines of evidence implicate the participation of additional cell types in the generation of this mediator. When dispersed human lung cells are sensitized and then challenged with specific antigen, the yield of SRS-A relative to histamine approximates that for fragments, but is markedly reduced with increasing purity of the mast-cell-enriched population (Paterson *et al.*, 1976b). With the ionophore A23187 as a stimulus, leukemic human basophils are capable of generating and releasing SRS-A (Lewis *et al.*, 1975), but normal human peripheral leukocyte and basophil-poor, granulocyte-rich fractions also generate SRS-A-like activity (Conroy *et al.*, 1976). In the rat, three pathways leading to SRS-A generation and release are recognized: an IgE-mediated mast-cell-dependent process occurs in the peritoneal cavity (Orange *et al.*, 1970); an IgG_a-mediated complement- and neutrophil-dependent generation also occurs in the peritoneal space (Orange *et al.*, 1968, 1969); and a calcium ionophore (A23187)-induced release from peritoneal macrophagelike cells has been noted *in vitro* (Bach and Brashler, 1974; Brashler and Bach, 1976). The yield of SRS-A from isolated rat peritoneal mast cells (Yecies *et al.*, 1978) or dispersed rat lung mast cells (Paterson *et al.*, 1976a) following challenge with anti-rat IgE or calcium ionophore is inordinately low for the observed histamine release, again suggesting a role for a second cell type in achieving appreciable SRS-A generation and release. In mice treated with intraperitoneal injection of distilled water to deplete mast cells, the subsequent peritoneal cell harvest is over 80% macrophages; these cells release SRS-A when stimulated *in vitro* by A23187 in the presence of 10 mM L-cysteine. In the same system, the presence of mast cells in the peritoneal lavage from untreated mice reduce SRS-A generation and release (Orange, 1977). The reduced SRS-A yield from mast-cell-containing rodent cell populations may reflect mediator inactivation by endogenous arylsulfatases, especially that of released arylsulfatase A (Orange and Moore, 1976a; MacDonald-Lynch *et al.*, 1978).

SRS-A activities obtained from human lung fragments (IgE-mediated), rat peritoneal cavities (hyperimmune serum-mediated) (Orange *et al.*, 1973), normal and leukemic basophils and granulocytes (ionophore-induced) (Conroy *et al.*, 1976; Lewis *et al.*, 1975), and mixed rat peritoneal cells (ionophore-mediated) (Bach and Brashler, 1974) have comparable chromatographic elution profiles and are inactivated by arylsulfatases. The SRS-A-like activities released from rat mast cells and perfused cat paws subsequent to stimulation by 48/80 differ from the above in their solubility and elution profiles from DEAE columns (Änggård *et al.*, 1963; Strandberg and Uvnäs, 1971).

In contrast to the preformed mediators such as histamine and ECF-A, SRS-A is generated only after an appropriate stimulus to the responsible cells (Brocklehurst, 1960; Lewis *et al.*, 1974; Orange, 1974). There is a clear difference in the kinetics of release of SRS-A and the preformed mediators. In human lung fragments and dispersed cells, intracellular accumulation of SRS-A occurs within 0.5 min of IgE-dependent activation and reaches a plateau by 2 min, whereas release is not apparent until 2–5 min and continues 15–30 min; this indicates that SRS-A continues to be generated after the release of preformed mediators has ceased (Lewis *et al.*, 1974). With a minimal IgE-dependent direct or reversed anaphylactic activation, intracellular SRS-A accumulation occurs without the release of any mediators (Lewis *et al.*, 1974), indicating that cellular formation may be a highly sensitive marker of an immediate hypersensitivity reaction. When rat peritoneal cells are stimulated with A23187, the kinetics of SRS-A generation are similar to those of SRS-A generated from lung cells (Orange, 1977).

The immunological pathways leading to the release of the preformed mediators and to the generation and release of SRS-A involve both shared and independent steps. An antigen-independent "activated" serine esterase is involved in SRS-A generation (Orange *et al.*, 1971b), while an "activatable" serine esterase (see below) appears to be an early step in histamine release (Austen and Brocklehurst, 1961). Diethylcarbamazine has been shown to selectively suppress the release of SRS-A, but not histamine, from challenged rat peritoneal cavities prepared with IgG_a (Orange and Austen, 1968). A further dissociation of the two pathways is evident when human lung fragments are subjected to IgE-dependent mediator release in the presence of cytochalasins. Cytochalasin B reversibly suppresses the release of SRS-A while exerting a variable effect on histamine release; cytochalasin A irreversibly suppresses the release of SRS-A while enhancing that of histamine (Orange, 1975). It has also been established that SRS-A generation and release are more susceptible to inhibition and enhancement by agents capable of increasing cellular levels of cyclic AMP and cyclic GMP, respectively, than is histamine release from human lung (Kaliner *et al.*, 1973; Orange *et al.*, 1971a,b,c). Preincubation of human lung fragments with certain thiols including L-cysteine, thioglycollate, and sodium sulfide results in a selective enhancement of the formation of SRS-A (Orange and Chang, 1975). While L-cysteine also selectively increases the formation of SRS-A in human peripheral leukocytes (IgE-mediated), monkey lung fragments (IgE-mediated), guinea pig lung slices (IgG_1-mediated), and rat peritoneal cells (ionophore-mediated) (Orange and Moore, 1976a,b), D-cysteine even at high doses has little effect. Another sulfur-containing compound D,L-penicillamine, while demonstrating a similar dose-dependent enhancement of SRS-A release (twelvefold) from human lung, also increases the release of histamine (threefold) (Orange, 1977). This enhancement of SRS-A generation observed in different tissues and species suggests a common enzymatic step and supports the likelihood that SRS-As from different species are close chemical relatives.

Since both SRS-A and arachidonic acid metabolites such as prostaglandins and thromboxanes (Piper and Vane, 1971) are now postulated to be generated *de novo* in membrane perturbation, their relationships are of interest. Prostaglandins and thromboxane A_2 (TXA_2) are readily released from guinea pig lung fragments by mechanical as well as by antibody-dependent reactions (Palmer *et al.*, 1973), while formation and release of SRS-A from lung fragments require a specific immunological stimulus. Several of the prostaglandins (Tauber *et al.*, 1973) and TXB_2 (Boot *et al.*, 1977) modulate the release of SRS-A. Indeed, partially purified SRS-A, as well as histamine, injected directly into the pulmonary artery releases TXA_2 and various prostaglandins from guinea pig lungs (Piper and Vane, 1969a; Engineer *et al.*, 1977) but does not release SRS-A. The release of both SRS-A and prostaglandins is suppressed by disodium cromoglycate (Dawson and Tomlinson, 1974). Pretreatment of human lung fragments with the prostaglandin synthetase (cyclooxygenase) inhibitor indomethacin enhances the immunological release of SRS-A (Walker, 1973), and pretreatment of immunized calves with nonsteroidal antiinflammatory drugs enhances the *in vitro* antigen-induced release of SRS-A from lung fragments of these animals (Burka and Eyre, 1974). It has therefore been suggested by Walker (1973) that PGs and SRS-A might be formed from a limited common precursor. Indomethacin does not affect the ionophore-induced release of SRS-A from rat peritoneal monocytes (Bach *et al.*, 1977). With the rat basophil leukemic cell line RBL-1, arachidonic acid enhances the release of SRS-A, while eicosatetraynoic acid (ETYA), a competitive inhibitor of arachidonic acid, is inhibitory (Jakschik *et al.*, 1977). ETYA apparently does not affect SRS-A release from immunologically challenged guinea pig lungs (Dawson and Tomlinson, 1974), but it does prevent its generation from human lung fragments (Lewis and Austen, unpublished observations). Finally, in the presence of radiolabeled arachidonic acid, SRS-A bioactivity generated by ionophore from RBL-1 cells (Jakschik *et al.*, 1977) or rat peritoneal monocytes (Bach *et al.*, 1977) appears to cochromatograph with the radioactivity. Taken together, the data could indicate that SRS-A is a unique product of arachidonate oxidative metabolism via the lipoxygenase pathway or that, alternatively, its generation is directly modulated by oxidative metabolites of arachidonic acid.

Human pulmonary smooth muscle is exquisitely sensitive to SRS-A (Brocklehurst, 1962; Herxheimer and Stresemann, 1963; Sheard and Blair, 1970), whereas guinea pig bronchial smooth muscle appears to be about 20 times less sensitive (Brocklehurst, 1962). Because the bovine pulmonary vein is at least 10 times more reactive to SRS-A on a dose basis than is the guinea pig ileum (Burka and Eyre, 1974), the former may be another target tissue for SRS-A *in vivo*. *In vivo* studies in unanesthetized guinea pigs injected intravenously with a highly purified preparation of SRS-A demonstrated a marked decrease in pulmonary compliance (peripheral airway effect) with only a slight increase in pulmonary resistance (central airway effect) (Drazen and Austen, 1975); in contrast to the effect of histamine, that of SRS-A on peripheral airways was not opposed by atropine. In anesthetized, artificially ventilated guinea pigs, aerosol administration of SRS-A was more active on an estimated weight basis (1 unit equals 1 ng) than either $PGF_{2\alpha}$ or histamine in raising tracheal insufflation pressure (Strandberg and Hedqvist, 1975). Further, in a recent study of systemic anaphylaxis in monkeys, FPL55712 was the most effective pharmacological antagonist, prompting the investigator to implicate SRS-A as the major active mediator (Pavek, 1977). SRS-A has also been isolated from guinea pig serum during anaphylactic shock (Stecheschulte *et al.*, 1973). Additionally, a slow-reacting substance was detectable in the plasma of asthmatic children following bronchial provocation (Orange and Langer, 1974). It reached maximal levels 20 min after aerosol administration of specific allergen and was accompanied by a 50% fall in FEV_1. Furthermore, when these patients were retested while protected with disodium cromoglycate, no SRS-A activity could be recovered from their plasma. In addition, SRS-A was shown to have marked activity on vascular permeability when injected intracutaneously into the skin of guinea pigs and monkeys, as reviewed by Orange and Austen (1969), and thus may play a role in plasma extravasation into the pulmonary microvasculature. Finally, SRS-A-like activity noted in asthmatic sputum (Harkavy, 1930) has now been shown to be susceptible to inactivation by arylsulfatase (L. S. Turnbull *et al.*, 1977).

2.2.2. Platelet-Activating Factors (PAFs)

PAFs are a family of platelet-activating mediators from various mammalian species which are newly generated subsequent to IgE-dependent immunological reactions. PAF from IgE-sensitive and antigen-challenged rabbit basophils induced not only secretion of platelet vasoactive amines and nucleotides but aggregation as well (Henson, 1977). These activities are apparently independent of each other, since a concentration of PAF deactivating the platelets for secretion does not prevent aggregation. The mechanism of PAF-induced activation–secretion in platelets involves uncovering of a serine protease, influx of extracellular calcium, and energy utilization (Henson and Oades, 1976). PAF increases vascular permeability secondary to the platelet release reaction (Benveniste *et al.*, 1973) and *in vivo* also induces platelet aggregation (Fésüs *et al.*, 1977) and a coagulopathy (Pinckard *et al.*, 1975). PAF, by definition, is assayed by measuring the release of histamine or radiolabeled serotonin from homologous platelets.

PAFs are released by IgE-dependent mechanisms from rabbit (Henson, 1970) and human (Benveniste, 1974) leukocyte suspensions and from rabbit (Kravis and Henson, 1975) and human (Bogart and Stechschulte, 1974) lung fragments. Furthermore, leukemic human basophils release a PAF subsequent to interaction with the calcium ionophore A23187 (Lewis *et al.*, 1975). While PAFs are newly generated in most preparations, they have been extracted in lesser amounts directly from human leukocyte suspensions (Benveniste, 1974) and human lung fragments (Bogart and Stechschulte, 1974) without undergoing immunological activation.

The PAF generated in rat peritoneal cavities prepared with hyperimmune serum and challenged with specific antigen can be deproteinated with 80% ethanol and eluted, after a water wash, from XAD with 80% ethanol. This PAF coelutes with SRS-A from silicic acid in the more polar lipid solvents and filters on Sephadex LH-20 with a molecular mass of approximately 700 daltons (Kater *et al.*, 1976). Further, PAF and SRS-A are resolved into separate peaks by chromatography on acetylated DEAE cellulose eluted with a sequence of solvents from chloroform–methanol (7:1, v:v) to methanol–0.3 M ammonium carbonate (1:1, v:v). Rat PAF is differentiated from SRS-A by their separable biological activities, differential elution from DEAE cellulose, and the inactivation of the former by phospholipase D from both human eosinophils and cabbage, but not by arylsulfatase (Kater *et al.*, 1976). PAF is distinguishable from prostaglandins by its elution characteristics on silicic acid chromatography as well as its inability to contract the gerbil colon. PAF binds avidly to albumin, which acts as a carrier without loss of PAF biological activity, but its binding to neutrophils and platelets decreases its recovery (Benveniste *et al.*, 1973).

Three lines of evidence indicate chemical differences among PAFs of different sources. PAF from rabbit peripheral leukocytes exhibits a higher molecular weight on Sephadex LH-20 gel filtration, approximately 1100 (Benveniste, 1974), than that from the rat peritoneal cavity (Kater *et al.*, 1976); PAF derived from human or rabbit leukocytes is inactivated by phospholipase A and C (Benveniste and Polonsky, 1976) in contrast to that from the rat peritoneal cavity (Kater *et al.*, 1976); finally, PAFs derived by IgE reactions in rabbit lung and rabbit leukocytes fail to cross-deactivate homologous platelets (Kravis and Henson, 1975).

2.2.3. Prostaglandins and Other Metabolites of Arachidonic Acid

The prostaglandins are 20-carbon unsaturated hydroxy acids which are synthesized in virtually all mammalian tissues thus far examined (Christ and Van Dorp, 1973). They are generated from fatty acids, mainly arachidonic acid (20:4), and, to a minor extent, dihomo-γ-linolenic acid (20:3). The fatty acids are made available from phospholipid membrane stores subsequent to membrane perturbation induced by mechanical, hormonal, or immunological stimuli. Membrane perturbation allows the expression of the enzymatic activity of phospholipase A_2 on phospholipid substrates, with resultant arachidonic acid release (Coceani *et al.*, 1969; Kunze and Vogt, 1971; Lands and Samuelsson, 1968; Flower and Blackwell, 1976). The released arachidonic acid may be metabolized to a variety of products by two independent pathways. The cyclooxygenase pathway initially generates cyclic endoperoxides (PGG_2 and PGH_2), which are rapidly metabolized to other products: PGE_2 and PGD_2 by separate isomerases, $PGF_{2\alpha}$ by a reductase, TXA_2 and 12-L-hydroxy-5,8,10-heptadecatrienoic acid (HHT) by the "thromboxane synthetase," and PGI_2 by "prostacyclin synthetase." The lipoxygenase pathway generates a 12-L-hydroperoxy derivative of arachidonic acid (HPETE) and, subsequently, 12-L-hydroxy-5,8,11,14-eicosatetraenoic acid (HETE) (reviewed by Vane, 1976). PGAs, Bs, and Cs are all derivatives of the corresponding PGEs (Douglas, 1975b).

While the cyclooxygenase is exquisitely sensitive to inhibition by indomethacin and other nonsteroidal antiinflammatory compounds (Vane, 1971), thromboxane synthetase is less so (Moncada *et al.*, 1976), and the lipoxygenase is not inhibited at all (Hamberg *et al.*, 1974). The inhibitory effects of corticosteroids on arachidonic acid metabolism are expressed either on the release of prostaglandins from cells (Lewis and Piper, 1975) or on the bioavailability of precursor arachidonic acid (Hong and Levine, 1976). PGEs and PGFs are degraded by tissue-bound 15-hydroxyprostaglandin dehydrogenase, a particularly rapid process in the lung (Piper *et al.*, 1970); PGAs and Bs are catabolized more slowly.

Antigen challenge of sensitized human lung fragments has been shown to release prostaglandins E_1, E_2, and $F_{2\alpha}$, but no detectable TXA_2 (then designated "rabbit aorta-contracting substance," Piper and Vane, 1969b); contrastingly, sensitized and antigen-challenged perfused guinea pig lungs release TXA_2 as well as various prostaglandins (Palmer *et al.*, 1973). Similar products are released when sensitized guinea pig spleen slices are either challenged with antigen or merely mechanically vibrated (Flower and Blackwell, 1976). A lipid chemotactic factor, apparently an arachidonic acid metabolite, is generated immunologically from both the IgG_a-prepared rat peritoneal cavity and human lung fragments sensitized with IgE (Valone and Goetzl, 1978), and is active predominantly on neutrophils.

The prostaglandins and other arachidonic acid metabolites have several biological effects in immediate hypersensitivity models. Arachidonic acid, at concentrations of 30–100 μM, elicits the release of rat mast cell granule-associated mediators; in the same model, arachidonic acid enhances the effects of Con A and the calcium ionophore A23187 (Sullivan and Parker, 1979). PGG_2, PGH_2, and TXA_2 initiate platelet aggregation, contraction of guinea pig tracheal strips *in vivo* (reviewed by Moncada, 1977). In unanesthetized guinea pigs and medicated dogs, the bronchoconstrictor effects of $PGF_{2\alpha}$ are reduced in both central and peripheral airways by pretreatment with atropine, suggesting participation of a cholinergic reflex (Drazen and Austen, 1975; Wasserman, 1975). In contrast, the significantly greater but analogous effects of PGD_2 on canine airways are atropine-sensitive only centrally (M. Wasserman *et al.*, 1977). PGE_1 and PGE_2 cause bronchodilatation in some asthmatic humans (Cuthbert, 1969), while $PGF_{2\alpha}$ is a bronchoconstrictor (Mathé and Hedqvist, 1975; Newball, 1976). The prostaglandins A_1, A_2, B_1, and particularly

B_2 all contract human bronchial smooth muscle strips *in vitro* (Lo *et al.*, 1976). The lipoxygenase product, HETE, is chemoattractive to human granulocytes, most specifically for eosinophils (Goetzl *et al.*, 1977), and the cyclooxygenase product HHT has analogous effects at higher concentrations (Goetzl and Gorman, 1978).

As reviewed by Vane (1976), PGE_1 and $PGF_{2\alpha}$, at high doses, cause vasodilatation and are thus implicated in the production of erythema. PGE_1, PGE_2, and PGA_2 may participate in causing edema, pruritus, and pain by potentiating the effects of histamine, serotonin, and bradykinin (reviewed by Flower, 1977). The pyrogenic effects of prostaglandins E_1, E_2, and $F_{2\alpha}$ are attributed to direct action on the central nervous system.

3. Mast Cell Degranulation: Biochemical Mechanisms and Controls

That IgE-dependent degranulation of mast cells and basophils with attendant mediator release is a noncytotoxic secretory process has been firmly established. Basophils retain their capacity for motility and mast cells exclude trypan blue dye and retain ^{42}K subsequent to antigen-induced degranulation (Hastie, 1971; Kaliner and Austen, 1974). However, the sequence of biochemical events involved in target cell degranulation is not yet defined. Definitive kinetics and inhibition studies will require large numbers of homogeneous cells responding with significant granule secretion to an IgE-dependent stimulus.

Degranulation of mast cells is temperature- and pH-sensitive (Moran *et al.*, 1962; Baxter and Adamik, 1975), has an absolute requirement for calcium (Kaliner and Austen, 1973; Foreman and Mongar, 1972a), and proceeds only in the presence of an intact glycolytic pathway (Kaliner and Austen, 1973), analogous to secretion from other exocrine as well as endocrine cells (Becker and Henson, 1973; Cochrane and Douglas, 1974). In contrast, the modulation of mast cell mediator release by cyclic AMP best fits the bidirectional mode of control proposed by Berridge (1975), vs. the monodirectional cyclic AMP-regulated control apparent in many other secretory cells (see below). Further, the activation of a serine esterase early in the stepwise sequence leading to mast cell degranulation (Austen and Brocklehurst, 1961; Becker and Austen, 1964; Kaliner and Austen, 1973) has not been described as a general characteristic of the nonimmunological secretory process (Becker and Henson, 1973). With respect to modulation by cyclic nucleotides and a role for a serine esterase, a parallelism exists among the immunological effector cells: mast cells, lymphocytes, neutrophils, and platelets (Becker and Henson, 1973). High-affinity receptors for monomeric IgE (Tomioka and Ishizaka, 1971) are specific for mast cells and basophils, and susceptibility to inhibition of activation by disodium cromoglycate (Cox *et al.*, 1970) is mast cell specific.

In this section, the biochemical pathways involved in mast cell degranulation will be discussed. Both immunological and nonimmunological initiating events and those elements which modulate the release of mediators of immediate hypersensitivity will be considered. Finally, a theoretical model will be used to integrate current knowledge of the components of the mast cell degranulation reaction.

3.1. Agents Which Initiate Mast Cell Degranulation

A broad spectrum of agents with varied chemical structures degranulates mast cells, as demonstrated in the rat peritoneal mast cell model. A few agents such as complement-dependent anti-mast cell antibody, hypotonic solutions, and Triton X effect mast cell degranulation by inducing cytolysis, and thus will not be further discussed. Noncytolytic mast cell degranulation initiated by the several described agents is morphologically identical in the fusion of perigranular and cell membranes and subsequent granule extrusion (Lawson *et al.*, 1976). Kinetic studies reveal that the secretory reaction initiated by most agents occurs rapidly, with a peak rate occuring within 60 sec of cell challenge, followed by completion in 5 min (Kaliner and Austen, 1974; Bloom *et al.*, 1967; Baxter and Adamik, 1975; Dahlquist, 1974a). The only known exceptions occur with the anaphylatoxins C3a and C5a (Morrison *et al.*, 1975), which act over a longer time course. The biochemical requirements in terms of a serine esterase, extracellular calcium, and an energy source vary somewhat with the specific initiating agent (Diamant, 1975). These apparent biochemical differences presumably reflect different points of entry into the stepwise pathway of degranulation. In the following discussion, the degranulating agents are classified as immunological factors, enzymes, and other nonimmunological substances. While the immunological agents are presumably more clinically relevant, the enzymatic and other nonimmunological agents provide additional insights into the biochemistry of degranulation.

3.1.1. Enzymatic Agents

Crude phospholipase A from cobra venom has been recognized to induce histamine and SRS release since the early studies with perfused guinea pig lung (Feldberg and Kellaway, 1938). Subsequent observations on guinea pig lung fragments (Middleton and Phillips, 1964; Phillips and Middleton, 1965), rat mesenteric mast cells (Högberg and Uvnäs, 1957; Uvnäs and Antonsson, 1963), and mixed rat peritoneal cells (Bach *et al.*, 1971b) have confirmed the capability of this lipolytic carboxylesterase to release mediators from the target cells. Release so initiated requires both calcium ions and metabolic energy (Uvnäs and Antonsson, 1963). Purified phospholipase A, when injected intradermally into living rats, degranulates the subcutaneous mast cells (Orr and Cox, 1969) in a reaction that is blocked by disodium cromoglycate.

Chymotrypsin, but not trypsin, has also been shown to degranulate rat mast cells (Uvnäs and Antonsson, 1963; Bach *et al.*, 1971a) with requirements for calcium ions and energy similar to those of the phospholipase A mechanism. Notably, however, of the 18 additional proteases, phospholipases, and polysaccharidases studied by Bach *et al.* (1971a) and many more examined by Högberg and Uvnäs (1957), only pronase, phospholipase C, and sialidase were effective mast cell degranulators at the experimental concentrations used.

The significance of the releasing capability of these exogenous enzymes lies in the possibility that they bypass the activation of their endogenous mast cell membrane counterparts. Indeed, the uncovering of a serine esterase of chymotryptic specificity (Austen and Brocklehurst, 1961; Becker and Austen, 1966), phospholipase A (Ho and Orange, 1978), and probably phospholipase C is indirectly implicated during mast cell degranulation. As will be discussed, release is blocked both reversibly and irreversibly by inhibitors of chymotrypsin (Austen and Brocklehurst, 1961) and is associated with the appearance of defined oxidative metabolites of arachidonic acid (Roberts *et al.*, 1978). Sialidase, by removing negatively charged sialic acid moieties from the cell membrane, obviates electrostatic repulsion and so may facilitate contact of perigranular and cell membranes with subsequent fusion (Poste and Allison, 1973).

3.1.2. Nonimmunological Agents

a. Polycationic Amines and Polypeptides. In the group of polycationic amines and polypeptides are included 48/80, a polymerization product of *p*-methoxy-*N*-methylphenethylamine with equimolar formaldehyde (Baltzly *et al.*, 1949), polymyxin B, colistin, gramicidin, mellitin from bee venom, poly-L-lysine, protamine, stilbamidine, *d*-tubocurarine, morphine, and corticotropin (Stanworth, 1973). On the basis of the structural similarities in this list, it has been proposed that any molecule in which two basic groups are separated by an aliphatic chain of five carbon atoms or more or by a corresponding aromatic skeleton is likely to be a mast cell histamine liberator (Paton, 1958). Thon and Uvnäs (1967) speculated that the mechanism of degranulation involves alteration in electrostatic charges on the mast cell surface. Such changes may affect membrane permeability (Gingell, 1967) and displace membrane-bound calcium (reviewed by Seeman, 1972). Because the concentration of calcium in the membrane is about 10–20 times higher than that in the cytoplasm (Chau-Wong and Seeman, 1971), calcium influx from the cell membrane to the cytoplasm may achieve the same effect as intracellular injection of calcium through micropipettes, which initiates exocytosis of rat mast cell granules (Kanno *et al.*, 1973). Band 2 protein, a lysosomal cationic protein from neutrophils (Ranadive and Cochrane, 1971), and the anaphylatoxins C3a and C5a (Müller-Eberhard, 1976) are also strongly basic. They are of considerably larger size and more complex configuration, but could possibly fit with this general mechanism of action for cationic principles.

The anaphylatoxins C3a and C5a are formed from the complement components C3 and C5, respectively, by both the classical and the alternative complement pathways (Müller-Eberhard, 1976). Chemically, C3a and C5a are basic (cationic) peptides of approximately 8900 and 12,000 molecular weight, respectively. Anaphylatoxins degranulate mast cells *in vitro* (Morrison *et al.*, 1975) as well as *in vivo,* but the mechanism of target cell degranulation is unknown. The guinea pig ileum *in vitro* shows no cross-desensitization between C3a and C5a (Müller-Eberhard and Vallota, 1971). When the ileum of a guinea pig, immunized with two different antigens, is cross-desensitized to the antigens, it is still reactive to both anaphylatoxins and *vice versa* (Broder, 1973). The minimal dose of C3a that causes wheal-and-flare formation when injected into the human skin is 2×10^{-12} M and that of C5a, 1×10^{-15} M (Wuepper *et al.*, 1972). The wheal-and-flare responses are markedly diminished by simultaneous injections of an H-1 antihistamine. Skin biopsies from the site of a positive reaction show mast cell degranulation and extracellular disintegration of metachromatic granules. The capacity of the anaphylatoxins to degranulate mast cells allows the potential recruitment of the mediator cells in nonatopic inflammatory processes involving complement activation.

b. Ionophores. Ionophores are compounds which are able to interact stoichiometrically with cations and translocate them across an organic phase separating two aqueous phases (Tyson *et al.*, 1976). One such compound, A23187, specifically complexes with calcium and magnesium (Foreman *et al.*, 1973); another, X537A, is not specific for divalent cations but also transports monovalent cations and some amines (Pressman, 1972). Both induce mast cell degranulation provided that exogenous calcium is present. Although phosphatidylserine does not itself induce mast cell granule release, it enhances the degranulation of mast cells induced by antigen-IgE reaction, dextran, or concanavalin A and inhibits that caused by 48/80, polymyxin B, phospholipase C, and ATP (Read *et al.*, 1977). It forms complexes with calcium (Hauser *et al.*, 1976) and acts to an extent as an ionophore (Tyson *et al.*, 1976).

c. Adenosine-5′-triphosphate (ATP). Exogenous ATP, but not other phosphonucleotides (AMP, ADP, CTP, GTP, ITP, and UTP), induces histamine release from mast cells (Dahlquist, 1974a). Because this release is calcium-dependent, it is difficult to differentiate ATP from the Ca–ATP complex as the active agent. High concentrations of magnesium ion inhibit the reaction, probably by complexing with ATP. The earliest event appears to be calcium flux into the cell, occurring partly by an increase in the rate of calcium exchange and partly by increased net calcium entry (Dahlquist, 1974b). There is also an associated increased permeability to sodium. The complete reaction is energy-dependent (Dahlquist, 1974a), rendering it unlikely that ATP is acting merely as an energy donor (reviewed by Peterson, 1974).

d. Lectins. The lectins (plant seed proteins) express a range of specificities in binding to different sugars. For example, concanavalin A binds to α-linked glucose or mannose. Concanavalin A and other lectins have been shown not only to degranulate mast cells but also to desensitize the cells to a subsequent IgE-dependent immunological challenge (Bach and Brashler, 1975). Since the carbohydrate moieties of glycoproteins and glycolipids reside exclusively on the outer cell membranes (ectomembranes) (reviewed by Rothman and Lenard, 1977) and the lectins possess multivalent binding sites, a "bridging" phenomenon similar to that effected by antigen on membrane-bound IgE (see below) or by antireceptor antibody (Ishizaka *et al.*, 1978) may take place.

e. Fusogenic Agents. Phillips and Middleton (1965) demonstrated that lysolecithin releases histamine and SRS from guinea pig lung fragments. Sydbom and Uvnäs (1976) found that lysolecithin was at least twice as active as phosphatidylserine in enhancing anaphylactic histamine release from isolated rat mast cells. It is now established that lysolecithin functions as a "fusogen" (Lucy, 1970; Poole *et al.*, 1970): that is, it acts to favor membrane fusion by facilitating the transition of the cell membrane from a bimolecular leaflet (bilayer) to aggregates of radially oriented molecules (micelles). Most other lysophospholipids as well as phosphatidylserine, an acidic phospholipid carrying a net charge, may share this mode of action (Haydon and Taylor, 1963). While lysolecithin has also been regarded as a surface-active detergent, it does not induce cytolysis at low concentrations (3–13 μM) (Sydbom and Uvnäs, 1976) or when it is applied in microdroplets rather than in a dispersed form (Lucy, 1975). Dextran of molecular weight ranging from 4×10^4 to 2×10^6 has been used to induce histamine release from isolated rat mast cells (Read *et al.*, 1977; Baxter, 1973; Foreman and Mongar, 1972b), and its action is enhanced by phosphatidylserine. Dextran of 90,000 molecular weight has been shown to greatly facilitate sucrose- and glycerol-induced fusion of hen erythrocytes, and high-molecular-weight dextran (2×10^6) is itself fusogenic in this cell after long incubations (Ahkong *et al.*, 1975).

3.1.3. Immunological Agents

a. IgE. It is now established that the antibodies in atopic sera capable of mediating the antigen-induced release of chemical mediators from various tissues belong to the IgE immunoglobulin class (Ishizaka *et al.*, 1970; reviewed by Orange, 1976). Because IgE forms the topic of another chapter, by Ishizaka and Ishizaka, it will not be discussed here.

b. Homocytotropic IgG. Studies in several lower mammalian species and in humans indicate that a homologous immunoglobulin class distinctly different from IgE may also demonstrate homocytotropic binding to mast cells. The IgG_a antibody of the rat (Stechschulte *et al.*, 1967; Morse *et al.*, 1968), the IgG_1 antibody of the mouse (Prouvost-Danon *et al.*, 1966; Mota *et al.*, 1969) and of the guinea pig (Baker *et al.*, 1964), and an IgG antibody in the rabbit (Henson and Cochrane, 1969) are each capable of mediating *in vitro* and *in vivo* antigen-induced release of mediators. In the human, an IgG antibody capable of mediating the *in vitro* antigen-induced release of mediators from homologous lung and leukocytes has also been appreciated but not well characterized (Parish, 1973). Further, Bryant *et al.* (1975) demonstrated a specific homocytotropic IgG antibody in allergic asthmatic patients with cutaneous and bronchial reactivity to the allergen and low total and specific serum IgE. That IgG, as well as IgE, may reside on the surface of human basophils is supported by the observation that anti-IgG_4 induces histamine release from human leukocytes (Vijay and Perlmutter, 1977). The human homocytotropic antibodies have been differentiated from the IgE antibodies on the basis of physicochemical differences such as size, sensitivity to heat and reducing agents, specific immunosorption, and optimal latent periods of sensitization for passive cutaneous anaphylaxis. However, the amounts are small and the assays are very insensitive as compared to those for lower animal IgG homocytotropic antibodies.

Homologous IgG_a may competitively inhibit the interaction of IgE with mast cell membrane receptors in the rat (Bach *et al.*, 1971b). However, rat IgG_a binds weakly to mast cells and is readily removed by washing the sensitized cells in physiological buffers (Bach *et al.*, 1971c). Human homocytotropic IgG also has a low avidity for target cells (Petersson, 1975). Studies with rat IgG_a suggest that mast cell activation depends on the action of relatively large amounts of an immune complex and that the ratio of antigen to specific IgG_a is more critical than for IgE. It seems likely that homocytotropic IgG represents a relatively inefficient mechanism for perturbation of mast cell membrane (Bach *et al.*, 1971a,b).

3.2. Biochemical and Morphological Aspects of Degranulation

The biochemical sequence culminating in mast cell degranulation has been examined by manipulating the concentrations of various essential constituents of the incubation medium, introducing inhibitors of enzymes, and employing pharmacological agonists and antagonists. Such studies are supplemented by direct ultrastructural examination of the cellular events from membrane perturbation to granule extrusion.

3.2.1. Membrane Perturbation

Since the introduction of the fluid mosaic model of cell membrane structure by Singer and Nicholson (1972), the plasma membrane is no longer regarded as an inert protective cell covering; instead, its protein constituents are believed to function as receptors for specific chemical messengers and as enzymes while its lipid bilayer participates in membrane fusion. IgE receptors on mast cell and basophil surface plasma membranes were appreciated using [^{125}I]-anti-IgE (Ishizaka *et al.*, 1970; Tomioka and Ishizaka, 1971) and fluoresceinated anti-IgE (Feltkamp-Vroom *et al.*, 1975). Recently, the monovalent IgE receptor (Mendoza and Metzger, 1976) has been isolated following solubilization of the plasma membrane of rat basophilic leukemia cells and identified as a glycoprotein with an apparent molecular weight of 60,000 (Kulczycki *et al.*, 1976; Conrad and Froese, 1978; Newman *et al.*, 1977). The affinity constant of IgE for its receptor is high ($K \sim 10^9$ M^{-1}) (Conrad *et al.*, 1975). Bridging of adjacent receptor-bound IgE molecules by specific antigen or anti-IgE initiates degranulation (Metzger, 1977; Newman *et al.*, 1977), and the quantitative relationship between antigen concentration and degranulation is dose-dependent with high-dose inhibition. Subsequent to bridging of IgE and, secondarily, the receptors, the immediate biochemical consequences presumably involve the uncovering of several enzymes. Interpretation of these initial steps is aided by applying the mobile receptor hypothesis of Cuatrecasas (1974) to the relationship of IgE receptors and mast cell surface enzymes. The central feature of the hypothesis is that the receptors and enzymes on cell membranes, although discrete and separate structures, acquire the affinities to form complexes with each other after occupation of the receptors by specific messengers or substrates. The fluidity of the cell membrane allows the interposition of receptors and enzymes, and their increased coaffinities facilitate complexing. While the binding sites of the receptors are externally oriented, the enzyme catalytic sites face inward toward the cytoplasm. The IgE receptor on rat peritoneal mast cells is indeed mobile as has been demonstrated by the fluorescent photobleaching recovery technique (Schlessinger *et al.*, 1976). This receptor mobility in the fluid phospholipid matrix does not require metabolic energy and is inhibited by both colchicine and cytochalasin B. The observed latent period for sensitization of mast-cell-rich tissues is theoretically compatible with a time requirement for coupling of IgE receptors to appropriate enzyme subunits. Activation of several different mast cell enzymes subsequent to immunological challenge at the cell surface may occur either in parallel or, alternatively, in sequence.

3.2.2. Membrane Fusion

Mast cell granules serve not only to store and segregate the preformed mediators from the rest of the cytoplasm but also as the sites from which the mediators are released. Secretion involves the fusion of the perigranular membrane with the plasma membrane, thereby exteriorizing granule contents. Membrane fusion is now widely appreciated as a common mechanism underlying secretion or exocytosis from exocrine, endocrine, and neuronal cells (reviewed by Poste and Allison, 1973). Membrane fusion in degranulating rat mast cells follows a well-defined sequence, whether induced by antigen, Con A, 48/80, or polymyxin B. Just prior to fusion, the cell membrane bilayer becomes disarrayed, giving rise to micelles, forming an intermediate hexagonal phase (Cullis and Hope, 1978) laterally displacing membrane-associated protein molecules (Ahkong *et al.*, 1975). Lateral protein displacement, including that of IgE receptors, has been demonstrated by freeze-fracture and by transmission electron microscopy using ferritin-labeled antibodies directed against IgE, Con A, and phytohemagglutinin (Lawson *et al.*, 1977). Such membrane disorganization may be produced *in vivo* by fusogenic lysophosphatides and is accompanied by translocation of calcium from the membrane (Poste and Allison, 1973) and by membrane–membrane opposition. The repulsion of the membranes needs to be overcome (Poste and Allison, 1973); this may be achieved by an active cytoskeletal contractile process acting on the granules (Orr *et al.*, 1972; Chi *et al.*, 1976). Dense bands of microfilaments have been observed around mast cell granules, particularly during degranulation (Trotter and Orr, 1973). A pentalaminar structure is formed by fusion of the perigranular and plasma membranes (Lagunoff, 1973; Lawson *et al.*, 1977). Further outward egression of the granules produces bulges on the surface membrane which are delimited by a single central dense lamina devoid of intramembranous particles (Chi *et al.*, 1976). As shown by the scanning electron photomicrograph in Figure 1, openings then appear, which become channels to the exterior and widen to allow passage of the granules (Lagunoff, 1973). Once fully formed, these channels are delimited by membrane with the normal distribution of intramembranous particles (Chi *et al.*, 1976), suggesting stabilization by reversal of the inductive fusion event. Finally, reversion of the membrane to the bilayer state takes place (Lucy, 1975) and calcium ions and ATP are reassociated to their original binding sites in the membrane. This is believed to require energy utilization and is blocked by factors that limit the availability of calcium and ATP (Poste and Allison, 1973).

Although these morphological events all relate to the peripherally located granules, other changes occur in the granular structure of both peripheral and deep granules prior to extrusion. These include loss of electron density, swelling, and loosening of granular structure into a fibrous mesh-work (Uvnäs, 1973). Using lanthanum as an extracellular tracer (Uvnäs, 1973) and freeze-fracture studies (Chi *et al.*, 1976), fusion of several perigranular membranes with resultant formation of labyrinthine channels has been described. Whether the granules are physically extruded or are connected to the exterior via channels, certain of the preformed primary mediators are released from the granule matrix (Thon and Uvnäs, 1967; Wasserman *et al.*, 1974a). Despite the fact that most of the granules in maximally stimulated rat mast cells are ultrastructurally altered, the cells retain their original shape and the cytoplasmic organelles are morphologically unaltered (Uvnäs, 1973), further supporting the noncytolytic nature of degranulation.

On scanning electron microscopy, an unstimulated rat mast cell surface is relatively smooth except for the presence of ridges and folds up to 1 μm in length and 100–200 nm in thickness and a few short microvilli (Sturgess, Jeffrey, and Orange, unpublished observations). After maximal challenge with anti-IgE, there is a rapid increase in cell size which is evident in photomicrographs (Thon and Uvnäs, 1967; Bloom *et al.*, 1967); the diameter increases by 25%, indicating a doubling of volume and a 60% increment in cell surface area, assuming the mast cell to be a perfect sphere. Kinsolving *et al.* (1975) estimated an even greater increase in cell surface area, up to 3.5-fold. Since it is unlikely that an unaltered plasma membrane can tolerate such a sudden expansion, extra membrane material presumably must be incorporated to maintain cell integrity. When [^{3}H]glycerol is added to incubating mast cells as a marker for *de novo* synthesis of phospholipid during anti-IgE challenge, no increase in incorporation into phosphatidylcholine or phosphatidylethanolamine is observed (Ho and Orange, 1979); this suggests that the additional membrane material is derived from perigranular membrane brought into physical continuity with the plasma membrane during exocytosis.

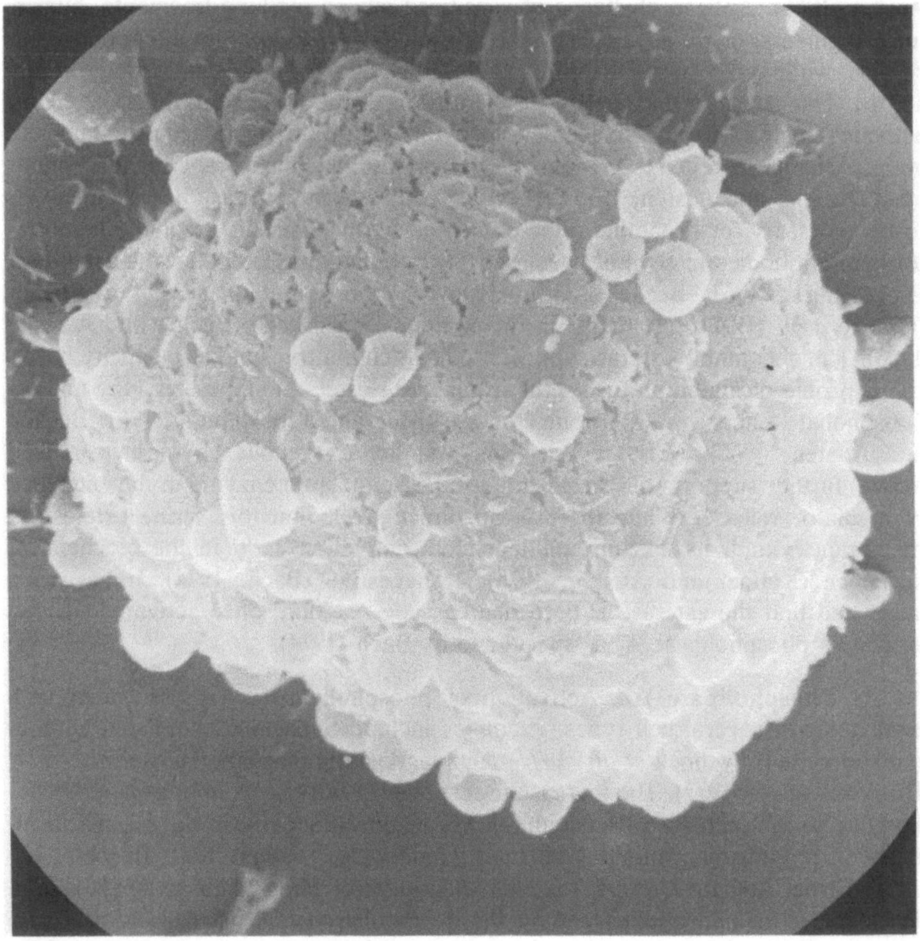

Figure 1. Scanning electron micrograph of an isolated rat mast cell undergoing IgE-mediated degranulation. Egressing granules are adherent to the plasma membrane, and membrane-delimited channels penetrate the cell surface as open pores. 21,500×. Reduced 35% for reproduction. Courtesy of Sturgess, Jeffrey, and Orange, Department of Immunology, Hospital for Sick Children, Toronto.

3.2.3. Activation of Membrane-Bound Enzymes

Indirect evidence of a requirement for enzymatic activities in mediator release has been previously obtained by the use of various nonspecific enzymatic blockers (Högberg and Uvnäs, 1957, 1960; Moran *et al.*, 1962; Uvnäs and Antonsson, 1963). Among these are reagents which act on sulfhydryl groups (iodoacetic acid, *N*-ethylmaleimide, allicin, phenol, *O*-iodobenzoate) and amino groups (ninhydrin, acetic anhydride, dinitrofluorobenzene, formaldehyde, phenylisocyanate).

a. Serine Esterases. Diisopropylfluorophosphate (DFP) irreversibly phosphorylates sterically available serine residues in peptides and proteins, thus inactivating enzymes with active-center serine moieties (Hartley, 1960). Involvement of a serine esterase in mast cell degranulation was first postulated from the inhibitory activity of synthetic ester substrates and DFP (Austen and Brocklehurst, 1961; Becker and Austen, 1966). Antigen challenge of sensitized guinea pig lung fragments, human lung fragments, or rat mast cells in the presence of DFP does not effect histamine release, while removal of DFP prior to challenge allows full release (Orange *et al.*, 1971b). This suggests that a DFP-resistant form of the esterase in the mast cell is activated by bridging of adjacent homocytotropic antibody molecules. Further, antigen challenge requires calcium to convert the esterase to a DFP-susceptible state (Kaliner and Austen, 1973). This activatable serine esterase has been shown to be necessary for histamine release initiated by mechanisms involving homocytotropic antibodies in several species: IgG_1 in guinea pig lung slices (Austen and Brocklehurst, 1961; Becker and Austen, 1964), IgE in human lung fragments (Orange *et al.*, 1971b), and IgE in rat peritoneal màst cells (Becker and Austen, 1966). The activatable esterase appears to have chymotrypsinlike specificity based on its profile of inhibition by synthetic substrate esters in guinea pig lung and by phosphonate esters in rat peritoneal cells (Austen and Brocklehurst, 1961; Becker and Austen, 1966). Mast cell degranulation by exogenous chymotrypsin (see above) further supports the suggestion of a chymotryptic enzyme in the sequence of mediator release. While there is no direct proof that this serine esterase is membrane-bound, its calcium-ion-dependent activation early in the biochemical sequence (Kaliner and Austen, 1973) is suggestive (Bach, 1974). It has been suggested that the esterase is part of a cascade reaction; once activated, it may activate a phospholipase A, as speculated by Bach (1974).

b. Phospholipase A. Activation of phospholipase A_2 is associated with exocytosis in several cell types; examples include Synacthen-stimulated adrenocortical cells (Laychock *et al.*, 1977), and aggregating platelets (Bills *et al.*, 1977; Blackwell *et al.*, 1977). The increase in turnover of fatty acids in phosphatidylcholine due to the increased lysolecithin-acyltransferase activity in the plasma membrane of phytohemagglutinin-stimulated lymphocytes (Ferber, 1971; Resch *et al.*, 1972; Ferber and Resch, 1973) is also suggestive of phospholipase A activation. Participation of phospholipase A in the degranulation of mast cells is based on several observations, including the capacity of exogenous enzyme to induce noncytotoxic release of histamine from mast cells (Höberg and Uvnäs, 1960; Bach *et al.*, 1971a). Giacobini *et al.* (1965), using a modified cartesian diver technique, demonstrated that isolated mast cells hydrolyze lecithin and that this activity is enhanced by activation with 48/80. Mastocytoma cells also have a high degree of intrinsic phospholipase A activity (Koren *et al.*, 1971). Further evidence of intrinsic phospholipase A_2 activation during anaphylaxis is derived from observations of release of [^{14}C]arachidonic acid from prelabeled phospholipids in guinea pig spleen slices (Flower and Blackwell, 1976) and hydrolysis of radiolabeled phophatidylcholine perfused into guinea pig lungs (Blackwell *et al.*, 1978).

Deacylation and reacylation are closely coupled reactions. Hydrolysis of phospholipids by phospholipase A yields lysophosphatides which, in the presence of acylcoenzyme A, are readily reverted to phospholipids by the action of acyltransferase. Although this intrinsic regulatory mechanism prevents excess lysocompounds from accumulating, an appropriate concentration of lysocompounds should be fusogenic and may have a function in degranulation. It is therefore pertinent that in recent investigations the amount of [^{3}H]oleic acid incorporated into isolated rat mast cell phosphatidylethanolamine was shown to increase during reverse anaphylactic challenge, indicating reacylation of the corresponding lysophosphatide (Ho and Orange, 1978). Since in the same experiments the concentration of lysophosphatidylethanolamine remained unchanged in the challenged cells, enhanced turnover of the parent phospholipid by an increase in phospholipase A activity is implied. The reacylation of the lysophosphatidylethanolamine occurred rapidly, in agreement with the general kinetics of mast cell degranulation (Bloom *et al.*, 1967; Dahlquist, 1974a), and was not accompanied by reacylation of lysophosphatidylcholine. Similar observations have been made in platelets activated by the calcium ionophore A23187 (Pickett *et al.*, 1977). If the observations on asymmetrical membrane distribution of phospholipids in mammalian red cells and virus coat (Rothman and Lenard, 1977) hold true for rat mast cells, phosphatidylethanolamine should be located in the endomembrane and phosphatidylcholine in the ectomembrane. This implies that the active catalytic site of the enzyme is endomembrane-oriented. Since membrane fusion takes place between the inner layer of the plasma membrane and the outer perigranular membrane layer, selective hydrolysis of phosphatidylethanolamine, providing a transient localized elevation of lysophosphatidylethanolamine, would enhance the fusion process.

Supportive evidence for phospholipase A activation during mast cell degranulation has been derived from preliminary studies on the effect of phospholipase A inhibitors and the elaboration of oxidative metabolites of arachidonic acid. Both a phosphinate analogue of phosphatidylcholine (Rosenthal and Han, 1970; Frye and Frion, 1976) and *p*-bromophenacyl bromide (Volwerk *et al.*, 1974) were shown to inhibit anti-IgE-induced histamine release from isolated rat mast cells in a dose-dependent fashion (Jeffrey and Orange, unpublished observations). Additionally, mast cells activated by anti-F(ab′)$_2$ and the calcium ionophore A23187 form arachidonic acid metabolites via both the cyclooxygenase and lipoxygenase pathways (Roberts *et al.*, 1978), indirectly implicating release of the substrate fatty acid from its phospholipid stores. Consistent with the role of phospholipase A_2 in endoperoxide and prostaglandin biogeneration is the finding that rat mast cell phosphatidylethanolamine contains a higher concentration of arachidonic acid than any other phospholipid species (Strandberg and Westerberg, 1976).

Our present knowledge of the putative mast cell membrane phospholipase A is necessarily derived by analogy with like enzymes in or extracted from other cells. Phospholipase A in the rat liver plasma membrane is of A_2 specificity (Victoria *et al.*, 1971), requires calcium for optimal activity, is resistant to heat, DFP, and *N*-ethylmaleimate, and demonstrates a substrate preference for phosphatidylethanolamine over phosphatidylcholine. If the properties of membrane-bound phospholipase A_2 reflect those more readily studied in the exogenous enzyme, their modes of activation may be similar. For example, *Crotalus adamanteus* phospholipase A_2 is a dimer in its active form (Wells, 1973); by analogy, membrane-bound phospholipase A_2 may be activated by dimerization, subsequent to the dimerization of the IgE receptors. It is also known that exocrine phospholipase A_2 exists as a proenzyme (Pieterson *et al.*, 1974a,b; Rothman and Lenard, 1977) and that, on cleavage of its *N*-terminal amino acid residues, the enzymatic activity is revealed. Again, by analogy, mast cell membrane-bound phospholipase A_2 might be activated by the serine esterase in an enzymatic cascade. It remains to be established whether either or both of these mechanisms participate in mast cell phospholipase A_2 activation.

c. Phospholipase C. Turnover of phosphatidylinositol has been documented in a variety of cell activation phenomena, including endocrine and exocrine secretions, lymphocyte transformation, platelet aggregation, and neutrophil phagocytosis (Michell, 1975). This is executed by a phosphatidylinositol-specific phospholipase C which hydrolyzes its substrate to yield cyclic inositol monophosphate and 1,2-diacylglycerol. The latter product, at the expenditure of ATP, is converted to phosphatidic acid, which subsequently combines with *myo*inositol to re-form the parent phospholipid. Since phosphatidylinositol catabolism is an early event in cellular responses, and phosphatidic acid exhibits ionophoric activity (Tyson *et al.*, 1976), turnover of this phospholipid has been postulated to control calcium movement across membranes either by liberating membrane-bound calcium or by opening the "calcium gate" (Michell, 1975; Jefferji and Michell, 1976). Another speculated role of phosphatidylinositol turnover is regulation of cyclic nucleotides, because this phospholipid (and/or phosphatidylserine) is essential to the activity of adenylate cyclase (Levey, 1971).

Phospholipase C elicits histamine release from rat mast cells (Bach *et al.*, 1971a), and its activation during reverse anaphylaxis in isolated rat mast cells has recently been demonstrated. When [^{32}P]*ortho*-phosphate is preincubated with rat mast cells, a consistent two- to three-fold increased incorporation into phosphatidylinositol occurs, while incorporation into lecithin, phosphatidylethanolamine, and phosphatidylserine is more variable (Chang, Ho, and Orange, unpublished observations). Similar findings have also been reported by others (Kennerly *et al.*, 1979).

3.2.4. Role of Divalent Cations

Calcium influx forms an essential segment of the "stimulus–secretion coupling" hypothesis, first proposed by Douglas and Rubin (1961) and later extended to cover most if not all secretory phenomena (Douglas, 1968). Release of mediators from human lung (Kaliner and Austen, 1973), human basophils (Lichtenstein, 1973), and rat mast cells (Foreman and Mongar, 1972a) has an absolute requirement for extracellular calcium ions which cannot be replaced efficiently by other divalent cations. Only at much higher concentrations do strontium or barium ions allow rat mast cell degranulation (Foreman and Mongar, 1972a), whereas magnesium, beryllium, lead, copper, and zinc ions competitively inhibit the effect of calcium (Högberg and Uvnäs, 1960; Diamant *et al.*, 1974). Influx of ^{45}Ca into isolated mast cells has been shown during mediator release induced by antigen challenge

(Foreman *et al.*, 1975), ATP (Dahlquist, 1974b), or ionophore A23187 (Johnson and Bach, 1975). Kanno *et al.* (1973) elicited mast cell exocytosis by injecting calcium ions directly into the cells with micropipettes, whereas injection of magnesium or potassium was without any effect. In IgE-dependent mast cell degranulation, a cell membrane "calcium gate," postulated from demonstrations of induced cellular uptake of ionic ^{45}Ca (Foreman and Gomperts, 1975), is opened after IgE bridging and closed by an increase in intracellular cyclic AMP; phosphatidylserine is held to enhance granule release by prolonging calcium entry (Foreman *et al.*, 1975). Calcium entry appears energy-independent because antimycin A concentrations which effectively inhibit endogenous ATP production do not block influx of the cation (Foreman *et al.*, 1975; Dahlquist, 1974a).

In IgE-dependent mediator release from human lung fragments, calcium is required in at leaset two stages (Kaliner and Austen, 1973). An early stage is associated with the uncovering of a serine esterase and might also be involved in phospholipase A activation. The late stage follows an energy-requiring step and may be equated with calcium requirements for microfilament contraction (Kaliner and Austen, 1973), membrane fusion, or regulation of cellular levels of cyclic AMP. Rat mast cells in calcium-free media develop increased basal cyclic AMP levels (Sullivan *et al.*, 1975a), which may relate to interaction of the cation with a regulator protein controlling adenylate cyclase, guanylate cyclase, or phosphodiesterase activities (Brostrom *et al.*, 1975).

3.2.5. Requirements for Metabolic Energy

Release of mediators from isolated rat mast cells requires an intact glycolytic pathway. Mediator release is inhibited in the absence of glucose by anoxia (Diamant, 1975), cyanide, which inhibits cytochrome oxidase, 2,4-dinitrophenol, which uncouples oxidative phosphorylation (Högberg and Uvnäs, 1960), and antimycin A, which interrupts electron transfer from cytochrome *b* to cytochrome *c* (Kaliner and Austen, 1974). Further, both phlorizin, an inhibitor of glucose transport, and 2-deoxyglucose, a competitive inhibitor of phosphoglucose isomerase, reduce histamine release from isolated mast cells (Kaliner and Austen, 1974); both 2-deoxyglucose and iodoacetic acid, which blocks 3-phosphoglyceraldehyde dehydrogenase, inhibit release of histamine and SRS-A from antigen-challenged human lung fragments (Orange *et al.*, 1971b). Energy consumption during histamine release is reflected in the fall of endogenous mast cell ATP levels during reversed anaphylaxis (Kaliner and Austen, 1974) and 48/80-induced histamine release (Diamant, 1975). Since rat mast cells are relatively poor in mitochondria (Smith, 1963), high ATP turnover requires glycolysis (Diamant, 1975). ATP from glycolysis may be utilized through a calcium-dependent ATPase to activate actinomyosinlike contractile proteins in the microfilaments (Peterson, 1974; Kaliner and Austen, 1973).

3.3. Modulating Agents

3.3.1. Cyclic Nucleotides

Cyclic AMP, cyclic GMP, and calcium modulate specific functions in a diverse group of cell types (Robison *et al.*, 1971; Berridge, 1975). Berridge has proposed monodirectional and bidirectional models for these controls. In monodirectional systems, the control mechanism is an on-off signal and external agonists cause an increase in intracellular cyclic AMP or cytoplasmic calcium concentrations which mediate the cell function. Examples include secretion from the adrenal medulla (Douglas, 1968), pancreatic β-cells (Brisson *et al.*, 1972), and salivary glands (Thorn, 1974). In bidirectional control systems, cellular function is enhanced by increased cytoplasmic calcium and inhibited by increased cyclic AMP. Examples are found in smooth muscle (Rasmussen, 1975) and platelets (Henson and Oades, 1976). In this broad classification, mast cells conform best to a bidirectional model. Additionally, modulating effects of cyclic GMP may oppose cyclic AMP effects in the mast cell as they do in some other cells (Goldberg, 1975).

In human lung fragments, agents that stimulate adenylate cyclase such as β-adrenergic agonists (Orange *et al.*, 1971a) and some prostaglandins (Tauber *et al.*, 1973) increase tissue concentrations of cyclic AMP and inhibit mediator generation and/or release. Phosphodiesterase inhibitors such as aminophylline also block mediator release and are synergistic with β-adrenergic agonists. Conversely, imidazole, which stimulates phosphodiesterase activity with a resultant lowering of tissue concentrations of cyclic AMP, enhances the mediator release (Kaliner and Austen, 1974). α-Adrenergic agonists also decrease tissue concentrations of cyclic AMP and enhance the release of chemical mediators (Orange *et al.*, 1971a; Kaliner *et al.*, 1972). There is thus an inverse relationship between tissue concentrations of cyclic AMP and the degree of mediator release observed. These observations imply the presence of receptors for β- and α-adrenergic agents and for specific prostaglandins on human lung mast cells. Some of these observations have been corroborated in purified rat mast cells: PGE_1 and theophylline inhibit histamine release by 48/80 and by IgE-dependent mechanisms (Kaliner and Austen, 1974), while adenine and diazoxide, which lower the intracellular cyclic AMP concentration, potentiate the release (Sullivan *et al.*, 1975a,b). However, in this model, epinephrine does not inhibit histamine release even though it raises the cyclic AMP level, and isoproterenol has no effects.

Incubation of human lung fragments with acetylcholine, carbamylcholine chloride, and $PGF_{2\alpha}$ increases tissue concentrations of cyclic GMP (Kaliner, 1977) and enhances IgE-dependent mediator release without decreasing cyclic AMP (Kaliner *et al.*, 1972). The cholinergic stimulation is blocked by atropine, suggesting the presence of a muscarinic receptor in human lung mast cells. This reciprocal relationship between cyclic AMP and cyclic GMP has been observed in other tissues and cells (Schultz *et al.*, 1973; Hadden *et al.*, 1974) and may be due either to competition of the cyclic nucleotides for the same protein kinase or to activation of the cyclic-AMP-specific phosphodiesterase by cyclic GMP (Goldberg *et al.*, 1973; Goldberg, 1975). In addition, intracellular cyclic AMP, via protein kinase, may affect the degree of phosphorylation of protein associated with microtubules (Sloboda *et al.*, 1975), thus regulating their assembly.

3.3.2. Cytoskeletal-Active Agents

The cytochalasins A and B are fungal products which bind to microfilaments and prevent their contractile action. Their effects on the immunological release of mediators from human tissues and cells vary with the target. Anti-IgE- or antigen-mediated histamine release from human peripheral leukocytes is either enhanced or inhibited by cytochalasin B depending on the source of the cell donor (Gillespie and Lichtenstein, 1972). Cytochalasin B inhibits the *in vitro* antigen-induced release of histamine from sensitized human skin slices (Yamamoto *et al.*, 1973). In human lung fragments, both cytochalasins enhance the release of histamine while inhibiting the concomitant formation of SRS-A (Orange, 1975). In the latter tissue, the enhancement of histamine release may be due to removal of a cytochalasin-sensitive barrier to granule exocytosis (Colten and Gabbay, 1972; Davies *et al.*, 1973; Zurier *et al.*, 1974) by interference with microfilament function (McGuire and Moellmann, 1972; Axline and Reaven, 1974), while the inhibition of SRS-A generation may be related to inhibition of certain membrane transport systems (Bloch, 1973; Mizel, 1973).

Microtubules presumably form a cytoskeleton in many cells and they have been specificially demonstrated in rat mast cells (Lagunoff and Chi, 1976). Colchicine binds to the disaggregated microtubular subunit, tubulin, and prevents microtubule assembly. Morphologically, it causes the tubules to disappear and deforms the rat mast cells, with concomitant inhibition of histamine release. In human lung fragments, colchicine inhibits IgE-dependent histamine and SRS-A release (Orange, 1976) but permits the generation of at least limited amounts of intracellular SRS-A without release (Orange, 1974). Deuterium oxide (D_2O), which opposes the effects of colchicine, presumably by stabilizing assembled microtubules, does not independently effect the release of either histamine or SRS-A from human lung. D_2O enhances IgE-mediated histamine release from human basophils (Gillespie and Lichtenstein, 1972), especially from poorly responding cells (Patterson *et al.*, 1975), and its effect in this model is reversed by colchicine (Gillespie and Lichtenstein, 1972).

3.4. A Conceptual Model for Cell Activation

The delineation of the biochemical steps involved in the release of mediators as described above suggests the conceptual model depicted in Figures 2a to 2c. Membrane receptors bound to IgE may be coupled to enzymatic subunits which dimerize subsequent to IgE bridging by specific antigen or anti-IgE. The concomitant membrane perturbation leads to increased permeability to calcium, which then participates in the activation of a chymotrypsinlike esterase and of phospholipase A. The latter hydrolyzes endomembrane phospholipids in the presence of calcium, thus liberating lysophosphatides and fatty acids. Some of the free fatty acids are metabolized via cyclooxygenase to prostaglandins and thromboxanes, and to lipoxygenase products, while the lysophosphatides may facilitate membrane fusion (Figure 2a). At the final stage of fusion, channels are formed between the perigranular and plasma membranes, as well as between adjacent perigranular membranes. Where intracytoplasmic movement of granules occurs, this follows the cytoskeletal network laid down by the microtubules and is facilitated by an actinomyosinlike contraction of the microfilaments requiring calcium and metabolic energy in the form of ATP. The state of microtubule aggregation is presumably controlled by protein kinases, whose activity, in turn, is intimately related to cytosol cyclic AMP and perhaps cyclic GMP levels (Figure 2b). Granules in contact with the surrounding medium, whether by physical exteriorization or via

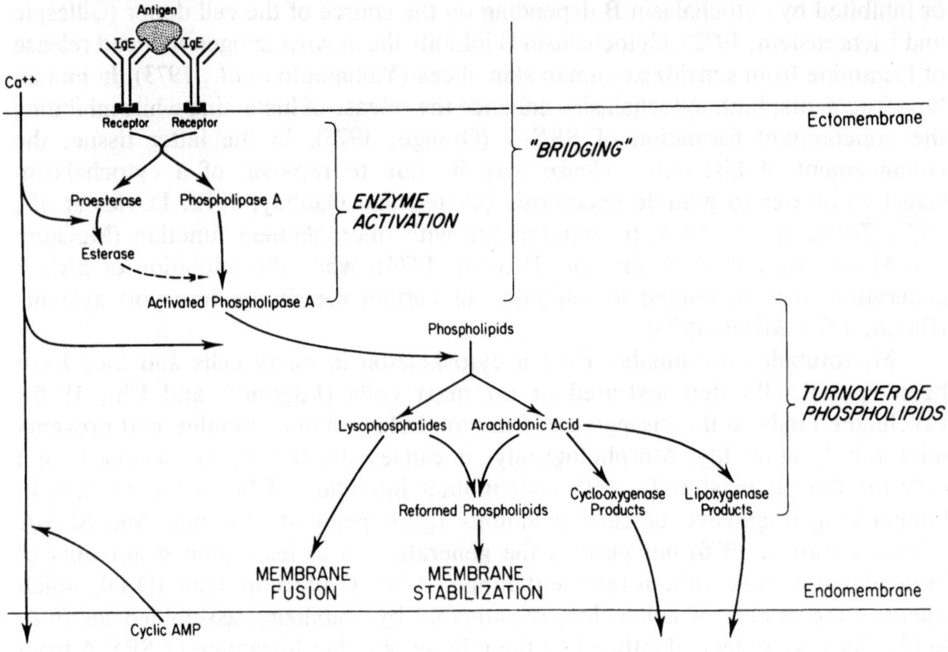

Figure 2a. Cell membrane events initiating IgE-dependent mast cell degranulation.

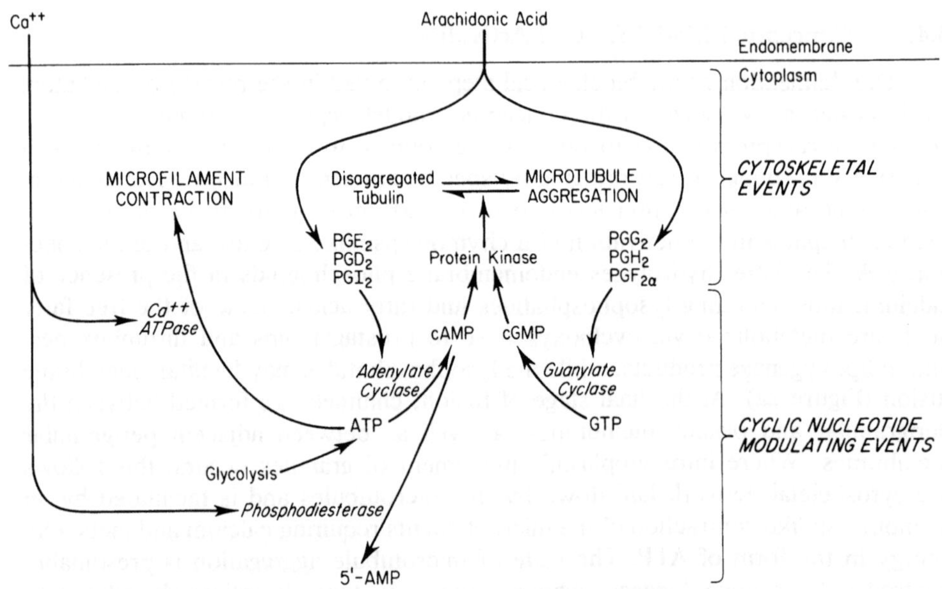

Figure 2b. Cytoplasmic events during mast cell degranulation.

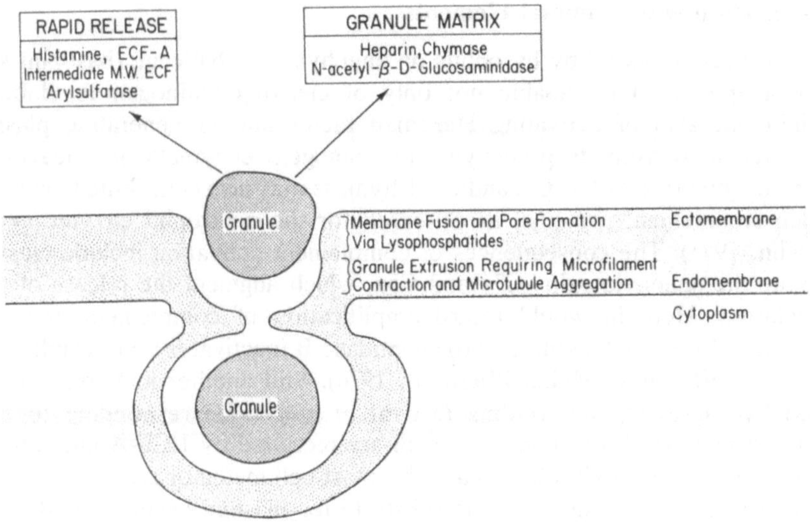

Figure 2c. Mast cell granule extrusion and the release of preformed mediators of immediate hypersensitivity.

communicating channels, discharge certain preformed mediators such as histamine and ECF-A by ion exchange (Figure 2c), while retaining others.

4. Interaction of the Mediators of Immediate Hypersensitivity with Humoral and Cellular Elements of the Immune System

Mast cells have a role not only in effecting signs and symptoms of allergic disease but also in host defense. By virtue of their mucosal and cutaneous locations, these cells are in contact with noxious agents (including specific allergens) before the latter penetrate to deeper tissues. The mediators of immediate hypersensitivity, once released, may recruit other immunological defenses to the local areas. Vasoactive mediators such as histamine, SRS-A, and PAF (via release of platelet amines) increase vascular permeability, allowing an influx of plasma proteins, including immunoglobulins and complement components, into local tissue sites. Additionally, an ingress of phagocytes occurs in response to chemotactic and chemokinetic factors such as ECF-A, intermediate-molecular-weight ECF(s), and histamine. The combined local recruitment of antibody, complement, and phagocytes allows enhanced clearance of the noxious invading agents. Failure to terminate the humoral phase of the response to vasoactive mast cell mediators results in those pathological states recognized clinically as urticaria, angioedema, acute exacerbations of rhinitis and asthma, and systemic anaphylaxis. Similarly, an inability to regulate the cellular response leads to evolution of the local inflammatory state from the acute stage to subacute and chronic phases. This is reflected experimentally in late pulmonary reactions to inhaled antigens by allergic asthmatics (Pepys and Hutchcroft, 1975) and late dermal reactions to intradermally injected antigens (Solley *et al.*, 1976) or to intradermal anti-IgE (Dolovitch *et al.*, 1973).

4.1. Interaction with Humoral Elements

The tryptase released by basophils on anaphylactic challenge (basophil kallikrein of anaphylaxis) is capable not only of cleaving kininogen to elaborate bradykinin but also of activating Hageman factor and of generating plasmin. Plasmin, activated from its proenzyme plasminogen, enzymatically cleaves the complement components C1, C3, and C5. Chymase may also contribute to cleavage of certain complement proteins, as observed for the neutrophil enzyme (Venge and Olsson, 1975). The consequences of complement activation include cleavage to generate the anaphylatoxins C3a and C5a, which augment the release of mast cell mediators. Heparin would retard amplification of complement activation (Weiler *et al.*, 1978), and serum carboxypeptidase B inactivates both anaphylatoxins with high efficiency (Müller-Eberhard, 1976). Still another kallikrein may be provided by ingressing neutrophils (Movat *et al.*, 1973) responding to high-molecular-weight NCF. Eosinophils, which are recruited by ECF-A and intermediate-molecular-weight ECF(s), also amplify mast cell mediator release by providing another source of plasminogen as substrate for plasmin generation (Barnhart and Riddle, 1963).

4.2. Interaction with Cellular Elements

Eosinophils are frequently encountered at the site of allergic reactions, having been specifically mobilized by ECF-A, intermediate-molecular-weight ECF(s), and histamine. Although they could contribute to the inflammatory response by the release of lysosomal enzymes during phagocytosis, the bulk of evidence gives them a role in damping the inflammatory effects of mast cell mediator release. The eosinophil is rich in arylsulfatase B, which inactivates SRS-A; phospholipase D, which inactivates PAF; and diamine oxidase (histaminase). This cell also ingests the granule matrix with its heparin and protein enzymes (Wintroub *et al.*, 1978). While mast-cell-derived high-molecular-weight NCF and ECF-A can account for the attraction of neutrophils into tissue sites, HETE (Goetzl *et al.*, 1977), HHT (Goetzl and Gorman, 1978), split products of complement proteins (Ward, 1967; Ward and Hill, 1970), and fibrinogen (McKenzie *et al.*, 1975) may also contribute. Neutrophils are generally proinflammatory and provide an array of acid hydrolases and neutral proteases (Movat *et al.*, 1973; Cochrane and Aikin, 1966; Scherer and Janoff, 1968; Ohlsson and Olsson, 1973, 1974) while participating in the phagocytosis of pathogens and degraded cells and tissues. Platelet aggregation and release reactions caused by PAF would have a procoagulant effect, and released ATP might further degranulate local mast cells. Arachidonic acid metabolites may also be important either as additional platelet-aggregating agents (thromboxane A_2) or as messengers affecting mast cell cyclic nucleotide levels.

4.3. Regulation of the Immediate Hypersensitivity Response in Tissue

Regulation of IgE-dependent phenomena can be visualized to occur at six levels: by the nature and intensity of activation; intracellular regulation of secretion of granules; release of mediators from granules and action of granule-retained mediators; generation of secondary mediators; composite action of mediators on common target cells; and mediator biodegradation.

At the first level, studies with human lung have shown that limited IgE-dependent activation can initiate intracellular accumulation of SRS-A without release of either SRS-A or histamine (Lewis *et al.*, 1974). Atopic sera from different donors may have differing capacities for sensitizing target tissue for SRS-A and histamine release, independent of their antigen-specific IgE concentrations or specific/total IgE ratios (Lewis and Austen, 1977). Additionally, differences in the capacities of different tissues to generate and release mediators have been noted: antigen-challenged sensitized lung tissue releases more SRS-A per unit release of histamine than do comparably sensitized and challenged nasal polyps (Kaliner *et al.*, 1973). Finally, there appears to be no correlation between the absolute amounts of histamine and SRS-A released from different human lung specimens sensitized with the same atopic serum and then challenged with specific antigen or anti-IgE (Orange and Langer, 1974).

At the second level, endogenous modulation of mediator release by intracellular cyclic nucleotides has already been discussed. Intracellular cyclic AMP and GMP levels would presumably respond, respectively, to exogenous sympathetic and parasympathetic regulation *in vivo,* as do tissue cyclic nucleotide levels in lung fragments incubated with adrenergic and cholinergic agonist *in vitro.* As noted above, some arachidonic acid metabolites are also potent modulators of cytosol cyclic nucleotide levels.

Histamine increases the cyclic AMP level in human peripheral leukocytes by binding to an H-2 receptor (Bourne *et al.*, 1971) and is therefore believed to exert a damping effect *in vivo* on ongoing mediator release. The other major evidence of intracellular regulation of mediator generation and release is derived from observations that arylsulfatases, which inactivate SRS-A, are found in the mast cells (Orange and Moore, 1976a) and basophils (Wasserman and Austen, 1977). This may explain the findings that SRS-A yields from isolated rat mast cells are inordinately low for the observed histamine release and that the presence of mast cells is associated with significantly less detectable SRS-A in the supernatants of mouse macrophages challenged with ionophore (Orange, 1977).

The third level relates to the evolving appreciation that only certain mediators leave the discharged granule. The residual mediators, such as chymase and heparin, have proteolytic and anticomplementary actions (Yurt and Austen, 1978; Weiler *et al.*, 1978), but granule solubilization increases proteolytic function markedly and uncovers the antithrombin III cofactor function. At the fourth level is the generation of unstored mediators from mast cells and especially from other local cell types. Target tissue responses often lead to generation of prostaglandins and related products as has been demonstrated by perfusing guinea pig lungs with histamine, SRS-A, or bradykinin (Palmer *et al.*, 1973).

At the fifth level are the synergistic or antagonistic effects of primary mediators on the same target cell. Smooth muscle contractile response to histamine is potentiated by SRS-A (Brocklehurst, 1960), although the *in vivo* demonstration of this effect has not been achieved. Via different receptors, histamine facilitates (H-1) and inhibits (H-2), respectively, the chemotactic response of eosinophils to ECF-A tetrapeptides (Goetzl and Austen, 1976b) and of neutrophils to C5 fragments (Goetzl, 1978).

At the sixth and final level of regulation, inactivation or biodegradation of the mediators regulates the time courses of their activities. The lung, which is frequently studied as a shock organ, is particularly active in degrading a number of mediators, including serotonin, PGs, bradykinin, and probably histamine, because of the almost ubiquitous presence of histaminase in tissues. Human lung also contains arylsulfatases A and B, which inactivate SRS-A. Mediator inactivation by humoral factors may be important since altered vascular permeability would allow an influx of various plasma proteins. In this respect, the various carboxypeptidases in plasma hydrolyze bradykinin and possibly ECF-A and ECF oligopeptides. Kallikrein is inhibited by α_2-macroglobulin, and the nonspecific adsorption of PAF and SRS-A to plasma proteins may reduce their activities. Specific destruction of the mediators by eosinophil arylsulfatase, histaminase, and phospholipase D has already been noted.

5. References

Åborg, C., and Uvnäs, B., 1971, A mucopolysaccharide–protein complex with amine binding properties in rat thrombocytes, *Acta Physiol. Scand.* **81**:568–570.

Ahkong, Q. F., Fisher, D., Tampion, W., and Lucy, J. A., 1975, Mechanisms of cell fusion, *Nature (London)* **253**:194–195.

Änggård, E., Berqvist, U., Högberg, B., Johansson, K., Thon, J. L., and Uvnäs, B., 1963, Biologically active principles occurring in histamine release from cat paw, guinea pig lung, and isolated rat mast cells, *Acta Physiol. Scand.* **59**:97–110.

Anwar, A. R. E., and Kay, A. B., 1977, The ECF-A tetrapeptides and histamine selectively enhance human eosinophil complement receptors, *Nature (London)* **269**:522–524.

Ash, A. S. F., and Schild, H. O., 1966, Receptors mediating some actions of histamine, *Br. J. Pharmacol. Chemother.* **27**:427–439.

Augstein, J., Farm., J. B., Lee, T. B., Sheard, P., and Tattersall, M. L., 1973, Selective inhibitor of slow reacting substance of anaphylaxis, *Nature (London) New Biol.* **245**:215–217.

Austen, K. F., 1976, Assay of histamine, in: *Methods in Immunology and Immunochemistry*, Vol. 5 (C. A. Williams and M. W. Chase, eds.), pp. 126–129, Academic, New York.

Austen, K. F., 1979, Biological implications of the structural and functional characteristics of the chemical mediators of immediate type hypersensitivity, in: *The Harvey Lectures*, Academic, New York (in press).

Austen, K. F., and Becker, E. L., 1966, Mechanisms of immunologic injury of rat peritoneal mast cells. II. Complement requirement and phosphonate ester inhibition of release of histamine by rabbit anti-rat gamma globulin, *J. Exp. Med.* **124**:397–416.

Austen, K. F., and Brocklehurst, W. E., 1961, Anaphylaxis of chopped guinea-pig lung. I. Effect of peptidase substrates and inhibitors, *J. Exp. Med.* **113**:521–539.

Axline, S. G., and Reaven, E. P., 1974, Inhibition of phagocytosis and plasma membrane motility of the cultivated macrophage by cytochalasin B: Role of subplasma laminal microfilaments, *J. Cell Biol.* **62**:647–659.

Bach, M. K., 1974, A molecular theory to explain the mechanisms of allergic histamine release, *J. Theor. Biol.* **45**:131–151.

Bach, M. K., and Brashler, J. R., 1974, *In vivo* and *in vitro* production of a slow reacting substance in the rat upon treatment with calcium ionophores, *J. Immunol.* **113**:2040–2044.

Bach, M. K., and Brashler, J. R., 1975, Inhibition of IgE and compound 48/80-induced histamine release by lectins, *Immunology* **29**:371–386.

Bach, M. K., Brashler, J. R., Bloch, K. J., and Austen, K. F., 1971a, Studies in the receptor site for IgE antibody in the peritoneal mast cell of the rat, in: *Biochemistry of the Acute Allergic Reactions* (K. F. Austen and E. L. Becker, eds.), pp. 65–89, Blackwell, Oxford.

Bach, M. K., Bloch, K. J., and Austen, K. F., 1971b, IgE and IgG_a antibody-mediated release of histamine from rat peritoneal cells. II. Interaction of IgG_a and IgE at the target cell, *J. Exp. Med.* **133**:772–784.

Bach, M. K., Bloch, K. J., and Austen, K. F., 1971c, IgE and IgG_a antibody-mediated release of histamine from rat peritoneal cells. I. Optimal conditions for *in vitro* preparation of target cells with antibody and challenged with antigen, *J. Exp. Med.* **133**:752–771.

Bach, M. K., Brashler, J. R., and Gorman, R. R., 1977, On the structure of slow reacting substance of anaphylaxis: Evidence of biosynthesis from arachidonic acid, *Prostaglandins* **14**:21–38.

Baker, A. R., Bloch, K. J., and Austen, K. F., 1964, *In vitro* passive sensitization of chopped guinea pig lung by guinea pig 7 S antibodies, *J. Immunol.* **93**:525–531.

Baltzly, R., Buck, J. S., DeBeer, E. J., and Webb, F. J., 1949, A family of long acting depressors, *J. Am. Chem. Soc.* **71**:1301–1305.

Barnhart, M. I., and Riddle, I. M., 1963, Cellular localization of profibrinolysin (plasminogen), *Blood* **21**:306–321.

Baxter, J. H., 1973, Role of Ca^{2+} in mast cell activation, desensitization and histamine release by dextran, *J. Immunol.* **111**:1470–1473.

Baxter, J. H., and Adamik, R., 1975, Control of histamine release: Effect of various conditions on rates of release and rate of cell desensitization, *J. Immunol.* **114**:1034–1041.

Beall, G. N., and VanArsdel, P. P., Jr., 1960, Histamine metabolism in human disease, *J. Clin. Invest.* **39**:676–683.

Beaven, M. A., 1976, Histamine, *New Engl. J. Med.* **294**:30–36, 320–325.

Becker, E. L., and Austen, K. F., 1964, A comparison of the specificity of inhibition by phosphonate esters of the first component of complement and the antigen-induced release of histamine from guinea-pig lung, *J. Exp. Med.* **120**:491–506.

Becker, E. L., and Austen, K. F., 1966, Mechanisms of immunologic injury of rat peritoneal mast cells. I. The effect of phosphonate inhibitors on the homocytotropic antibody-mediated histamine release and the first component of rat complement, *J. Exp. Med.* **124**:379–395.

Becker, E. L., and Henson, P. M., 1973, *In vitro* studies of immunologically induced secretion of mediators from cells and related phenomena, *Adv. Immunol.* **17**:93–193.

Benditt, E. P., Wong, R. L., Arase, M., and Roeper, E., 1955, 5-Hydroxytryptamine in mast cells, *Proc. Soc. Exp. Biol. Med.* **90**:303–304.

Benveniste, J., 1974, Platelet activating factor, a new mediator of anaphylaxis and immune complex deposition from rabbit and human basophils, *Nature (London)* **249**:581–582.

Benveniste, J., and Polonsky, J., 1976, Characterization of platelet activating factor (PAF), *Fed. Proc.* **35**:516 (abstr.).

Benveniste, J., Henson, P. M., and Cochrane, C. G., 1973, A possible role for IgE in immune complex disease, in: *The Biological Role of the Immunoglobulin E System* (K. Ishizaka and D. H. Dayton, eds.), pp. 187–205, U.S. Department of Health, Education and Welfare, Washington, D.C.

Berridge, M. G., 1975, The interaction of cyclic nucleotides and calcium in the control of cellular activity, *Adv. Cyclic Nucleotide Res.* **6**:1–98.

Bills, T. K., Smith, J. B., and Silver, M. J., 1977, Selective release of arachidonic acid from the phospholipids of human platelets in response to thrombin, *J. Clin. Invest.* **60**:1–6.

Black. J. W., Duncan, W. A. M., Durant, C. J., Ganellin, C. R., and Parsons, E. M., 1972, Definition of antagonism of histamine H_2-receptors, *Nature (London)* **236**:385–390.

Blackwell, G. J., Duncombe, W. G., Flower, R. J., Parsons, M. F., and Vane, J. R., 1977, The distribution and metabolism of arachidonic acid in rabbit platelets during aggregation and its modification by drugs, *Br. J. Pharmacol.* **59**:353–366.

Blackwell, G. J., Flower, R. J., Nijkamp, F. P., and Vane, J. R., 1978, Phospholipase A_2 activity of guinea-pig isolated perfused lungs, *Br. J. Pharmacol.* **62**:79–89.

Bloch, R., 1973, Inhibition of glucose transport in the human erythrocyte by cytochalasin B, *Biochemistry* **12**:4799–4801.

Bloom, G. D., Foldholm, B., and Haegermark, O., 1967, Studies on the time course of histamine release and morphological changes induced by histamine liberators in rat peritoneal mast cells, *Acta Physiol. Scand.* **71**:270–282.

Bogart, D. B., and Stechschulte, D. J., 1974, Release of platelet activating factor from human lung, *Clin. Res.* **22**:652(abstr.).

Boot, J. R., Brockwell, A. D. J., Dawson, W., and Sweatman, W. J. F., 1977, The relationship between prostaglandin-like substances and SRS-A released from immunologically challenged lungs, *Br. J. Pharmacol.* **59**:444p.

Boswell, R. N., Austen, K. F., and Goetzl, E. J., 1976, A chemotactic receptor for Val-(Ala)-gly-ser-glu on human eosinophil polymorphonuclear leukocytes, *Immunol. Commun.* **5**:469–479.

Boswell, R. N., Austen, K. F., and Goetzl, E. J., 1978, Intermediate molecular weight eosinophil chemotactic factors in rat peritoneal mast cells: Immunologic release, granule association, and demonstration of structural heterogeneity, *J. Immunol.* **120**:15–20.

Bourne, H. R., Melmon, K. L., and Lichtenstein, L. M., 1971, Histamine augments leukocyte cyclic AMP and blocks antigenic histamine release, *Science* **173**:743–745.

Brashler, J. R., and Bach, M. K., 1976, Production of slow reacting substance of anaphylaxis (SRS-A) *in vitro:* Involvement of phagocytes in an ionophore A23187-induced reaction, *Fed. Proc.* **35**:864 (abstr.).

Brisson, G. R., Malaisse-Lagore, F., and Malaisse, W. J., 1972, The stimulus-secretion coupling of glucose-induced insulin release. VII. A proposed site of action for adenosine-3′,5′-cyclic monophosphate, *J. Clin, Invest.* **51**:232–241.

Brocklehurst, W. E., 1958, The action of 5-hydroxytryptamine on smooth muscle, in: *5-Hydroxytryptamine* (G. P. Lewis, ed.), pp. 172–176, Pergamon, Oxford.

Brocklehurst, W. E., 1960, The release of histamine and formation of a slow-reacting substance (SRS-A) during anaphylactic shock, *J. Physiol. (London)* **151**:416–435.

Brocklehurst, W. E., 1962, Slow reacting substance and related compounds, *Progr. Allergy* **6**:539–558.

Brocklehurst, W. E., and Lahiri, S. C., 1962, Formation and destruction of bradykinin during anaphylaxis, *J. Physiol. (London)* **160**:15–16.

Broder, I., 1973, Appraisal of anaphylatoxin as an intermediary of anaphylactic histamine release, in: *Mechanisms in Allergy* (L. Goodfriend, A. H. Sehon, and R. P. Orange, eds.), pp. 481–493, Dekker, New York.

Brostrom, C. O., Huang, Y., Breckenridge, B. M., and Wolff, D. J., 1975, Identification of a calcium-binding protein as a calcium-dependent regulator of brain adenylate cyclase, *Proc. Natl. Acad. Sci. USA* **72**:64–68.

Bryant, D. H., Burns, M. W., and Lazarus, L., 1975, Identification of IgG antibody as a carrier of reaginic activity in asthmatic patients, *J. Allergy Clin. Immunol.* **56**:417–428.

Burka, J. F., and Eyre, P., 1974, The immunological release of slow reacting substance of anaphylaxis in bovine lung, *Can. J. Physiol. Pharmacol.* **52**:1201–1204.

Chau-Wong, M., and Seeman, P., 1971, The control of membrane-bound Ca^{2+} by ATP, *Biochim, Biophys. Acta* **241**:473–482.

Chi, E., Lagunoff, D., and Koehler, J. K., 1976, Freeze-fracture study of mast cell secretion, *Proc. Natl. Acad. Sci. USA* **73**:2823–2827.

Christ, E. J., and Van Dorp, D. A., 1973, Comparative aspects of prostaglandin biosynthesis in animal tissue, in: *Advances in the Biosciences International Conference on Prostaglandins* (S. Bergstrom and S. Bernhard, eds.), pp. 35–38, Pergamon, Oxford.

Clark, R. A. F., Gallin, J. I., and Kaplan, A. P., 1975, Selective eosinophilic chemotactic activity of histamine, *J. Exp. Med.* **142**:1462–1476.

Clark, R. A. F., Sandler, J. A., Gallin, J. I., and Kaplan, A. P., 1977, Histamine modulation of eosinophil migration, *J. Immunol.* **118**:137–145.

Coceani, F., Dreifuss, J. J., Puglisi, L., and Wolfe, L. S., 1969, Prostaglandins and membrane function, in: *Prostaglandins, Peptides and Amines* (P. Mantagazza and E. W. Horton, eds.), pp. 73–82, Academic, New York.

Cochrane, C. G., and Aikin, B. S., 1966, Polymorphonuclear leykocytes in immunologic reactions: The destruction of vascular basement membrane *in vivo* and *in vitro*, *J. Exp. Med.* **124**:733–752.

Cochrane, D. E., and Douglas, W. W., 1974, Calcium-induced extrusion of secretory granules (exocytosis) in mast cells exposed to 48/80 or the ionophores A-23187 and X-537A, *Proc. Natl. Acad. Sci. USA* **71**:408–412.

Colten, H. R., and Gabbay, K. H., 1972, Histamine release from human leukocytes: Modulation by a cytochalasin B-sensitive barrier, *J. Clin. Invest.* **51**:1927–1931.

Conrad, D. H., and Froese, A., 1978, Characterization of the target cell receptor for IgE. III. Properties of the receptor isolated from rat basophilic leukemia cells by affinity chromatography, *J. Immunol.* **120**:429–437.

Conrad, D. H., Bazin, H., Sehon, A. H., and Froese, A., 1975, Binding parameters of the interaction between rat IgE and rat mast cell receptors, *J. Immunol.* **114**:1688–1691.

Conroy, M. C., Orange, R. P., and Lichtenstein, L. M., 1976, Release of slow reacting substance of anaphylaxis (SRS-A) from human leukocytes by the calcium ionophore A23187, *J. Immunol.* **116:**1677–1681.

Cox, J. S. G., Beach, J. E., Blaire, A. M. J. N., Clarke, A. J., King, J., Lee, T. B., Loveday, D. E. G., Moss, G. F., Orr, T. S. C., Ritchie, J. T., and Sheard, P., 1970, Disodium cromoglycate (Intal), in: *Advances in Drug Research,* Vol. 5 (N. J. Harper and A. B. Simmonds, eds.), pp. 115–196, Academic, New York.

Cullis, P. R., and Hope, M. J., 1978, Effects of fusogenic agents on membrane structure of erythrocyte ghosts and the mechanism of membrane fusion, *Nature (London)* **271:**672–674.

Cuatrecasas, P., 1974, Membrane receptors, *Annu. Rev. Biochem.* **43:**169–214.

Cuthbert, M. F., 1969, Effect of airway resistance of prostaglandin E given by aerosol to healthy and asthmatic volunteers, *Br. Med. J.* **4:**723–726.

Czarnetski, B. M., König, W., and Lichtenstein, L. M., 1976, Eosinophil chemotactic factor (ECF). I. Release from polymorphonuclear leukocytes by the calcium ionophore A23187, *J. Immunol.* **117:**229–234.

Dahlquist, R., 1974a, Relationship of uptake of sodium and ^{45}calcium to ATP-induced histamine release from rat mast cells, *Acta Pharmacol. Toxicol.* **35:**11–22.

Dahlquist, R., 1974b, Determination of ATP-induced ^{45}calcium uptake in rat mast cells, *Acta Pharmacol. Toxicol.* **35:**1–10.

Davies, P., Fox, R. I., Polyzonis, M., Allison, A. C., and Haswell, D., 1973, The inhibition of phagocytosis and facilitation of exocytosis in rabbit polymorphonuclear leukocytes by cytochalasin B, *Lab. Invest.* **28:**16–22.

Dawson, W., and Tomlinson, R., 1974, Effect of cromoglycate and eicosatetraynoic acid on the release of prostaglandins and SRS-A from immunologically challenged guinea-pig lungs, *Br. J. Pharmacol.* **52:**107–108.

Diamant, B., 1975, Energy production in rat mast cells and its role for histamine release, *Int. Arch. Allergy Appl. Immunol.* **49:**155–171.

Diamant, B., Grosman, N., Skov, P. S., and Thomle, S., 1974, Effect of divalent cations and metabolic energy in the anaphylactic histamine release from rat peritoneal mast cells, *Int. Arch. Allergy Appl. Immunol.* **47:**412–424.

Dolovitch, J., Hargreave, F. E., Chalmers, R., Shier, K. J., Gauldie, J., and Bienenstock, J., 1973, Late cutaneous allergic responses in isolated IgE-dependent reactions, *J. Allergy Clin. Immunol.* **52:**38–46.

Douglas, W. W., 1968, Stimulus-secretion coupling: The concept and clues from chromaffin and other cells, The First Gaddum Memorial Lecture, *Br. J. Pharmacol.* **34:**451–474.

Douglas, W. W., 1975a, Histamine and antihistamines; 5-hydroxytryptamine and antagonists, in: *The Pharmacological Basis of Therapeutics,* 5th ed. (L. S. Goodman and A. Gilman, eds.), pp. 590–629, Macmillan, New York.

Douglas, W. W., 1975b, Polypeptides—angiotensin, plasma kinins and other vasoactive agents; prostaglandins, in: *The Pharmacological Basis of Therapeutics,* 5th ed. (L. S. Goodman and A. Gilman, eds.), pp. 630–652, Macmillan, New York.

Douglas, W. W., and Rubin, R. P., 1961, The role of calcium in the secretory response of the adrenal medulla to acetylcholine, *J. Physiol. (London)* **159:**40–57.

Drazen, J. M., and Austen, K. F., 1975, Atropine modification of the pulmonary effects of chemical mediators in the guinea pig, *J. Appl. Physiol.* **38:**834–838.

Drazen, J. M., Lewis, R. A., Wasserman, S. I., and Austen, K. F., 1978, Effects of histamine and slow reacting substance of anaphylaxis (SRS-A) on central and peripheral airway function *in vitro, Am. Rev. Resp. Dis.* **117**(Suppl.):63 (abstr.).

Engineer, D. M., Piper, P. J., and Sirois, P., 1977, Release of prostaglandins and rabbit aorta contracting substance (RCS) from guinea-pig lung by slow reacting substance of anaphylaxis (SRS-A), *Br. J. Pharmacol.* **59:**444P.

Engleberg, H., 1963, Metabolism of heparin, in: *Heparin,* pp. 20–41, Charles C. Thomas, Springfield, Ill.

Farmer, J. B., Richards, I. M., Sheard, P., and Woods, A. M., 1975, Mediators of passive lung anaphylaxis in the rat, *Br. J. Pharmacol.* **55:**57–64.

Feldberg, W., and Kellaway, C. H., 1938, Liberation of histamine from the perfused lung by snake venom, *J. Physiol. (London)* **90:**257–279.

Feltkamp-Vroom, T. M., Stallman, P. J., Aalberse, R. C., and Reerink-Brongers, E. E., 1975,

Immunofluorescent studies on renal tissue, tonsils, adenoids, nasal polyps, and skin of atopic and non-atopic patients with special reference to IgE, *Clin. Immunol. Immunopathol.* **4**:392–404.

Ferber, E., 1971, Membrane phospholipid metabolism during cell activation and differentiation, in: *The Dynamic Structure of Cell Membrane* (D. F. H. Wallach and H. Fischer, eds.), pp. 129–147, Springer-Verlag, Berlin.

Ferber, E., and Resch, K., 1973, Phospholipid metabolism of stimulated lymphocytes: Activation of acyl-CoA:lysolecithin acyltransferase in microsomal membranes, *Biochim. Biophys. Acta* **296**:335–349.

Fésüs, L., Csaba, B., and Muszbek, L., 1977, Platelet activating factor, the trigger of haemostatic alterations in rat anaphylaxis, *Clin. Exp. Immunol.* **27**:512–515.

Fillion, G. M. D., Slorach, S. A., and Uvnäs, B., 1970, The release of histamine, heparin, and granule protein from rat mast cells treated with compound 48/80 *in vitro, Acta Physiol. Scand.* **78**:547–560.

Flower, R. J., 1977, The role of prostaglandins in inflammatory reactions, *Nauyn-Schmiedeberg's Arch. Pharmacol.* **297**:577–579.

Flower, R. J., and Blackwell, G. J., 1976, The importance of phospholipase-A_2 in prostaglandin biosynthesis, *Biochem. Pharmacol.* **25**:285–291.

Foreman, J. C. and Gomperts, B. D., 1975, The relationship between anaphylactic histamine secretion and the permeability of the mast cell membrane to calcium, *Int. Arch. Allergy Appl. Immunol.* **49**:179–182.

Foreman, J. C., and Mongar, J. L., 1972a, The role of the alkaline earth ions in anaphylactic histamine secretion, *J. Physiol. (London)* **224**:753–769.

Foreman, J. C., and Mongar, J. L., 1972b, Effect of calcium in dextran-induced histamine release from isolated mast cells, *Br. J. Pharmacol.* **46**:767–769.

Foreman, J. C., Mongar, J. L., and Gomperts, B. D., 1973, Calcium ionophores and movement of calcium ions following the physiological stimulus to a secretory process, *Nature (London)* **245**:249–251.

Foreman, J. C., Hallett, M. B., and Mongar, J. L., 1975, ^{45}Calcium uptake in rat peritoneal mast cells, *Br. J. Pharmacol.* **55**:283P–284P.

Frye, L., and Frion, G., 1976, K cell cytotoxicity: Studies into nature of kill phase, in: *Leukocyte Membrane Determinants Regulating Immune Reactivity* (V. P. Eijsvoogel, D. Roos, and W. P. Zeijlemaker, eds.), p. 653, Academic, London.

Gershon, M. D., and Ross, L. L., 1962, Studies on the relationship of 5-hydroxytryptamine and the enterochromaffin cell to anaphylactic shock in mice, *J. Exp. Med.* **115**:367–381.

Giacobini, E., Sedvall, G., and Uvnäs, B., 1965, Phosphatidase A activity of isolated rat mast cells, *Exp. Cell Res.* **37**:368–375.

Gillespie, E., and Lichtenstein, L. M., 1972, Histamine release from human leukocytes: Studies with deuterium oxide, colchicine and cytochalasin B, *J. Clin. Invest.* **51**:2941–2947.

Gingell, D., 1967, Membrane surface potential in relation to a possible mechanism for intercellular interactions and cellular responses: A physical basis, *J. Theor. Biol.* **17**:451–482.

Goetzl, E. J., 1978, Regulation of the polymorphonuclear leukocyte chemotactic response by immunologic reactions, in: *Leukocyte Chemotaxis, Methodology, Physiology, Clinical Implications* (J. I. Gallin and P. G. Quie, eds.), pp. 161–177, Raven, New York.

Goetzl, E. J., and Austen, K. F., 1975, Purification and synthesis of eosinophilotactic tetrapeptides of human lung tissue: Identification as eosinophil chemotactic factor of anaphylaxis, *Proc. Natl. Acad. Sci. USA* **72**:4123–4127.

Goetzl, E. J., and Austen, K. F., 1976a, Structural determinants of the eosinophil chemotactic activity of the acidic tetrapeptides of eosinophil chemotactic factor of anaphylaxis, *J. Exp. Med.* **144**:1424–1437.

Goetzl, E. J., and Austen, K. F., 1976b, Specificity and modulation of the eosinophil polymorphonuclear leukocyte response to eosinophil chemotactic factor of anaphylaxis (ECF-A), in: *Molecular and Biological Aspects of the Acute Allergic Reactions* (S. G. O. Johansson, K. Strandberg, and B. Uvnäs, eds.), pp. 417–435, Plenum, London.

Goetzl, E. J., and Gorman, R. R., 1978, Chemotactic and chemokinetic stimulation of human eosinophil and neutrophil polymorphonuclear leukocytes by 12-L-hydroxy-5,8,10-heptadecatrienoic acid (HHT), *J. Immunol.* **120**:526–531.

Goetzl, E. J., Woods, J. M., and Gorman, R. R., 1977, Stimulation of human eosinophil and neutrophil polymorphonuclear leukocyte chemotaxis and random migration by 12-L-hydroxy-5,8,10,14-eicosatetraenoic acid, *J. Clin. Invest.* **59**:179–183.

Goetzl, E. J., Tashjian, A. H., Jr., Rubin, R. H., and Austen, K. F., 1978, Production of a low molecular weight eosinophil polymorphonuclear leukocyte chemotactic factor by anaplastic squamous cell carcinomas of human lung, *J. Clin. Invest.* **61**:770–780.

Gold, M., LaPierre, J. G., Levison, H., Bryan, A. C., and Orange, R. P., 1976, Changes in lung mechanics induced by antigen or by infusion of mediators via the pulmonary or bronchial artery, *J. Allergy Clin. Immunol.* **57**:214 (abstr.).

Goldberg, N. D., 1975, Cyclic nucleotides and cell function, in: *Cell Membrane* (B. Weissmann and R. Claiborne, eds.), pp. 185–201, Hospital Practice Publisher, New York.

Goldberg, N. D., O'Dea, R. F., and Haddox, M. K., 1973, Cyclic GMP, in: *Advances in Cyclic Nucleotide Research,* Vol. 3 (P. Greengard and G. A. Robison, eds.), pp. 155–223, Raven, New York.

Grant, J. A., and Lichtenstein, L. M., 1974, Release of slow reacting substance of anaphylaxis from human leukocytes, *J. Immunol.* **112**:897–904.

Greaves, M. W., Yamamoto, S., and Fairley, V. M., 1972, IgE-mediated hypersensitivity in human skin studied using a new *in vitro* method, *Immunology* **23**:239–248.

Hadden, J. W., Hadden, E., and Goldberg, N. D., 1974, Cyclic GMP and cyclic AMP in lymphocyte metabolism and proliferation, in: *Cyclic AMP, Cell Growth and the Immune Response* (W. Braun, L. M. Lichtenstein, and C. W. Parker, eds.), pp. 237–246, Springer-Verlag, New York.

Hällgren, R., and Venge, P., 1976a, Cationic proteins of human granulocytes: Enhancement of phagocytosis of staphylococcus protein A–IgG complexes, *Inflammation* **1**:237.

Hällgren, R., and Venge, P., 1976b, Cationic proteins of human granulocytes: Effects on human platelet aggregation and serotonin release, *Inflammation* **1**:359.

Hamberg, M., Svensson, J., and Samuelsson, B., 1974, Prostaglandin endoperoxides. A new concept concerning the mode of action and release of prostaglandins. *Proc. Natl. Acad. Sci. USA* **71**:3824–3828.

Harkavy, J., 1930, Spasm-producing substance in the sputum of patients with bronchial asthma, *Arch. Intern. Med.* **45**:641–646.

Hartley, B. S., 1960, Proteolytic enzymes, *Annu. Rev. Biochem.* **29**:45–72.

Hastie, R., 1971, The antigen-induced degranulation of basophil leukocytes from atopic subjects, studied by phase-contrast microscopy, *Clin. Exp. Immunol.* **8**:45–61.

Hauser, H., Darke, A., and Phillips, M. C., 1976, Ion-binding to phospholipids—Interaction of calcium with phosphatidylserine, *Eur. J. Biochem.* **62**:335–344.

Haydon, D. A., and Taylor, J., 1963, The stability and properties of bimolecular lipid leaflets in aqueous solutions, *J. Theor. Biol.* **4**:281–296.

Henson, P. M., 1970, Release of vasoactive amines from rabbit platelets induced by sensitized mononuclear leukocytes and antigen, *J. Exp. Med.* **131**:287–304.

Henson, P. M., 1977, Activation of rabbit platelets by platelet-activating factor derived from IgE-sensitized basophils, *J. Clin. Invest.* **60**:481–490.

Henson, P. M., and Cochrane, C. G., 1969, Immunological induction of increased vascular permeability. I. A rabbit passive cutaneous anaphylactic reaction requiring complement, platelets and neutrophils, *J. Exp. Med.* **129**:153–165.

Henson, P. M., and Oades, Z., 1976, Activation of platelets by platelet-activating factor (PAF) derived from IgE-sensitized basophils. II. The role of serine proteases, cyclic nucleotides, and contractile elements in PAF-induced secretion, *J. Exp. Med.* **143**:953–968.

Herxheimer, H., 1955, The 5-hydroxytryptamine shock in the guinea-pig, *J. Physiol. (London)* **128**:435–445.

Herxheimer, H., and Stresemann, E., 1963, The effect of slow reacting substance (SRS-A) in guinea pigs and in asthmatic patients, *J. Physiol. (London)* **165**:78–79.

Ho, P. C., and Orange, R. P., 1978, Indirect evidence of phospholipase A activation in purified rat mast cells during reverse anaphylactic challenge, *Fed. Proc.* **37**:1667 (abstr.).

Ho, P. C., and Orange, R. P., 1979, Phospholipid metabolism in rat mast cells during reverse anaphylactic challenge. I. Release and *de novo* synthesis, submitted for publication.

Högberg, B., and Uvnäs, B., 1957, The mechanism of the disruption of mast cells produced by compound 48/80, *Acta Physiol. Scand.* **40**:345–369.

Högberg, B., and Uvnäs, B., 1960, Further observations on the disruption of rat mesentery mast cells caused by compound 48/80, antigen-antibody reaction, lecithinase A and decylamine, *Acta Physiol. Scand.* **48:**133–145.

Hong, S., and Levine, L., 1976, Inhibition of arachidonic acid release from cells as the biochemical action of anti-inflammatory corticosteroids, *Proc. Natl. Acad. Sci. USA* **73:**1730–1734.

Ishizaka, K., Tomioka, H., and Ishizaka, T., 1970, Mechanisms of passive sensitization. I. Presence of IgE and IgG molecules on human leukocytes, *J. Immunol.* **105:**1459–1467.

Ishizaka, T., Ishizaka, K., Conrad, D. H., and Froese, A., 1978, Histamine release from rat mast cells by antibodies againt IgE-receptors, *J. Allergy Clin. Immunol.* **61:**153 (abstr.).

Jakschik, B. A., Falkenheim, S., and Parker, C. W., 1977, Precursor role of arachidonic acid in release of slow reacting substances from rat basophilic leukemic cells, *Proc. Natl. Acad. Sci. USA* **74:**4577–4581.

Jefferji, S. S., and Michell, R. J., 1976, Effects of calcium-antagonistic drugs on the stimulation by carbamoylcholine and histamine of phosphatidyl-inositol turnover in longitudinal smooth muscle of guinea pig ileum, *Biochem. J.* **160:**163–169.

Johnson, H. G., and Bach, M. K., 1975, Prevention of calcium ionophore-induced release of histamine in rat mast cells by disodium cromoglycate, *J. Immunol.* **114:**514–516.

Jonasson, O., and Becker, E. L., 1966, Release of kallikrein from guinea pig lung during anaphylaxis, *J. Exp. Med.* **123:**509–522.

Kaliner, M., 1977, Human lung tissue and anaphylaxis. I. The role of cyclic GMP as a modulator of the immunologically induced secretory process, *J. Allergy Clin. Immunol.* **60:**204–211.

Kaliner, M., and Austen, K. F., 1973, A sequence of biochemical events in the antigen-induced release of chemical mediators from sensitized human lung tissue, *J. Exp. Med.* **138:**1077–1094.

Kaliner, M., and Austen, K. F., 1974, Cyclic AMP, ATP, and reversed anaphylactic histamine release from rat mast cells, *J. Immunol.* **112:**664–674.

Kaliner, M., Orange, R. P., and Austen, K. F., 1972, Immunologic release of histamine and slow-reacting substance of anaphylaxis from human lung. IV. Enhancement by cholinergic and alpha-adrenergic stimulation, *J. Exp. Med.* **136:**556–567.

Kaliner, M., Wasserman, S. I., and Austen, K. F., 1973, Immunologic release of chemical mediators from human nasal polyps, *N. Engl. J. Med.* **289:**277–281.

Kanno, T., Cochrane, D. E., and Douglas, W. W., 1973, Exocytosis (secretory granule extrusion) induced by injection of calcium into mast cells, *Can. J. Physiol. Pharmacol.* **51:**1001–1004.

Kaplan, A. P., Gray, L., Shaff, R. E., Horakova, Z., and Beavan, M. A., 1975, *In vivo* studies of mediator release in cold urticaria and cholinergic urticaria, *J. Allergy Clin. Immunol.* **55:**394–402.

Kaplan, A. P., Hunt, K. J., Sobotka, A. K., Smith, P., Horakova, Z., Gralnick, H., and Lichtenstein, L. M., 1977, Human anaphylaxis: A study of mediator systems, *Clin. Res.* **25:**361 (abstr.).

Kater, L. A., Austen, K. F., and Goetzl, E. J., 1976, Isolation of human eosinophil phospholipase D, *J. Clin. Invest.* **57:**1173–1180.

Kay, A. B., and Austen, K. F., 1971, The IgE-mediated release of an eosinophil leukocyte chemotactic factor from human lung, *J. Immunol.* **107:**899–902.

Kay, A. B., Stechschulte, D. J., and Austen, K. F., 1971, An eosinophil leukocyte chemotactic factor of anaphylaxis, *J. Exp. Med.* **133:**602–619.

Kay, A. B., Roberts, E. M., and Jones, D. G., 1976, Tissue inactivation of slow reacting substance of anaphylaxis, *Immunology* **30:**83–87.

Kennerly, D. A., Sullivan, T. J., and Parker, C. W., 1979, Activation of phospholipid metabolism during mediator release from stimulated red mast cells, *J. Immunol.* **122:**152–159.

Kinsolving, C. R., Johnson, A. R., and Moran, N. C., 1975, The uptake of a substituted acridone by rat mast cells in relationship to histamine release: A possible indicator of exocytosis-induced expansion of the plasma membrane, *J. Pharmacol. Exp. Ther.* **192:**654–669.

König, W., Czarnetski, B. M., and Lichtenstein, L. M., 1976, Eosinophil chemotactic factor (ECF). II. Release during phagocytosis of human polymorphonuclear leukocytes, *J. Immunol.* **117:**235–241.

Koren, H. S., Terber, E., and Fischer, H., 1971, Changes in phospholipid metabolism of a tumor target cell during a cell-mediated cytotoxic reaction, *Biochim. Biophys. Acta* **231:**520–526.

Kravis, T. C., and Henson, P. M., 1975, IgE-induced release of a platelet activating factor from rabbit lung, *J. Immunol.* **115:**1677–1681.

Kulczycki, A., Jr., McNearney, T. A., and Parker, C. W., 1976, The rat basophilic leukemia cell receptor for IgE. I. Characterization as a glycoprotein, *J. Immunol.* **117:**661–665.

Kunze, H., and Vogt, W., 1971, Significance of phospholipase A for prostaglandin formation, *Ann. N.Y. Acad. Sci.* **180:**123–125.
Lagunoff, D., 1972, The mechanism of histamine release from mast cells, *Biochem. Pharmacol.* **21:**1889–1896.
Lagunoff, D., 1973, Membrane fusion during mast cell secretion, *J. Cell Biol.* **57:**252–259.
Lagunoff, D., and Benditt, E. P., 1963, The proteolytic enzymes of mast cells, *Ann. N.Y. Acad. Sci.* **103:**185–198.
Lagunoff, D., and Chi, E. Y., 1976, Effect of colchicine on rat mast cells, *J. Cell Biol.* **71:**182–195.
Lagunoff, D., and Pritzl, P., 1976, Characterization of rat mast cell granule proteins, *Arch. Biochem. Biophys.* **173:**554–563.
Lagunoff, D., Pritzl, P., and Mueller, L., 1970, *N*-Acetyl-beta-glucosaminidase in rat mast cell granules, *Exp. Cell Res.* **61:**129–132.
Lands, W. E. M., and Samuelsson, B., 1968, Phospholipid precursors of prostaglandins, *Biochim. Biophys. Acta* **164:**426–429.
LaPierre, J. G., Gold, M., Levison, H., and Orange, R. P., 1976, The effect on lung mechanics of infusion of chemical mediators to the bronchial and pulmonary arteries, *Fed. Proc.* **35:**395 (abstr.).
Lawson, D., Raff, M. C., Gomperts, B., Fewtrell, C., and Gilula, N. B., 1976, Molecular events in membrane fusion occurring during mast cell degranulation, in: *Molecular and Biological Aspects of the Acute Allergic Reaction* (S. G. O. Johansson, K. Strandberg, and B. Uvnäs, eds.), pp. 279–291, Nobel Foundation Symposium, Plenum, New York.
Lawson, D., Raft, M. C., Gomperts, B., Fewtrell, C., and Gilula, N. B., 1977, Molecular events during membrane fusion. *J. Cell Biol.* **72:**242–259.
Laychock. S. G., Franson, R. C., Weglicki, W. B., and Rubin, R. P., 1977, Identification and partial characterization of phospholipases in isolated adrenocortical cells, *Biochem. J.* **164:**753–756.
Lecomte, J., 1957, Liberation of endogenous histamine in man, *J. Allergy* **28:**102–112.
Levey, G. S., 1971, Restoration of norepinephrine responsiveness of solubilized myocardial adenylate cyclase by phosphatidylinositol, *J. Biol. Chem.* **246:**7405–7407.
Lewis, G. P., and Piper, P. J., 1975, Inhibition of release of prostaglandins as an explanation of some of the action of anti-inflammatory corticosteroids, *Nature (London)* **254:**308–311.
Lewis, R. A., and Austen, K. F., 1977, Non-respiratory functions of pulmonary cells: The mast cell, *Fed. Proc.* **36:**2676–2683.
Lewis, R. A., Wasserman, S. I., Goetzl, E. J., and Austen, K. F., 1974, Formation of SRS-A in human lung tissue and cells before release, *J. Exp. Med.* **140:**1133–1146.
Lewis, R. A., Goetzl, E. J., Wasserman, S. I., Valone, F. H., Rubin, R. H., and Austen, K. F., 1975, The release of four mediators of immediate hypersensitivity from human leukemic basophils, *J. Immunol.* **114:**87–92.
Lichtenstein, L. M., 1973, The pharmacologic control of allergic reactions, in: *Mechanisms in Allergy* (L. Goodfriend, A. J. Sehon, and R. P. Orange, eds.), pp. 395–412, Dekker, New York.
Lichtenstein, L. M., 1976, The interdependence of allergic and inflammatory processes, in: *Molecular and Biological Aspects of the Acute Allergic Reaction* (S. G. O. Johansson, K. Strandberg, and B. Uvnäs, eds.), pp. 233–254, Nobel Foundation Symposium, Plenum, New York.
Lindahl, U., Bäckström, G., Jansson, L., and Hallén, A., 1973, Biosynthesis of heparin. II. Formation of sulfamino groups, *J. Biol. Chem.* **248:**7234–7241.
Lloyd, A. G., Bloom, G. D., and Balazs, E. A., 1967, Evidence for the covalent association of heparin and protein in mast cell granules, *Biochem. J.* **103:**76P–77P.
Lo, P. Y., Adaikan, P. G., and Karim, S. M. M., 1976, Effects of PGA and PGB compounds on human respiratory tract smooth muscle *in vitro*, *Prostaglandins* **11:**531–536.
Lucy, J. A., 1970, The fusion of biologic membranes, *Nature (London)* **227:**815–817.
Lucy, J. A., 1975, The fusion of cell membranes, in: *Cell Membrane* (G. Weismann and R. Claiborne, eds.), pp. 75–83, Hospital Practice Publisher, New York.
MacDonald-Lynch, S., Austen, K. F., and Wasserman, S. I., 1978, Subcellular localization of rat mast cell arylsulfatases A and B, *J. Allergy Clin. Immunol.* **61:**154 (abstr.).
Majno, G., Shea, S. M., and Leventhal, M., 1969, Endothelial contraction induced by histamine-type mediators: An electron-microscopy study, *J. Cell Biol.* **42:**647–672.
Malemud, C. J., and Janoff, A., 1975, Identification of neutral proteases in human neutrophil granules that degrade articular cartilage proteoglycan, *Arthr. Rheum.* **18:**361–368.

Mathé, A. A., and Hedqvist, P., 1975, Effect of prostaglandins $F_{2\alpha}$ and E_2 on airway conductance in healthy subjects and asthmatic patients, *Am. Rev. Resp. Dis.* **111**:313–320.

McFadden, E. R., Jr., and Soter, N. A., 1977, A search for chemical mediators of immediate hypersensitivity and humoral factors in the pathogenesis of exercise-induced asthma, in: *Asthma: Physiology, Pharmacology, and Treatment* (L. M. Lichtenstein and K. F. Austen, eds.), pp. 351–364, Academic, New York.

McGuire, J., and Moellmann, G., 1972, Cytochalasin B: Effects on microfilaments and movement of melanin granules within melanocytes, *Science* **175**:642–644.

McKenzie, R., Pepper, D. S., and Kay, A. B., 1975, The generation of chemotactic activity for human leukocytes by the action of plasmin on human fibrinogen, *Thromb. Res.* **6**: 1–6.

Mendoza, G., and Metzger, H., 1976, Distribution and valency of receptor for IgE on rodent mast cells and related tumor cells, *Nature (London)* **264**:548–550.

Metcalfe, D. D., Lewis, R. A., Silbert, J. E., Rosenberg, R. D., Wasserman, S. I., and Austen, K. F., 1978, Isolation, identification and characterization of heparin from human lung, *Fed. Proc.* **37**:1776 (abstr.).

Metzger, H., 1977, The cellular receptor for IgE, in: *Receptors and Recognition*, Ser. A., Vol. 4 (P. Cuatrecasas and M. F. Greaves, eds.), pp. 75–102, Chapman and Hall, London.

Michell, R. H., 1975, Inositol phospholipids and cell surface receptor function, *Biochim. Biophys. Acta* **415**:81–147.

Middleton, E., Jr., and Phillips, B. G., 1964, Distribution and properties of anaphylactic and venom-induced slow-reacting substance and histamine in guinea pigs, *J. Immunol.* **93**:220–227.

Mizel, S. B., 1973, Differential effect of cytochalasin B on the two possible modes of 2-deoxyglucose transport in HeLa cells, *Nature (London)* **243**:125–126.

Moncada, S., 1977, Prostaglandin endoperoxides and thromboxanes: Formation and effects, *Naunyn-Schmiedeberg's Arch. Pharmacol.* **297**:581–584.

Moncada, S., Needleman, P., Bunting, S., and Vane, J. R., 1976, Prostaglandin endoperoxide and thromboxane generating systems and their selective inhibition, *Prostaglandins* **12**:323–329.

Moran, N. C., Uvnäs, B., and Westerholm, B., 1962, Release of 5-hydroxytryptamine and histamine from rat mast cells, *Acta Physiol. Scand.* **56**:26–41.

Morrison, D. C., Roser, J. F., Cochrane, C. G., and Henson, P. M., 1975, Two distinct mechanisms for the initiation of mast cell degranulation, *Int. Arch. Allergy Immunol.* **49**:172–178.

Morse, H. C., Bloch, K. J., and Austen, K. F., 1968, Biologic properties of rat antibodies. II. Time-course of appearance of antibodies involved in antigen-induced release of slow reacting substance of anaphylaxis (SRS-A^{rat}): Association of this activity with rat IgG_a, *J. Immunol.* **101**:658–663.

Mota, I., Wong, D., and Sauden, E. H., 1969, Separation of mouse homocytotropic antibodies by biological screening, *Immunology* **17**:295–301.

Movat, H. A., Steinberg, S. G., Habal, F. M., and Ranadive, N. S., 1973, Demonstration of a kinin-generating enzyme in the lysosomes of human polymorphonuclear leukocytes, *Lab. Invest.* **29**:669–684.

Müller-Eberhard, H. J., 1976, The anaphylatoxins: Formation, structure, function and control, in: *Molecular and Biological Aspects of the Acute Allergic Reaction* (S. G. O. Johansson, K. Strandberg, and B. Uvnäs, eds.), pp. 339–352, Nobel Foundation Symposium, Plenum, New York.

Müller-Eberhard, H. J., and Vallota, E. H., 1971, Formation and inactivation of anaphylatoxins, in: *Biochemistry of the Acute Allergic Reactions* (K. F. Austen and E. L. Becker, eds.), pp. 217–228, Blackwell, Oxford.

Newball, H. H., 1976, Effects of chemical mediators on asthmatic airways, in: *Lung Cells in Disease* (A. Bouhuys, ed.), pp. 261–264, Elsevier/North-Holland, Amsterdam.

Newball, H. H., Lichtenstein, L. M., and Talamo, R. C., 1975a, Leukocyte arginine esterase—a potential new mediator of allergic reactions, *J. Allergy Clin. Immunol.* **55**:72 (abstr.).

Newball, H. H., Lichtenstein, L. M., and Talamo, R. C., 1975b, Basophil kallikrein of anaphylaxis (BK-A), *Fed. Proc.* **34**:1045 (abstr.).

Newman, S. A., Rossi, G., and Metzger, H., 1977, Molecular weight and valence of the cell surface receptor for immunoglobulin E, *Proc. Natl. Acad. Sci. USA* **74**:869–872.

Odeberg, H., and Olsson, I., 1975, Antibacterial activity of cationic proteins from human granulocytes, *J. Clin. Invest.* **56**:1118–1124.

Ögren, S., and Lindahl, U., 1975, Cleavage of macromolecular heparin by an enzyme from mouse mastocytoma, *J. Biol. Chem.* **250**:2690–2697.

Ögren, S., and Lindahl, U., 1976, Metabolism of macromolecular heparin in mouse neoplastic mast cells, *Biochem. J.* **154**:605–611.

Ohlsson, K., and Olsson, I., 1973, The neutral proteases of human granulocytes. Isolation and partial characterization of two granulocyte collagenases, *Eur. J. Biochem.* **36**:473–481.

Ohlsson, K., and Olsson, I., 1974, The neutral proteases of human granulocytes. Isolation and partial characterization of granulocyte elastases, *Eur. J. Biochem.* **42**:519–527.

Orange, R. P., 1974, The formation and release of slow reacting substance of anaphylaxis in human lung tissues, in: *Progress in Immunology II,* Vol. 4 (L. Brent and J. Holborow, eds.), pp. 29–39, North-Holland, Amsterdam.

Orange, R. P., 1975, Dissociation of the immunologic release of histamine and slow reacting substance of anaphylaxis from human lung using cytochalasins A and B, *J. Immunol.* **114**:182–186.

Orange, R. P., 1976, The immunological release of chemical mediators from human lung: Approaches to pharmacological antagonisms, in: *The Role of Immunological Factors in Infections, Allergic and Autoimmune Processes* (R. F. Beers, Jr., and E. G. Bassett, eds.), pp. 223–235, Raven, New York.

Orange, R. P., 1977, The formation and release of slow reacting substance of anaphylaxis, in: *Monographs in Allergy,* Vol. 12 (K. Rother and A. de Weck, eds.), pp. 231–240, Karger, Basel.

Orange, R. P., and Austen, K. F., 1968, Pharmacologic dissociation of immunologic release of histamine and slow-reacting substance of anaphylaxis in rats, *Proc. Soc. Exp. Biol. Med.* **129**:836–841.

Orange, R. P., and Austen, K. F., 1969, Slow reacting substance of anaphylaxis, *Adv. Immunol.* **10**:106–144.

Orange, R. P., and Austen, K. F., 1976, The biological assay of slow reacting substances—SRS-A, bradykinin and prostaglandins, in: *Methods in Immunology and Immunochemistry* (C. A. Williams and M. W. Chase, eds.), pp. 145–149, Academic, New York.

Orange, R. P., and Chang, P. L., 1975, The effect of thiols on the immunologic release of slow reacting substance of anaphylaxis. I. Human lung, *J. Immunol.* **115**:1072–1077.

Orange, R. P., and Langer, H., 1974, Bronchial asthma: Hyperreactivity of airways and target cells, in: *Proceedings of the VIII International Congress of Allergology,* pp. 325–333, Excerpta Medica, Amsterdam.

Orange, R. P., and Moore, E. G., 1976a, Functional characterization of rat mast cell arylsulfatase activity, *J. Immunol.* **117**:2191–2196.

Orange, R. P., and Moore, E. G., 1976b, The effect of thiols on immunologic release of slow reacting substance of anaphylaxis. II. Other *in vitro* and *in vivo* models, *J. Immunol.* **116**:392–397.

Orange, R. P., Valentine, M. D., and Austen, K. F., 1968, Antigen-induced release of slow-reacting substance of anaphylaxis ($SRS\text{-}A^{rat}$) in rats prepared with homologous antibody, *J. Exp. Med.* **127**:767–782.

Orange, R. P., Stechschulte, D. J., and Austen, K. F., 1969, Cellular mechanisms involved in the release of slow reacting substance of anaphylaxis, *Fed. Proc.* **28**:1710–1715.

Orange, R. P., Stechschulte, D. J., and Austen, K. F., 1970, Immunochemical and biologic properties of rat IgE. II. Capacity to mediate the immunologic release of histamine and slow reacting substance of anaphylaxis (SRS-A), *J. Immunol.* **105**:1087–1095.

Orange, R. P., Austen, W. G., and Austen, K. F., 1971a, Immunological release of histamine and slow reacting substance of anaphylaxis from human lung. I. Modulation by agents influencing cellular levels of cyclic 3′,5′-adenosine monophosphate, *J. Exp. Med.* **134:** 136s–148s.

Orange, R. P., Kaliner, M. A., and Austen, K. F., 1971b, The immunological release of histamine and slow-reacting substance of anaphylaxis from human lung. III. Biochemical control mechanisms involved in the immunologic release of chemical mediators, in: *Second International Symposium on the Biochemistry of the Acute Allergic Reactions* (K. F. Austen and E. L. Becker, eds.), pp. 189–204, Blackwell, Oxford.

Orange, R. P., Kaliner, M. A., LaRaia, P. J., and Austen, K. F., 1971c, Immunological release of histamine and slow reacting substance of anaphylaxis from human lung. II. Influence of cellular levels of cyclic AMP, *Fed. Proc.* **30**:1725–1729.

Orange, R. P., Murphy, R. C., Karnovsky, M. L., and Austen, K. F., 1973, The physicochemical characteristics and purification of slow reacting substance of anaphylaxis, *J. Immunol.* **110:**760–770.

Orange, R. P., Murphy, R. C., and Austen, K. F., 1974, Inactivation of slow reacting substance of anaphylaxis (SRS-A) by arylsulfatases, *J. Immunol.* **113:**316–322.

Orenstein, N. S., Galli, S. J., Hammond, M. E., Smith, G. N., Silbert, J. E., and Dvorak, H. F., 1977, Mucopolysaccharides synthesized by guinea pig basophilic leukocytes, *Fed. Proc.* **36:**1329 (abstr.).

Orr, T. S. C., and Cox, J. S. G., 1969, Disodium cromoglycate, an inhibitor of mast cell degranulation and histamine release induced by phospholipase A, *Nature (London)* **223:**197–198.

Orr, T. S. C., Hall, D. E., and Allison, A. C., 1972, Role of contractile microfilaments in the release of histamine from mast cells, *Nature (London)* **236:**350–351.

Palmer, M. A., Piper, P. J., and Vane, J. R., 1973, Release of rabbit aorta contracting substance (RCS) and prostaglandins induced by chemical or mechanical stimulation of guinea pig lungs, *Br. J. Pharmacol.* **49:**226–242.

Parish, W. E., 1973, Reaginic and non-reaginic antibody reactions in anaphylactic participating cells, in: *Mechanisms in Allergy* (L. Goodfriend, A. H. Sehon, and R. P. Orange, eds.), pp. 197–219, Dekker, New York.

Paterson, N. A. M., Leid, R. W., Said, J. W., Wasserman, S. I., and Austen, K. F., 1976a, Release of chemical mediators from dispersed and partially purified human and rat lung mast cells, in: *Lung Cells in Disease* (A. Bouhuys, ed.), pp. 223–238, Elsevier/North-Holland, Amsterdam.

Paterson, N. A. M., Wasserman, S. I., Said, J. W., and Austen, K. F., 1976b, Release of chemical mediators from partially purified human lung mast cells, *J. Immunol.* **117:**1356–1362.

Paton, W. D. M., 1958, The release of histamine, *Progr. Allergy* **5:**79–148.

Patterson, R., Suszko, I. M., and Harris, K. E., 1975, Potentiation of IgE-mediated cutaneous reactivity and blood leukocyte histamine release by deuterium oxide, *Clin. Exp. Immunol.* **19:**335–342.

Pavek, K., 1977, Anaphylactic shock in the monkey: Its hemodynamics and mediators, *Acta Anaesthesiol. Scand.* **21:**293–307.

Pepys, J., and Hutchcroft, B. J., 1975, Bronchial provocation tests in etiologic diagnosis and analysis of asthma, *Am. Rev. Resp. Dis.* **112:**829–859.

Peterson, C., 1974, Role of energy metabolism in histamine release—A study on isolated rat mast cells, *Acta Physiol. Scand. Suppl.* **413:**5–34.

Petersson, B. A., 1975, Induction of histamine release and desensitization in human leukocytes—IgG-mediated histamine release, *Scand. J. Immunol.* **4:**774–784.

Phillips, G. B., and Middleton, E., Jr., 1965, Release of histamine and slow-reacting substance activities from guinea pig lung, *Proc. Soc. Exp. Biol. Med.* **119:**465–470.

Pickett, W. C., Jesse, R. L., and Cohen, P., 1977, Initiation of phospholipase A_2 activity in human platelets by the calcium ion ionophore A23187, *Biochim. Biophys. Acta* **486:**209–213.

Pieterson, W. A., Vidal, J. C., Volwerk, J. J., and deHaas, G. H., 1974a, Zymogen-catalysed hydrolysis of monomeric substrates and the presence of a recognition site for lipid water interfaces on phospholipase A_2, *Biochemistry* **13:**1455–1460.

Pieterson, W. A., Volwerk, J. J., and deHaas, G. H., 1974b, Interaction of phospholipase A_2 and its zymogen with divalent metal ions, *Biochemistry* **13:**1439–1445.

Pinckard, R. N., Tanigawa, C., and Halonen, M., 1975, IgE-induced blood coagulation alterations in the rabbit: Consumption of coagulation Factors XII, XI, and IX *in vivo, J. Immunol.* **115:**525–532.

Piper, P. J., and Vane, J. R., 1969a, The release of prostaglandins during anaphylaxis in guinea pig isolated lungs, in: *Prostaglandins, Peptides and Amines* (P. Mantegassa and E. W. Horton, eds.), pp. 15–19, Academic, New York.

Piper, P. J., and Vane, J. R., 1969b, Release of additional factors in anaphylaxis and its antagonism by anti-inflammatory drugs, *Nature (London)* **223:**29–35.

Piper, P. J., and Vane, J. R., 1971, The release of prostaglandins from lung and other tissues, *Ann. N.Y. Acad. Sci.* **180:**363–385.

Piper, P. J., Vane, J. R., and Wyllie, J. H., 1970, Inactivation of prostaglandins by the lungs, *Nature (London)* **225:**600–604.

Plaut, M., Lichtenstein, L. M., Gillespie, E., and Henney, C. S., 1973, Studies on the mechanism of lymphocyte-mediated cytolysis. IV. Specificity of the histamine receptor on effector T cells, *J. Immunol.* **111**:389–394.

Poole, A. R., Howell, J. I., and Lucy, J. A., 1970, Lysolecithin and cell fusion, *Nature (London)* **227**:810–814.

Poste, G., and Allison, A. C., 1973, Membrane fusion, *Biochim. Biophys. Acta* **300**:421–465.

Pressman, B.C., 1972, Carboxylic ionophores as mobile carriers for divalent ions, in: *The Role of Membranes in Metabolic Regulation* (M. A. Mehlman and R. W. Hanson, eds.), pp. 149–157, Academic, New York.

Prouvost-Danon, A., Javierre, M. Q., and Lima, M. S., 1966, Passive anaphylactic reaction in mouse peritoneal mast cells *in vitro, Life Sci.* **5**:1751–1760.

Ranadive, N. S., and Cochrane, C. G., 1971, Mechanism of histamine release from mast cells by cationic protein (band 2) from neutrophilic lysosomes, *J. Immunol.* **100**:506–516.

Rasmussen, H., 1975, Ions as "second messengers," in: *Cell Membrane* (G. Weissmann and R. Claiborne, eds.), pp. 203–212, Hospital Practice Publisher, New York.

Read, G. W., Knoohuizen, M., and Goth, A., 1977, Relationship between phosphatidylserine and cromolyn in histamine release, *Eur. J. Pharmacol.* **42**:171–177.

Resch, K., Gelfand, W. E., Hanoen, K., and Ferber, E., 1972, Lymphocyte activation: Rapid changes in the phospholipid metabolism of plasma membrane during stimulation, *Eur. J. Immunol.* **2**:598–601.

Roberts, L. J., II, Lewis, R. A., Hansbrough, R., Austen, K. F., and Oates, J. A., 1978, Biosynthesis of prostaglandins, thromboxanes, and 12-hydroxy-5,8,11,14-eicosatetraenoic acid by rat mast cells, *Fed. Proc.* **37**:384 (abstr.).

Robison, G. A., Butcher, R. W., and Sutherland, E. W., 1971, *Cyclic AMP,* Academic, New York.

Rosenthal, A. F., and Han, S. C., 1970, A study of phospholipase A inhibition by a glycerophosphatide analog in various systems, *Biochim. Biophys. Acta* **218**:213–220.

Rothman, J. E., and Lenard, J., 1977, Membrane asymmetry, *Science* **195**:743.

Rothschild, A. M., Castania, A., and Cordeiro, R. S. B., 1974, Consumption of kininogen, formation of kinin, and activation of arginine ester hydrolase in rat plasma by rat peritoneal fluid cells in the presence of L-adrenaline, *Naunyn-Schmeideberg's Arch. Pharmacol.* **285**:243–256.

Rouser, G., Bauman, A. J., Kritchevsky, G., Heller, D., and O'Brien, J. S., 1961, Quantitative chromatographic fractionation of complex lipid mixtures: Brain lipids, *J. Am. Oil Chemists' Soc.* **38**:544–555.

Sanyal, R. K., and West, G. B., 1958, Relationship of histamine and 5-HT to anaphylactic shock in different species, *J. Physiol.* **144**:525–531.

Schayer, R. W., 1952, Biogenesis of histamine, *J. Biol. Chem. (London)* **199**:245–250.

Scherer, J., and Janoff, A., 1968, Mediators of inflammation in leukocyte lysosomes. VII. Observations on mast cell-rupturing agents in different species, *Lab. Invest.* **18**:196–202.

Schild, H. O., Hawkins, D. F., Mongar, J. L., and Herxheimer, H., 1951, Reactions of isolated human asthmatic lung and bronchial tissue to a specific antigen, *Lancet* **2**:376–382.

Schlessinger, J., Metzger, H., Webb, W. W., and Elson, E. L., 1976, Lateral motion and valence of Fc receptors in rat peritoneal mast cells, *Nature (London)* **264**:550–552.

Schultz, G., Hardman, J. G., and Sutherland, E. W., 1973, Cyclic nucleotides and smooth muscle function, in: *Asthma: Physiology, Immunopharmacology and Treatment* (K. F. Austen and L. M. Lichtenstein, eds.), p. 123, Academic, New York.

Seeman, P., 1972, The membrane actions of anaesthetics and tranquilizers, *Pharmacol. Rev.* **24**:583–655.

Sheard, P., and Blair, A. M. J. N., 1970, Disodium cromoglycate. Activity in three *in vitro* models of immediate hypersensitivity reaction in lung, *Int. Arch. Allergy Appl. Immunol.* **38**:217–224.

Shore, P. A., 1976, Fluorometric assay of histamine, in: *Methods in Immunology and Immunochemistry*, Vol. 5 (C.A. Williams and M.W. Chase, eds.), pp. 129–131, Academic, New York.

Silva, M. G., and Dietrich, C. P., 1975, Structure of heparin, *J. Biol. Chem.* **250**:6841–6846.

Singer, S. J., and Nicholson, G. L., 1972, The fluid mosaic model of the structure of cell membrane, *Science* **175**:720–731.

Sjoerdsma, A., Weissbach, H., and Udenfriend, S., 1956, A clinical, physiologic, and biochemical study of patients with malignant carcinoid (argentaffinoma), *Am. J. Med.* **20**:520–532.

Sjoerdsma, A., Waalkes, T. P., and Weissbach, H., 1957, Serotonin and histamine in mast cells, *Science* **125**:1202–1203.

Sloboda, R. D., Rudolph, S. A., Rosenbaum, J. L., and Greengard, P., 1975, Cyclic AMP-dependent endogenous phosphorylation of a microtubule-associated protein, *Proc. Natl. Acad. Sci. USA* **72**:177–181.

Slorach, S. A., and Uvnäs, B., 1968, Amine formation by rat mast cells *in vitro*, *Acta Physiol. Scand.* **73**:457–470.

Smith, D. E., 1963, Electron microscopy of normal mast cells under various experimental conditions, *Ann. N.Y. Acad. Sci.* **103**:40–52.

Snyder, S. H., and Taylor, K. M., 1976, Enzymatic-isotopic microassay of histamine, in: *Methods in Immunology and Immunochemistry*, Vol. 5 (C. A. Williams and M. W. Chase, eds.), pp. 135–139, Academic, New York.

Solley, G. O., Gleich, G. J., Jordon, R. E., and Schroeter, A. L., 1976, The late phase of the immediate wheal and flare skin reaction—Its dependence upon IgE antibodies, *J. Clin. Invest.* **58**:408–420.

Soter, N. A., Wasserman, S. I., and Austen, K. F., 1976, Cold urticaria: Release of histamine and ECF-A during cold challenge, *N. Engl. J. Med.* **294**:687–690.

Spector, S., 1976, Assay of serotonin, in: *Methods in Immunology and Immunochemistry*, Vol. 5 (C. A. Williams and M. W. Chase, eds.), pp. 139–144, Academic, New York.

Stanworth, D. R., 1973, Mechanism of release of mediators of immediate hypersensitivity, in: *Immediate Hypersensitivity in Frontiers of Biology Series*, Vol. 28, p. 290, North-Holland/Elsevier, Amsterdam.

Stechschulte, D. J., Austen, K. F., and Bloch, K. J., 1967, Antibodies involved in antigen-induced release of slow-reacting substance of anaphylaxis in the guinea pig and rat, *J. Exp. Med.* **125**:127–147.

Stechschulte, D. J., Orange, R. P., and Austen, K. F., 1973, Detection of slow-reacting substance of anaphylaxis (SRS-A) in plasma of guinea pigs during anaphylaxis, *J. Immunol.* **111**:1585–1589.

Strandberg, K., and Hedqvist, P., 1975, Airway effects of slow reacting substance, prostaglandin $F_{2\alpha}$ and histamine in the guinea-pig, *Acta Physiol. Scand.* **94**:105–111.

Strandberg, K., and Uvnäs, B., 1971, Purification and properties of slow reacting substance formed in cat paw perfused with compound 48/80, *Acta Physiol. Scand.* **82**:358–374.

Strandberg, K., and Westerberg, S., 1976, Composition of phospholipids and phospholipid fatty acids in rat mast cells, *Mol. Cell. Biochem.* **11**:103–107.

Sullivan, T. J., and Parker, C. W., 1979, Possible role of arachidonic acid and its metabolites in mediator release from rat mast cells, *J. Immunol.* **122**:431–436.

Sullivan, T. J., Parker, K. L., Stenson, W., and Parker, C. W., 1975a, Modulation of cyclic AMP in purified rat mast cells. I. Responses to pharmacologic, metabolic and physical stimuli, *J. Immunol.* **114**:1473–1479.

Sullivan, T. J., Parker, K. L., Eisen, S. A., and Parker, C. W., 1975b, Modulation of cyclic AMP in purified rat mast cells. II. Studies on the relationship between intracellular cyclic AMP concentrations and histamine release, *J. Immunol.* **114**:1480–1485.

Sydbom, A., and Uvnäs, B., 1976, Potentiation of anaphylactic histamine release from isolated rat pleural mast cells by rat serum phospholipids, *Acta Physiol. Scand.* **97**:222–232.

Tauber, A. I., Kaliner, M., Stechschulte, D. J., and Austen, K. F., 1973, Immunological release of histamine and slow-reacting substance of anaphylaxis from human lung. V. Effect of prostaglandins in release of histamine, *J. Immunol.* **111**:27–32.

Thon, I. L., and Uvnäs, B., 1967, Degranulation and histamine release, two consecutive steps in the response of rat mast cells to compound 48/80, *Acta Physiol. Scand.* **71**:303–315.

Thorn, N. A., 1974, Role of calcium in secretory processes, in: *Secretory Mechanisms of Exocrine Glands* (N. A. Thorn and O. H. Peterson, eds.), pp. 305–326, Munksgaard, Copenhagen.

Tomioka, H., and Ishizaka, K., 1971, Mechanisms of passive sensitization. II. Presence of receptors for IgE on monkey mast cells, *J. Immunol.* **107**:971–978.

Trotter, C. M., and Orr, T. S. C., 1973, A fine structure study of some cellular components in allergic reactions. 1. Degranulation of human mast cells in allergic asthma and perennial rhinitis, *Clin. Allergy* **3**:411–425.

Turnbull, L. S., Turnbull, L. W., Leitch, A. G., Crofton, J. W., and Kay, A. B., 1977, Mediators of immediate-type hypersensitivity in sputum from patients with chronic bronchitis and asthma, *Lancet* **2**:526–529.

Turnbull, L. W., Evans, D. P., and Kay, A. B., 1977, Human eosinophils, acidic tetrapeptides (ECF-A) and histamine—Interactions *in vitro* and *in vivo*, *Immunology* **32**:57–63.

Tyson, C. A., Vande Zande, H., and Green, D. E., 1976, Phospholipids as ionophores, *J. Biol. Chem.* **251**:1326–1332.

Ungar, G., and Damgaard, E., 1955, Tissue reactions to anaphylactoid stimuli: Proteolysis and release of histamine and heparin, *J. Exp. Med.* **101**:1–15.

Uvnäs, B., 1971, Quantitative correlation between degranulation and histamine release in mast cells, in: *Biochemistry of the Acute Allergic Reactions: Second International Symposium* (K. F. Austen and E. L. Becker, eds.), pp. 175–188, Blackwell, Oxford.

Uvnäs, B., 1973, Correlation between morphological and biochemical events on antigen-induced histamine release from mast cells, in: *Mechanisms in Allergy* (L. Goodfriend, A. H. Sehon, and R. P. Orange, eds.), pp. 369–383, Dekker, New York.

Uvnäs, B., and Antonsson, J., 1963, Triggering action of phosphatidase A and chymotrypsins on degranulation of rat mesentery mast cells, *Biochem. Pharmacol.* **12**:867–873.

Valone, F. H., and Goetzl, E. J., 1978, Immunologic release in the rat peritoneal cavity lipid chemotactic and chemokinetic factors for polymorphonuclear leukocytes, *J. Immunol.* **120**:102–108.

Vane, J. R.., 1969, The release and fate of vasoactive hormones in the circulation. The Second Gaddum Memorial Lecture, *Br. J. Pharmacol.* **35**:209–242.

Vane, J. R., 1971, Inhibition of prostaglandin synthesis as a mechanism of action for aspirin-like drugs, *Nature (London) New Biol.* **231**:232–235.

Vane, J. R., 1976, The mode of action of aspirin and similar compounds, *J. Allergy Clin. Immunol.* **58**:691–712.

Venge, R., and Olsson, I., 1975, Cationic proteins of human granulocytes. VI. Effects on the complement system and mediation of chemotactic activity, *J. Immunol.* **115**:1505–1508.

Victoria, E., Van Golde, L. M. G., Hostetler, K. Y., Scherphof, G. L., and Van Deenan, L. L. M., 1971, Some studies on the metabolism of phospholipids in plasma membranes from rat liver, *Biochim. Biophys. Acta* **239**:443–457.

Vijay, H. M., and Perlmutter, L., 1977, Inhibition of reagin-mediated PCA reactions in monkeys and histamine release from human leukocytes by human IgG_4, *Int. Arch. Allergy Appl. Immunol.* **53**:78–87.

Volwerk, J. J., Pieterson, W. A., and deHaas, G. H., 1974, Histidine at the active site of phospholipase A_2, *Biochemistry* **13**:1446–1454.

Walker, J. L., 1973, The regulatory function of prostaglandins by the release of histamine and SRS-A from passively sensitized human lung, *Adv. Biosci.* **9**:235–240.

Ward, P. A., 1967, A plasmin-split fragment of C3 as a new chemotactic factor, *J. Exp. Med.* **126**:189–206.

Ward, P. A., and Hill, J. H., 1970, C5 chemotactic fragments produced by an enzyme in lysosomal granules of neutrophils, *J. Immunol.* **104**:535–543.

Wasserman, M., 1975, Bronchopulmonary responses to prostaglandin $F_{2\alpha}$, histamine, and acetylcholine in the dog, *Eur. J. Pharmacol.* **32**:146–155.

Wasserman, M., DuCharme, D. W., Griffin, R. L., and Robinson, F. G., 1977, Bronchopulmonary and cardiovascular effects of prostaglandin D_2 in the dog, *Prostaglandins* **13**:255–269.

Wasserman, S. I., and Austen, K. F., 1976, Arylsulfatase B of human lung: Isolation, characterization and interaction with slow reacting substance of anaphylaxis, *J. Clin. Invest.* **57**:738–744.

Wasserman, S. I., and Austen, K. F., 1977, Identification and characterization of arylsulfatase A and B of the rat basophil leukemic tumor, *J. Biol. Chem.* **252**:7074–7080.

Wasserman, S. I., Goetzl, E. J., and Austen, K. F., 1974a, Preformed eosinophil chemotactic factor of anaphylaxis, *J. Immunol.* **112**:351–358.

Wasserman, S. I., Goetzl, E. J., Ellman, L., and Austen, K. F., 1974b, Tumor-associated eosinophilotactic factor, *N. Engl. J. Med.* **290**:420–424.

Wasserman, S. I., Goetzl, E. J., and Austen, K. F., 1975, Inactivation of slow reacting substance of anaphylaxis by human eosinophil arylsulfatase, *J. Immunol.* **114**:645–649.

Wasserman, S. I., Soter, N. A., Center, D. M., and Austen, K. F., 1977, Cold urticaria: Recognition and characterization of a neutrophil chemotactic factor which appears in serum during experimental cold challenge, *J. Clin. Invest.* **60**:189–196.

Webster, M. E., Horakova, Z., Beaven, M. A., Takahashi, H., and Newball, H. H., 1974, Release of arginine esterase and histamine from human lung passively sensitized with ragweed antibody, *Fed. Proc.* **33**:761 (abstr.).

Weiler, J. M., Yurt, R. W., Fearon, D. T., and Austen, K. F., 1978, Modulation of the formation of the amplification convertase of complement, C3b,Bb, by native and commercial heparin, *J. Exp. Med.* **147**:409–421.

Weiss, S., Robb, G. B., and Ellis, L. B., 1932, Systemic effects of histamine in man with special reference to the responses of the cardiovascular system, *Arch. Int., Med.* **49**:360–396.

Wells, M. A., 1973, Effects of chemical modification on the activity of *Crotalus adamanteus* phospholipase A_2—Evidence for an essential amino group, *Biochemistry* **12**:1086–1093.

Wilhelm, D. L., 1973, Mechanisms responsible for increased vascular permeability in acute inflammation, *Agents Actions* **3**:297–306.

Wintroub, B. U., Goetzl, E. J., and Austen, K. F., 1974, A neutrophil-dependent pathway for the generation of a neutral peptide mediator, *J. Exp. Med.* **140**:812–824.

Wintroub, B. U., Mihm, Jr., M. C., Goetzl, E. J., Soter, N. A., and Austen, K. F., 1978, Morphologic and functional evidence for release of mast cell products in bullous pemphigoid, *N. Engl. J. Med.* **298**:417–421.

Wuepper, K. D., Bokisch, V. A., Müller-Eberhard, H. J., and Stoughton, R. B., 1972, C3 anaphylatoxin in human skin, *Clin. Exp. Immunol.* **11**:13–20.

Yamamoto, S., Greaves, M. W., and Plummer, V., 1973, Inhibition of human cutaneous anaphylaxis by cytochalasin B, *Immunology* **24**:1007–1012.

Yecies, L. D., Wedner, H. J., Johnnson, S. M., and Parker, C. W., 1978, Polar metabolites of arachidonic acid in rat mast cells, *J. Allergy Clin. Immunol.* **61**:131 (abstr.).

Yurt, R. W., and Austen, K. F., 1977, Preparative purification on the rat mast cell chymase: Characterization and interaction with granule components, *J. Exp. Med.* **146**:1405–1419.

Yurt, R. W., and Austen, K. F., 1979, Cascade events in mast cell activation and function, in: *Proteolysis, Demineralization, and Other Degradative Processes* (I. Lepow, ed.), Academic, New York (in press).

Yurt, R. W., Leid, Jr., R. W., Austen, K. F., and Silbert, J. E., 1977a, Native heparin from rat peritoneal mast cells, *J. Biol. Chem.* **252**:518–521.

Yurt, R. W., Leid, Jr., R. W., Spragg, J., and Austen, K. F., 1977b, Immunologic release of heparin from purified rat peritoneal mast cells, *J. Immunol.* **118**:1201–1207.

Zurier, R. B., Weissman, G., Hoffstein, S., Kammerman, F., and Tai, H. H., 1974, Mechanisms of lysosomal enzyme release from human leukocytes. II. Effects of cAMP and cGMP, autonomic agonists and agents which affect microtubule function, *J. Clin, Invest.* **53**:297–309.

7

The Genetics of Allergy

C. EDWARD BUCKLEY, III

1. Introduction

Allergic disorders exhibit a familial prevalence. Coca and Cooke observed similarities among the allergic diseases exhibited by family members and defined this predisposition as atopy (Cooke and Vander Veer, 1916; Coca, 1920; Coca and Cooke, 1923). Anaphylaxis, hay fever, asthma, angioedema, certain gastrointestinal disorders, and hypersensitivity reactions associated with infection are all included among the atopic diseases. Coca and Cooke (1923) suggested that an innate predisposition toward hypersensitiveness might be involved. A familial prevalence of atopy has been confirmed in many epidemiological studies of allergic disease (Ratner and Silberman, 1952). These findings suggest that an inherited capacity to respond to allergens may contribute to the pathogenesis of the atopic diseases.

The genetic control of the capacity to respond to antigen has been subjected to extensive study in experimental animals (Shreffler and David, 1975; Klein, 1975; Goetze, 1977). Animal studies have been facilitated by (1) the use of synthetic polypeptides (McDevitt and Sela, 1965; Pinchuck and Maurer, 1965) and low doses (Green *et al.*, 1970) of naturally occurring antigens exhibiting restricted heterogeneity (Blumberg *et al.*, 1972), (2) the availability of highly inbred animal strains (Klein, 1975), and (3) the ability to test hypotheses in the most informative progeny. Initial studies focused on the genetic control of mechanisms regulating the induction of immune cell proliferation (Paul *et al.*, 1966). The genetic control of the ability to respond to antigenic stimuli is well documented. Less attention has been directed toward the information content of the antigenic stimulus (Gunther and Rude, 1976) and how this information relates to the genetic control of the specificity of the antibody response (Di Pauli, 1973). The conceptual and methodological issues needed to extend these elegant genetic studies of animal models to purposeful naturally occurring immunity in man has received much less attention.

Despite this problem, a large number of provocative positive reports suggest that similar genetic mechanisms exist in man. Early studies of human hypersensi-

C. Edward Buckley, III • Department of Medicine, Duke University School of Medicine, Durham, North Carolina 27710.

tivity to allergens provide the first compelling evidence that similar genetic mechanisms probably control human responsiveness (Levine *et al.*, 1972; Marsh *et al.*, 1973; Buckley *et al.*, 1973; Blumenthal *et al.*, 1974). Similar mechanisms may be important in many kinds of immunological diseases (Goodfriend *et al.*, 1976; Buckley and Roseman, 1976; Svejgaard and Ryder, 1977; Buckley *et al.*, 1977; Allen *et al.*, 1977; Sasazuki *et al.*, 1978). An understanding of the cognitive function of the immune system and the complexities of human genetics is an important part of this general problem. This chapter reviews selected aspects of cognitive function important in immunity. Pragmatic emphasis is placed on how these concepts and methods can be applied to the study of the genetic control of naturally occurring immunity in man. Current knowledge of the genetics of immunity is summarized with emphasis on understanding the atopic diseases.

Historical Considerations: Uncertainty about the importance of heredity in the allergic diseases stems from the obvious contribution of environmental allergens to hypersensitivity reactions. A shared exposure to the same source of allergens could account for the tendency of allergic diseases to cluster in families. An awareness of innate differences in susceptibility to infection in mice has existed for many years (Gorer and Schutze, 1938). With the exception of Chase's perceptive experimental studies of the effect of inbreeding on the size of contact hypersensitivity reactions in guinea pigs (Chase, 1941), little effort was directed toward resolution of the genetic control of sensitization until studies initiated by Benaceraff and his colleagues (Benacerraf *et al.*, 1967; Benacerraf and Dorf, 1974). These investigators studied the responsiveness of guinea pigs to synthetic antigens composed of haptens conjugated to polymers of single amino acids. Certain animals were unable to be sensitized with simple haptens conjugated to an L-lysine polymer. Selective inbreeding yielded responder and nonresponder strains of animals. Tests of responsiveness in prospectively bred progeny of appropriate crosses and backcrosses revealed segregation of the capacity to respond as a single Mendelian codominant trait. Subsequent studies by Benaceraff and his colleagues established that the poly-L-lysine carrier and any of several conjugated haptens sufficed to stimulate immune cell proliferation and the production of antibody in responder animals. The antibody exhibited specificity for the particular hapten conjugated to the poly-L-lysine carrier. The allelic genes coding, respectively, for the responder or nonresponder status of guinea pigs represent an immune response (Ir) polymorphism. These observations, coupled with ongoing studies of the inheritance of responsiveness to tissue antigens, prompted an expansion of investigative efforts and clinical interest in immunogenetics.

2. Immunogenetics

Immunogenetics is concerned with the inheritance of the ability to respond to antigens. Historically, immunogenetics began with the study of tissue antigens, particularly those antigens important in blood transfusions (Landsteiner, 1928). This primitive understanding was subsequently extended into transplantation biology and our present knowledge of histocompatibility. These focused areas of inquiry provided a foundation for the current thrust toward a holistic understanding of how innate differences in the responsiveness of the immune system relate to the environment.

Studies of the genetic control of the immune response have been facilitated by the availability of inbred strains of mice. Initially, these mouse strains were bred for their ability to accept engraftment with spontaneously occurring neoplasms from other animals of the same strain (Klein, 1975). Studies of this phenomenon led to the discovery of histocompatibility antigens (Gorer, 1927, 1959). The ability to reject transplanted tumors or normal tissues is controlled by a cluster of genes located on chromosome number 17 of the mouse (Klein, 1975). This gene cluster is known as a "major histocompatibility complex" (MHC) or the H-2 complex of the mouse. Analogous gene clusters exist in other species (Goetze, 1977). The major histocompatibility complex gene cluster of man is known as the "histocompatibility antigen" (HLA) complex and is located on chromosome number 6. Similarities exist between the major histocompatibility complex regions of chromosomes of man, mouse, and other species of experimental animals. Multiallelic genes can occur at several loci within the major histocompatibility complex. These genes code for polymorphic cell surface products of certain tissues and/or the ability to respond to the tissue antigens of other individuals of the same species. The cell surface gene products and the responder ability coded by the several loci of the major histocompatibility complex are unique for each individual member of the species. At the HLA-A, B, C, and D loci of man, there are, respectively, a minimum of 8, 17, 5, and 7 well-documented public alleles (Kissmeyer-Nielsen *et al.*, 1977). A public allele is a genetically determined difference found generally among members of the species. These public alleles can give rise to a minimum of 4760 possible combinations of alleles. Private alleles detectable in comparisons among closely related members of the same species or families also exist. Collectively, these genetic differences account for a major portion of the tissue diversity responsible for transplantation reactions.

The transplantation of tissues between members of the same species is dependent on the presence of syngeneic or genetically identical major histocompatibility complex gene products. Genetically different or allogeneic tissues from members of the same species are rejected. Cell surface products of allelic genes at one locus within the major histocompatibility complex stimulate the proliferation of immune cells bearing dissimilar gene products. Cell surface stimulatory gene products are innate constitutive components of the cell. These gene loci are known as "stimulator" or "mitogenic" loci and are detected by measures of cell proliferation (Goetze, 1977). Allelic genes located at the mitogenic HLA-D locus of man code for the main cell surface product responsible for the mixed-leukocyte reaction. The mixed-leukocyte reaction can be used to identify the genetic polymorphism of the HLA-D locus of the human major histocompatibility complex.

The initiation of a mitogen response by the HLA-D locus gene product permits the proliferation of immunocompetent cells. The antibody generated by immune cell stimulation is directed toward alloantigens located on the stimulator cell. The most important alloantigens in transplantation are genetically determined cell surface products coded by other genes in the major histocompatibility complex. These specific alloantigens are characteristic of each individual member of the species. Major histocompatibility complex coded alloantigens are expressed on the surface of thymus-derived (T) lymphocytes. In man, two multiallelic series of alloantigens are coded by genes located at the HLA-A and HLA-B loci of the HLA complex. The gene loci detected by alloantisera are called the "serologically detectable" loci. Antisera can be raised against lymphocyte alloantigens by immunization of human volunteers with lymphocytes from a genetically different individual. Alloantisera are also generated by the transplacental passage of lymphocytes during the course of multiple pregnancies. Both sources of antisera can be used to type tissues by measures of antibody-induced cytolysis of appropriate human target cells (Amos *et al.*, 1970). The serologically detectable leukocyte alloantigens coded by the HLA-A and HLA-B loci are used to type human tissues prior to transplantation. The multiallelic genes coding for the antibody response of humans immunized with allogeneic cells represent a human Ir polymorphism. Unlike the HLA-D locus, this response polymorphism involves the permissive selection of specific genetic information by the responding individual's antibody-producing cells.

Experimental searches with synthetic antigens and other antigens exhibiting restricted heterogeneity among different histocompatible mouse strains quickly revealed evidence of an impressive number of additional immune response polymorphisms (Shreffler and David, 1975; Klein, 1975). Elegant genetic studies of recombinant mouse strains soon led to the identification of genes located in an immune response (Ir) region proximate to the major histocompatibility complex of the mouse. Analogous major histocompatibility complex associated Ir regions have been detected in other species of animals (Goetze, 1977). Ir polymorphisms unassociated with the major histocompatibility complex have also been detected in the mouse (Klein, 1975). Collectively, these exciting studies suggest that a similar major histocompatibility complex associated Ir region may exist in man. This analogy has prompted studies of the possible role of major histocompatibility complex gene products in the genetic control of human immune function. In these studies, the HLA-A and HLA-B serologically detectable loci and other loci within the HLA complex have been used as independent markers of the segregation of the chromosome bearing the human major histocompatibility complex.

2.2. Cell Cooperation and Genetic Restriction

In the mouse, allelic genes within an Ir gene region of the major histocompatibility complex code for immune response associated (Ia) cell surface products. Ia antigens are found on antibody-producing bone-marrow-derived lymphocytes (B cells), macrophages, and a small number of T cells (David, 1976). The antibody-producing B cell also generates a surface product which shares antigenic similarities with humoral immunoglobulins. These immunoglobulinlike cell surface products are called "surface immunoglobulin" (SIg) receptors (Goding *et al.*, 1977). B-cell Ia and SIg cell surface receptors change as the cell matures and disappear when the antibody-producing cell becomes a plasma cell.

Certain antigens can activate the synthesis of antibodies by mouse B cells without the cooperation of macrophages and T cells (Coutinho and Moller, 1975). Examples of "thymus-independent" antigens in the mouse include type III pneumococcal polysaccharide, lipopolysaccharide endotoxin, and dextran. Other antigens require macrophages and T cells to activate B cells. Like the induction of an antibody response to allogeneic lymphocytes, the response to these foreign antigens is "thymus dependent." The antigen-induced sequence of cell cooperation leading to a thymus-dependent immune response involves syngeneic or histocompatible cell surface products. Much evidence supports a role of the major histocompatibility complex gene-controlled cell surface products on macrophages. T cells, and B cells in the cooperative mechanisms leading to the immune response. The presence of syngeneic or major histocompatibility complex identical cells appears necessary for the immune cell cooperation leading to the response to thymus-dependent antigens. For example, syngeneic macrophages are needed to induce maximum proliferation of antigen-primed T cells (Rosenthal and Shevach, 1973; Yano *et al.*, 1977). Soluble factors from syngeneic mouse macrophages are needed to generate helper T cells (Erb and Feldmann, 1975; Pierce *et al.*, 1976). Identity at the major histocompatibility complex is necessary for the transfer of delayed-type hypersensitivity with T cells (Miller *et al.*, 1975, 1977). The cytolytic activity of T cells toward target cells is dependent on the presence of syngeneic antigens in the mouse (Schrader and Edelman, 1976) and can be blocked by antisera directed toward major histocompatibility complex gene controlled antigens (Nabholz *et al.*, 1974; Germain *et al.*, 1975; Shearer *et al.*, 1976; Zinkernagel and Doherty, 1975; Doherty *et al.*, 1976). In contrast, the activation of T cells by soluble protein antigens can be blocked by antisera to the particular Ia antigen (Shevach *et al.*, 1972, 1974; Schwartz *et al.*, 1976). The antibody response of B cells induced by a polyclonal activator can be blocked by specific anti-Ia antisera (Niederhuber *et al.*, 1976). Evidence suggests that a close functional relationship exists between the Ia cell surface receptor and the immunoglobulin Fc receptor of the B cell (Dickler and Sachs, 1974) even though the two cell surface products are located on different parts of the cell surface (Dickler *et al.*, 1978). I-region genetic restrictions control interactions between T and B cells (Katz *et al.*, 1973a, b, 1976), and quantitative evidence suggests that B-cell Ia gene products appear to interact in the process of initiating antibody production (Henry *et al.*, 1978). These observations establish a restrictive role of major histocompatibility complex gene products on macrophages, T cells, and B cells in guiding the cell cooperation necessary for normal immune function.

Genetic mechanisms controlling responsiveness to allergens have been detected in experimental animals. A major histocompatibility complex associated Ir polymorphism to an allergen from ragweed pollen has been detected in the mouse (Dorf *et al.*, 1974a). In contrast, the genetic control of IgE suppressor T cells and inhibition of IgE antibody production is not located within the major histocompatibility complex of the mouse (Wanatabe *et al.*, 1976, 1977; Chiorazzi *et al.*, 1977). Experimental treatment which ablates IgE suppressor T-cell activity converts low IgE producer animals to high-responder animals (Tada *et al.*, 1975). Finally, it is important to note that, within highly inbred mouse strains differing only at the major histocompatibility complex, the capacity of mitogens to initiate cell proliferation is age dependent (Meredith and Walford, 1977). Genetic differences in the ability to respond and initiate immune-cell cooperation may change with age.

2.3. Antibody Diversity

Each immunoglobulin molecule is composed of a pair of heavy (H) polypeptide chains and a pair of light (L) polypeptide chains. The polypeptide chains are composed of a variable (V) region and a constant (C) region. The V regions of immunoglobulin polypeptide chains are responsible for the ability of the antibody to react with antigen. The C region of the polypeptide chain contributes those attributes of the antibody molecule characteristic of the biological activity of the particular type of immunoglobulin. The C region of IgE is responsible for the cytophilic nature and hypersensitivity reactions initiated by reaginic antibodies. Structural studies of the amino acid sequence of immunoglobulins suggest that the genetic information coding for the variable portion of the heavy and light polypeptide chains of the antibody molecule (V-region genes) is united with the genetic information controlling the constant portion of the polypeptide chains (C-region genes) during T- and B-cell differentiation (Hood *et al.*, 1975). This event probably involves splicing genetic information contained in separate segments of the DNA content of the cell—an irreversible differentiation step (Milstein *et al.*, 1974; Kohler *et al.*, 1976). Genes coding for the linear sequence of amino acids in the V region control the ability of antibodies of each immunoglobulin class to react with a specific antigen (Gearhart *et al.*, 1975; Slege *et al.*, 1976; Bleux *et al.*, 1977). Differences among the genes coding for the approximately 110 amino acids within the V region account for the specificity and diversity of antibodies to naturally occurring antigens.

Specific antibodies can be generated to synthetic antigens not found in nature as well as the extraordinarily large number of antigens found in the natural environment. While it is not possible to know the actual diversity of the genes coding for antibody molecules, structural studies provide a basis for estimates of the possible information content of V-region genes. The potential complexity of the V region is enormous. For example, genes coding for any one of 16 amino acids at each of the 110 positions in the linear amino acid sequence could give rise to more than 10^{132} different V-region genes. Assuming a molecular weight of 6×10^{15}, this amounts to 10^{114} g of nucleic acid per cell—a quantity far in excess of the capacity of the cell nucleus. This suggests that the potential structural diversity of V-region genes is limited more by the physical constraints of cell size than by the structure of the V-region polypeptide chain.

A large portion of the polypeptide chain amino acid sequence of the V region is concerned with maintaining the conformation of the protein structure about the complementary region of the antibody. The complementary region is the site responsible for antigen bindings. Only a small portion of the amino acid sequence is located in the complementary region. When comparisons are made of the V regions of many different H and L chains, segments of the amino acid sequence in the complementary region of antibody appear hypervariable (Kabat *et al.*, 1976). Three hypervariable regions have been identified in studies of L chains; of the four hypervariable regions identified in studies of H chains, three lie in the complementary region. Studies of the amino acid sequence of homogeneous antibodies suggest that occasional differences in sequences can be detected at approximately 50 of the 110 positions in the V region of the L chain (Haber *et al.*, 1977). Many fewer than 16 amino acids are involved. At a minimum, 10–25 nucleotide base changes and a smaller number of amino acids could account for the observed variability among sequenced antibody L chains. Figure 1 illustrates the relationship between the relative contribution of the number of hypervariable amino acid sequence positions and the number of amino acid substitutions at each sequence position to the maximum diversity of the V region. The diagonal line across the center of Figure 1 identifies intersections where minimum numbers of sequence alterations and amino acid substitutions would yield maximum diversity. For example, as few as seven hypervariable sequence positions and seven amino acids could generate nearly 10^6 different V-region genes. This number of V-region genes would require picogram quantities of nucleic acid per cell. Figure 1 shows the relationship between the number of hypervariable sequence positions and the number of amino acids involved in minimum estimates of V-region diversity. Many fewer amino acid substitutions are needed as the number of involved hypervariable sequence positions is increased. Germ line differences can account for a large part of antibody diversity.

A mechanism for the somatic mutation of germ line V-region genes has been postulated. This mechanism is thought to operate during the differentiation of antibody-producing cells (Jerne, 1971). Somatic mutation provides a mechanism for increasing the diversity of antibodies generated from a smaller number of germ line genes. The extent to which somatic mutation contributes to the diversification of V-region genes and the potential repertoire of antibodies is uncertain (Secher *et al.,* 1977). Estimates based on nucleic acid hybridization indicate the existence of fewer germ line genes than the number of V-region genes revealed by study of myeloma proteins (Rabbits, 1977). Cell clones producing V-region genes potentially

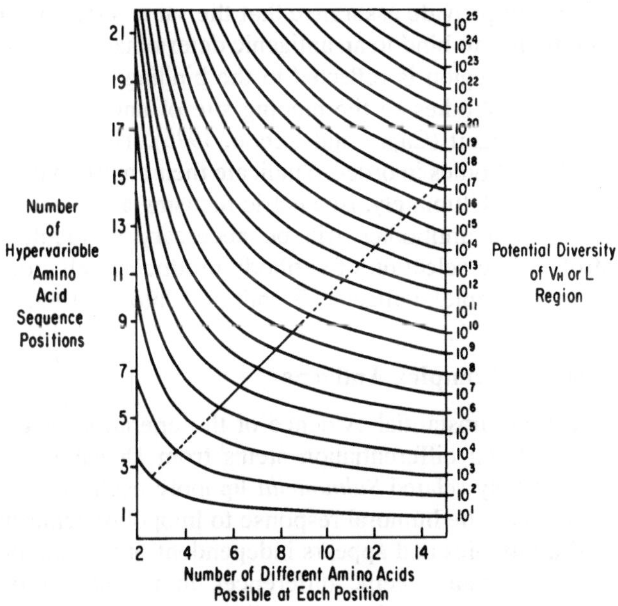

Figure 1. Minimum estimate of the diversity of antibody V regions. The actual number of V-region genes is unknown. The diagram illustrates the relationship between the number of amino acids substituted at involved sequence positions and the number of sequence positions. The diagonal line intersects the number of V regions possible with equivalent numbers of substituted amino acids and sequence positions. Current estimates suggest as many as a million genes could code for different antibody light (L) chain V regions. As few as six to eight substituted amino acids and six to eight sequence positions could account for this estimate of V-region diversity.

appropriate for specific structural attributes of an antigen are thought to differentiate and mutate within the limitations imposed by the repertoire of germ line genes. The attribute of antigen which is recognized in this process is the antigenic determinant. Several unique differentiated immunocyte clones can become committed to one antigenic determinant. Expansion of the clones of antibody-producing cells results in detectable levels of polyclonal or heterogenous antibodies. The persistence of clones of committed antibody-producing cells is responsible for long-lasting immune memory.

Very little is known about the genetic control of the selection of a particular V-region gene expressed by an expanded clone of antibody-producing cells. In contrast to evidence of the genetic control of the immune response to an antigenic determinant, much less is known about the genetic control of the selection of the set of V-region genes ultimately expressed in clones of antibody-producing cells. Potentially informative studies have focused on the genetic control of the response to closely related natural antigens. These include studies of the cellular and humoral response to multiple determinants on a single antigen. An unambiguous answer to this problem is not available.

Despite this uncertainty, these studies emphasize the importance of evaluating the genetic control of V-region diversity in relation to a single antigenic determinant. The multiplicity of antigenic determinants on naturally occurring antigens can obscure genetic polymorphisms. Closely related specificity controls provide the best initial immunoserological or immunochemical assessment of this problem. This assessment does not provide assurance that the same V-region genes account for the ability of antibodies to bind to an antigenic determinant. The genetic control of the structure of the V region is reflected in the binding site of the antibody. It is possible to prepare antibodies to the binding site of antibodies generated to a specific antigenic determinant (Capra and Kehoe, 1975). These antiantibodies are called "antiidiotype" antibodies in order to indicate their ability to detect structures coded by V-region genes. Ultimately, isoelectric focusing and structural studies of the V regions of isolated antibodies will be necessary to identify the genetic mechanisms controlling the selection of antibody-producing cell clones in relation to the fine structure of complex antigens (Brandt and Jaton, 1978a,b).

2.4. Polymorphisms to Complex Antigens

Possibly the best circumstantial evidence of the operation of genetic mechanisms at the level of B-cell differentiation stems from Di Pauli's studies of the immune response to closely related *Salmonella* lipopolysaccharide endotoxins (Di Pauli, 1973). In the mouse, the humoral response to lipopolysaccharide endotoxins is composed of IgM antibodies and appears independent of the function of T cells. A single gene controls strain-specific differences in the ability of Balb/c and DBA/2 mice to generate IgM antibodies to *S. anatum* lipopolysaccharide. Inherited differences in the antibodies produced by the two strains can be detected by evaluating their capacity to cross-react with a closely related lipopolysaccharide from *S. strassbourg*. The DBA/2 antibodies fail to cross-react with the lipopolysaccharide from *S. strassbourg*. Both mouse strains exhibit the ability to generate equivalent antibody responses when immunized with the *S. strassbourg* lipopolysaccharide. A difference in cross-reactivity to two closely related antigens detects a difference in the humoral responses of the two mouse strains. The lack of dependence of the lipopolysaccharide endotoxin response on T-cell function suggests the possible existence of a genetic mechanism controlling selective access to V-region genes. The genetic control of the observed response difference is not known to be associated with the H-2 complex. The apparent segregation of the difference in cross-reactivity does not provide information about the structure of the V regions responsible for the observed difference. Despite these limitations, this study suggests that differences in cross-reactivity to closely related antigens can be used to evaluate the genetic control of the immune response to thymus-independent antigens (Di Pauli, 1973).

This same general deduction is suggested by studies of the response to naturally occurring thymus-dependent antigens. Sensitization of strain 2 and strain 13 inbred guinea pigs with porcine insulin yields lymphocytes which respond differently to *in vitro* antigen challenge (Barcinski and Rosenthal, 1977). Cells from strain 2 animals exhibit about 60% of the cell proliferation observed with cells from strain 13 animals. Sensitization of strain 2 guinea pigs with bovine insulin yields an *in vitro* cell proliferation response which is about 25% of the response detected with lymphoid cells from bovine-insulin-sensitized strain 13 animals. Native insulin is composed of A and B polypeptide chains. Sensitization with porcine insulin and *in vitro* stimulation with the A chain yields a low level of cell proliferation with cells from strain 2 and 13 guinea pigs. Stimulation with the B chain yields no significant response with cells from strain 2 guinea pigs and approximately 50% of the cell proliferation produced by intact insulin with cells from strain 13 guinea pigs. This suggests strain 13 guinea pigs recognize an antigenic specificity on the isolated B chain of insulin. Comparisons between the *in vitro* proliferation of cells from porcine-insulin-sensitized strain 2 guinea pigs stimulated with insulins from a large number of animal species and the primary amino acid sequence of the respective insulins suggest residues 8–10 of the A chain account for the low level of observed cell proliferation. This suggests the modest level of responsiveness of cells from strain 2 guinea pigs to the intact porcine insulin is directed toward an A- and B-chain-dependent conformational antigen. Despite this evidence of the contribution of two distinct antigenic determinants to the difference in responsiveness, isoelectric focusing and antiidiotype inhibition studies of antibodies isolated from the strain 2 and strain 13 guinea pigs revealed similar patterns. This suggests different genes induced the recruitment of similar V-region genes in the antibody responses of both animal strains (Barcinski and Rosenthal, 1977).

In the mouse, an initial assessment of the response to staphylococcal nuclease suggested the existence of an Ir gene closely linked to the H-2 major histocompatibility complex (Lozner *et al.*, 1974). On closer study, the genetic control of the mouse antinuclease response appears complex (Berzofsky *et al.*, 1977a,b). A tenfold difference exists in the antibody response to intact nuclease among A/J and B10.A responder strains bearing the same H-2 haplotype (Berzofsky *et al.*, 1977a). This suggests non-H-2-associated genetic differences are also important in the control of the magnitude of the response. Repetitive immunization with the intact nuclease in the low-responder C57BL10 strain and the H-2 congenic B10.A high-responder strain ultimately yielded comparable levels of antibody activity. This suggests the existence of additional complexities regulating the H-2-linked control of the antinuclease response. Studies of the response to polypeptide chain fragments of staphylococcal nuclease indicate that responsiveness to as little as a third of the intact molecule (residues 99–149) is under the same apparent genetic control as the primary response to the intact protein (Berzofsky *et al.*, 1977a). Although A/J and SJL mice responded similarly to immunization with intact staphylococcal nuclease, they responded differently to immunization with residue 1–126 and residue 99–149 fragments of the whole nuclease (Berzofsky *et al.*, 1977a). Repetitive immunization with the polypeptide chain fragment yielded no significant response in low responder C57BL/10 mice, which developed responsiveness comparable to that of the B10.A strain when repetitively stimulated with the intact nuclease. Repetitive immunization of the same mouse strains with another fragment of the nuclease molecule (residues 1–126) yielded a significant response in the congenic low- and high-responder strains but not in a third nonresponder mouse strain (DBA/1) bearing a different H-2 haplotype. This suggests the existence of an additional H-2-linked Ir gene.

A multivariate comparison of the time course of the response of all five mouse strains to the residue 1–126 and residue 99–149 fragments of nuclease revealed highly significant differences (Berzofsky *et al.*, 1977a). The selective detection of response differences appeared highly dependent on the antigenic determinants on the respective fragments of the nuclease molecule. Despite the similarity of the H-2-linked genetic control of the response to the intact molecule and the control of the responses to antigenic determinants formed by residues 99–149, antibody raised to the respective fragments of the nuclease molecule reacted poorly with the intact nuclease (Berzofsky *et al.*, 1977b). This suggests the clonal expansion of antibody-producing cells bearing V-region genes appropriate for the conformation of the fragments as opposed to the conformation of the native nuclease molecule. In contrast, antibodies raised to the intact nuclease molecule reacted with the fragments. Studies of the avidity and the magnitude of the response to the several antigenic specificities represented on the fragments of the nuclease molecule suggested that different H-2-associated Ir genes can control the time course of the antibody response to different antigenic determinants on the same molecule separately from one another (Berzofsky *et al.*, 1977b).

Antiidiotype antisera raised in rats against A/J and SJL antibodies to staphylococcal nuclease have the ability to block approximately half of the capacity of the respective homologous antibodies' ability to inhibit the activity of the enzyme (Fathman *et al.*, 1977). Nonhomologous blocking was not detected. A large portion of the antibody activity generated by each mouse strain involved different idiotypes. This suggests that different V-region genes accounted for similar antinuclease activity in the two mouse strains. The segregation of the A/J antinuclease idiotype was independent of the segregation of genes in the H-2 region (Fathman *et al.*, 1977) and appeared linked with a high recombination frequency to a C-region allotypic marker (Pisetsky and Sachs, 1977). This suggests localization of the V-region genes coding for antinuclease activity on another chromosome which also bears genes coding for the C region of the antibody molecule. These findings suggested that the complexity of the immune response to multideterminant antigens can mask the genetic control of the response to the antigen. Restriction of experimental comparisons to antigenic determinants found on a small part of the intact antigen facilitated detection of thymus-dependent Ir gene coded response differences.

Although the genetic control of the ability to respond to the antigenic determinants of staphylococcal nuclease is H-2 linked, the genetic control of a large portion of the V-region genes coding for antinuclease activity is linked to non-H-2 genes coding for other portions of the structure of antibody molecules. While H-2-linked genes are not known to exert an influence over the selection of specific V-region genes, the possibility exists that T-suppressor cells may regulate the quantity of V-region genes selected. With highly restricted synthetic antigens, experimental impairment of suppressor T-cell function increases the average number of clonally expanded V-region genes from 2.8 to 7 populations of antibody-producing cells (Kipps *et al.*, 1978).

Several other naturally occurring antigens are also under H-2-linked Ir gene control (Young and Ebringer, 1976; Hill and Sercarz, 1975; Nowack *et al.*, 1977). Among the most complex is sperm whale myoglobin. Studies of the humoral response of inbred mouse strains to varying doses of sperm whale myoglobin revealed a plateau effect in the antibody level as antigen dose was increased (Young and Ebringer, 1976). Maximum differences between strain-specific antibody responses were detected at high antigen doses. The antibody response to sperm whale myoglobin is controlled by H-2-linked and non-H-2-linked genes (Berzofsky, 1978). The T-lymphocyte-dependent proliferative response appears to be under similar Ir gene control (Okuda *et al.*, 1978).

When these lines of inquiry are viewed from the perspective of the genetic control of the transfer of biological information involved in the immune response, several important concepts emerge. First, the genetic control of mitogen and carrier recognition and stimulation or cell proliferation is well established. Second, induced immune cell proliferation and differentiation are necessary permissive events for the generation of specific responsiveness. Third, the transfer of the information involved in the genetically controlled cognitive event is dependent on major histocompatibility complex gene products which control the cooperation of macrophages, T cells, and B cells. Fourth, the genetically controlled initiation of the proliferative response may be age dependent; this suggests that the initiating cues provided to the immune system may be a part of a developmental or life cycle process. This attribute is of special importance in view of the phenomena of the age-dependent penetrance of many genetic diseases and disorders of immunity. Fifth, although present evidence does not document a role of major histocompatibility complex genes in the selection of the V-region genes represented in the antibody response, H-2-linked T-lymphocyte suppressor effects may have a regulatory function in determining the number of V-region genes represented in expanded clones of antibody-producing cells directed toward a particular antigenic determinant. Finally, a mechanism not associated with the major histocompatibility complex can suppress IgE production and could have an important role in the genetic control of the expression of immediate hypersensitivity. This mechanism is independent of the particular antigen involved in the IgE-mediated response.

3. Cognitive Function

"Cognition" can be defined as the act or process of knowing. Higher levels of cognition can include the qualities of awareness or judgment. The cognitive function of the immune sytem does not exist in a biological void. Similar recognition abilities exist among other plant and animal species. For example, a cognitive system permissively controls the selection of pollen strains for the fertilization of flowering plants (Heslop-Harrison, 1975). Cell surface gene products within the internal environment of complex life forms may provide the cognitive signals leading to the development and integration of the form and function of the organism (Hood *et al.*, 1977). Cognitive functions in lower and higher forms of animal life range in complexity from those involved in nutrient acquisition and assimilation through the recognition of interspecific and intraspecific differences to the adaptive capacity of the responses controlled by the central nervous system.

Among the physiological systems concerned with the recognition of stimuli, differences exist in the ways afferent stimuli are received and among the ways efferent responses are expressed. Despite these differences, remarkable similarities exist among the mechanisms concerned with cognitive function. When the relative complexity of the adaptive purpose of each system is taken into consideration, the number of similarities exceed the differences. Similar concepts are applicable to all forms of cognitive function. Principles applicable to the study of cognitive function in one physiological system are often applicable to the study of other physiological systems. Intuitively, many of these principles are applicable to the study of the immune system. Important precedents for the study of the immune system exist in our knowledge of the acquisition and assimilation of nutrients, the pollenization of flowering plants, and the function of the central nervous system. Many of the precedents steming from the study of the central nervous system have been recently reviewed and summarized in the *Handbook of Perception* (Carterette and Friedman, 1973–1976). Portions of this literature, classic essays (Pavlov, 1927; Piaget, 1969; Sokolov, 1963, 1975), and recent theories about brain function (Edelman and Mountcastle, 1978) provide a rich source of information for the biologist concerned with the genetic control of cognitive function.

The responsive processing of biological information can be conceptualized in general terms as a series of mechanisms (Roberts, 1973). It is possible to identify and define these mechanisms within the context of the sequence in which they occur. Information processing begins with the stimulus. A source of environmental information outside the cognitive system provides the stimulus. Differences in the magnitude and coherence of the physiochemical attributes of the stimulus distinguish its information content from that of other stimuli and from the environmental level of physiochemical background noise. The stimulus impinges on an appropriate biological transducer which is sensitive to the particular physiochemical attributes of the stimulus. For example, the taste buds of the tongue are transducers which change the attributes of nutrient chemicals into internally represented nerve impulses (Wenzel, 1973). The transducer changes the information in the stimulus into a signal that can be carried and processed within the particular biological system. During this transformation, logarithmic increments of change in stimulus intensity are represented additively in the internal signal (Stevens, 1951, 1974; Jones, 1974; Carroll and Wish, 1974; Green and Swets, 1966). The internal representation of levels of signal change may be considerably less than the levels of significant change in the external stimulus. For example, approximately seven levels of difference can be independently identified by the human ear. This contrasts with the ability to distinguish many more levels of difference in dependent comparisons of two tones. The transformed and internally represented information contained in the signal is conveyed within the biological system through a channel.

The channel identifies the route by which the information reaches other parts of the biological system. The external auditory canal and the globe of the eye, as well as their neural connections, represent examples of channels. The channel can exert a selective influence on the primary source of responsive information recruited from within the system. The information content of the signal is used to selectively recruit one or more responses from among the several innate alternatives available within the biological system (Sutherland, 1973). The use of the information content of the signal to select alternatives distinguishes higher forms of cognitive function from less complex and more predictable stimulus–response relationships. There are three general levels of physiological function at which an innate deficiency of cognitive function could contribute to an observed response polymorphism. Opportunities exist for polymorphic variation in transducers, in channels, and in the innate alternatives available within the biological system (Thomas, 1973).

Informative comparisons can be made between the cognitive functions of different physiological systems. Similarities exist among the mechanisms responsible for the genetic control of (1) the adaptive acquisition and digestion of nutrients, (2) self and nonself distinctions in sexual reproduction in plants, (3) specific adaptive immunity, and (4) the specific adaptive behavior permitted by the central nervous system. Teleological considerations permit the speculation that all forms of cognitive function may have evolved from some common primitive cellular feeding mechanism. This suggestion is prompted by many kinds of circumstantial evidence. An exhaustive summary of this evidence is beyond the purpose of this chapter. An intuitive appraisal of this proposition and a comparison of a few cognitive systems are useful. This speculation and a brief summary of the comparative biology of cognition provide an assessment of biochemical and physiological mechanisms of potential importance in the genetic control of the cognitive function of the immune system.

3.1. Nutrient Recognition

Selective pressures favor the survival and evolution of single-celled organisms able to biochemically identify and manipulate potential nutrients in the natural environment During evolution, the polymeric products of other living organisms probably provided the most abundant source of nutrients. Foreign biopolymers probably exerted a profound influence on the development and selection of cognitive processes important in nutrition. Intuitively, nutrient sources provide the most plausible basis for the early development of cognitive mechanisms capable of distinguishing self and nonself. The ability of evolving organisms to recognize and use a wide range of nonself biopolymers represents an important nutritional advantage. A selection advantage would accrue to those species of organisms able to generate cell surface receptors capable of adhering to and using the largest number of foreign nutrient biopolymers prevalent in the environment.

With respect to cognitive control mechanisms, there are two hypothetical ways an evolving organism can manage the innate information necessary to distinguish between self and nonself (Figure 2). One mechanism requires the evolution of an innate capacity to generate selective cell surface receptors capable of binding and initiating feeding on specific foreign biopolymers. Specific innate information about each potential nutrient is needed to code for receptors for each nutrient. This mechanism is sufficient when the number of primitive potential nutrients in the environment is restricted to a small number of biopolymers. This mechanism becomes inefficient with increased diversification of competitive foreign life forms. This positive control mechanism physically restricts the range of potentially useful nonself nutrients to the number of cell surface receptor products that can be coded by the germ line resources. Cognition coupled with a positive control mechanism imposes a finite limit on the nutrient resources available to the cell. Biological economy dictates a need to conserve the amount of germ line information dedicated to performance of cognitive tasks.

A second hypothetical mechanism (Figure 2) requires the evolution of an innate germ line capacity to generate cell surface receptors capable of binding most biopolymers. When this mechanism is coupled with innate information coding for the specific ability to recognize and suppress feeding on self biopolymers, the range of potential nutrients is increased. Figure 2 compares the adaptive potential for nutrient assimilation and the germ line resources needed for both kinds of control mechanisms. Equal quantities of innate germ line information dedicated to distinguishing self and nonself are illustrated. When the organism's capacity to retain innate information is invested in a positive control mechanism, the range of potential nutrients is limited. When the same amount of germ line information is coupled with the ability to selectively not respond to a small number of self biopolymers, the organism can adapt to an almost unlimited range of nonself nutrients. Figure 2 illustrates the power of coupling cognitive germ line information with a negative control mechanism which suppresses the performance of an important adaptive task. The underlying principle in this comparison of two hypothetical mechanisms governing the recognition of self and nonself is the

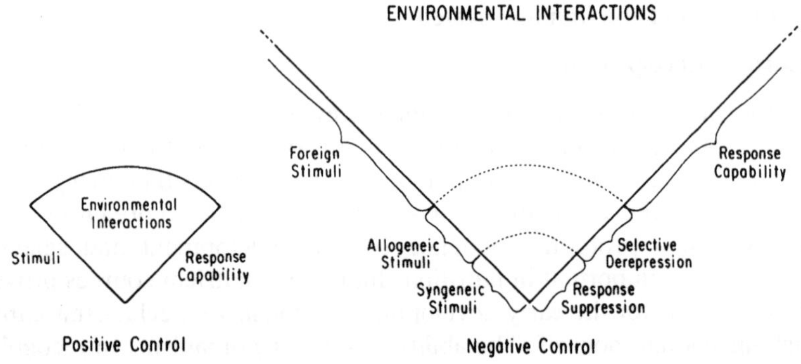

Figure 2. A remarkable difference exists between the advantages provided by positive and negative control of cognitive mechanisms coded by information in the genome (see text). This distinction may be important in nutrient assimilation and in immune function. The diagram on the left illustrates the relative quantity of cognitive environmental interactions permitted by genes coding for an explicit response to a finite set of environmental stimuli. Self-recognition is avoided by the absence of genes coding for self biopolymers. The diagram on the right illustrates the potential advantages of using the same quantity of germ line information to explicitly recognize self biopolymers and suppress the response to syngeneic and certain allogeneic biopolymers. A small number of genes coding for self recognition and suppression of responsiveness coupled with an innate general capacity to respond greatly increases the capacity for adaptive cognitive interactions.

biological economy of using a smaller number of cues to prompt appropriate biological function.

In the absence of self recognition, the binding of foreign biopolymers activates energy-dependent mechanisms for pinocytosis or phagocytosis (Pearsall and Weiser, 1970; Gordon and Cohn, 1973). These mechanisms incorporate the substrate into a phagosome, which fuses with a lysosome. The constitutive enzymes produced by the lysosome degrade the biopolymer into simple compounds. One level of cognitive function is involved in the selective nonassimilation of bound self biopolymers through the surface of the feeding cell. A second level of cognitive function exists in the way assimilated nonself biopolymers are processed within the cell. In the competitive arena of selective evolutionary pressures, growth, replication, and survival of the organism are favored by the rapidity with which an engulfed substrate can be converted into simple nutrients. A competitive advantage lies in the cell's ability to generate enzymes capable of yielding the maximum nutrition in the least amount of time. This implies a selective advantage for those organisms capable of expanding and diversifying the content of this part of their genome. Replication and redundancy of the genetic information in the cell provide an opportunity for the organism to survive chance mutations of the genome. Advantageous mutations can also code for the ability to depolymerize additional substrates. A selective advantage would accrue to those organisms which develop novel genes coding for enzymes capable of increasing the range and rapidity of substrate depolymerization. The selection of surviving organisms on the basis of fitness for the efficient biochemical manipulation of a wide range of biopolymers implies the development of an applicable spectrum of specific enzymes. This suggests that the organism's past history of nutritive successes with foreign biopolymers would be recorded in genes coding for specific enzymes in the organism's germ line memory. An enriched germ line history of nutritive successes provides a basis for competitive adaptive capacity in the face of changing environmental nutrients. The cognitive mechanisms by which cells respond to the biochemical attributes of specific polymeric nutrients through the augmented generation of specific enzymes provide a model of cybernetic mechanisms for accessing highly specific germ line information.

A highly developed ability to generate hydrolyases capable of depolymerizing biopolymers is a part of the function of cells. The lysosome contains a basic repertoire of hydrolyases which assures the ultimate utilization of most engulfed biopolymers. Important exceptions exist in this capacity for site-specific enzymatic activity. In primitive phagocytic cells, nondegradable substrates are expelled from the cell by a process called "exocytosis" (Gordon and Cohn, 1973). In higher animals, phagocytized nondegradable polymers can accumulate and persist in the form of intracellular inclusions. The retarded enzymatic degradation of cell wall polymers from group A streptococci probably represents the best-studied example of this type of deficiency of germ line information (Smialowcz and Schwab, 1977). The failure of the organism to degrade substrate implies the existence of a deficiency in the germ line information available for specific site binding. This polymorphism differs from a transducer polymorphism in that the organism is unable to act on the basis of the content of the channeled signal as opposed to the stimulus which initiated the signal.

Even though this hypothetical primitive form of substrate recognition and coupled permissive generation of specific enzymes does not approach the presumed complexity of the function of the immune or central nervous systems, several useful concepts are suggested. Portions of these concepts can be identified in the function of other cognitive systems. Perhaps the most important concept is the notion that the response to a stimulus is divided into two parts. The first part of the response can involve a permissive congitive event in which the organism exhibits the constitutive ability to respond in the absence of specific information. This innate cognitive event is constitutive in that the product of the germ line gene is avilable prior to the presentation of the stimulus. The ability to respond to the presentation of the substrate is immediately available to the organism. The second part of the response involves a second cognitive event in which the unique content of the signal is used to recruit a portion of the germ line history of the organism. The product of these genes is a specific adaptive ability not ordinarily exhibited by the organism. The two components of the response are permissively coupled in that the first cognitive mechanism permits selection of the second part of the response.

3.2. Pollen Biology

A recognition system is responsible for the control of reproduction in plants (Knox *et al.,* 1976). The pollen grain is composed of an outer exine layer which encloses an intine layer. Male gametes are carried within the layers of the pollen grain. The exine and intine portions of the pollen also contain soluble proteins which provide cues necessary to initiate plant fertilization. These same proteins cause pollen allergy. Fertilization begins when the pollen grain lands on the stigma, the female portion of the plant. The surface of the stigma is sticky and can bind pollen grains from many plant families. In certain self-fertilizing plants, adherent pollen strains from plants belonging to species of the same family as the maternal plant stimulate the stigma to provide moisture at the point of pollen contact. Within 20 min following adherence, the pollen grain becomes hydrated and swells. Moisture is not provided to pollen grains from plants belonging to other plant families, and they fail to hydrate. Pretreatment of the stigma surface with a 0.5% solution of sodium deoxycholate, a detergent, does not prevent the adherence of pollen grains, but does prevent hydration of the pollen grains from plants of an acceptable genotype. This suggests that the surface properties of the stigma and the exine proteins of the pollen grain have an important role in the cognitive process responsible for initiating plant fertilization (Knox *et al.,* 1976). The fertilization process is initiated by a transducer mechanism which permits a positive response to the proper environmental stimulus.

A second cognitive process leads to fertilization. Adherent hydrated pollen grains generate a pollen tube. If the genotype of the pollen grain is compatible with the maternal genotype, the pollen tube penetrates the papilla cuticle of the stigma and the male gametes are transferred into the female portion of the plant. Pollen tubes generated by pollen grains from genetically similar but incompatible species of the same plant family generate a longer pollen tube which coils about the papilla of the stigma and fails to penetrate the cuticle. Pretreatment of the stigma surface with concanavalin A, a naturally occurring lectin, also prevents the penetration of pollen tubes generated by genetically compatible plants. This suggests that cues provided by the intine proteins of the pollen grain and a concanavalin-binding receptor on the stigma are both necessary for the generation of the enzymes which digest the cuticle of the papilla and permit penetration of the pollen tube into the stigma.

In certain plant species, an active proliferative response of cells on the surface of the stigma participates in the rejection of intergeneric and self matings. In contrast to the failure to activate the enzymes necessary for the penetration of the cuticle, plants belonging to the Cruciferae and Compositae families develop a callus at the site of fixation of the pollen tube, which prevents fertilization. This suggests that the information carried by the intine proteins of plant pollens can elicit one of two different kinds of responses leading to fertilization. In different plant species, either (1) the generation of enzymes capable of digesting the cuticle of the stigma or (2) the failure to proliferate cells and generate a callus can lead to fertilization. Both positive and negative effector control mechanisms can be used to facilitate the proper response to the appropriate pollen. The inhibition of pollen tube penetration by concanavalin A suggests that a specific lectin-binding structure on the stigma has an important role in conveying the genetic information provided by the pollen grain through physiological channels (Knox *et al.,* 1976).

3.3. The Immune System

Evolution has used cognitive mechanisms for the appraisal of polymeric components of the environment in many ways. The most prevalent natural biopolymers adhere readily to cell surfaces. For example, proteins and polysaccharides bind tightly to the cell surface of the macrophage (Gordon and Cohn, 1973). Biopolymer adherence initiates cognitive tasks other than nutrient assimilation in primitive life forms which are slightly more complex than a single cell. In invertebrates, adherence mechanisms initiate the selective aggregation of single cells belonging to members of the same species into a multicellular colony (Hildemann, 1974). This type of cognitive event in marine sponges is regulated by the presence of a cell surface biopolymer (Moscona, 1973). In other invertebrates, the same cognitive event has been adapted to elicit aggressive reactions between different members of the same invertebrate species (Theodor, 1970; Hildemann *et al.,* 1975). The expression of tissue incompatibility among members of the same species has been interpreted as evidence of multiple alleles at a monogenic histocompatibility locus (Hildemann, 1977). The multiple alleles of the polygenic loci of the major histocompatibility complex of higher life forms may have evolved from similar monogenic loci through the process of gene duplication. A tenable role of gene duplication has been postulated in the evolution of gene clusters and in families and subfamilies of genes for immunoglobulins (Hood *et al.,* 1975). A similar mechanism has been suggested as the origin of the several loci of the major histocompatibility complex of higher vertebrates (Hildemann, 1977; Klein, 1977).

From the perspective of cognitive function, the initial interaction of a stimulus with a native cell or cell surface component can be viewed as a biologically passive but chemically predictable event which triggers subsequent changes in cell form and function. The noncovalent adsorption of a mitogen or carrier to the surface of an immune system cell represents an example of this kind of chemical event. The cognitive response to the stimulus can be identified only after subsequent changes in cell structures or cell function. In the immune system, other cells cooperate and participate in the responsive changes. The cooperative responses of immune system cells are supported by the use of cell energy, and can vary from a simple reorganization of cell components through the production of new cell products to replication of the cell. In terms of cognitive processes, an immune cell surface receptor becomes a stimulus transducer when the information provided by the stimulus is transformed into a signal capable of activating other cell mechanisms. The innate ability of a immune cell to initiate a signal provides an opportunity for a genetic polymorphism. A genetic difference at this level of cognitive function can be properly considered a transducer polymorphism.

An important distinction can be made between response polymorphisms detected by measurements based on immune cell replication and polymorphisms detected by other measures of immune function. Cell proliferation *per se* replicates all of the genetic information contained in the nucleus of the sensitized cell. Penultimate measures of immune function are dependent on selective access to additional information contained in the cell nucleus. Sources of genetic variability other than the transducer mechanism can contribute to penultimate response variation. Measures of induced immune cell proliferation are not likely to detect the expression of innate information beyond that of the transducer polymorphism. Nonmitotic mechanisms are an essential part of the specific response to an antigenic stimulus.

Beyond the transducer mechanism, there are two additional levels of function at which the immune system could selectively recruit innate information. The second level is not specific and involves the selection of the channel and general kind of immune function eventuating from the antigenic stimulus. The third level of innate information is specific for the unique properties of the particular antigen. All three levels of cognitive function differ from a general capacity for cell proliferation and augmentation of the number of cells cooperating at each level of cognitive function.

The macrophage-transformed antigenic stimulus activates a signal which is routed to other cooperating cells of the immune system. Immune cell cooperation is the channel by which cognitive function is implemented. Syngeneic histocompatibility antigens are necessary for normal cooperation among the cells of the immune system (Shearer *et al.,* 1976; Zinkernagel and Doherty, 1975). These restrictions define the channel by which information is passed to other parts of the immune system. Opportunity exists for genetic differences in the regulation of the flow of this information. Innate differences regulating the general biological attributes of the kind (Wanatabe *et al.,* 1976, 1977; Chiorazzi *et al.,* 1977; Tada *et al.,* 1975) and the magnitude of the immune response represent another possible source of polymorphic variation. The possibility exists that inherited differences in regulatory genes controlling the flow of signals through the channels of the immune system could contribute to or obscure immune response polymorphisms. Differences in the context within which the antigen stimulus is presented, such as adjuvants and concurrent infections, are also important (Revolta and Ovary, 1969; Jarrett and Bazin, 1974; Ogilvie and Jones, 1973; Urban *et al.,* 1977). These nongenetic factors can alter channel selection and could obscure inherited differences in regulatory mechanisms.

Although the permissive nature of immune cell stimulus transduction and channel selection can impose genetic limitations on the immune response and the ability to generate antibody to the antigen, it is important to note that neither of these limitations is necessarily equivalent to the genetic control of the specific immune response. The genetic control of the specificity of antibodies resides at the level of the genes controlling the V region of antibody. Perhaps the best experimental illustration of this aspect of the problem can be found in the report of Gunther and Rude (1976), who studied the patterns of cross-stimulation of cell proliferation and humoral cross-reactivity to three synthetic polypeptide antigens under Ir gene control. Isocongenic rat strains differing in only the major histocompatibility complex were immunized with synthetic antigens differing in only one amino acid. Antibodies generated to each of the three homologous antigens exhibited extensive cross-reactivity toward the two respective nonhomologous synthetic antigens. In contrast, no cross-stimulation of antigen-primed cells could be elicited with one of the three antigens, and only unidirectional cross-stimulation could be elicited with the second synthetic antigen (Gunther and Rude, 1976). These observations suggest that the genetic control of the transducer of the carrier stimulus for cell proliferation differed from the genetic control of the information contained in the antibodies. In this experiment, the genetic control of the transducer mechanism responsible for sensitization, cell proliferation, and the generation of antibodies exhibited greater specificity than the cross-reacting antibodies. The use of congenic animals in these experiments suggests the transduced signal permitted access to identical V-region genes coding for an equivalent immunoserological outcome. Although the identification of an equivalent immunoserological outcome in congenic rats can be considered presumptive evidence of identical V regions, the possibility also exists that different V-region genes are actually involved in these observations. Different V-region genes coding for structurally different antibodies can exhibit similar ability to bind to the same antigen (Fathman *et al.*, 1977). This phenomenon is called "degeneracy." A degenerate response implies the innate ability to respond adequately to the information contained in a transduced signal with any of several components of the repertoire of information contained in the genome (Edelman and Mountcastle, 1978). The possibility exists that different V-region genes coded for equivalent serological cross-reactivity among the three antigens. A comparison of the results of structural studies of the antibodies produced by each congenic animal would be needed to ascertain whether or not identical V-region genes gave rise to the cross-reacting antibodies. Studies of the idiotype or structure of the antibody generated as the result of the transduction event are necessary to evaluate genetic differences at this level of the control of the cognitive function of the immune system (Brandt and Jaton, 1978a,b).

3.4. The Central Nervous System

The cognitive function of the immune system is probably intermediate in complexity between the control of specific enzyme induction and the responses controlled by the central nervous system. Certain aspects of the cognitive function of the central nervous system are similar to the responses of simpler cognitive systems. The cognitive function of the central nervous system differs from simpler systems in an important way. The complex responses of the nervous system are composed of a sequentially organized hierarchy of simpler responses leading to the selection of a specific outcome. Signals initiated by concurrent external stimuli and from innate resources within the central nervous system contribute to the context in which the specific stimulus is received. The context in which the specific stimulus is presented has an important influence on the response outcome.

Possibly the closest analogy between the cognitive function of the immune system and the central nervous system can be drawn at the level of the simple reflex. A simple reflex is a reaction which is reliably elicited by a stimulus (Pavlov, 1927). The patellar and corneal reflexes represent examples of simple reflexes. A simple reflex is initiated by the transduction of an appropriate external stimulus and is implemented by channeling the resulting signal through cooperating nerve cells leading to the specific response. Depending on the context in which the external stimulus is received, the simple reflex response can be augmented or depressed. The immune response to a single antigenic determinant shares similarities with the simple reflex. In addition to an appropriate stimulus transducer and the channeling of the signal through cooperating cells, the magnitude of both kinds of responses can be altered by concurrent suppression. The simple reflex and the immune response differ in two important ways. First, the immune system signal can be channeled through several paths, thus leading to different kinds of immune responses. Second, diversity exists in the degenerate but specific outcome of the humoral immune response. In contrast, the outcome of the simple reflex is restricted to a single outcome. Variation in channel selection and diversity of the response outcome are attributes of more complex levels of central nervous system cognitive function.

Complex central nervous sytem reflexes are composed of a hierarchy or cascade of simpler responses in which a part of the response outcome of the intermediate simple response is channeled within the system. One simple response leads to another and eventually to the response outcome. Portions of this type of response sequence can be identified in the organization of complex reflexes. The psychophysiologist describes a nonspecific "arousal" component of the central nervous system response followed by a hierarchy of sequential responses which selectively adapt the organism to the particular external situation (Deutsch and Deutsch, 1963). For example, the Moro response of the newborn infant can be viewed as an example of the initial segment of a hierarchy of responses. Exposure of the sleeping infant to a loud noise, sudden movement, or almost any significant stimulus elicits awakening and purposeless movements. This innate, nonspecific capacity to respond is characteristic of healthy newborn infants. The purposeless portions of the Moro response become suppressed as the infant matures and the capacity for arousal becomes linked to useful activities. The sucking response of the infant represents an example of a complex response in which several simpler responses can be identified. This response can be elicited by gentle stimulation of the face of the sleeping infant. The infant awakens and, once aroused, turns the head toward the stimulus, takes the offered object into the mouth, and begins repetitive sucking movements. This complex response is composed of a sequence of simple responses which lead from one to another and to purposeful muscular efforts, a response repertoire designed to serve the best interests of the infant. In the absence of arousal, the specific behavior does not occur. Arousal directs or permits the sequence of responses. The important concept in this simple comparison is the relatively nonspecific nature of the Moro response and the important role of the arousal portion of the initial response in the permissive selection of a sequence of responses leading to specific purposeful function. Suppression has an important role in the modulation of complex orienting reflexes which operate at a subconscious level (Sokolov, 1963, 1975). Reinforcement or suppression can result from the selective channeling of signals within the system and from signals generated by associations maintained in central nervous system memory. At even higher levels of central nervous system cognitive function, reentrant or cyclic channeling of internal signals has been postulated in the organization of consciousness and complex behavior (Edelman and Mountcastle, 1978).

Cell surface receptors which direct the synaptic connections necessary for signal transmission within the central nervous system may have an important role in cognitive function. Potentially important similarities exist between antigenically similar cell surface structures found on immune system T cells and on cells from the liver and the brain (Reif and Allen, 1964). The cerebral cortex of man is composed of minicolumns containing approximately 260 cells (Edelman and Mountcastle, 1978). An average of thirty neurons per minicolumn are connected with other portions of the brain. The innate and selective influences which determine these connections are not known. Other portions of the central nervous system modulate and suppress the activity of the cerebral cortex. The total number of neurons in a single minicolumn is close to the number of penultimate possibilities that would be expected from combinations arising from two alternatives among eight units of information taken at one time.

Examples of inherited differences in the perception of color and taste provide examples of polymorphic variation in specially adapted neural transducers of environmental stimuli (Thomas, 1973). Like the immune system, transducer polymorphisms are easily detected. At the level of differences in the repertoire of innate response information within the genome, the repetitive expression of malapropisms (Fromkin, 1971), deficiencies in visual pattern recognition (Sutherland, 1973), and other errors in internal information provide possible opportunities to identify central nervous system polymorphisms analogous to V-region gene differences in the immune system. Studies of immune system V-region genes and amino acid sequences provide one source of information leading to current hypotheses about the higher levels of the cognitive function of the central nervous system (Edelman and Mountcastle, 1978). These hypotheses include concepts about conscious awareness of the environment and memory.

Complex cognitive processes involve memory. A primitive form of memory is a part of the cognitive function of the immune system. Memory can be defined as the facilitated selective access to associated units of information. It is possible to design experimental paradigms to evaluate the relationship between cognitive process and central nervous system memory (Anderson, 1973). A conceptual understanding of the amount of information transferred is important in the design of experimental studies. Psychophysiological studies of central nervous system memory provide an important estimate of the size and the characteristics of the memory information transferred during cognitive processes. The unit of responsive information involved in this process is called a "chunk" (Miller, 1956; Simon, 1974). It is intuitively possible to relate the principles and attributes of a chunk of central nervous system information to experimentally identifiable components of the information involved in immune system memory. Because of the probability that the number of units of information in a chunk of immune system memory are fewer than the number of units involved in the transfer of central nervous system memory, estimates of chunk size are important. Concepts about chunk size and repetitive stimulation provide a basis for fashioning paradigms designed to evaluate the cognitive function and memory of the immune system.

By definition, a "chunk" of information is the largest piece of information that can be transferred as a single entity. The size of a chunk is equal to or greater than the smallest unit of information possessed by the biological system. Chunk size can be increased by repetitive stimulation. Temporally related stimuli and repetitive access to units of information can result in a useful response outcome and lead to the associated processing of information as a collective unit or chunk. Subsequent restimulation results in the processing of all of the units of information and a response outcome characteristic of the chunk. Even though chunk size can be increased by training, the maximum size is limited. The maximum complexity of the information processed by biological systems is limited by chunk size. Estimates of chunk size in the central nervous sytem reveal an average of seven units of information (Miller, 1956). Training can increase chunk size in exceptional individuals (Simon, 1974).

The possibility exists that more than coincidence may account for the numerical similarities between (1) the six to eight amino acid sequence positions and six to eight amino acid substitutions that might account for the current postulate of a million germ line V-region genes (Figure 1), (2) the increase from an average of 2.8–7 monoclonally expanded antibodies to a single antigenic determinant following pharmacological abrogation of suppressor T-cell function (Kipps *et al.*, 1978), (3) the eight binary units necessary to code or account for the 260 selective channels offered by the neurons of each minicolumn of the human cerebral cortex (Edelman and Mountcastle, 1978) and, (4) psychophysiological estimates of average chunk size (Miller, 1956). It seems intuitively reasonable to postulate that the average size of the chunk of information processed by the immune system is not larger than the seven units of information processed by the central nervous system. This suggests that the complexity of the cognitive function of the normal human immune system may be accessible to clinical study.

4. Problem Solving in Clinical Immunogenetics

Experimental studies in animals suggest that Ir genes control the ability to recognize antigens and permit the production of antibodies (Shreffler and David, 1975; Klein, 1975; Goetze, 1977). These experiments have been facilitated by the well-characterized inbred animal strains (Klein, 1975) which enable the investigator to rigorously test a single hypothesis in informative prospectively bred progeny. Certain Ir genes appear closely linked to the major histocompatibility complex of the animal species (McDevitt and Sela, 1965). Ir polymorphisms have been detected following immunization with synthetic antigens (McDevitt and Sela, 1965; Pinchuck and Maurer, 1965) and with low doses of a few naturally occurring antigens of restricted heterogeneity (Green *et al.*, 1970). Because of the experimental options provided by inbred experimental animals and the availability of useful test antigens, much information has been acquired about Ir genes in animals. These findings suggest that HLA-linked Ir genes should be detectable in man.

Studies of the genetic control of immunity in man are more difficult. Despite the leads provided by animal studies, similar experimental opportunities do not exist in man. In studies of naturally occurring immunity in healthy subjects, reliance must be placed on the probability of chance sensitization to complex common antigens or to induced responsiveness to equally complex ethical antigens. The atopic allergens and antigens prepared from common infectious agents provide ideal probes for health-related studies of natural immunity in man. Ethical antigens can be used to study the response to immunization. Adequate numbers of patients with relevant diseases and concerned families are available. Despite these opportunities, a major problem handicaps disease-oriented genetic studies. This problem stems from the multifactorial nature of most human diseases. Complex disease mechanisms can contribute to the same diagnosis and obscure measurable genetic variation in patients. An awareness of this problem and the need for an adequate clinical phenotype is important. Sampling limitations impose another problem in human studies. Despite these limitations and the complexity of naturally occurring antigens, evidence suggests that immune response polymorphisms can be detected in nuclear families and selected human populations.

4.1. Multifactorial Diseases

Clinically, it is tempting to study the formal genetics of a specific disease. Precedent exists for this approach in past studies of metabolic diseases. Available evidence suggests that allergic and infectious diseases are more complex. Even when the disease can be clinically evaluated and treated in terms of a single factor, additional sources of complexity are present. A simple approach to an allergic or infectious disease is convenient only when a single remedial factor predicts the occurrence and clinical outcome of treatment. Certain infectious diseases provide examples of clinical simplification of a multifactorial disease process. The efficacy of antibiotic therapy for pneumonococcal pneumonia represents an example of this type of clinical simplification. Because of the predictable effectiveness of penicillin therapy, interactions between the products of the pneumococcus and the host can be ignored. The complexity of the host's interaction with the infectious agent is important only in the exceptional patient (Siber *et al.,* 1978).

Epidemiological studies suggest that changes in ventilation associated with allergic and infectious airways disease are more prevalent in certain families than in the general population (Higgins and Keller, 1975). Despite the possible genetic contribution to this prevalence of airways disease, a simple approach to this problem is not possible. Even when irreversible changes in ventilation are excluded, shared exposure to allergens, infectious agents, chemicals, and nonspecific environmental factors as well as innate differences in responsiveness to each respective factor could contribute to the familial prevalence of reversible ventilatory dysfunction.

Asthma is a severe form of nontoxic, noninfectious reversible airways disease. A clinical diagnosis of asthma can be applied to any disease characterized by recurring episodes of paroxysmal wheezing and shortness of breath. Asthma can also be caused by pulmonary embolization and congestive heart failure. Restriction of the diagnosis of asthma to exposure-induced reversible airways disease is helpful but does not solve the multifactorial complexity of the problem. Exposure-related asthma can be induced by at least three major mechanisms. First, bronchospasm and excessive airway mucus secretion can be induced by allergen exposure. Allergen-initiated, IgE-mediated permease release from bronchial mast cells is the most prevalent cause of reversible airways disease.

Second, oxidant gas exposure (Golden *et al.*, 1978), chemical (Zeiss *et al.*, 1977) or drug exposure (Chafee and Settipane, 1974), and certain infections (Hall *et al.*, 1978; Little *et al.*, 1978) can predispose patients to subsequent nonspecific provocation of episodes of bronchospasm and mucus secretion. Oxidant gases injure airway cells through the generation of free radicals. This effect may be very similar to the action of alkylating drugs such as cyclophosphamide, which impair the function of T-suppressor cells and augment IgE production in experimental animals (Wanatabe *et al.*, 1976, 1977; Chiorazzi *et al.*, 1977; Tada *et al.*, 1975). A pathological synergism between pollutant-induced augmentation of airways responsiveness and augmented local IgE production cannot be excluded. Other chemicals such as aspirin and yellow food dyes have a direct effect on prostaglandin production and can also cause asthma (Chafee and Settipane, 1974). Nonspecific provocative causes of asthma include temperature change, exercise, and nonantigenic irritants. Responsiveness of the airways can be detected by an assessment of the response to inhaled methacholine (Townley *et al.*, 1975; Barter and Campbell, 1976) and histamine (Gold, 1977). Nonspecific airways responsiveness can be separated from the response to allergen exposure. The allergen-induced airways response persists, while methacholine responsiveness is blocked by atropine treatment (Townley *et al.*, 1975). Innate attributes controlling the ability to develop augmented airways responsiveness add another dimension of complexity to this problem. Genetic factors contribute to the occurrence of exercise-induced bronchospasm (Konig and Godfrey, 1974; Godfrey and Konig, 1975), and a genetic contribution to methacholine responsiveness cannot be excluded (Townley *et al.*, 1976).

Third, inhalation exposure to organic dusts and noninfectious components of fungal allergens can specifically and nonspecifically induce bronchospasm, mucus secretion, and airways inflammation (Marx and Flaherty, 1976; Olenchock and Burrell, 1976). In addition to acting as antigens, components of certain microorganisms can directly activate the properiden pathway of the complement system and initiate inflammation and permease release. Genetic differences in the function of the complement system are well documented (Agnella *et al.*, 1972; Alper *et al.*, 1972; Day *et al.*, 1973; Wolski *et al.*, 1975; Hoppe *et al.*, 1978; Yamamura and Valdimarsson, 1977) and could contribute to the complexity of this problem. Another source of complexity is suggested by the apparent need for concurrent mitogen and antigen exposure to induce the tissue changes associated with organic dust-induced respiratory disease (Willoughby *et al.*, 1976; Willoughby and Willoughby, 1977). More than one organic dust- or fungal product-initiated mechanism can cause airways disease in the same patient.

Finally, multiple interacting causes of asthma are especially difficult to exclude in patients who are unduly susceptible to infection. All three mechanisms plus an innate impairment of specific responsiveness to infectious agents could contribute to this complexity. The possible role of multiple interacting environmental causes and host factors in reversible allergic airways disease emphasizes the need for multifactorial appraisal. The use of a multifactorial appraisal in disease-oriented genetic studies is based on the premise that more than one factor may be responsible for the disease process. A simultaneous evaluation of several factors and their interactions can predict the occurrence and severity of the disease better than the sum of predictions based on an assessment of each factor. Without a multifactorial appraisal of complex disease processes, naive interpretations are possible.

4.2. Clinical Phenotypes

The multifactorial nature of disease-oriented immunogenetic studies has been encountered in past studies of the atopic diseases. The central problem is the selection of an adequate clinical phenotype. A phenotype is the identifiable expression of an inherited trait. The diagnosis of an allergic or immunological disease is not likely to provide a reliable phenotype. A clinical diagnosis summarizes variable symptoms and signs which can be provoked by more than one mechanism and/or etiological agent. Several etiological agents and mechanisms can produce the same pathophysiological changes. Exposure-related hay fever or bronchospasm can provide a basis for a diagnosis but may not provide an adequate clinical phenotype for studies of the inheritance of allergic diseases.

One intuitive solution of this problem stems from Coca and Cooke's assessment of allergic diseases. Coca and Cooke (1923) noted the many clinical manifestations of the immediate hypersensitivity diseases and observed that several organs or organ systems could be involved by a similar pathophysiological process. The varied signs and symptoms of patients depended on the particular organ or tissues involved. Involvement of different organs and tissues by the same type of unusual responsiveness resulted in the diagnosis of different diseases. Members of the same family exhibited different diseases but shared the same capacity to exhibit cutaneous reaginic hypersensitivity to otherwise harmless antigens. Similar cutaneous responses could be demonstrated in family members who did not have an allergic disease. Coca and Cooke deduced that an innate predisposition toward altered responsiveness was shared by family members, and they called this trait "atopy." An assessment of reaginic responses provides a better clinical phenotype than the diagnosis of a specific allergic disease. Intuitively, reliable measurements of the immune response to relevant antigens can provide a better clinical phenotype than the diagnosis of the allergic disease.

4.3. Environmental Interactions

Another important problem is an assessment of the relative importance of environmental and genetic components of a familial disease. Familial diseases can be caused by (1) genetic effects, (2) environmental effects, and (3) a combination of genetic and environmental effects. For example, phenylketonuria is predominantly caused by a genetically determined metabolic inability to tolerate the quantity of phenylalanine normally found in the diet (Stanbury *et al.*, 1972). Although an environmental dietary contribution is important, the underlying cause of the disease is the innate inability to generate an enzyme capable of metabolizing the amino acid. Familial disease can also be caused by shared exposure to the same harmful environmental agent. The tendency of tuberculosis to occur in several members of the same family provides an example of a shared environmental cause of a familial disease. Tuberculosis is clearly a consequence of exposure to an infectious agent. Even though shared exposure to the tubercle bacillus is necessary for the familial occurrence of tuberculosis, recent studies suggest that inherited differences may exist in the ability to respond to the antigens of the tubercle bacillus (Buckley *et al.*, 1977). Both environmental and genetic effects could contribute to the familial prevalence of tuberculosis. These simple illustrations suggest that the categorization of a disease as environmental or genetic is based on the relative importance of each possible cause. Intuitively, an interaction between environmental antigen exposure and the genetic control of responsiveness is likely in familial allergic and infectious disorders.

4.4. Antigens

A number of ethical antigens are used in routine clinical testing and in immunoprophylaxis. A need exists for an assessment of genetic contributions to the variability of responsiveness to ethical antigens in man. An even greater need exists for studies of the possible genetic component of instances of the failure of immunoprophylaxis (Siber *et al.*, 1978; Hirszfeld and Hirszfeld, 1928; Schneibel, 1943; Fink and Quinn, 1953). Ethical antigens can be used to study the genetic control of human immunity. Antigens associated with a unique infectious disease present a different ethical problem. When the possible benefit of immunization with the unique antigen outweighs the risk of harm in an exposed family or patient population, an ethical need also exists for studies of the genetic control of immunity. With informed consent, relevant antigens can be used in patients with a familial disease and among family members. Studies of the response to other natural antigens which are unrelated to disease entail the risk of a subsequent chance encounter and an adverse reaction. Studies of the immune response to novel synthetic antigens may circumvent this problem, but it is ethically difficult to reconcile the possible discomfort and risks involved with the relevance of the information to a disease or to the normal protective function of the human immune system. Ethical considerations limit the antigens and opportunities to study the genetic control of the response to immunization in man.

Natural immunity develops to many common antigens. It is possible to evaluate natural immunity. Most naturally occurring antigens are complex molecules. The antigens responsible for inducing the normal protective function of the immune system differ considerably from the synthetic polypeptides and antigens of restricted heterogeneity used to detect Ir genes in inbred experimental animals. The complexity of naturally occurring antigens precludes a simple approach to the detection of Ir genes in man. Problems related to antigen complexity can be circumvented. Structural redundancy exists among the products of living organisms. Remarkable similarities often exist among the macromolecular components of cells and tissues serving similar biological functions. These similarities are most prevalent in macromolecules serving the same function in closely related species. This type of structural similarity among living organisms is used by the taxonomist to identify phyla, genera, and families. The antigenic similarities and differences of macromolecules from closely related species can be used to select antigen panels which provide useful probes of the genetic control of normal protective immunity. An assessment of the response to the cross-reacting or the non-cross-reacting portion of the compared responses provides a probe of a response increment which is less complex than the individual response to either antigen.

4.5. Sampling Problems

Unlike inbred experimental animals, human populations are genetically heterogeneous. Inbred animal strains provide an opportunity for replicate observations of the segregation of a gene product located on chromosomes which are identical by descent through successive generations of progeny. A similar incidence of identical chromosomes does not exist in most human populations. Experimental opportunities for replicate observations in man do exist in nuclear families and isolated human populations. A nuclear family is composed of the immediate kin of the propositus—the individual used to select the family for study. Studies in families can be limited by family size, the number of available generations, and necessity to rely on the chance occurrence of informative progeny. Appropriate replicate observations in informative progeny are not always available. This problem can be lessened by selection of large families or by studies in population isolates where the chance of consanguinity exists. A final possible opportunity for replicate observations in human populations exists among families whose probands share the same HLA-associated disease (Svejgaard *et al.*, 1975). Observations in populations selected on the basis of an HLA-associated disease cannot be extrapolated to a general population. This limitation is compensated by the opportunity to identify relationships of possible importance in the particular disease.

4.6. Models and Solutions

Hypothetical models of the genetic control of inherited traits are necessary to elucidate genetic mechanisms. An adequate mathematical model is needed to evaluate the genetic control of the human immune response to complex antigens. A number of analytical models can be devised to test the possible association of the magnitude of the immune response with independently identified gene products of the HLA complex. The adequacy of each model can be evaluated by application to experimental data. When a model fits the observed experimental variation and predicts more specific response associations than would be expected by chance, the model provides a close approximation of how the genetic control of the immune response may work.

Mathematical models designed to evaluate the associated segregation of the magnitude of the immune response and independently identified genetic markers are generally similar to conventional models of genetic mechanisms used to evaluate categorically defined traits. A recent review of this general problem is available (Elston and Rao, 1978). A recent effort has been made to apply methods devised for the study of categorical traits to the study of metric traits (Lange *et al.*, 1976). Despite these efforts, currently available mathematical models of categorical traits do not adequately account for the probable complexity of the immune response. Animal studies indicate a need for models capable of simultaneously evaluating multiple metric traits and the gene products of the histocompatibility complex. A clinical need exists for models applicable to the study of nuclear human families, patient populations, and pseudopopulations composed of nuclear families.

Fisher (1918) was the first to point out that the genetic contribution to a quantitative or metric trait could be made up of the sum of many small independent additive effects. The mathematical use of a metric model of a trait imposes requirements beyond those applicable to conventional categorical traits. The use of a metric trait entails a consideration of whether or not the magnitude of variation of the presumed polymorphism is greater than measurement error. This consideration is comparable to determining whether or not differences actually exist in the trait in the family or population under scrutiny. The distribution of the metric trait must also be evaluated in order to assure that it is additive over the range of variation to be evaluated. This is comparable to resolving whether or not the trait is dominant, codominant, or recessive. Scaling or a suitable transformation can be used to assure that the increments of change attributed to the postulated gene product are additive or codominant (Mather and Jinks, 1971). Animal studies suggest that Ir gene products are usually codominant (Ebringer *et al.,* 1976).

Mathematical models can be devised to detect the segregation of response increments among simultaneously compared responses to closely related test antigens. The rationale behind this approach to the study of responsiveness to complex antigens is important. The immune system is capable of recognizing similarities and differences among antigens. Immunization with an antigen from one species often induces a response to a closely related antigen from other species. This phenomenon is called "cross-reactivity." The detection of cross-reactivity implies the existence of similar structures on both antigens. It is experimentally possible to use the redundant information shared by closely related antigens to detect and exploit less complex differences and similarities among responses to the antigens. The response increments detected among measured responses to cross-reacting antigens represent units of biological information which are less complex than the responses to each antigen. This comparison of the responses to several antigens is analogous to the classic immunoserological use of a closely related specificity control.

Figure 3 illustrates the simplest set of circumstances in which carefully designed studies can exploit the redundant information shared by two complex naturally occurring antigens. Figure 3 illustrates hypothetical responses to antigen X and antigen Y in 16 subjects. The scaled responses on the left (A) represent the responses to each antigen. By inspection, it is not possible to identify similarities or differences among the 16 subjects on the basis of an independent evaluation of the response to either antigen. A conventional evaluation of the relationship between antigen responses is presented on the right (B) side of Figure 3. By inspection, the magnitude of the response to antigen X appears related to the magnitude of the response to antigen Y. Subjects who exhibit a large response to antigen X also exhibit a large response to antigen Y. The high degree of correlation between each subject's responsiveness to the two antigens provides presumptive evidence of cross-reactivity.

The diagonal line in the center of the right side of Figure 3 represents the best-fitting regression line for the hypothetical observations. Actually, this line is an estimate of the relationship which best separates two discrete groups of subjects. The basis for this difference is in the ability of subgroups of the subjects to respond to the two test antigens. One or more antigenic determinants could account for this difference. Despite uncertainty about the number of antigenic determinants responsible for the experimental difference, the basis of the observed difference is intuitively less complex than the total response to either antigen. The 16 subjects can be divided into two groups, one of which exhibits proportionately more responsiveness to antigen X than to antigen Y. The observations belonging to the two groups of subjects can be projected on the X axis along a line parallel to the regression line. This removes the portion of responsiveness shared to antigens X and Y. By inspection, no overlap exists between the distribution of the two groups of subjects. In this illustration, the difference in the response to the two antigens represents a "response increment" which separates the subjects. The response increment can be demonstrated only when responses to both antigens are simultaneously evaluated. The importance of the response increment becomes apparent when the cross-reacting portion of the responses is removed. The cross-reacting and the non-cross-reacting portions of the compared responses represent a reduction in the complexity of the observed responses. Either portion of the compared responses could segregate as a genetic difference in the immune response in family and population studies.

This approach can be extended to include additional closely related antigens. Even though more than one antigenic determinant could be involved in an experimentally identified response increment, the response increment can be

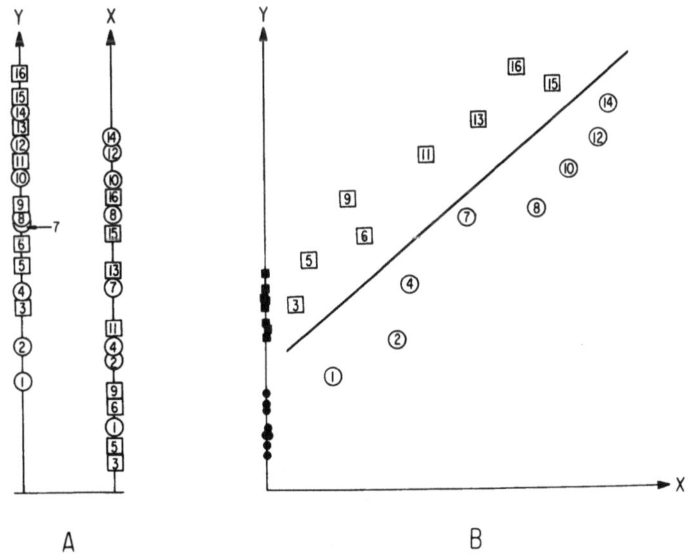

Figure 3. Simultaneous evaluation of two related sets of observations can yield more information than the separate evaluation of each set of observations (see text). This illustration represents responses to hypothetical cross-reacting antigens X and Y in 16 subjects. Inspection of the responses on the left (A) reveals no discernible differences between the responding subjects. When both sets of responses are simultaneously evaluated (B), inspection reveals evidence of cross-reactivity and important differences between the responding subjects.

attributed to a single antigenic determinant in the experimental context in which it is described. This concept is adequate for purposes of description. Consider a group of closely related antigens which share three antigenic determinants on a common antigenic background (Figure 4). Responsiveness to the background antigenic determinants shared by all test antigens can be ignored. Assume that an additive measurable relationship exists between the response increments attributed to each antigenic determinant. Among three antigenic determinants, there are eight possible combinations capable of eliciting different levels of responsiveness in sensitized subjects. Each one of the eight possible unique test antigens can elicit varying degrees of cross-reactivity with the other seven test antigens.

Figure 4 illustrates all eight possible combinations of three antigenic determinants. Figure 4 also presents the 28 possible comparisons among the responses to any two of the eight hypothetical test antigens. Ignoring higher-order comparisons, 12 of the 28 hypothetical response comparisons would be expected to yield a difference equivalent to the response increment shown in Figure 3. The probability of detecting a simple first-order response increment with a panel of closely related test antigens sharing three antigenic determinants is 12/28 or 0.4285. Figure 4 suggests that the use of measured responses to closely related cross-reacting test antigens yields a finite probability of detecting differences which are much less complex than the responses to the individual test antigens. This suggests that the

TEST ANTIGENS AND COMPARISONS WITH 3 ANTIGEN DETERMINANTS

Test Antigen Number	Combinations of Antigenic Determinants A	B	C	Possible Test Antigen
1	+	+	+	ABC
2	+	+	−	AB
3	+	−	+	AC
4	−	+	+	BC
5	+	−	−	A
6	−	+	−	B
7	−	−	+	C
8	−	−	−	−

POTENTIAL COMPARISONS BETWEEN ALL POSSIBLE TEST ANTIGENS

Antigens	ABC	AB	AC	BC	A	B	C	−
ABC	I							
AB	C*	I						
AC	B*	B/C	I					
BC	A*	A/C	A/B	I				
A	BC	B*	C*	BC/A	I			
B	AC	A*	AC/B	C*	A/B	I		
C	AB	AB/C	A*	B*	A/C	B/C	I	
−	ABC	AB	AC	BC	A*	B*	C*	I

Figure 4. Informative comparisons can be made between responses to sets of test antigens which share antigenic determinants. This illustration shows all possible antigenic combinations of three antigenic determinants and the potential comparisons that can be made between the cross-reacting responses (see text). Immunogenetic studies with cross-reacting antigens provide a reasonable expectation of informative simple comparisons between the observed responses. *Informative comparisons, 12/28 = 0.4285.

antigenic structure of closely related antigens can be used to design antigen panels capable of detecting the segregation of response increments.

It is possible to extend this logical approach to the detection of response increments to test antigen panels containing larger numbers of antigenic determinants. Figure 5 summarizes the relationship among antigenic determinants, cross-reacting test antigens, and the probability of detecting simple informative response increments with two to nine antigenic determinants. The number of response increments increases as the number of antigenic determinants and number of possible test antigens increase. The increase in the number of response increments is not proportionate to the maximum number of possible test antigens. Comparisons based on test panels composed of antigens sharing more than seven antigenic determinants have less than 1 chance in 20 of yielding a simple response increment (Figure 5). With less than seven antigenic determinants, an appreciable probability of finding an informative comparison exists among cross-reacting test antigens. This suggests that studies of responsiveness with small numbers of closely related test antigens sharing a small number of antigenic determinants have a reasonable chance of detecting simple response increments. An evaluation of the antigenic structure of naturally occurring test antigens and selection of cross-reacting antigens can be used to design antigen panel probes which simulate the restricted antigenic heterogeneity of the synthetic antigens used in studies of experimental animals.

Clinical immunogenetic problems usually present in the form of a patient with an unusual family history. If the nuclear family is sufficiently large and available, an opportunity exists to evaluate whether or not some portion of the immune response to clinically relevant antigens segregates with independently identified chromosomes shared by family members. The null hypothesis of this assessment is the independent assortment of the two traits—Mendel's first law of inheritance. Rejection of the null hypothesis is interpreted as evidence of lack of evidence for the independent assortment of genes coding for the traits. The rejection of the null

Number of Antigenic Determinants	Maximum Number of Test Antigens	Total Number of Possible Comparisons	Informative Simple Comparisons	Probability of an Informative Comparison,
2	4	6	4	.6667
3	8	28	12	.4285
4	16	120	32	.2666
5	32	496	80	.1612
6	64	2016	192	.0952
7	128	8128	448	.0551
8	256	32640	1024	.0314
9	512	130816	2304	.0176
⋮	⋮	⋮	⋮	⋮
n	2^n	$(2^{2n}-2^n)/2$	$\int_{k=0}^{n}(k(nCk))$*	$n/(2^n-1)$

Figure 5. The chance of obtaining an informative simple comparison between any two cross-reacting test antigens decreases as the number of antigenic determinants is increased. The probability of an informative comparison is less than 1 in 20 when more than seven antigenic determinants are involved. An *a priori* assessment of cross-reactivity among closely related test antigens is important in the design of studies of the genetic control of the immune response to complex antigens. *nCk= n!/k!(n-k)!

hypothesis in a single nuclear family cannot be interpreted as evidence that the traits are linked. This semantic uncertainty is usually avoided by interpreting rejection of the null hypothesis as evidence of the associated segregation of the two traits. When subsequent studies in additional informative families identify the same association, it is possible to deduce that linkage accounts for the finding. Studies of the frequency of recombination between the traits are necessary to define linkage relationships.

In order to apply a model to experimental data, a multiallelic system of genes is needed to identify the segregation of chromosomes among family members. The large number of human histocompatibility antigen (HLA) alleles of the several loci of the major histocompatibility complex provide ideal markers of the segregation of HLA complex. The polymorphic nature of the alleles of the HLA complex optimizes opportunities for resolution of genetic differences. The several loci of the HLA complex and other linked genes increase the opportunity to study recombination between different parts of the chromosome. A mathematical model has been devised for the evaluation of a possible HLA-associated disease susceptibility gene shared by family members (Day and Simons, 1976). Related models can be applied to variation in the magnitude of the immune response among family members. Figure 6 illustrates the use of this type of model.

Dorf *et al.* (1974b) evaluated the immune response to a glutamic acid–alanine copolymer in rhesus monkey families. Allelic genes coding for RhLA haplotypes, which are analogous to the HLA haplotypes of man, were used to identify the independent segregation of the major histocompatibility complex. A sensitive antigen-binding assay was used to measure the antibody response to synthetic antigens. By inspection, the investigators were able to deduce that an RhLA-linked Ir gene could account for the observed difference in antibody responses. Figure 6 illustrates a model which can be used to statistically evaluate their deduction. A similar model can be applied to observations in the families of patients (Buckley and Roseman, 1976).

Figure 6 illustrates the main steps in the identification of RhLA-associated responses. This model tests the null hypothesis that variation in the magnitude of the primary antibody response to the synthetic antigen is not associated with the RhLA haplotypes of the monkey family members. There are five steps in this analysis: (1) an assessment of response variation among family members in relation to measurement error in order to determine whether the family is informative; (2) if necessary, a transformation of the observed responses to some scale on which the measured responses are normally distributed and additive over the range of response variation; (3) formulation of an algebraic relationship between the hypothesized increments of the response associated with each RhLA haplotype and the measured response; (4) a least-squares estimate of the magnitude of the response associated with each RhLA haplotype; and (5) an estimation of the portion of the observed response among all monkey family members predicted by the least-squares solution. The null hypothesis is rejected when the portion of the immune response variation predicted by this simple model is large in relation to residual or error variation. When the residual within-haplotype variation is small and equivalent to measurement error, it is possible to deduce from the goodness of the fit that the model closely approximates how the genetic control of the immune response to the antigen actually works.

The dashed line about the central boxed portion of Figure 6 encloses 17 simultaneous equations. These equations state the postulated algebraic relationship between the RhLA haplotypes and the measured responses. Symbols designating the paternal monkey, his three monkey spouses, and the progeny of each respective conjugal combination are shown at the left outside the box. Observed antibody responses are shown on the right. Each equation relates the two unknown RhLA haplotype-associated responses of a single monkey to the log-transformed antibody response. Log-transformed antibody responses closely approximate a normal distribution and meet the requirement for additivity over the observed range of response variation. In Figure 6, the value of 1 pmole/m is arbitrarily substituted for the antibody activity of nonresponders; this precaution avoids the use of the log of zero—an undefined number. This precaution does not alter the statistical evaluation of the data. The RhLA haplotypes shared by the monkey family are listed at the top of Figure 6. The presence or absence of a particular haplotype in each equation is indicated, respectively, by a value of 1 or 0 under the appropriate column.

PRIMARY ANTIBODY RESPONSE OF RELATED RHESUS MONKEYS TO A GLUTAMIC ACID-ALANINE COPOLYMER

ANIMAL	RhL-A Genotype: 6,R24	10,2	9,b	R22,R18	6,b	9,11	R21,b	R3,11	Error	Log_e of Response	Antibody Response pM/ml
♂600	1 +	1 +	0 +	0 +	0 +	0 +	0 +	0	+ 0.92	= 2.94	19
♀669	0 +	0 +	1 +	1 +	0 +	0 +	0 +	0	+- 1.08	= 3.82	46
AC	1 +	0 +	0 +	1 +	0 +	0 +	0 +	0	− 0.36	= 0.00	1*
BI	1 +	0 +	0 +	1 +	0 +	0 +	0 +	0	− 0.36	= 0.00	1*
CR	1 +	0 +	0 +	1 +	0 +	0 +	0 +	0	− 0.36	= 0.00	1*
EL	0 +	1 +	1 +	0 +	0 +	0 +	0 +	0	− 0.30	= 4.11	61
FS	0 +	1 +	1 +	0 +	0 +	0 +	0 +	0	− 0.78	= 3.63	38
♀597	0 +	0 +	0 +	0 +	1 +	1 +	0 +	0	− 0.63	= 4.48	89
CG	1 +	0 +	0 +	0 +	0 +	1 +	0 +	0	− 0.26	= 0.00	1*
DW	1 +	0 +	0 +	0 +	1 +	0 +	0 +	0	+ 0.42	= 4.55	95
AB	0 +	1 +	0 +	0 +	1 +	0 +	0 +	0	+ 0.21	= 7.08	1190
BF	0 +	1 +	0 +	0 +	0 +	1 +	0 +	0	+ 0.89	= 3.89	49
♀603	0 +	0 +	0 +	0 +	0 +	0 +	1 +	1	+ 0.46	= 4.70	111
T	0 +	1 +	0 +	0 +	0 +	0 +	0 +	1	− 0.14	= 4.11	61
DF	0 +	1 +	0 +	0 +	0 +	0 +	0 +	1	− 0.73	= 3.52	34
FO	0 +	1 +	0 +	0 +	0 +	0 +	0 +	1	+ 0.41	= 4.66	106
GY	0 +	1 +	0 +	0 +	0 +	0 +	1 +	0	− 0.46	= 4.30	74

ANALYSIS OF VARIANCE

	Sum of Squares	d.f.	Mean Squares	F
Regression	245.19	7	35.02	55.12
Error	5.72	9	0.63	
Total	250.92	16		$p \leq 0.001$

RhL-A Genotype Associated Responses

6,R24	−0.36
10,2	2.38
9, b	2.02
R22,R18	0.72
6, b	4.49
9,11	0.62
R21,10	2.37
R3,11	1.86

Figure 6. A simple mathematical model for excluding the independent segregation of RhLA-associated responses in monkey families. This paradigm can be constructed from measures of the magnitude of the immune response and independently determined haplotypes (see text). Adapted from Table II, Dorf *et al.* (1974b), *Transplant. Proc.* **6**:119–123. A similar model can be applied to the clinical evaluation of human families and patient populations. *Value 0.1 set equal to 1 for calculation.

A least-squares solution yields the RhLA haplotype-associated responses tabled on the lower right of Figure 6. The error term in each equation is the difference between the sum of each monkey's two RhLA-associated responses and the log-transformed measured response of the animal. The error terms are squared and summed to provide the residual or error sum of squares—an estimate of the response variation not predicted by the model. The regression sum of squares represents the "between-RhLA-haplotype" response variation. The error variation respresents the "within-RhLA-haplotype" variation. Invalid assumptions about the segregation of the genetic control of the observed responses and several additional sources of variation could contribute to the within-haplotype variation. These additional sources of variation include inappropriate assignment of RhLA haplotypes and extraneous sources of response variation such as the age and sex of the animal and response contributions by genes on other chromosomes. The analysis presented in Figure 6 suggests that these sources of variation are small. The within-haplotype variation in the study of Dorf and his colleagues probably does not differ from measurement error. The null hypothesis—the independent assortment of RhLA haplotypes and the immune response—can be rejected. This suggests that an association exists between the genetic control of the response to the synthetic polypeptide antigen and the RhLA haplotypes of the monkeys. Dorf and his colleagues deduced that RhLA-linked Ir genes coding for responsiveness to the synthetic polypeptide exist in the monkey family.

4.7. Multivariate Analysis

Because of the complexity of naturally occurring antigens, the most useful assessment of possible Ir genes in human families and populations depends on a simultaneous evaluation of dependent relationships among carefully selected test antigens. An infeasible alternative is an assessment of responses to fragments of complex antigens which exhibit reduced heterogeneity. The power of this general type of model can be augmented by incorporating replicate estimates of measured responses to each antigen. This provides a direct assessment of the relationship between error variation and within-haplotype variation—a simultaneous assessment of the goodness of the fit. Because of the use of multiple measured responses, a parametric multidimensional method is needed. A linear method for multivariate analysis of variance is suitable if the measured responses are normally distributed and additive over the range of response variation (Morrison, 1967; Van de Geer, 1974). Available multivariate models are not capable of evaluating pedigrees or providing a formal evaluation of linkage similar to conventional genetic models (Elston and Rao, 1978; Lange *et al.,* 1976). These deficiencies are more than compensated by the resolving power of the multivariate assessment of responses to a panel of closely related test antigens. Multivariate methods have been developed for application to similar quantitative genetic problems (Felsenstein, 1977) and have proven useful in the evaluation of responses to antigenic fragments of a naturally occurring protein antigen in inbred experimental animals (Berzofsky *et al.,* 1977a). These studies confirm the applicability of multivariate models in studies of the immune response to complex antigens in man (Buckley *et al.,* 1973).

There are several ways the associated segregation of metric immune response phenotypes and independently identified chromosomes can be evaluated by multivariate analysis. A relatively simple model can be devised from the general method of multivariate analysis described by Starmer and Grizzle (1968). In this model (Figure 7) of the genetic control of the immune system, multivariate regression takes the form

$$\underset{(n\times p)}{E(R)} = \underset{(n\times m)}{H} \; \underset{(m\times p)}{\beta}$$

where H is a $(n \times p)$ matrix composed of known coefficients determined by the m genotypes of n family members. The R matrix is composed of the n observed immune responses to p cross-reacting antigens. β is a parameter matrix composed of m elements for the p antigens. Hypotheses are tested using the general relationship

$$H_0: \quad \underset{(s\times m)}{C} \; \underset{(m\times p)}{\beta} \; \underset{(p\times u)}{U} = \underset{(s\times u)}{0}$$

where C is an $(s \times m)$ matrix and U is an $(p \times u)$ matrix and are arbitrarily designed to yield appropriate hypotheses. The C matrix is structured to form linear combinations of the rows of the β matrix. The U matrix is structured for linear combinations of the columns of the β matrix. The mathematics of multivariate regression and similar general methods of hypothesis testing have been described in an available textbook (Morrison, 1967). The rationale behind the use of the C and U matrices in Figure 7 is also described by Starmer and Grizzle (1968), but differs from other applications of multivariate analysis.

A short description may be of interest. The use of the C and U matrices is independent of the number of variables considered. For simplicity, Figure 7 illustrates an analysis of responses to one antigen. The diagram at the top of Figure 7 presents the pedigree of a ten-member two-generation family in whom responses (r_{1-10}) were measured to the same antigen. In this pedigree, only similarities between family members who share the same chromosome are considered. Within the family, the categorization of members is independent of the particular alleles used to independently identify chromosomes A through D. The chromosomes and immune responses are identified in the circles symbolizing each family member. Six combinations of the four chromosomes exist among members of a two-generation family. Two unique combinations of genotypes occur in the parents; the remaining genotypes are shared by the sibship. The family in Figure 7 is composed of the parental AB and CD genotypes, and four AD, two AD, one BC, and one BD genotypes among the siblings; replicate observations within each sibship are not always possible. Genotypes, numbers of family members, and numbers of chromosomes in the family are summarized beneath the pedigree.

The H matrix is composed of known coefficients determined by the six genotypes of the ten family members. The R matrix column vector is composed of the ten measured immune responses. The β matrix column vector is composed of six elements associated with each genotype. Each element represents the best linear estimate of the response associated with each genotype. The midportion of Figure 7 presents the H matrix and the R and β column vectors applicable to one of the p antigen responses applicable to the family. The information available in

Figure 7 is sufficient to design a set of vectors which accounts for the four chromosome-associated effects within the family. In Figure 7, a total of 20 chromosomes are distributed among the ten family members. Seven chromosomes contribute to the A effect; three, six, and four chromosomes contribute, respectively, to the B, C, and D effects. Contrast vectors containing factor loadings applicable to the A, B, C, and D haplotype effects of the particular family are illustrated near the bottom of Figure 7. Collectively, these contrast vectors account for the responses associated with all the chromosomes in the family. The elements of these vectors are factors proportionate to the incidence of each chromosome among the six genotypes.

The design contrast vectors at the bottom of Figure 7 are obtained by subtracting the vectors for appropriate haplotype-associated effects. There are three differences among four chromosomes. The design contrast vectors shown at the bottom of Figure 7 are orthogonal with respect to each contrasted haplotype-associated effect; this means the factor loadings for each design contrast vector sums to zero. Simultaneous use of all three comparisons at the bottom of Figure 7 provides an assessment of the observed variation in the immune responses

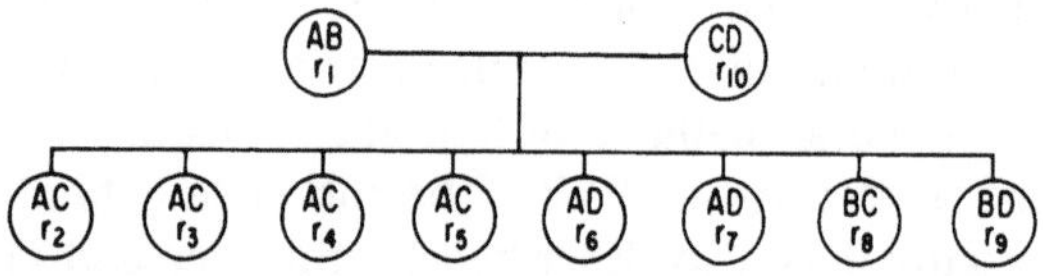

Haplotype Catagories	AB	AC	AD	BC	BD	CD
No. of Family Members	1	4	2	1	1	1
No. of Haplotype Chromosomes	2	8	4	2	2	2

Response Vector / Coefficient Matrix / Parameter Vector

$$R = \begin{bmatrix} r_1 \\ r_2 \\ r_3 \\ r_4 \\ r_5 \\ r_6 \\ r_7 \\ r_8 \\ r_9 \\ r_{10} \end{bmatrix} \quad H = \begin{bmatrix} 1 & 0 & 0 & 0 & 0 & 0 \\ 0 & 1 & 0 & 0 & 0 & 0 \\ 0 & 1 & 0 & 0 & 0 & 0 \\ 0 & 1 & 0 & 0 & 0 & 0 \\ 0 & 1 & 0 & 0 & 0 & 0 \\ 0 & 0 & 1 & 0 & 0 & 0 \\ 0 & 0 & 1 & 0 & 0 & 0 \\ 0 & 0 & 0 & 1 & 0 & 0 \\ 0 & 0 & 0 & 0 & 1 & 0 \\ 0 & 0 & 0 & 0 & 0 & 1 \end{bmatrix} \quad \hat{\beta} = \begin{bmatrix} \beta_{AB} \\ \beta_{AC} \\ \beta_{AD} \\ \beta_{BC} \\ \beta_{BD} \\ \beta_{CD} \end{bmatrix}$$

	β_{AB}	β_{AC}	β_{AD}	β_{BC}	β_{BD}	β_{CD}
HAPLOTYPE VECTORS						
A Effect	1/7	4/7	2/7	0	0	0
B Effect	1/3	0	0	1/3	1/3	0
C Effect	0	4/6	0	1/6	0	1/6
D Effect	0	0	2/4	0	1/4	1/4
DESIGN CONTRAST VECTORS USED TO TEST ASSOCIATION						
C(A−B)	−.19	.57	.28	−.33	−.33	0
C(A−C)	.14	−.09	.28	−.17	0	−.17
C(A−D)	.14	.57	−.21	0	−.25	−.25

Figure 7. Multivariate methods are necessary for the evaluation of the independent segregation of genetic markers and the magnitude of the immune response. This diagram illustrates the type of hypotheses that can be tested in studies of human families (see text). The limitations of this general model are not different from those applicable to more conventional methods for the analysis of the segregation of genetic traits.

among all family members. When used as a design contrast or C matrix, the design contrast vectors test the null hypothesis that the magnitude of the differences in immune responsiveness associated with the chromosomes is not different from residual or error variation. When applied to p immune responses, the hypothesis tested becomes

$$H_0: \ \beta_1 = \beta_2 = \beta_3 = \ \ldots \beta_p = 0$$

In testing this hypothesis, the best unbiased estimates of the parameter matrix β, the matrix sum of products due to error, and the matrix sum of products due to hypothesis are obtained. Classic univariate F or multivariate test statistics can be computed from the error sum of products and the hypothesis sum of products. The multivariate statistics obtained include the Wilkes likelihood ratio, the Hotelling T2 trace, and Roy's largest root, each with the appropriate number of degrees of freedom. The null hypothesis is rejected when the hypothesis that responsiveness to the test antigens is not associated with the chromosomes has a small chance of being correct ($p<0.05$).

Each multivariate statistic provides an assessment of the relationship between the variation due to the hypothesis and the residual or error variation. Shared variation or cross-reacting responsiveness is evaluated and compensated in the process of making the multivariate comparison. Differences exist in the way cross-reacting responsiveness is evaluated by the three multivariate statistics. The Wilkes ratio assesses the proportionate contribution of all sources of shared variation among the set of observations in an overall test of the hypothesis. The Hotelling statistic is based on a profile of the variance, in which the main components of cross-reacting responsiveness are represented. The relative contribution of the major sources of cross-reacting responsiveness is greater. Comparisons based on Roy's largest root focus on the main component of cross-reacting responsiveness—the dominant specificity shared by the test antigens. Conceptually, the different assessments provided by these three multivariate statistics are much like a comparison of two mountains. The Wilkes ratio assesses differences in the mass of the mountains and ignores the profile of the peaks. The Hotelling statistic evaluates a view of differences in the profile of the peaks of the mountains. Roy's largest root assesses differences related to the largest peak of each respective mountain. Intuitively, rejection of the null hypothesis on the basis of Roy's largest root and, to a lesser degree, the Hotelling statistic and the Wilkes ratio suggests differences in the relative importance of less immunodominant cross-reacting responses to the test antigens.

Several comments about possible limitations of this analytic method are important. These limitations stem from (1) the small number of observations usually available within human families and (2) the confounded nature of the two haplotype-associated effects attributed to each family member. Multivariate linear models are based on the assumption that equal numbers of observations are available among the contrasted categories. This assumption is not valid in families. Only two parental genotypes are available. The occurrence of sibling genotypes is a matter of chance. Imbalanced observations are internally compensated in this multivariate analytic method. Slight imbalances among contrasted categories are compensated and tolerated without difficulty. Proportionate compared categories are better tolerated than those which are disproportionate in sample size. A severe imbalance could weaken this analytical method. For example, in the family illustrated in Figure 7, the contributions of the A and B haplotypes of the parent balance one another out in the comparison of the A and B haplotype-associated effects. The A vs. B comparison is based on response variation among the sibship. Information pertaining to the parent is lost in the comparison. The effect of the imbalanced sampling within family genotype categories on the comparison is not known.

The design contrast matrix shown in Figure 7 is a first-order interaction. Two haplotype effects occur in each family member; second-order interactions are confounded in these contrasts. An example of a second-order interaction would be the influence of one haplotype chromosome on the magnitude of the response associated with another chromosome. Large second-order interactions could obscure the additive nature of the model and handicap detection of associated segregation of responses. Conversely, second-order interactions could contribute to the apparent associated segregation of responsiveness.

These same limitations are shared with other methods for evaluation of the immune response in families. The problems related to sample size and imbalance become less severe when this method of analysis is applied to large families and pseudopopulations composed of closely related families. The ability to detect the similar immune response associations in populations composed of families who share identical chromosomes by descent and in individual families drawn from the population suggests that the sampling limitations within families may not be severe. The detection of many highly significant response associations with this method of analysis of family data suggests that second-order interactions (epistaxis) may not limit the application of this method of analysis to studies of the human immune response. In the absence of multivariate methods applicable to the formal analysis of pedigrees or linkage between genes coding for cross-reacting metric traits and a categorical trait, this general method of analysis provides an extremely useful method for the study of responses to complex antigens in man.

5. HLA-Associated Diseases

The prevalence of HLA phenotypes is altered in certain diseases. The frequency of an HLA phenotype in unrelated patients sharing the same disease can differ from the frequency of the same phenotype in healthy unrelated subjects. Statistical tests, such as Fisher's exact test or the χ^2 analysis, are used to evaluate the chance occurrence of the observed difference. When a difference exceeds chance expectations, the disease and the HLA antigen are considered associated. Diseases in which the frequency of one or more HLA phenotypes is significantly increased are called "HLA-associated" diseases. The detection of this type of association between an independently identified genetic marker and a disease suggests that inherited attributes of the patients predispose to the disease.

5.1. Disease Associations

The relative risk of a disease in individuals who possess an HLA phenotype provides a clinically useful formulation of this phenomenon (Svejgaard *et al.*,

1975). The relative risk of an HLA-associated disease can be estimated from the incidence of the HLA antigen in unrelated patients and in the general population from which the patients were drawn:

$$\text{relative risk} = f_p[1\text{-}f_c]/f_c[1\text{-}f_p]$$

The decimal fractions f_p and f_c represent the frequencies of the HLA antigen in patients and controls respectively. A large number of diseases are associated with specific HLA phenotypes. Table 1 summarizes the majority of known risks of nonmalignant HLA-associated diseases (Svejgaard and Ryder, 1977). Although the magnitude of the estimates of relative risk in Table 1 are small, each estimate is statistically significant. When a single disease is considered alone, most estimates of risk are relatively unimportant in the evaluation of the individual patient. An 88-fold increase in the risk of ankylosing spondylitis in individuals with HLA-B27 represents an important exception. Approximately 90% of patients with ankylosing spondylitis have HLA-B27. The detection of HLA-B27 can be used to corroborate the clinical diagnosis in instances of uncertainty.

Table 1 illustrates two clinically important aspects of HLA-associated diseases.

TABLE 1. Nonmalignant HLA Disease Associations[a]

	HLA antigens							
	A1	A2	A3	B7	B8	B13	B27	BW19
Pernicious anemia				2.2				
Paralytic poliomyelitis				1.9				
Multiple sclerosis		0.2	1.5	1.6				
Celiac disease	4.2			0.4				
Dermatitis herpetiformis	4.4				9.2			
Recurrent herpes labialis	3.7				2.5			
Chronic active hepatitis	1.8				3.0			
Myasthenia gravis	2.4			0.4	4.4			
Thyrotoxicosis					2.5			
Idiopathic Addison's disease					3.9			
Juvenile diabetes mellitus				0.5	2.1			
Idiopathic hemachromatosis			9.5		8.8			
Sjogren's sicca syndrome					3.2			
Psoriasis vulgaris				0.4	0.5	4.6		4.9
Psoriasis, nonspecific		1.5		0.4		3.9		5.4
Peripheral psoriatic arthritis						2.2	2.5	5.8
Central psoriatic arthritis						4.8	8.6	2.5
Rheumatoid arthritis							1.9	
Psoriasis, pustular							3.7	
Juvenile arthritis		1.9					4.7	
Acute anterior uveitis							15.4	
Salmonella arthritis							17.6	
Yersina arthritis		3.1					24.3	
Reiter's syndrome							35.9	
Ankylosing spondylitis		1.5		0.6	0.6		87.8	

[a] Adapted from Svejgaard and Ryder (1977). The data in this table account for 25 of the 31 (80%) HLA-associated nonmalignant diseases and 41 of the 68 (60%) statistically significant increases in relative risk. Significant decreases in relative risk are identified by ratios less than 1.0.

First, the HLA associations in Table 1 are arranged in clusters. A spectrum of diseases prevails among patients with a specific HLA phenotype. A high degree of relatedness may exist among diseases clustered in relation to a specific HLA phenotype. This suggests a common etiological or pathogenetic mechanism among these diseases. Second, varied diagnoses exist within each cluster of HLA-associated diseases. The particular clinical diagnosis is determined by factors other than those intimately related to the specific HLA antigen within each clustered group of diseases. This suggests that non-HLA-associated factors contribute to the clinical diversity of the clustered diseases.

HLA-B27 is associated with a large clustered group of unexplained inflammatory diseases (Table 1). These diseases include peripheral and central psoriatic arthritis, rheumatoid arthritis, pustular psoriasis, juvenile arthritis, acute anterior uveitis, salmonella and yersina arthritis, Reiter's syndrome, and ankylosing spondylitis. HLA-associated susceptibility to rheumatism or unexplained inflammation and destruction of connective tissue may provide a better clinical phenotype than the diagnosis of a specific rheumatic disease. This same deduction about mechanisms arose from Coca and Cooke's (1923) consideration of the basis of the immediate hypersensitivity diseases.

Another large group of diseases is associated with HLA-B8. Idiopathic hemachromatosis, dermatitis herpetiformis, chronic active hepatitis, recurrent herpes labialis, myasthenia gravis, idiopathic Addison's disease, Sjogren's sicca syndrome, and insulin-dependent diabetes mellitus make up the HLA-B8-associated group of diseases. Although exceptions exist, an apparent predilection for inflammation of glandular tissues best characterizes this group of diseases. Viruses can exhibit trophism for infection of glandular tissues. Herpes labialis is caused by a virus. A possible relationship exists between viral trophism for pancreatic tissue in juvenile diabetes mellitus (Gamble *et al.*, 1973). This same possibility has been considered important in idiopathic Addison's disease and in certain instances of polyglandular endocrinopathy (Eisenbarth *et al.*, 1978). Susceptibility to virus-induced inflammation of glandular tissues may provide a clinical phenotype for these diseases.

Another clinically important aspect of HLA-associated diseases is also illustrated in Table 1. A decrease in the relative risk of certain diseases (ratios less than 1.0) is associated with certain HLA antigens. The risk of celiac disease, myasthenia gravis, juvenile diabetes mellitus, psoriasis vulgaris, nonspecific psoriasis, and ankylosing spondylitis is decreased in HLA-B7 subjects. A decrease in the relative risk of an HLA-associated disease is more difficult to identify, but may be equally important. Both kinds of estimates of risk provide a basis for prospective patient evaluation.

The association of specific HLA phenotypes with an increase or decrease in the risk of a specific disease implies the possible enrichment of other HLA antigens in individuals who survive to the end of a normal life span. While this seems possible (Bender *et al.*, 1973; Gerkins *et al.*, 1974; Magurova *et al.*, 1975), available evidence suggests that selective effects of mortality on the late life enrichment specific HLA phenotypes can be identified only within populations exhibiting restricted genetic heterogeneity (Bender *et al.*, 1973; Magurova *et al.*, 1975). An enrichment of heterozygous individuals is a more prevalent finding in surviving older individuals (Gerkins *et al.*, 1974). This suggests the possible importance of hybrid vigor in survival.

Table 2 focuses on another aspect of decreased HLA relative risks. The relationships of estimates of risk to the respective control populations for each disease have been removed by calculating the ratios of relative risk applicable in a comparison of the two respective diseases. This comparison makes use of the estimates of decreased and increased risk to detect differences between the two diseases. When applied to clinical problems, this comparison can be more informative than the estimates of relative risk presented in Table 1. Assume that the clinical problem is a patient who presents with unexplained focal weakness. For purposes of illustration, assume that preliminary diagnostic studies have not been helpful and further studies are needed. The identification of HLA-B8 in the patient would suggest that studies of the function of the myoneural junction would be 5 times more likely to be helpful than studies focused on other neurological causes of weakness. Alternately, the identification of HLA-AW32 in the same patient

TABLE 2. Comparison of the Relative Risks of HLA Associations in Multiple Sclerosis and Myasthenia Gravis[a]

HLA	Multiple sclerosis	Myasthenia gravis
A1		2.41
A2		1.67
A3	3.26	
A9	1.55	
A10	1.00	1.00
A11	1.65	
A28		1.59
AW32	5.27	
B5		1.98
B7	3.69	
B8		5.14
B12	1.19	
B13	1.14	
B14	2.96	
B18	1.18	
B27		1.36
BW15		1.37
BW17	1.13	
BW35	1.82	
BW40	1.21	

[a] Adapted from Bertrams and Kuwert (1978) and Van den Berg-Loonen *et al.* (1977). The ratios presented were obtained by dividing the larger relative risk associated with either disease by the relative risk associated with the second disease. Only positive risks are shown.

would suggest that studies of the composition of the spinal fluid would be 5 times more likely to produce useful information. This formulation of risk in relation to a particular clinical situation is not apparent in the data presented in Table 1. Compared estimates of relative risk between plausible clinical alternatives provide a better basis for making clinical decisions.

Compared estimates of relative risk can be used in another important way. Uncertainty exists about the mechanisms responsible for HLA-associated diseases. Compared estimates of relative risk similar to those illustrated in Table 2 can be used to design experimental tests of postulated genetic mechanisms. A viral etiology has been suggested in patients with multiple sclerosis (Haire *et al.*, 1973). For purposes of illustration, assume that defective antiviral immunity is a valid hypothesis in multiple sclerosis and myasthenia gravis. Also assume that uncertainty exists about the relative importance of several viruses and the role of several kinds of immune mechanisms in the pathogenesis of each disease. The compared estimates of relative risk illustrated in Table 2 suggest that maximum genetic variation in immune function toward a panel of viruses would be expected in a two-way comparison between (1) multiple sclerosis patients and controls with HLA-AW32 and (2) myasthenia gravis patients and controls with HLA-B8. Useful deductions about hypothetical mechanisms and viruses could be made from comparisons of antiviral humoral and cellular immunity to each virus with this type of multifactoral two-way disease by control experimental design. The strength of this design stems from the *a priori* optimization of possible HLA-associated genetic variation and the selection of appropriate controls within the two compared levels of genetic stratification. A failure to find reliable experimental differences would provide reasonable evidence that a particular virus or immune mechanism is not responsible for the HLA association. Optimally designed studies of hypothetical genetic disease mechanisms can be based on comparisons of the relative risk between appropriately selected HLA-associated diseases.

5.2. Hypothetical Mechanisms

The possibility exists that immunogenetic and nonimmunogenetic mechanisms can contribute to the occurrence of HLA-associated diseases. Postulated immunogenetic mechanisms can be conveniently grouped in relation to the three mechanisms responsible for cognitive function. Polymorphisms can exist in (1) the transducer of the antigen-carrier stimulus, (2) the regulation of the channels through which the transduced signal is transmitted, and (3) the innate information selected on the basis of the content of the signal. Although the variability of HLA-associated diseases directs attention toward the potential diversity of structural genes as opposed to polymorphic variation in regulatory function, neither possibility can be excluded.

The first immunogenetic category includes polymorphisms responsible for the transduction of the antigen-carrier stimulus into a signal. This category includes defective Ir genes which permit a failure of immune protection and accelerated toxin-induced injury. Disease mechanisms in this category also include defective cell surface receptors which bind environmental substances without transducing a signal for an immune response. One plausible pathogenetic mechanism involved "molecular mimicry" between an invasive pathogen and host, leading to pathogen binding and facilitation of infection. Another possible mechanism involves binding of a noninfectious potential antigen, leading to "self-modification" of the cell surface and the induction of an autoaggressive immune response.

The second immunogenetic category includes polymorphisms regulating the transmission of the transduced signal within the immune system. This category includes hypothetical mechanisms responsible for the genetic control of differentiation antigens (Hood, 1978), immune cell cooperation (Shearer *et al.*, 1976; Zinkernagel and Doherty, 1975; Doherty *et al.*, 1976), enzyme generation, and production of products important in the metabolic support of cell proliferation and the immune response. Genetic mechanisms controlling the preferential production of reaginic antibodies and an augmented capacity for permease release are included in this general category. Conceptually, this type of hypothetical polymorphism is responsible for the general type of biological outcome of the immune response, as opposed to the degenerate selection of appropriate V-region genes on the basis of the content of the transduced signal.

The third immunogenetic category of polymorphic variation involves V-region genes. Even though the structural genes coding for the V regions of antibodies are not linked to HLA, the possibility exists that a deficiency in V-region genes could lead to an HLA-associated disease. A failure of immune function resulting from the lack of appropriate V-region genes would be expected to result in antigen persistence and continued transducer stimulation. Continued stimulation would be expected to lead to compensatory overactivity of less specific immune mechanisms controlled by genes linked to HLA. The most obvious clinical attribute of this hypothetical mechanism would be an apparently unexplained alteration in an HLA-associated immune function. Diseases characterized by unexplained inflammation and production of antibodies which bear little or no relationship to the disease process are included in this category. Defective V-region genes cannot be excluded as a possible cause of HLA-associated diseases.

Nonimmunogenetic mechanisms can also contribute to HLA-associated diseases. Allelic genes controlling the generation of complement components exist within the HLA complex (Agnella *et al.*, 1972; Alper *et al.*, 1972; Day *et al.*, 1973; Wolski *et al.*, 1975) and could contribute to variation in the inflammatory process. A recessive gene for 21-hydroxylase deficiency and congenital adrenal hyperplasia is closely linked to the HLA-B locus (Dupont *et al.*, 1977). A fascinating and clinically important pharmacogenetic polymorphism is also associated with the HLA complex. Atopic symptoms and HLA-B12 are both more common among children with the steroid-responsive nephrotic syndrome (Thomson *et al.*, 1976). HLA-B12 is associated with increased *in vitro* responsiveness to steroids. Mitogen-stimulated cultured lymphocytes from HLA-B12 patients with primary open-angle glaucoma are suppressed by a lower dose of prednisone than cells from HLA-B7 glaucoma patients and normal controls (Becker *et al.*, 1976). Both immunogenetic and nonimmunogenetic mechanisms could contribute to the occurrence of HLA-associated diseases.

5.3. Predictions and Prevention

Studies of disease associations in relation to other HLA loci suggest many of the estimates of risk in Table 1 can be improved. Certain disease associations appear more closely related to the D locus than to the A or B locus. Linkage disequilibrium between genes located near the D locus accounts for the improvement in estimates of relative risk. Recombination normally occurs between distant loci on homologous chromatids during meiosis. The frequency of crossing over and recombination between distant loci usually meets chance expectations and is said to exhibit linkage equilibrium. The closeness of the A, B, C, and D loci of the HLA complex prevents this type of random assortment of traits among progeny. These loci tend to segregate together during meiosis. This phenomenon is called "linkage disequilibrium." The degree of linkage disequilibrium is a measure of the closeness of the loci. Linkage disequilibrium between genes responsible for disease and the A and B loci probably accounts for most of the associations listed in Table 1. It is unlikely that the serologically detectable HLA alloantigens cause the disease. The finding that other loci lie closer to genes responsible for a disease is not unexpected. These additional loci provide a means for mapping the HLA complex. Because of this relationship among the loci of the HLA complex, the clinical determination of a complete HLA phenotype is likely to prove more useful in the ultimate care of patients than a serological assessment of alloantigens at a single locus.

For example, multiple sclerosis is more closely associated with a D locus mitogenic marker, the HLA-DW2 allele, than the A and B loci (Jersilid *et al.*, 1973). The apparent association between celiac disease and HLA-B8 in Table 1 is related to linkage disequilibrium between HLA-B8 and HLA-DW3 (Keuning *et al.*, 1976). Intrinsic or nonreaginic bronchial asthma appears associated with a high incidence of homozygosity at the HLA-CW6 locus, another serologically defined alloantigen (Brostoff *et al.*, 1976). Of interest, approximately half of the patients in this informative study had complement component defects, particularly involving C2.

An additional genetic marker, which segregates with genes located in the HLA complex, is expressed on B cells. These alloantigens are presumed to be analogous to the Ia alloantigens of the mouse. Between 80% and 90% of multiple sclerosis patients carry a unique alloantigen which is found on B lymphocytes (Compston *et al.*, 1976; Terasaki *et al.*, 1976). A closer association also exits between gluten-sensitive enteropathy and dermatitis herpetiformis and another B-cell alloantigen than the association between these diseases and HLA-B8 (Mann *et al.*, 1976). Finally, a close association has been reported between B-cell alloantigens and bronchial asthma (Rachelefsky *et al.*, 1976).

The current thrust toward identification and localization of additional genetic markers within the HLA complex seems likely to improve and extend our understanding of HLA-associated diseases. Refinements and better understanding of the mechanisms responsible for increased relative risk, along with technological improvements in automated immunoserology, may eventually enable prospective clinical appraisal of disease susceptibility in healthy subjects as well as in patients. The eventual goal of this understanding is preventive clinical intercession prior to the onset of disabling disease.

6. Human Immune Response Genes

Genetic controls of specific cognitive function exist in man. Human metabolic diseases provide evidence of genetic polymorphisms which control the biochemical recognition of specific substrates and generation of specific enzymes (Stanbury *et al.*, 1972). The inheritance of taste perception for phenylthiocarbamide and the visual perception of specific wavelengths of light is well documented (Thomas, 1973). Genetic differences also exist in the perception of odors (Patterson and Lauder, 1948; Whissell-Buechy and Amoore, 1973). This observation assumes new importance because of the recent report of a possible role of the H-2 complex on mating behavior in experimental animals (Yamazaki *et al.*, 1976). Much evidence suggests that similar, less easily defined genetic mechanisms control the cognitive function of the human immune system.

Immunogenetic studies in man lack the simplistic clarity and high degree of experimental predictability inherent in studies of inbred animals. Controversy exists about the value of immunogenetic inquiries in man. This uncertainty stems from reservations about the applicability of available methods for the study of complex human immunogenetic mechanisms. Although exceptions may exist, methods applicable to the study of traits coded by monogenic loci are not applicable to the multifactorial complexity of human immunity. Improved models and methods are needed. The resolution of this uncertainty will depend on the reproducibility of the predictions provided by methods applicable to multifactorial problems and the eventual reconciliation of these methods with formal analysis of the segregation and linkage of complex human traits.

Early speculations about the inheritance of tuberculosis (Spencer, 1888) and susceptibility to diphtheria (Hirszfeld and Hirszfeld, 1928) antedated past studies of the familial prevalence of atopy (Coca and Cooke, 1923; Ratner and Silberman, 1952) and of drug (Polak and Turk, 1969) and contact hypersensitivity (Walker *et al.*, 1967; Forsbeck *et al.*, 1971). These early reports identified illnesses associated with an interesting source of variation in the immune response. Although a role of heredity was suggested in reports of early family studies, this possibility remained unexplored for many years. Recent work has not excluded the postulated role of genetic mechanisms. Prior studies of the familial prevalence of allergic and infectious diseases provide useful leads for the study of human immune response polymorphisms.

Because of ethical limitations on the experimental use of immunization in man, variability in natural immunity provides the best available opportunity for immunogenetic studies of large numbers of people. This opportunity is handicapped by an important assumption which is implicit in genetic studies of immunity to ubiquitous pollens, common microorganisms, and other antigens responsible for natural immunity. Studies of polymorphic variation in natural immunity are based on the assumption that the magnitude of the individual's response is limited by the ability to respond as opposed to the probability of prior antigen exposure. While this assumption is plausible for pollens and for many common microorganisms, a certain knowledge of prior exposure exists only in studies of the response to ethical antigens and known infection.

The uncertainty about prior antigen exposure in clinical studies of natural immunity may be more than compensated by other important considerations. The possibility exists that important immune response polymorphisms may be more easily detected in studies of natural immunity. Two logical considerations support this suggestion. First, selective evolutionary pressures would be expected to operate on genetic differences in natural specific adaptive immunity and not on the response to artificial immunization. Intuitively, genetic mechanisms capable of providing protection following repetitive minimal natural antigen exposure are probably necessary for the survival of a healthy breeding population. If this reasonable assumption is valid, a high incidence of polymorphic variation in natural immunity is most likely to be found in immunogenetic studies of natural immunity in relation to disease.

Second, a proportionate relationship exists between the magnitude of the antigen stimulus and the recruitment of available genes and gene products yielding the response phenotype. Large doses of antigen are likely to recruit a complex degenerate response coded by a larger number of V-region genes. This type of response is inefficient in that it diminishes the organism's opportunity to selectively invest energy in the generation of the most specific responsive function. It seems plausible to suggest that unique immune transducer polymorphisms may be more detectable at the lower limits of antigen stimulation and induced responsiveness. These considerations and the prevalence of natural low-dose exposure to pollens and common microorganisms provide a strong rationale for studies of the genetic control of natural immunity in man.

6.1. Allergic Diseases

Studies of the familial prevalence of the atopic diseases span more than six decades (Coca and Cooke, 1923). Early assessments of possible genetic mechanisms were limited to the use of the clinical diagnosis as a phenotype (Ratner and Silberman, 1952). Although a variety of genetic mechanisms have been postulated, most critical assessments of observations suggest a recessive mode of inheritance (Wiener *et al.*, 1935; Tips, 1954; Van Arsdel and Motulsky, 1959). Postulated recessive genetic mechanisms have varied from a single gene with irregular expressivity of atopy in the heterozygous individual (Wiener *et al.*, 1935) through three gene pairs with alleles coding, respectively, for asthma, hay fever, and atopic eczema (Tips, 1954). The most recent critical assessment reconciled available observations with either an incompletely recessive gene or a polygenic mode of inheritance (Van Arsdel and Motulsky, 1959). In addition to problems related to the inadequacy of the clinical phenotype, the estimates of gene frequencies in these studies may be at risk because of the bias induced by the socioeconomic status of allergic individuals (Barbee *et al.*, 1976) in samples composed of college students and families gleaned from private practice.

6.2. Immunoglobulin E

A recessive mode of inheritance is also suggested by studies of IgE levels in families. Studies of IgE levels in normal infants and mothers (Bazaral *et al.*, 1971), twins (Kalff and Hijmans, 1969), and families (Turner *et al.*, 1974) have consistently revealed a high degree of heritability. A closer relationship exists between serum IgE levels in parents and progeny of the opposite sex than of the same sex (Turner *et al.*, 1974). A similar relationship has been described for serum IgM concentrations (Grundbacher, 1972, 1974) and suggests that sex-linked genetic mechanisms may control the inheritance of serum levels of IgM and IgE.

Serum IgE levels exhibit a bimodal distribution. This distribution has been used to identify plausible phenotypes which reveal a recessive mode of inheritance when compared to serum IgE levels in families (Marsh *et al.*, 1974). The recessive gene coding for high serum levels of IgE segregates independently of the HLA complex. A path and segregation analysis of similar observations in a large number of families has confirmed the high heritability of serum levels of IgE and provided evidence of significant polygenic heritability in addition to a major recessive regulatory gene which codes for high serum levels of IgE (Gerrard and Morton, 1978). When viewed from the perspective of the cognitive function of the immune system, these observations suggest the existence of a recessive regulatory gene which channels immune system signals into the production of IgE.

6.3. Allergen Response Polymorphisms

A large number of HLA-associated responses have been detected in studies of families and patient populations (DeWeck *et al.*, 1977). The deduction that HLA-linked immune response genes account for these associations is based on family studies. Population studies provide less compelling evidence of HLA-linked Ir genes, but can be used to extend information about possible polymorphisms associated with the HLA complex. The first evidence of the existence of HLA-linked human Ir genes was detected with a ragweed pollen allergen. Studies in a remarkable series of seven ragweed hay fever families revealed a highly significant association between intense cutaneous wheal-and-flare responses to a purified antigen from ragweed pollen (antigen E) and the HLA haplotypes shared by family members (Levine *et al.*, 1972). Responder family members also had IgG antibodies to the same purified antigen. Skin tests with relatively impure cat dander and timothy grass allergens revealed no evidence of an HLA haplotype association. The HLA haplotype associated responses detected in these seven families were associated with seven different haplotypes. This suggested a low level of linkage disequilibrium between an Ir gene for antigen E and the HLA complex.

Studies in an extended family, composed of related nuclear families, revealed evidence of a similar association between cutaneous responses to ragweed antigen E and a different HLA haplotype (Blumenthal *et al.*, 1974). On the basis of one identified and two assumed HLA recombinant or "transmitter" family members, the postulated ragweed immune response gene appeared closely linked to the HLA-B locus. This report has been criticized because of the lack of a formal analysis of linkage and the postulated recombinant individuals or "transmitters" of ragweed hypersensitivity (Bias and Marsh, 1975). An extension of these studies based on an analysis of the HLA-D locus of recombinant family members suggests the postulated "Ir E" gene lies outside the D locus (Yunis *et al.*, 1975). A formal assessment of the linkage of Ir E has been presented (Blumenthal *et al.*, 1977). The existance of an HLA-linked gene controlling the response to purified ragweed antigen E in certain informative families seems plausible.

A simultaneous evaluation of the magnitude of responses to several closely related antigens can be much more informative than the evaluation of responses to single antigens (Figure 7). A multivariate assessment of the magnitude of reaginic skin test responses to fungal and bacterial antigens in three informative families also failed to exclude a close association between genes controlling several cutaneous allergen responses and the HLA haplotypes of family members (Buckley *et al.*, 1973). In a related simpler analysis (Figure 6) of the magnitude of individual skin test responses and serum antibody titers to viruses, the existence of HLA-linked Ir genes could not be excluded in a fourth family. While this method of analysis is not capable of identifying high and low responses associated with HLA haplotypes in two-generation nuclear families, it has the advantage of being clinically applicable to the evaluation of small unique informative families (Buckley and Roseman, 1976).

A close association can also be detected between HLA antigens and allergen responses in patient populations. An association has been described between cutaneous hypersensitivity to a second purified ragweed allergen (Ra5) and HLA-B7 in a group of highly allergic individuals (Marsh *et al.*, 1973). Although a few of these subjects had received immunotherapy and specificity controls were lacking, this response association is probably specific; HLA-B7 patients tend to exhibit decreased wheal-and-flare responses when tested with a large number of control allergens (Buckley *et al.*, 1977). A selective comparison of cutaneous responses and HLA phenotypes among individuals with low serum IgE levels has revealed a close association between HLA-A2 and B12 and responses to a third purified ragweed pollen allergen (Ra3) (Marsh *et al.*, 1977). In a related study, the cutaneous response to a purified allergen from rye grass (Rye I) was found associated with HLA-B8 and A1 (Marsh and Bias, 1977). No evidence of an immune response polymorphism to ragweed antigen E was detected in these studies. Response polymorphisms were detectable only among individuals with serum IgE levels in the lowest quartile of the normal range. These findings are also consistent with a role of a recessive IgE regulator gene in the facilitated expression of many V-region genes in reaginic antibodies. This same phenomenon could also account for the large amount of IgE that can be adsorbed from the sera of certain individuals with specific allergens such as antigen E (Gleich and Jacob, 1975). The presence of homozygous recessive regulatory genes permitting the clonal expansion of many populations of IgE antibodies could obscure the expression of HLA-linked transducer genes. An assessment of the individual's overall ability to mount a reaginic response is an appropriate covariable in studies of HLA-associated allergen responses.

Analyses of cutaneous responses in a pseudopopulation composed of members of healthy, closely related Amish families with an extended multivariate regression model (Roseman *et al.*, 1976) suggest that HLA-associated responses can also be detected by direct skin tests with a large number of conventional skin test allergens. Severe allergic disorders were not prevalent in this population. A large number of cutaneous hyperresponders were not detected. Scratch tests were used to induce and measure the size of the wheal-and-flare response to panel of 40 allergens. Replicate measures of the flare responses induced by scratch tests with the same dose and allergen in the same individual at different times have a coefficient of variation of 3–5%. This reproducibility compares with a minimum coefficient of variation of 7% based on estimates to the nearest 0.5 log unit in a 7-log-unit range in intradermal endpoint titrations (Marsh and Bias, 1977) and a coefficient of variation of 17–21% in the *in vitro* RAST inhibition assay (Yman *et al.*, 1975). The direct skin test remains the most reliable investigative tool in studies of reaginic hypersensitivity. In the analysis of responses to scratch tests, all HLA-A and -B locus tissue antigens in the population were simultaneously used as independent genetic markers. The between-HLA antigen response variation was significantly greater than the within-HLA antigen response variation. Inspection of the multivariate statistics suggested that cross-reacting components of the measured responses to the panel of allergens accounted for the response associations.

A second sample of the same population was studied with the same allergens several months later. At the time of the second study, potential subjects with seasonal hay fever had gone as a group to a clinic in a nearby state for treatment. Skin tests in remaining untested volunteers were accomplished and a multivariate analysis was made of these observations. A large number of the same response associations was detected. This suggests that the observed response associations were reproducible (Table 3). Like the simple regression model illustrated in Figure 6, this method of analysis does not provide estimates of levels of responsiveness associated with specific HLA antigens; available estimates are limited by the degree to which cross-reacting responses account for the multivariate assessment. Despite this limitation, this observation suggests analyses of responses to relatively impure allergens can be informative. A prior assessment of HLA-associated responsiveness to crude allergens avoids the biochemical isolation of uninteresting purified allergens. The allergens listed in Table 3 provide a source of information

TABLE 3. HLA-Associated Allergen Scratch Test Responses[a]

	Sample 1	Sample 2
Families	8	11
Subjects	62	98
Associated with A locus[b]	Blue grass Orchard grass[c] Russian thistle Cottonwood[c]	Red oak Red maple
HLA-A phenotypes	1,2,11,28,29,W32	1,2,3,9,10,11,28,29
Associated with both loci	Sage Staphylococcus Sheep sorrell[c] Hormodendrum[c]	Corn pollen[c] Marsh elder Black walnut Aspergillus Trichophytin Hormodendrum[c]
HLA-B phenotypes	5,7,8,12,27,W17, W35,blank	5,7,8,12,27,W15, W17,W35,W40,blank
Associated with B locus[b]	Corn pollen[c] Short ragweed[c] Cocklebur River birch White ash Mimosa Lambs quarter[c]	Orchard grass[c] Sweet vernal Red top grass Sheep sorrel[c] Plantain Lambs quarter[c] Alfalfa Short ragweed[c] Cottonwood[c] American beech

[a] The tabled allergen responses did not segregate independently of the HLA phenotypes in univariate analysis ($P<.05$) in two sequential samples of a population composed of closely related Amish families.
[b] Hotelling T2 trace $P<.0001$, Wilkes ratio not significant.
[c] HLA-associated responses in both subject samples.

for possible investigative studies. This type of analysis can be used to identify allergens for biochemical purification and use as probes in subsequent inquiries. Possible relationships between genes controlling responses to a few of these allergens and the HLA complex are summarized in Figure 8. These relationships are based on the inability to exclude independent assortment of the responses to the allergens with respect to one or another HLA locus.

Genetic factors are also important in contact allergy. A familial aggregation of contact hypersensitivity to dinitrochlorobenzene and paranitrosodimethylaniline has been detected in prospectively sensitized and challenged family members (Walker *et al.*, 1967). A dependent relationship was detected between the ability to become sensitized to the two contact allergens. A high incidence of atopy (atopic dermatitis, asthma, hay fever) has been reported among the daughters of male probands with contact dermatitis and among contact allergen reactors who did not have active dermatitis (Forsbeck *et al.*, 1971). This pattern shares similarities with the inheritance of high serum IgE levels and suggests a possible role of sex-linked genetic factors in contact dermitits.

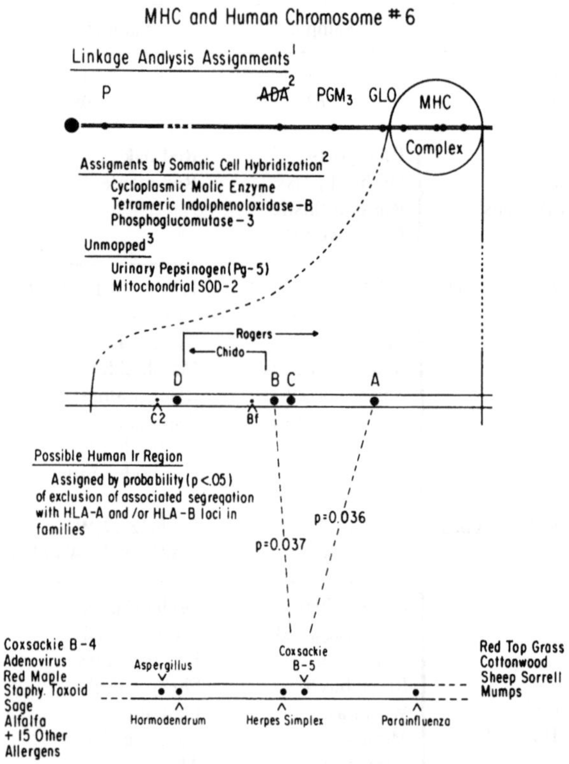

Figure 8. Configuration of some of the genes located on human chromosome 6. The relative certainty of the relationships decreases from the top to the bottom of the figure (see text). The relative location of the postulated loci controlling antibody responses to viruses and the reaginic responses to fungi and pollen allergens are based on the exclusion of independent segregation with either the HLA-A, HLA-B, or both loci by multivariate analysis of observations in pseudopopulations composed of closely related families. [1]Edwards *et al.* (1973). [2]Gerald and Bruns (1975). [3]Bijnen *et al.* (1976).

Hypersensitivity is an important part of most infections. Conversely, infection frequently complicates allergic respiratory diseases. Virus infections can potentiate the responsive state associated with allergic disorders (Hall *et al.*, 1978; Little *et al.*, 1978). The antigenic products of microorganisms can act as allergens and/or induce immune protection. A role of genetic mechanisms controlling the host's response to microbiological antigens is another aspect of the genetics of allergy. HLA-associated responses to microbiological antigens have also been detected.

Stimulation of cultured lymphocytes with optimal doses of streptococcal antigens reveals a close association between hyporesponsiveness and HLA-B5 (Greenberg *et al.*, 1975). Delayed cutaneous responses to a standard dose of tuberculin are decreased in HLA-B7 BCG-treated melanoma patients (Buckley *et al.*, 1977). Family studies of dimorphic leprosy revealed an increase in the segregation of similar HLA haplotypes among siblings who share the same kind of leprosy and decreased segregation of similar haplotypes among siblings with different dimorphic forms of leprosy (DeVries *et al.*, 1976).

Genetic factors have been detected in studies of the serum antibody titer to measles vaccine and diphtheria toxoid in monozygotic and dizygotic twins (Haverkorn *et al.*, 1975). Evidence of possible linkage with HLA was detected with the response to the measles vaccine. An association has been detected between an HLA-D allele (DHO) and hyporesponsiveness to immunization with diphtheria toxoid in healthy Japanese medical students (Sasazuki *et al.*, 1978). Following measles virus vaccination, children with HLA-B14 and BW22 had higher geometric mean titers than other recipients of the vaccine; HLA-A28 was detected in four of nine children with the highest anti-measles virus titers, and HLA-B12 and BW17 were detected in three of six children who did not undergo seroconversion (Spencer *et al.*, 1977). An increased response to vaccination with influenza type A virus has been described in HLA-BW16 individuals (Spencer *et al.*, 1976). These observations suggest that HLA-associated responses can be detected following immunization with ethical antigens. Family studies of the response to immunization with ethical antigens are feasible.

Apparent antibody-mediated polymorphisms can also be detected following other types of antigen exposure. Among insulin-dependent diabetics, HLA-BW15 is associated with generation of high levels of antibody activity to insulin. Hyporesponsiveness is associated with the presence of HLA-B8 and absence of HLA-B7 (Bertrams *et al.*, 1976; Bertrams and Gruneklee, 1977). The prevalence and magnitude of antibody titers to gluten and milk antigens are associated with HLA-B8 in patients with various diseases and in healthy controls (Scott *et al.*, 1974). When both antibodies are considered together, good discrimination between B8 and non-B8 individuals is possible. Studies in informative families are needed to clarify the genetic mechanisms responsible for these potential immune response polymorphisms.

Finally, alleleic genes coding for various complement components important in infection are also linked to HLA. Linkage relationships have been defined for C2 (Wolski *et al.*, 1975; Fu *et al.*, 1975), properidin factor B (Bf) (Rittner *et al.*, 1975), and C4 (Raum *et al.*, 1976; Ochs *et al.*, 1977) in family studies.

Collectively, these studies suggest that it is not possible to exclude the existence of HLA-linked immune response genes to allergens and other natural antigens. Potentially important polymorphisms can be detected with ethical antigens. A summary of available information about the possible configuration of the human major histocompatibility complex (Bijnen *et al.*, 1976) is presented in Figure 8. Several levels of confidence in the postulated linkage relationships are illustrated. The assignments at the top of the figure are based on conventional methods for the analysis of possible genetic mechanisms. The postulated relationships at the bottom of the figure are based on less conventional methods of assessment of genetic probabilities.

Conventional genetic methods of probability analysis clearly offer the most confidence in the assignment of linkage relationships. The relative reliability of these methods must be balanced against their applicability to the particular human immunogenetic trait. Hazards exist in the use of both conventional and unconventional methods of analysis. For example, a Lod score analysis of possible genetic markers in relation to HLA suggested that the gene coding for adenosine deaminase was closely linked to HLA (Edwards *et al.,* 1973). This result could not be confirmed by studies of somatic cell hybridization (Gerald and Bruns, 1975). An element of uncertainty exists in all probability methods of analysis of the segregation and linkage of genetic traits. Studies of the expression of gene products at a cellular level provide the most reliable way to avoid this problem.

Available evidence of the existence of HLA-linked immune response genes in man consists of repetitive ability to reject the independent segregation of immune responsiveness and genetic markers in informative families and populations. Although the current findings in man are not so extensive as in experimental animals, the possibility that these observations do not represent human HLA-linked immune response genes is remote. Further studies of human families and populations are likely to resolve current uncertainties and lead to the development of methods applicable to the study of many complex genetic problems. Ultimately, these relationships may help guide prospective efforts for prevention of allergic and immunological diseases.

7. References

Agnella, V., deBarco, M. M. E., and Kunkle, H. G., 1972, Hereditary C2 deficiency with some manifestations of systemic lupus erythematosus, *J. Immunol.* **108**:837–840.

Allen, D. H., Basten, A., Woolcock, A. J., and Guinan, J., 1977, HLA and bird breeder's hypersensitivity pneumonitis, *Monogr. Allergy* **11**:45–54.

Alper, C. A., Colten, H. R., Rosen, F. S., Rabson, A. R., McNab, G., and Gear, J. S. S., 1972, Homozygous deficiency of the third component of complement (3) in a patient with repeated infections, *Lancet* **2**:1179–1181.

Amos, D. B., Cabrera, G., Bias, W. B., MacQueen, M., Lancaster, S., Southworth, J., and Ward, F. E., 1970, The inheritance of human leukocyte antigens. III. The organization of specificities, in: *Histocompatibility Testing*, pp. 259–275, Munksgaard, Copenhagen.

Anderson, J. A., 1973, A theory for the recognition of items from short memorized lists, *Psychol. Rev.* **30**:417–438.

Barbee, R. A., Lebowitz, M. D., Thompson, H. C., and Burrows, B., 1976, Immediate skin test reactivity in a general population sample, *Ann. Intern. Med.* **84**:129–133.

Barcinski, M. A., and Rosenthal, A. S., 1977, Immune response gene control of determinant selection. I. Intramolecular mapping of the immunogenic sites on insulin recognized by guinea pig T and B cells, *J. Exp. Med.* **145**:726–742.

Barter, C. E., and Campbell, A. H., 1976, Relationship of constitutional factors and cigarette smoking to decrease in 1-second forced expiratory volume, *Am. Rev. Respir. Dis.* **113**:305–314.

Bazaral, M., Orgel, H. A., and Hamburger, R. N., 1971, IgE levels in normal infants and mothers and an inheritance hypothesis, *J. Immunol.* **107**:794–801.

Becker, B., Shin, D. H., Palmberg, P. F., and Waltman, S. R., 1976, HLA antigens and corticosteroid response, *Science* **194**:1427–1428.

Benacerraf, B., and Dorf, M. E., 1974, Genetic control of specific immune responses, in: *Proceedings of the Second International Congress of Immunology*, Vol. 2 (E. J. Holbrow and L. Brent, eds.), pp. 181–190, Elsevier, New York.

Benacerraf, B., Green, I., and Paul, W. E., 1967, The immune response to hapten-poly-L-lysine conjugates as an example of the genetic control of the recognition of antigenicity, *Cold Spring Harbor Symp. Quant. Biol.* **32**:569–575.

Bender, K., Ruter, G., Mayerova, A., and Hiller, C., 1973, Studies on the heterozygosity at the HLA gene loci in young and old individuals, in: *International Symposium on HL-A Reagents* (R. H. Ragsmey and J. V. Sprack, eds.), pp. 287–290, Karger, Basel.

Bertrams, H. J., and Gruneklee, D., 1977, Association between HLA-B27 and allergic reactions to insulin in insulin-dependent diabetes mellitus, *Tissue Antigens* **10**:273–277.

Bertrams, H. J., and Kuwert, E. K., 1978, Association of histocompatibility haplotype HLA-A3-B7 with multiple sclerosis, *J. Immunol.* **117**:1906–1912.

Bertrams, H. J., Jansen, F. K., Gruneklee, D., Reis, H. E., Drost, H., Beyer, J., Gries, F. A., and Kuwert, E., 1976, HLA antigens and immunoresponsiveness to insulin in insulin-dependent diabetes mellitus, *Tissue Antigens* **8**:13–19.

Berzofsky, J. A., 1978, Genetic control of the immune response to mammalian myoglobins in mice. I. More than one I-region gene in H-2 controls the antibody response, *J. Immunol.* **120**:360–369.

Berzofsky, J. A., Schecter, A. N., Shearer, G. M., and Sachs, D. H., 1977a, Genetic control of the immune response to staphylococcal nuclease. III. Time-course and correlation between the response to native nuclease and the response to its native polypeptide fragments, *J. Exp. Med.* **145**:111–122.

Berzofsky, J. A., Schechter, A. N., Shearer, G. M., and Sachs, D. H., 1977b, Genetic control of the immune response to staphylococcal nuclease. IV. H-2-linked control of the relative proportions of antibodies produced to different determinants of native nuclease, *J. Exp. Med.* **145**:123–135.

Bias, W. B., and Marsh, D. G., 1975, HLA linked antigen E immune response genes: An unproved hypothesis, *Science* **188**:375–377.

Bijnen, A. B., Schreader, I., Khan, P. M., Allen, F. H., Giles, C. M., Los, W. R. T., Volkers, W. S., and Van Rood, J. J., 1976, Linkase relationships of the loci of the major histocompatibility complex in families with a recombination in the HLA region, *J. Immunogenet.* **3**:171–183.

Bleux, C., Ventura, M., and Liacpoulos, P., 1977, IgM-IgG switch-over among antibody forming cells in the mouse, *Nature (London)* **267**:709–711.

Blumberg, B. S., Geckler, W. R., and Weigart, M., 1972, Genetics of the antibody response to dextrans in mice, *Science* **177**:178–180.

Blumenthal, M. N., Amos, D. B., Noreen, H., Mendell, N. R., and Yunis, E. J., 1974, Genetic mapping of Ir locus in man. Linkage to second locus of HLA, *Science* **184**:1301–1303.

Blumenthal, M. N., Mendell, N. R., Yunis, E., Amos, D. B., Muscoplat, C., and Elston, R. C., 1977, HLA and ragweed allergy, *Monogr. Allergy* **11**:83–88.

Brandt, D. C., and Jaton, J.-C., 1978a, Occurrence of idiotypically identical antibodies in the sera of two outbred rabbits hyperimmunized with type II pneumonococcal vaccine, *J. Immunol.* **121**:1188–1193.

Brandt, D. C., and Jaton, J.-C., 1978b, Identical VI region sequences of two antibodies from two outbred rabbits exhibiting complete idiotypic cross-reactivity and probably the same antigen binding site fine structure, *J. Immunol.* **121**:1194–1198.

Brostoff, J., Mowbray, J. F., Kapoor, A., Hollowell, S., Rudolf, M., and Saunders, K. B., 1976, 80% of patients with intrinsic asthma are homozygous for HLA W6, *Lancet* **2**:872–873.

Buckley, C. E., and Roseman, J. M., 1976, Immunity and survival, *J. Am. Geriatr. Soc.* **24**:241–248.

Buckley, C. E., Dorsey, F. C., Corley, R. B., Ralph, W. B., Woodbury, M. A., and Amos, D. B., 1973, HLA linked immune response genes, *Proc. Natl. Acad. Sci. USA.* **70**:2157–2161.

Buckley, C. E., White, D. H., and Seigler, H. F., 1977, HLA-B7 associated tuberculin hyporesponsiveness in BCG treated melanoma patients, *Monogr. Allergy* **11**:97–105.

Capra, J. D., and Kehoe, J. M., 1975, Hypervariable regions, idiotypy and the antibody combining site, *Adv. Immunol.* **20**:1–40.

Carroll, J. D., and Wish, M., 1974, Multidimensional perceptual models and measurement methods in: *Handbook of Perception, Psychophysical Judgement and Measurement*, Vol. 3 (E. C. Carterette and M. P. Friedman, eds.), pp. 391–447, Academic, New York.

Carterette, E. C., and Friedman, M. P., eds, 1973-76. *Handbook of Perception*, Vols. 1–6, Academic, New York.

Chafee, F. H., and Settipane, G. A., 1974, Aspirin intolerance. I. Frequency in an allergic population, *J. Allergy Clin. Immunol.* **53**:193–199.

Chase, M. W., 1941, Inheritance in guinea pigs of the susceptibility to skin sensitization with simple chemical compounds, *J. Exp. Med.* **73**:711–726.

Chiorazzi, N., Fox, D. A., and Katz, D. H., 1977, Hapten-specific IgE antibody responses in mice. VII. Conversion of IgE "non-responder" strains to IgE "responders" by elimination of suppressor T cell activity, *J. Immunol.* **118**:48–54.

Coca, A. F., 1920, Hypersensitiveness, anaphylaxis and allergy, *J. Immunol.* **5**:363–372.

Coca, A. F., and Cooke, R. A., 1923, On the classification of the phenomena on hypersensitization, *J. Immunol.* **8**:163–182.

Compston, D. A. S., Batchelor, J. R., and McDonald, W. I., 1976, B-lymphocyte alloantigens associated with multiple sclerosis, *Lancet* **2**:1261–1265.

Cooke, R. A., and Vander Veer, A., 1916, Human sensitization, *J. Immunol.* **1**:201–205.

Coutinho, A., and Moller, G., 1975, Thymus-independent B-cell induction and paralysis, *Adv. Immunol.* **21**:114–236.

David, C. C., 1976, Serologic and genetic aspects of murine Ia antigens, *Transplant. Rev.* **30**:299–322.

Day, N. E., and Simons, M. J., 1976, Disease susceptibility genes—their identification by multiple case family studies, *Tissue Antigens* **8**:109–119.

Day, N. K., Geiger, H., Michael, R., and Good, R. A., 1973, C2 deficiency. Development of lupus erythematosus, *J. Clin. Invest.* **52**:1601–1607.

Deutsch, J. A., and Deutsch, D., 1963, Attention: Some theoretical considerations, *Psychol. Rev.* **70**:80–90.

DeVries, R. R. P., Fat, R. F. M. L. A., Nijenhuis, L. E., and Van Rood, J. J., 1976, HLA linked genetic control of host response to *Mycobacterium leprae, Lancet* **2**:1328–1330.

DeWeck, A. L., Blumenthal, M. N., Jeannet, M., and Yunis, E. L., 1977, HLA and allergy, in: *HLA and Disease* (J. Dauset, ed.), Munksgaard, Copenhagen.

Dickler, H. D., and Sachs, D. H., 1974, Evidence for identity or close association of the Fc receptor of B-lymphocytes and alloantigens determined by the Ir region of the H-2 complex, *J. Exp. Med.* **140**:779–796.

Dickler, H. D., Kubicek, M. T., Arbeit, R. D., and Shanow, S. O., 1978, Studies of the nature of the relationship between Ia antigens and Fc receptors on murine lymphocytes, *J. Immunol.* **119**:348–354.

Di Pauli, R., 1973, Genetics of the immune response. II. Inheritance of antibody specificity to lipopolysaccharides in mice, *J. Immunol.* **111**:82–84.

Doherty, P. C., Blanden, R. V., and Zinkernagel, R. M., 1976, Specificity of virus immune effector T cells for H-2k or H-2d compatible interactions: Implications for H antigen diversity, *Transplant. Rev.* **29**:89–124.

Dorf, M. E., Newburger, P. E., Hamoka, T., Katz, D. H., and Benacerraf, B., 1974a, Characterization of an immune response gene in mice controlling IgE and IgG antibody responses to ragweed pollen extract and its 2,4-dinitrophenylated derivative, *Eur. J. Immunol.* **4**:346–349.

Dorf, M. E., Balner, H., de Groot, M. L., and Benacerraf, B., 1974b, Histocompatibility-linked immune response genes in the rhesus monkey, *Transplant. Proc.* **6**:119–123.

Dupont, B., Oberfield, S. E., Smithwick, E. M., Lee, T. D., and Levine, L. S., 1977, Close genetic linkage between HLA and congenital adrenal hyperplasia (21-hydroxylase deficiency), *Lancet* **2**:1309–1312.

Ebringer, A., Deacon, N. J., and Young, C. R., 1976, Codominant inheritance in immunogenetic (Ir gene) systems, *J. Immunogenet.* **3**:401–409.

Edelman, G. M., and Mountcastle, V. B., 1978, *The Mindful Brain*, MIT Press, Cambridge, Mass.

Edwards, J. H., Allen, F. H., Glenn, K. P., Lamm, L. U., and Robson, E. B., 1973, The linkage relationships of HL-A in: *Histocompatibility Testing, 1972* (J. Dausset and J. Colombani, eds.), pp. 745–751, Munksgaard, Copenhagen.

Eisenbarth, G., Wilson, P., Ward, F., and Lebovitz, H. E., 1978, HLA type and occurrence of disease in familial polyglandular failure, *N. Engl. J. Med.* **298**:92–94.

Elston, R. C., and Rao, D. C., 1978, Statistical modeling and analysis in human genetics, *Annu. Rev. Biophys. Bioeng.* **7**:253–286.

Erb, P., and Feldmann, M., 1975, The role of macrophages in the generation of helper T-cells. II. The genetic control of the macrophage-T-cell interaction for helper cell induction with soluble antigens, *J. Exp. Med.* **142**:460–472.

Fathman, C. G., Pisetsky, D. S., and Sachs, D. H., 1977, Genetic control of the immune response to nuclease. V. Genetic linkage and strain distribution of anti-nuclease idiotypes, *J. Exp. Med.* **145**:569–577.

Felsenstein, J., 1977, Multivariate normal genetic models with a finite number of loci, in: *Proceedings of the International Conference on Quantitative Genetics* (E. Pollak, O. Kempthorne, and T. B. Bailey, eds.), pp. 227–246, Iowa State University Press, Ames.

Fink, M. A., and Quinn, V. A., 1953, Antibody production in inbred strains of mice, *J. Immunol.* **70**:61–67.

Fisher, R. A., 1918, The correlations between relatives on the supposition of Mendelian inheritance, *Trans. R. Soc. Edinburgh* **52**:399–433.

Forsbeck, M., Skog, K., and Ytterborn, K. H., 1971, Allergic diseases among relatives of patients with allergic contact dermatitis, *Acta Dermatol.* **51**:123–128.

Fromkin, V., 1971, The non-anomalous nature of anomalous utterances, in: *Speech Errors as Linguistic Evidence* (V. Fromkin, ed.), Mouton, The Hague.

Fu, S. M., Stern, R., and Kunkel, H. G., 1975, Mixed lymphocyte culture determinants and C2 deficiency: LD-7a associated with C2 deficiency in four families, *J. Exp. Med.* **142**:495–506.

Gamble, D. R., Taylor, K. W., and Cumming, H., 1973, Coxsackie viruses and diabetes mellitus, *Br. Med. J.* **4**:260–262.

Gearhart, P. J., Sigal, N. H., and Klinman, N. R., 1975, Production of antibodies of identical idiotype but diverse immunoglobulin classes by cells derived from a single stimulated B cell, *Proc. Natl. Acad. Sci. USA* **72**:1707–1711.

Gerald, P. S., and Bruns, G. A., 1975, Human chromosome mapping by somatic cell hybridization, in: *Combined Immunodeficiency and Adenosine Deaminase Deficiency* (H. J. Meuwissen, R. J. Pickering, B. Pollara, and I. H. Porter, eds.), pp. 91–101, Academic, New York.

Gerkins, V. R., Ting, A., Menck, H. T., Casagrande, J. T., Terasaki, P. I., Pike, M. C., and Henderson, B. E., 1974, HL-A heterozygosity as a marker of long term survival, *J. Natl. Cancer Inst.* **52**:1909–1911.

Germain, R. N., Dorf, M. E., and Benacerraf, B., 1975, Inhibition of T-lymphocyte-mediated tumor specific lysis by alloantisera directed against the H-2 serological specificities of the tumor, *J. Exp. Med.* **142**:1023–1028.

Gerrard, J. W., and Morton, R., 1978, A genetic study of immunoglobulin E, *Am. J. Human Genet.* **30**:46–58.

Gleich, G. J., and Jacob, G. L., 1975, Immunoglobulin E antibodies to pollen allergens account for high percentages of total immunoglobulin E protein, *Science* **190**:1106–1108.

Godfrey, S., and Konig, P., 1975, Exercise-induced bronchial lability in wheezing children and their families, *Pediatrics* **56(S)**:851–855.

Goding, J. W., Scott, D. W., and Layton, J. E., 1977, Genetics, cellular expression and function of IgD and IgM receptors, *Immunol. Rev.* **37**:152–186.

Goetze, D., ed, 1977, *The Major Histocompatibility System in Man and Animals,* Springer-Verlag, New York.

Gold, W., 1977, Neurohumoral interactions in airways, *Am. Rev. Resp. Dis.* **115**:127–137.

Golden, J. A., Nadel, J. A., and Boushey, H. A., 1978, Bronchial hyperirritability in healthy subjects after exposure to ozone, *Am. Rev. Respir. Dis.* **118**:287–294.

Goodfriend, L., Santilli, J., Schacter, B., Bias, W. B., and Marsh, D. G., 1976, HLA-B7 cross-reacting group and human IgE mediated sensitivity to ragweed allergen Ra-5, *Monogr. Allergy* **11**:80–82.

Gordon, S., and Cohn, Z. A., 1973, The macrophage, *Int. Rev. Cytol.* **36**:171–214.

Gorer, P. A., 1927, The genetic and antigenic basis of tumor transplantation, *J. Pathol. Bacteriol.* **44**:691–697.

Gorer, P. A., 1959, Some recent work in tumor immunity, *Adv. Cancer Res.* **4**:149–186.

Gorer, P. A., and Schutze, H., 1938, Genetic studies on immunity in mice. II. Correlation between antibody formation and resistance, *J. Hyg.* **38**:647–662.

Green, D., and Swets, J. A., 1966, *Signal Detection Theory and Psychophysics,* Wiley, New York.

Green, I., Inman, J., and Benacerraf, B., 1970, Genetic control of the immune response of guinea pigs to a limiting dose of bovine serum albumin, *Proc. Natl. Acad. Sci. USA* **66**:1267–1274.

Greenberg, L., Gray, E., and Yunis, E., 1975, Association of HL-A5 and immune responsiveness to streptococcal antigens, *J. Exp. Med.* **141**:935–943.

Grundbacher, F. J., 1972, Human X chromosome carries quantitative genes for immunoglobulin M, *Science* **176**:311–312.

Grundbacher, F. J., 1974, Heritability estimates and genetic and environmental correlations for the human immunoglobulins G, M and A, *Am. J. Hum. Genet.* **26**:1–12.

Gunther, E., and Rude, E., 1976, Cross-stimulation of antigens under separate histocompatibility linked Ir gene control, *Immunogenetics* **3**:261–269.

Haber, E., Margolis, M. N., and Cannon, L. E., 1977, Structure of the framework and complementary regions of elicited antibodies, in: *Antibodies in Human Diagnosis and Therapy* (E. Haber and R. M. Krause, eds.) pp. 45–77, Raven, New York.

Haire, M., Fraser, K. B., and Miller, J. H. D., 1973, Measles and other virus specific immunoglobulins in multiple sclerosis, *Br. Med. J.* **3**:612–615.

Hall, W. J., Hall, C. B., and Speers, D. M., 1978, Respiratory syncytial virus infection in adults. Clinical, virologic and serial pulmonary function studies, *Ann. Intern. Med.* **88**:203–205.

Haverkorn, M. J., Hofman, B., Masurel, N., and Van Rood, J. J., 1975, HLA linked genetic control of immune response in man, *Transplant. Rev.* **22**:120–124.

Henry, C., Chan, E. L., and Kodlin, D., 1978, Expression and function of I region products on immunocompetent cells. II. I region products in T-B interaction, *J. Immunol.* **119**:744–748.

Heslop-Harrison, J., 1975, Incompatibility and the pollen stigma interaction, *Annu. Rev. Plant Physiol.* **26**:403–425.

Higgins, M., and Keller, J., 1975, Familial occurrence of chronic respiratory disease and familial resemblance in ventilatory capacity, *J. Chronic Dis.* **28**:239–251.

Hildemann, W. H., 1974, Phylogeny of immune responsiveness in invertebrates, *Life Sci.* **14**:605–614.

Hildemann, W. H., 1977, Specific immunorecognition by histocompatibility markers: The original polymorphic system of immunoreactivity characteristic of all multicellular animals, *Immunogenetics* **5**:193–202.

Hildemann, W. H., Linthicum, D. S., and Vann, D. C., 1975, Transplantation and immunocompatibility reactions among reef building corals, *Immunogenetics* **2**:269–284.

Hill, S. W., and Sercarz, E. E., 1975, Fine specificity of the H-2 linked immune response gene for gallinaceious lysozymes, *Eur. J. Immunol.* **5**:317–324.

Hirszfeld, H., and Hirszfeld, L., 1928, Weitere Untersuchungen über die Vererbung der Empfänglichkeit für Infektionskrankheiten, *Z. Immunitaetsforsch. Exp. Ther.* **54**:81–104.

Hood, L., Campbell, J. H., and Elgin, S. C. R., 1975, The organization, expression and evolution of antibody genes and other multigene families, *Annu. Rev. Genet.* **9**:305–353.

Hood, L., Huang, H. V., and Dreyer, W. J., 1977, The area-code hypothesis: The immune system provides clues to understanding the genetic and molecular basis of cell recognition during development, *J. Supramol. Struct.* **7**:407–435.

Hoppe, H. H., Goedde, H. W., Agarwal, D. P., Benkmann, H.-G., Hirth, L., and Janssen, W., 1978, A silent gene (C3-) producing partial deficiency of the third component of human complement, *Hum. Hered.* **28**:141–146.

Jarrett, E. E. E., and Bazin, H., 1974, Elevation of total serum IgE in rats following helminth parasite infection, *Nature (London)* **251**:613–614.

Jerne, N. K., 1971, The somatic generation of immune recognition, *Eur. J. Immunol.* **1**:1–9.

Jersilid, C., Hanson, G. S., Svvejgaard, A., Fog, T., Thomsen, M., and Dupont, B., 1973, Histocompatibility determinants in multiple sclerosis with special reference to clinical course, *Lancet* **2**:1221–1225.

Jones, F. N., 1974, History of psychophysics and judgement, in: *Handbook of Perception, Psycho-*

physical Judgement and Measurement, Vol. 2 (E. C. Carterette and M. P. Friedman, eds.), pp. 2–33, Academic, New York.

Kabat, E. A., Wu, T. T., and Bilofsky, H., 1976, Variable regions of immunoglobulin chains. Tabulations and analysis of amino acid sequences, Medical Computer Systems, Bolt Beranek and Newman, Cambridge, Mass.

Kalff, M. W., and Hijmans, W., 1969, Serum immunoglobulin levels in twins, *Clin. Exp. Immunol.* **5:**469–477.

Katz, D. H., Hamaoka, T., Dorf, M. E., and Benacerraf, B., 1973a, Cell interactions between histoincompatible T and B lymphocytes. III. Demonstration that the H-2 gene complex determines successful physiologic lymphocyte interactions, *Proc. Natl. Acad. Sci. USA* **70:**2624–2628.

Katz, D. H., Hamaoka, T., Dorf, M. E., Maurer, P. H., and Benacerraf, B., 1973b, Cell interactions between histoincompatible T and B lymphocytes. IV. Involvement of the immune response (Ir) gene in the control of lymphocyte interactions in responses controlled by the gene, *J. Exp. Med.* **138:**734–739.

Katz, D. H., Chiarazzi, N., McDonald, J., and Katz, L. R., 1976, Cell interactions between histocompatible T and B lymphocytes. IX. The failure of histoincompatible cells is not due to suppression and cannot be circumvented by carrier priming T cells with allogeneic macrophages, *J. Immunol.* **117:**1853–1859.

Keuning, J. J., Pena, A. S., Van Leeuwen, A., Van Hooff, J. P., and Van Rood, J. J., 1976, HLA-DW3 associated with coeliac disease, *Lancet* **1:**506–508.

Kipps, T. J., Benacerraf, B., and Dorf, M. E., 1978, Regulation of antibody heterogeneity by suppressor T cells: Diminishing suppressor T cell activity increases the number of dinitrophenyl clones in mice immunized with dinitrophenyl-poly(Glu,Lys,Phe) or dinitrophenyl-poly(Glu,Lys,Ala), *Proc. Natl. Acad. Sci. USA* **75:**2914–2817.

Kissmeyer-Nielsen, F., Ehlers, N., Kristensen, T., and Lamm, L. U., 1977, The HLA system, serology and transplantation, in: *HLA Systems: New Aspects* (G. B. Ferrara, ed.) pp. 69–91, North-Holland, Amsterdam.

Klein, J., 1975, *Biology of the Mouse Histocompatibility Complex*, Springer-Verlag, New York.

Klein, J., 1977, Evolution and function of the major histocompatibility system: Facts and speculations, in: *Major Histocompatibility System in Man and Animals* (D. Gotz, ed.), pp. 339–378, Springer-Verlag, New York.

Knox, R. B., Clark, A., Harrison, S., Smith, P., and Marchalonis, J. J., 1976, Cell recognition in plants: Determinants of the stigma surface and their pollen interactions, *Proc. Natl. Acad. Sci. USA* **73:**2788–2792.

Kohler, G., Howe, S. C., and Milstein, C., 1976, Fusion between immunoglobulin secreting and non-secreting myeloma cell lines, *Eur. J. Immunol.* **6:**292–295.

Konig, P., and Godfrey, S., 1974, Exercise induced bronchial lability in monozygotic (identical) and dizygotic (non-identical) twins, *J. Allergy Clin. Immunol.* **54:**280–287.

Landsteiner, K., 1928, Cell antigens and individual specificity, *J. Immunol.* **15:**589–600.

Lange, K., Spence, M. A., and Frank, M. B., 1976, Application of the lod method to the detection of linkage between a quantitative trait and a qualitative marker, *Am. J. Hum. Genet.* **28:**167–173.

Levine, B. B., Stember, R. H., and Fotino, M., 1972, Ragweed hay fever: Genetic control and linkage to HLA haplotype, *Science* **178:**1201–1203.

Little, J. W., Hall, W. J., Douglas, R. G., Mudholkar, G. S., Speers, D. M., and Patel, K., 1978, Airways hyperreactivity and peripheral airway dysfunction in influenza A infection, *Am. Rev. Respir. Dis.* **118:**295–303.

Lozner, E. C., Sachs, D. H., and Shearer, G. M., 1974, Genetic control of immune response to staphylococcal nuclease. I. Ir-nase: Control of the antibody response to nuclease by the Ir region of the mouse H-2 complex, *J. Exp. Med.* **139:**1204–1214.

Magurova, H., Ivanyl, P., Sajellova, H., and Trojan, J., 1975, HLA antigens in aged persons, *Tissue Antigens* **6:**269–271.

Mann, D. L., Katz, S. I., Nelson, D. L., Abelson, L. D., and Strober, W., 1976, Specific B-cell antigens associated with gluten sensitive enteropathy and dermatitis herpetiformis, *Lancet* **1:**110–111.

Marsh, D. G., and Bias, W. B., 1977, Basal serum IgE levels and HLA antigen frequencies in allergic subjects. II. Studies in people sensitive to rye grass group I and ragweed antigen E and postulated immune response (Ir) loci in the HLA region, *Immunogenetics* **5**:235–252.

Marsh, D. G., Bias, W. B., Hsu, S. H., and Goodfriend, L., 1973, Association of the HLA-7 cross-reacting group with a specific reaginic antibody response in allergic man, *Science* **179**:691–693.

Marsh, D. G., Bias, W. B., and Ishizaka, K., 1974, Genetic control of basal serum immunoglobulin E level and its effect on specific reaginic sensitivity, *Proc. Natl. Acad. Sci. USA* **71**:3588–3592.

Marsh, D. G., Goodfriend, L., and Bias, W. B., 1977, Basal serum IgE levels and HLA antigen frequencies in allergic subjects. I. Studies with ragweed allergen Ra3, *Immunogenetics* **5**:217–234.

Marx, J. J., and Flaherty, D. K., 1976, Activation of the complement sequence by extracts of bacteria and fungi associated with hypersensitivity pneumonitis, *J. Allergy Clin. Immunol.* **57**:328–334.

Mather, K., and Jinks, J. L., 1971, *Biometrical Genetics*, Cornell University Press, Ithaca, N.Y.

McDevitt, H. O., and Sela, M., 1965, Genetic control of the antibody response. I. The demonstration of determinant specific differences in response to synthetic polypeptide antigens in two strains of inbred mice, *J. Exp. Med.* **122**:517–531.

Meredith, P. J., and Walford, R. L., 1977, Effect of age on T- and B-cell mitogens in mice congenic at the H-2 locus, *Immunogenetics* **5**:109–128.

Miller, G. A., 1956, The magical number seven, plus or minus two: Some limits on our capacity for processing information, *Psychol. Rev.* **63**:81–97.

Miller, J. F. A. P., Vadas, M. A., Whitelaw, A., and Gamble, J., 1975, H-2 gene complex restricts transfer of delayed type hypersensitivity in mice, *Proc. Natl. Acad. Sci. USA* **72**:5095–5098.

Miller, J. F. A. P., Vadas, M. A., Whitelaw, A., Gamble, J., and Bernard, C., 1977, Histocompatibility linked immune responsiveness and restrictions imposed on sensitized lymphocytes, *J. Exp. Med.* **145**:1623–1628.

Milstein, C., Brownlee, G. G., Cartwright, E. M., and Jarvis, J. M., 1974, Sequence analysis of immunoglobulin light chain messenger RNA, *Nature (London)* **252**:354–358.

Morrison, D. F., 1967, *Multivariate Statistical Methods*, McGraw-Hill, New York.

Moscona, A. A., 1973, Cell aggregation, in: *Cell Biology in Medicine* (E. E. Bittar, ed.), pp. 571–591, Wiley, New York.

Nabholz, M., Vives, J., Young, H. M., Meo, T., Miggiano, V., Rijnbeck, A., and Schreffler, D. C., 1974, Cell mediated cell lysis *in vitro*: Genetic control of killer cell production and target specificities in the mouse, *Eur. J. Immunol.* **4**:378–387.

Niederhuber, J. E., Frelinger, J. A., Dugan, E., Coutinho, A., and Shreffler, D. C., 1976, The effects of anti-Ia serum on mitogenic responses. I. Inhibition of the proliferative response to B-cell mitogen LPS by specific anti-Ia sera, *J. Immunol.* **115**:1672–1676.

Nowack, H., Rohde, H., Gotze, D., and Timpl, R., 1977, Genetic control and carrier and suppressor effects in the antibody response of mice to procollagen, *Immunogenetics* **4**:117–125.

Ochs, H. D., Rosenfeld, S. I., Thomas, E. D., Giblett, E. R., Alper, C. A., Dupont, B., Schaller, J., Gilliland, B. C., Hansen, J. A., and Wedgewood, R. J., 1977, Linkage between the gene (or genes) controlling synthesis of the fourth component and the major histocompatibility complex, *N. Engl. J. Med.* **296**:470–475.

Ogilvie, B. M., and Jones, V. E., 1973, Immunity in the parasitic relationship between helminths and host, *Progr. Allergy* **17**:93–144.

Okuda, K., Christadoss, P. R., Twining, S., Atassi, M. Z., and David, C. S., 1978, Genetic control of immune response to sperm whale myoglobin in mice. I. T lymphocyte proliferative response under H-2 linked Ir gene control, *J. Immunol.* **121**:866–868.

Olenchock, S. A., and Burrell, R., 1976, The role of precipitins and complement activation in the etiology of allergic lung disease, *J. Allergy Clin. Immunol.* **58**:76–88.

Patterson, P. M., and Lauder, B. A., 1948, The incidence and probable inheritance of "small blindness," *J. Hered.* **39**:295–297.

Paul, W. E., Siskind, G. W., and Benacerraf, B., 1966, Studies of the effect of carrier molecules on anti-hapten antibody synthesis. II. Carrier specificity of anti-2,4-dinitrophenyl-poly-L-lysine antibodies, *J. Exp. Med.* **123**:689–705.

Pavlov, I. P., 1927, *Conditioned Reflexes: An Investigation of the Physiologic Activity of the Cerebral Cortex*, Oxford University Press, London.

Pearsall, N. N., and Weiser, R. S., 1970, *The Macrophage*, Lea and Febiger, Philadelphia.

Piaget, J., 1969, *The Mechanisms of Perception*, transl. by G. N. Seagrim, Basic, New York.

Pierce, C. W., Kapp, J. A., and Benacerraf, B., 1976, Regulation by the H-2 gene complex of macrophage-lymphoid cell interactions in secondary antibody response *in vitro*, *J. Exp. Med.* **144:**371–381.

Pinchuck, P., and Maurer, P. H., 1965, Antigenicity of polypeptides. XVI. Genetic control of immunogenicity of synthetic polypeptides in mice, *J. Exp. Med.* **122:**673–679.

Pisetsky, D. S., and Sachs, D. H., 1977, The genetic control of the immune response to staphylococcal nuclease. VI. Recombination between genes determining the A/J anti-nuclease idiotypes and heavy chain allotype locus, *J. Exp. Med.* **146:**1603–1612.

Polak, L., and Turk, J. L., 1969, Genetic background of certain immunological phenomena with particular reference to the skin, *J. Invest. Dermatol.* **52:**219–232.

Rabbits, T. H., 1977, A molecular hybridization approach for the determination of the immunoglobulin V-gene pool size, *Immunol. Rev.* **36:**29–50.

Rachelefsky, G., Terasaki, P. I., Park, M. S., Katz, R., Siegel, S., and Shoichiro, S., 1976, Strong association between B-lymphocyte group-2 specificity and asthma, *Lancet* **2:**1042–1044.

Ratner, B., and Silberman, D. E., 1952, Allergy—its distribution and the heredity concept, *Ann. Allergy* **10:**1–20.

Raum, D., Glass, D., Carpenter, C. B., Alper, C. A., and Schur, P. H., 1976, The chromosomal order of genes controlling the major histocompatibility complex and deficiency of the second component of complement, *J. Clin. Invest.* **58:**1240–1248.

Reif, A. E., and Allen, J. M. V., 1964, The AKR thymic antigen and its distribution in leukemias and nervous tissues, *J. Exp. Med.* **120:**413–433.

Revolta, R., and Ovary, Z., 1969, Preferential production of rabbit reaginic antibodies, *Int. Arch. Allergy Appl. Immunol.* **36:**282–289.

Rittner, C., Grosse-Wilde, H., and Bittner, B., 1975, Linkage group HL-A-MLC-Bf (properdin factor B): The site of the Bf locus at the immunogenetic linkage group on chromosome 6, *Humangenetik* **27:**173–183.

Roberts, T. D. M., 1973, Energy, transducers and sensory discrimination, in: *Handbook of Perception, Biology of Perceptual Systems*, Vol. 3 (E. C. Carterette and M. P. Friedman, eds.), pp. 2–20, Academic, New York.

Roseman, J., Buckley, C. E., and Amos, D. B., 1976, Human immune response (Ir) polymorphisms detected with 4 common allergens, *J. Allergy Clin. Immunol.* **57:**228A.

Rosenthal, A. S., and Shevach, E. M., 1973, Function of macrophages in antigen recognition by guinea pig T-lymphocytes. I. Requirement for histocompatible macrophages and lymphocytes, *J. Exp. Med.* **138:**1194–1212.

Sasazuki, T., Kohno, Y., Iwamoto, I, Tanimura, M., and Naito, S., 1978, Association between an HLA haplotype and low responsiveness to tetanus toxoid in man, *Nature (London)* **272:**359–361.

Schneibel, I. F., 1943, Hereditary differences in the capacity of guinea pigs for production of diphtheria antitoxin, *Acta Pathol. Microbiol. Scand.* **20:**464–484.

Schrader, J. W., and Edelman, G. M., 1976, Participation of the H-2 antigens of tumor cells in their lysis by syngeneic T-cells, *J. Exp. Med.* **143:**601–614.

Schwartz, R. H., David, C. S., Sachs, D. H., and Paul, W. E., 1976, T-lymphocyte-enriched murine peritoneal exudate cells. III. Inhibition of antigen-induced T-lymphocyte proliferation with anti-Ia antisera, *J. Immunol.* **117:**531–540.

Scott, B. B., Rajah, S. M., Swinburne, M. L., and Losowsky, M. S., 1974, HL-A8 and the immune response to gluten, *Lancet* **2:**374–377.

Secher, D. S., Milstein, C., and Adetugbo, K., 1977, Somatic mutants and antibody diversity, *Immunol. Rev.* **36:**51–72.

Shearer, G. M., Rehn, T. G., and Schmitt-Verhulst, A. M., 1976, Role of the murine major histocompatibility complex in the specificity of *in vitro* T-cell mediated lympholysis against chemically modified autologous lymphocytes, *Transplant. Rev.* **29:**222–248.

Shevach, E. M., Paul, W. E., and Green, I., 1972, Histocompatibility linked immune response gene functions in guinea pigs. Specific inhibition of antigen-induced lymphocyte proliferation by alloantisera, *J. Exp. Med.* **136:**1207–1221.

Shevach, E. M., Paul, W. E., and Green, I., 1974, Alloantiserum induced inhibition of immune response gene function. I. Cellular distribution of target antigens, *J. Exp. Med.* **139:**661–678.

Shreffler, D. C., and David, C. S., 1975, The H-2 major histocompatibility complex and the I immune response region. Genetic variation, function and organization, *Adv. Immunol.* **20:**125–195.

Siber, G. R., Weitzman, S. A., Aisenberg, A. C., Weinstein, H. J., and Shiffman, G., 1978, Impaired antibody response to pneumococcal vaccine after treatment of Hodgkin's disease, *N. Engl. J. Med.* **299**:442–448.

Simon, H. A., 1974, How big is a chunk? *Science* **183**:482–488.

Slege, C., Fair, D. S., Black, B., Kreuger, R. G., and Hood, L., 1976, Antibody differentiation: Apparent sequence identity between variable sequences shared by IgA and IgG immunoglobulins, *Proc. Natl. Acad. Sci. USA* **73**:923–927.

Smialowcz, R. J., and Schwab, J. H., 1977, Processing of streptococcal cell walls by rat macrophages and human monocytes *in vitro*, *Infect. Immun.* **17**:591–605.

Sokolov, E. N., 1963, *Perception and the Conditioned Reflex*, Pergamon, Oxford.

Sokolov, E. N., 1975, The neuronal mechanisms of the orienting reflex, in: *Neuronal Mechanisms and the Orienting Reflex* (E. N. Sokolov and O. S. Vinogradova, eds.), p. 217, Wiley, New York.

Spencer, H., 1888, *The Principles of Biology*, Vol. 1, p. 244, Appleton, New York.

Spencer, M. J., Cherry, J. D., and Terasaki, P. I., 1976, HLA antigens and antibody response after influenza A vaccination, *N. Engl. J. Med.* **294**:13–16.

Spencer, M. J., Cherry, J. D., Powell, K. R., Mickey, M. R., Terasaki, P. I., Marcey, S. M., and Sumaya, C. V., 1977, Antibody responses following Rubella immunization analyzed by HLA and ABO types, *Immunogenetics* **4**:365–372.

Stanbury, J. B., Wyngaarden, J. B., and Fredrickson, D. S., 1972, *The Metabolic Basis of Inherited Disease*, McGraw-Hill, New York.

Starmer, C. F., and Grizzle, J. E., 1968, *A Computer Program for Analysis of Data by General Linear Models*, Inst. Statistics Mimeo Series No. 560, University of North Carolina Press, Chapel Hill.

Stevens, S. S., 1951, Mathematics, measurement and psychophysics, in: *Handbook of Experimental Psychology*, (S. S. Stevens, ed.), pp. 1–41, Wiley, New York.

Stevens, S. S., 1974, Perceptual magnitude and its measurement, in: *Handbook of Perception, Psychophysical Judgement and Measurement*, Vol. 2 (E. C. Carterette and M. P. Friedman, eds.), pp. 361–389, Academic, New York.

Sutherland, N. S., 1973, Object recognition, in: *Handbook of Perception, Biology of Perceptual Systems*, Vol. 3 (E. C. Carterette and M. P. Friedman, eds.), pp. 157–185, Academic, New York.

Svejgaard, A., and Ryder, L. P., 1977, Associations between HLA and disease. Notes on methodology and a report from the HLA and disease registry, in: *HLA and Disease* (J. Dausset and A. Svejgaard, eds.), pp. 46–71, Williams and Wilkins, Baltimore.

Svejgaard, A., Platz, P., Nielson, L. S., and Thompson, M., 1975, HLA and disease associations—a survey, *Transplant. Rev.* **22**:3–43.

Tada, T., Tanguchi, M., and Takemori, T., 1975, Properties of primed suppressor T cells and their properties, *Transplant. Rev.* **26**:106–129.

Terasaki, P. I., Park, M. S., Opelz, G., and Ting, A., 1976, Multiple sclerosis and high incidence of a B lymphocyte antigen, *Science* **193**:1245–1247.

Theodor, J. L., 1970, Distinction between "self" and "non-self" in lower vertebrates, *Nature (London)* **227**:690–692.

Thomas, K. B., 1973, Genetic control, in: *Handbook of Perception, Biology of Perceptual Systems*, Vol. 3 (E. C. Carterette and M. P. Friedman, eds.), pp. 139–155, Academic, New York.

Thomson, P. D., Banatt, T. M., Stokes, C. R., Turner, M. W., and Soothill, J. F., 1976, HLA antigens and atopic features in steroid responsive nephrotic syndrome of childhood, *Lancet* **2**:765–768.

Tips, R. L., 1954, A study of the inheritance of atopic hypersensitivity in man, *Am. J. Hum. Genet.* **6**:328–343.

Townley, R. G., Ryo, U. Y., Kolokin, B. M., and Kang, B., 1975, Bronchial sensitivity to methacholine in current and former asthmatics and allergic rhinitis patients and control subjects, *J. Allergy Clin. Immunol.* **56**:429–442.

Townley, R. G., Gurgis, H., Bewtra, A., Watt, G., Burk, K., and Carney, K., 1976, IgE levels and methacholine inhalation responses in monozygous and dizygous twins, *J. Allergy Clin. Immunol.* **57**:227A.

Turner, K. J., Rosman, D. L., and O'Mahony, J., 1974, Prevalence and familial association of atopic disease and its relationship to serum IgE levels in 1061 school children and their families, *Int. Arch. Allergy Appl. Immunol.* **47**:650–664.

Urban, J. F., Ishizaka, T., and Ishizaka, K., 1977, IgE formation in the rat following infection with *Nipponstrongylus braziliensis*. III. Soluble factor for the generation of IgE bearing lymphocytes, *J. Immunol.* **119**:583–590.

Van Arsdel, P. P., and Motulsky, A. G., 1959, Frequency and hereditability of asthma and allergic rhinitis in college students, *Acta Genet.* **9**:101–114.

Van de Geer, J. P., 1974, *Introduction to Multiveriate Analysis for the Social Sciences.* Freeman, San Francisco.

Van den Berg-Loonen, E. M., Nijenhuis, L. E., Engelfriet, C. P., Feltkamp, T. E. W., Van Rossum, A. L., and Oosterhuis, H. J. G. H., 1977, Segregation of HLA haplotypes in 100 families with a myasthenia gravis patient, *J. Immunogenet.* **4**:331–340.

Walker, F. B., Smith, P. D., and Maibach, H. I., 1967, Genetic factors in human allergic contact dermatitis, *Int. Arch. Allergy* **32**:453–462.

Wanatabe, N., Kojima, S., and Ovary, Z., 1976, Suppression of IgE antibody production in SJL mice. I. Non-specific suppressor T cells, *J. Exp. Med.* **143**:833–845.

Wanatabe, N., Kojima, S., Shen, F., and Ovary, Z., 1977, Suppression of IgE antibody production in SJL mice. II. Expression of Ly-1 antigen on helper and non-specific suppressor T cells, *J. Immunol.* **118**:485–488.

Wenzel, B. M., 1973, Tasting and smelling, in: *Handbook of Perception, Biology of Perceptual Systems,* Vol. 3 (E. C. Carterette and M. P. Friedman, eds.), pp. 207–218, Academic, New York.

Whissell-Buechy, D., and Amoore, J. A., 1973, Odor blindness to musk: Simple recessive inheritance, *Nature (London)* **242**:271–273.

Wiener, A. S., Zieve, I., and Fried, J. H., 1935, The inheritance of an allergic disease, *Ann. Eugen.* **7**:141–164.

Willoughby, J. B., and Willoughby, W. F., 1977, *In vivo* responses to inhaled antigens. I. Quantitative analysis of antigen uptake, fate and immunogenicity in a rabbit model system, *J. Immunol.* **119**:2137–2146.

Willoughby, W. F., Barbaras, J. E.. and Wheelis, R., 1976, Hypersensitivity pneumonitis, *Chest* **69(2S)**:290–294.

Wolski, K. P., Schmid, F. R., and Mittal, K. K., 1975, Genetic linkage between the HLA system and a deficit of the second component (C2) of complement, *Science* **188**:1020–1021.

Yamamura, M., and Valdimarsson, H., 1977, Participation of C3 in intracellular killing of *Candida albicans*, *Scand. J. Immunol.* **6**:591–594.

Yamazaki, K., Boyse, E. A., Mike, V., Thaler, H. T., Mathieson, B. J., Abbott, J., Boyse, J., Zayas, Z. A., and Thomas, L., 1976, Control of mating preferences in mice by genes in the major histocompatibility complex, *J. Exp. Med.* **144**:1324–1335.

Yano, A., Schwartz, R. H., and Paul, W. E., 1977, Antigen presentation in the murine T-lymphocyte proliferative response. I. Requirement for genetic identity at the major histocompatibility complex, *J. Exp. Med.* **146**:828–843.

Yman, L., Ponterius, G., and Brandt, R., 1975, Rast-based allergen assay methods, *Dev. Biol. Stand.* **29**:151–165.

Young, C., and Ebringer, A., 1976, Genetic control of the immune response to sperm whale myoglobin in inbred mice, *Immunogenetics* **3**:299–304.

Yunis, E. J., Amos, D. B., and Blumenthal, M. N., 1975, Genetic mapping of IrE outside HL-A-MLRS complex, *Transplant. Proc.* **7**:49–51.

Zeiss, C. R., Patterson, R., Pruzansky, J. J., Miller, M. M., Rosenberg, M., and Levitz, D., 1977, Trimellitic anhydride-induced airway syndromes: Clinical and immunologic studies, *J. Allergy Clin. Immunol.* **60**:96–103.

Zinkernagel, R. M., and Doherty, P. C., 1975, H-2 compatibility requirement for T-cell mediated lysis of targets infected with lymphocytic choriomeningitis virus. Different cytotoxic T-cell specificities are associated with structures coded in H-2k or H-2d, *J. Exp. Med.* **141**:1427–1436.

8

Urticaria and Angioedema

ALLEN P. KAPLAN

1. Introduction

Urticaria and angioedema are common disorders affecting approximately 15–20% of the population at least once during their lifetime (Swinny, 1941; Sheldon *et al.*, 1954; McKee, 1966). Urticarial lesions result from localized dilatation and transudation of fluid from small venules, and in their simplest form are thought to represent the same sort of wheal-and-flare reaction observed when histamine is injected into the skin. Clinically, one observes the presence of pruritic, erythematous cutaneous wheals that blanch with pressure, reflecting the underlying edema and dilated blood vessels. The histopathological features of urticaria are dilatation of cutaneous blood vessels and lymphatics in the superficial dermis, widening of dermal papillae, flattening of rete pegs, and swelling of collagen fibers.

Acute urticaria is most frequently a self-limited disorder caused by an allergic reaction to a food or drug. When the urticaria exceeds six weeks, it rather arbitrarily is designated "chronic." Angioedema is caused by the same (or very similar) pathological alterations which occur in the deep dermis and subcutaneous tissue. Thus an area involved with angioedema has swelling as the prominent manifestation, and the external appearance of the skin may be normal. In this chapter we shall examine the biochemical mechanisms that lead to the development of urticaria and/or angioedema (Kaplan, 1977). The clinical presentation and pathogenesis of the various forms of each disorder and the diagnostic studies and treatment that are, in each instance, indicated will be discussed.

2. Mediator Pathways of Urticaria and Angioedema

The major noncytotoxic mechanisms by which histamine is known to be released requires the combination of an antigen with IgE antibody bound to

Allen P. Kaplan • Allergic Diseases Section, Laboratory of Clinical Investigation, National Institute of Allergy and Infectious Diseases, National Institutes of Health, Bethesda, Maryland. Present affiliation: Division of Allergy-Rheumatology, Health Sciences Center, State University of New York, Stony Brook, New York 11794.

basophils or tissue mast cells (Tomioka and Ishizaka, 1971; Ishizaka *et al.*, 1972). This reaction leads to the release of the various mediators that can cause a localized inflammatory response. Histamine is released from preformed granules as a consequence of this antigen–antibody interaction and is capable of eliciting the classical triple response (Lewis, 1927) consisting of vasodilatation (erythema), increased vascular permeability (edema), and an axon reflex which increases the extent of the erythema. Histamine itself has been shown to be selectively chemotactic for human eosinophils (Clark *et al.*, 1975, 1976) at a concentration between 10 and 300 ng/ml (peak activity at 120 ng/ml) while further increases in histamine concentration yield progressively less chemotactic response. Histamine can also modulate the eosinophil chemotactic response to other chemotactic factors (Clark *et al.*, 1977). In addition to histamine, tetrapeptides are released that are preferentially chemotactic for eosinophils (Goetzl and Austen, 1975). These had been previously referred to as the "eosinophil chemotactic factor of anaphylaxis" (ECF-A) (Kay *et al.*, 1971; Kay and Austen, 1971). Larger peptides are also released from such IgE-dependent reactions, which possess chemotactic activity for eosinophils but are apparently less potent or released in smaller quantities (Boswell *et al.*, 1978). Although eosinophil infiltration is commonly seen in allergic reactions, early, transient neutrophil infiltration is also observed. This may be secondary to the activity of these various peptides on neutrophils (histamine is not chemotactic for neutrophils) as well as a high-molecular-weight chemotactic factor which has greater specificity for neutrophils than eosinophils (Wasserman *et al.*, 1977). It is likely that the absolute quantities and ratio of these preformed mediators are responsible for the local accumulation of eosinophils in allergic reactions.

Other mediators are released as a consequence of this reaction; however, they are not preformed but rather are synthesized by the cell as a consequence of the allergic reaction. Slow-reacting substance of anaphylaxis, SRS-A, is a sulfated lipid (Orange and Austen, 1972; Orange *et al.*, 1973) of molecular weight 400 which causes a gradual and sustained contraction of bronchial smooth muscle. In addition, it can increase vascular permeability in primates (Orange and Austen, 1972) and therefore may contribute to the edema formation of IgE-mediated reactions. Another mediator called "platelet activating factor" (PAF) (Benveniste *et al.*, 1972, 1975; Kater *et al.*, 1975) is released from basophils and mast cells and causes degranulation of platelets, thereby releasing serotonin into the vicinity of the allergic reaction. However, serotonin does not increase vascular permeability in human skin; thus it is likely that if it contributes to a wheal-and-flare reaction, it does so indirectly in conjunction with other mediators.

A second pathway leading to the noncytotoxic release of histamine from basophils or mast cells involves the complement pathways. There are two fragments of complement components termed "C3a" and "C5a" (Cochrane and Müller-Eberhard, 1968) which act as anaphylatoxins, i.e., they interact directly with the cell surface in the absence of antibody to trigger histamine release. On a molar basis, C5a appears to be a more potent permeability factor than C3a as assessed by intradermal injection (Wuepper *et al.*, 1972). Since there is particularly rapid inactivation of C3a by the anaphylatoxin inactivator (Bokisch *et al.*, 1969; Vallota and Müller-Eberhard, 1973), only C5a is routinely isolated from serum after complement activation. C5a is also gradually destroyed by the same inhibitor. C5a or a derivative thereof also appears to function as a chemotactic factor and can attract neutrophils, eosinophils, or mononuclear cells to a site of inflammation (Fernandez *et al.*, 1978). The pathways by which C3a and C5a anaphylatoxins can be produced are shown in Figure 1, in which the classical and alternate complement pathways are shown diagrammatically. The classical pathway can be initiated by combination of antigen with either IgM antibody or the IgG_1, IgG_2, or IgG_3 subclasses of antibody. The immune complex then binds the C1q subunit of the first component of complement which leads to activation of the C1s subunit containing the active enzymatic site (Naff *et al.*, 1964). The activated first component of complement ($C\bar{1}$) can then act on its two substrates, C4 and C2, to form $C\overline{42}$, the C3-converting enzyme (Müller-Eberhard *et al.*, 1967) which releases C3a anaphylatoxin. The binding of C3b to this complex forms the C5-converting enzyme which cleaves C5 and liberates C5a.

The complement pathway can also be activated at the C3 step by an alternative route (Figure 1), originally called the "properdin pathway" (Pillemer *et al.*, 1954). This pathway can be directly activated by complex polysaccharides or lipopolysaccharides such as endotoxin (Gewerz *et al.*, 1968) with no apparent antibody requirement, but it can also be activated on combination of antigen with IgA antibody (Götze and Müller-Eberhard, 1971). Although the details of the steps leading to C3 activation in this pathway are not yet complete, critical proteins involved include C3 itself, factor B (Götze and Müller-Eberhard, 1971), factor D (Fearon *et al.*, 1974), and properdin (Götze and Müller-Eberhard, 1974). It has been shown that activators of C3 are generated in this pathway utilizing C3 as a critical factor. A magnesium-dependent combination of C3 and factor B can be acted on by activated factor D (designated $\bar{D}$) to form a C3-cleaving enzyme in which factor B has been digested to yield the active Bb fragment with the liberation of a smaller Ba fragment (Fearon and Austen, 1975a). Alternatively either activated

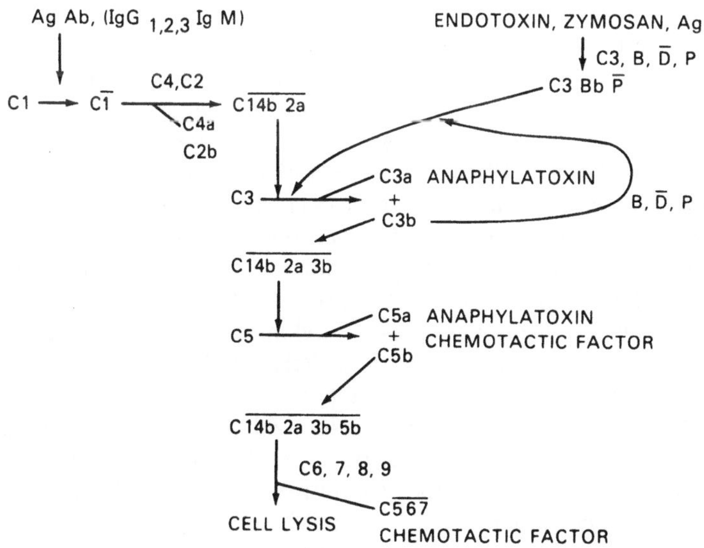

Figure 1. Classical and alternate complement pathways indicating the functionally active by-products of each reaction and the various C3-activating enzymes formed.

properdin ($\bar{P}$) or "C3 nephritic factor" (C3 Nef), an unusual antibody (Thompson, 1972; Davis *et al.*, 1977) present in patients with membranoproliferative glomerulonephritis, can combine with C3 and factor B to form a C3 activator by exposing an active site in B (indicated as $\bar{B}$) without cleaving it (Daha *et al.*, 1976b; Fearon and Austen, 1975b). This complex is then converted to a more efficient enzyme when $\bar{B}$ is converted to Bb by $\bar{D}$. The C3 is utilized in these reactions without conversion to C3b (Fearon and Austen, 1975a; Schreiber *et al.*, 1975). The product of the C3 reaction, i.e., C3b, can enter into the same series of reactions as C3 (Fearon and Austen, 1975c; Daha *et al.*, 1976a) with $\bar{P}$, C3 Nef, and $\bar{D}$ to yield the feedback loop of the alternative pathway. Thus it may be possible to recruit this alternate pathway secondary to activation of the classical complement pathway.

Direct formation of C5a in serum and the subsequent degranulation of basophils to release histamine have been described as a consequence of activation of the alternative complement pathway by zymosan (Grant *et al.*, 1975). Thus in situations in which there is an immune complex disease or nonimmune complement activation, histamine released into the skin could cause a wheal-and-flare reaction. In addition, studies of immune complex deposition in the rabbit suggest that the synthesis of IgE antibody to the immunizing antigen is a prerequisite for the deposition of IgG- and IgM-containing immune complexes into tissues. Such deposition is dependent on the release of vasoactive peptides such as histamine and serotonin which dilate small venules, thereby allowing the larger complexes to localize (Benveniste *et al.*, 1972). Thus IgE- and complement-dependent mechanisms of histamine release may operate simultaneously in immune complex diseases.

Another mediator pathway which can lead to the generation of inflammatory products is the plasma kinin-forming system (Figure 2) of the intrinsic coagulation pathway. One of its products is bradykinin, a nine-amino-acid peptide, which on a molar basis is as potent as histamine in increasing vascular permeability. Bradykinin is also a vasodilator and like histamine can cause hypotension when high systemic levels are reached. It does not cause pruritis on contact with sensory nerve endings but rather a burning-type pain. Activated Hageman factor initiates coagulation by activation of plasma thromboplastin antecendent (PTA or factor X1) (Ratnoff *et al.*, 1961). As shown in Figure 2, it also converts prekallikrein to kallikrein (Kaplan and Austen, 1970), which then digests the substrate kininogen to yield the vasoactive peptide bradykinin. However, the enzyme kallikrein and its substrate kininogen also have profound effects on the coagulation and fibrinolytic pathways. In Fletcher factor deficiency (Hathaway *et al.*, 1965; Hathaway and Alsever, 1970), in which there is congenital absence of prekallikrein (Wuepper, 1973), patients, as expected, cannot generate bradykinin. However, they also have a diminished rate of Hageman factor activation (Weiss *et al.*, 1973) as reflected by a diminished rate of surface-mediated coagulation and fibrinolysis. These latter defects can therefore be bypassed by reconstitution with *activated* Hageman factor (Weiss *et al.*, 1973) in the absence of a surface. Kallikrein has been shown to activate and fragment Hageman factor (Cochrane *et al.*, 1973); therefore, a feedback activation of Hageman factor by kallikrein may account for these abnormalities. However, kallikrein will not correct the Fletcher deficiency in the absence of a surface; thus the critical interaction occurs on the surface rather than in the fluid phase (Kaplan *et al.*, 1974). A deficiency of human kininogen has been found (Colman *et al.*, 1975; Wuepper *et al.*, 1975) which involves profound abnormalities of all Hageman-factor-dependent pathways. However, when normal plasma was fractionated to identify the corrective factor, a high-molecular-weight form of kininogen which constitutes about 15% of the total kininogen corrected each defect while the more abundant low-molecular form was not effective. High-molecular-weight kininogen acts as a cofactor for surface-mediated Hageman factor activation and function. It augments the function of activated Hageman factor on its substrates (Meier *et al.*, 1977) and augments the activation of Hageman factor by kallikrein (Griffin and Cochrane, 1976; Meier *et al.*, 1977). Furthermore, the substrates of activated Hageman factor, namely prekallikrein and factor XI, circulate bound to HMW kininogen (Mandle *et al.*, 1976; Thompson *et al.*, 1977). In the absence of kininogen, insufficient kallikrein is generated for its feedback effect to be evident. This Hageman-factor-dependent pathway also initiates fibrinolysis by activating one or more plasminogen proactivators to an activator which in turn converts plasminogen to the fibrinolytic enzyme plasmin (Kaplan and Austen, 1972). Kallikrein has been shown to function as one of these plasminogen activators (Mandle and Kaplan, 1977).

In general, negatively charged surfaces such as silicates initiate activation of Hageman factor upon binding the reactants. A conformational change in Hageman factor has been observed (McMillan *et al.*, 1974); however, no active-site generation has been detected in the absence of enzymatic cleavage of the Hageman factor (Griffin and Cochrane, 1976). The biological materials which can activate it include endotoxin (Morrison and Cochrane, 1974), sodium urate and pyrophosphate crystals (Kellermeyer and Breckenridge, 1965), and insoluble collagen (Niewiarowski *et al.*, 1965; Wilner *et al.*, 1968; Griffin *et al.*, 1975). In tissue injury, collagen–mucopolysaccharide complexes (Moskowitz *et al.*, 1970) or vascular basement membrane (Cochrane *et al.*, 1972) could serve as local activators of this pathway. Thus kinin formation may be a consequence of inflammation initiated by other pathways as well as being activated directly by certain negatively charged materials. Subsequent to initiation by surface activation, Hageman factor can be

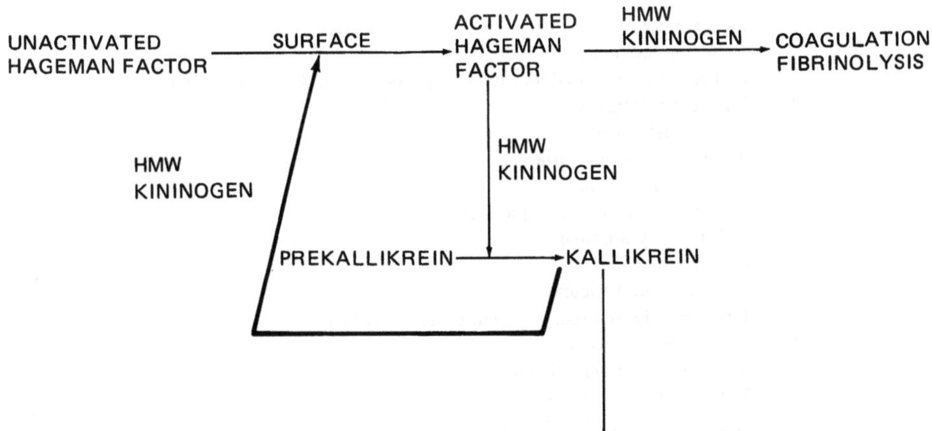

Figure 2. Hageman-factor-dependent pathways of coagulation, fibrinolysis, and kinin generation.

fragmented by proteolytic enzymes such as kallikrein (Cochrane *et al.*, 1973) or plasmin (Kaplan and Austen, 1971) to yield Hageman factor fragments (Kaplan and Austen, 1970), which, in the fluid phase, can continue to generate bradykinin and activate the fibrinolytic pathway. However, these fragments are ineffective in the coagulation pathway compared to the intact activated molecule. The reaction is then stopped when the various forms of activated Hageman factor are inactivated by plasma inhibitors.

In the next sections, the pathogenesis of specific diseases will be discussed in terms of these various inflammatory pathways.

3. Causes of Urticaria and Angioedema

Table 1 is a list of the major causes of urticaria and angioedema that should be considered when any patient is being evaluated. Urticaria may result from cytotoxic reactions, for example, after a blood transfusion; however, in such a case the cause is generally obvious and the symptoms are self-limited. Occasionally a patient may present with urticaria or angioedema which is recurrent with a seasonal pattern. One then has to consider the urticaria a manifestation of some allergen with a seasonal pattern that is either inhaled, ingested, or contacted. Such patients may have other manifestations of atopy such as allergic rhinitis or asthma to the same allergens; however, it is not known why, in some cases, skin manifestations of these presumably IgE-mediated reactions are evident (Waldbott and Merkle, 1952). Nevertheless, the route of administration of an allergen is an important determinant of the symptoms observed, and, in general, inhaled allergens

TABLE 1. Causes of Urticaria and Angioedema

1.	Drug reaction
2.	Foods, food additives, natural salicylates
3.	Inhalent antigens
4.	Transfusion reactions
5.	Infections—bacterial, fungal, viral
6.	Collagen vascular diseases
	a. Cutaneous vasculitis
	b. Serum sickness
7.	Malignancy—angioedema with acquired Cl and Cl INH depletion
8.	Physical urticarias
	a. Cold urticaria
	b. Cholinergic urticaria
	c. Dermographism
	d. Pressure urticaria (angioedema)
	e. Vibratory angioedema
	f. Solar urticaria
	g. Aquagenic urticaria
9.	Urticaria pigmentosa—systemic mastocytosis
10.	Hereditary diseases
	a. Hereditary angioedema
	b. Familial cold urticaria
	c. C3b inactivator deficiency
	d. Amyloidosis with deafness and urticaria
11.	Chronic idiopathic urticaria and chronic angioedema

cause respiratory symptoms while ingested allergens cause urticaria, angioedema, or gastrointestinal allergy.

Drug reactions are among the most commonly recognized causes of urticaria and angioedema. Almost any drug can be responsible, particularly antibiotics such as sulfa and penicillin as well as sedatives, tranquilizers, analgesics, laxatives, and diuretics. Certainly penicillin allergy is the best-studied drug allergy, and its most common presentation is urticaria. Urticaria may commence anywhere from minutes after administration of penicillin to 10 days later; the later reactions may be associated with a serum sickness-like picture. A syndrome of recurrent urticaria with arthralgias secondary to penicillin administration has been described that can last up to 7 weeks which also appears to be IgE mediated (Levine, 1966). One must remember that traces of penicillin may be present in various dairy products and can be a subtle cause of chronic urticaria. When a drug reaction is suspected, the diagnosis may be tested by eliminating the agent. If correct, gradual resolution of the urticaria is anticipated. All medications should be considered a potential cause of urticaria or angioedema and any unnecessary ones should be promptly eliminated. These include aspirin, vitamins, cold tablets, hemorrhoid suppositories, and birth control tablets. When a medication is required for treatment of some bona fide illness, a change to an alternative drug may be attempted. Although a variety of *in vitro* tests have been reported for use in drug reactions, e.g., observing migration inhibition factor release when the patient's leukocytes are challenged with the drug (Rocklin and David, 1971), most tests are not predictive of an allergic reaction. When positive tests are obtained, they usually indicate that the patient has developed an immune reaction to the drug, but there is often little correlation with any particular clinical manifestation. No routine tests are available which reliably can confirm or refute the diagnosis of drug-induced urticaria or angioedema, and an empirical approach is therefore indicated.

Recently we have become aware of patients who have urticaria secondary to ingestion of aspirin. The bulk of evidence suggests that these reactions are not immunological (Samter and Beers, 1967; Yurchak *et al.*, 1970). Such aspirin-sensitive patients frequently do not tolerate indomethacin, aminopyrine, or mefenamic acid, and also react to coal tar dye derivatives such as tartrazine yellow #5 used to color foods or medication capsules. Certainly when a patient gives a history of urticaria associated with a long list of medications, a search should be made for an alternative explanation such as an ingredient or an activity common to them which might account for such broad reactivity. All of the above drugs share the property of being inhibitors of prostaglandin synthetase (Vane, 1971; Szczeklik *et al.*, 1975) and aspirin may actually directly acetylate and thereby inactivate this enzyme (Roth *et al.*, 1975). Thus a susceptibility to the pharmacological or metabolic properties of these drugs may account for the urticaria. It is also possible that a subpopulation of patients react to aspirin anhydride by a true immune reaction (DeWeck, 1971); however, this observation has not yet been confirmed.

Foods are a common cause of urticaria, although their role in acute urticaria is much more important that their role in chronic urticaria. In some cases of urticaria secondary to foods such as nuts, fish, and eggs, an IgE-dependent mechanism appears to be operative (Golbert *et al.*, 1969) as assessed by passive transfer studies. When a food allergy is considered to be a cause of urticaria or angioedema, it is a common practice to do skin testing. Such tests have a high incidence of false-positive reactions which do not correlate with the patient's symptoms, as well as false-negative reactions which may fail to reveal allergy to a food metabolite. Their usefulness is at best controversial and, again, an empirical approach is indicated (Beall, 1964; Sheldon *et al.*, 1967). One may attempt to first eliminate common offenders from the patient's diet such as shellfish, chocolate, peanuts, and fresh fruits for a period of weeks. However, when dealing with urticaria which has been chronic for many months or years, a rigid elimination diet is most valuable. A diet consisting of rice, lamb, and water for a period of 1 week to 10 days will often yield an answer as to whether a food is responsible for the symptoms. Amelioration of the urticaria should be followed by adding one or two new foods to the patient's diet every 3 days. If the urticaria recurs, the incriminating food can be identified by adding and eliminating it from the diet two or three times to be sure that the observed association is not coincidental. Failure of the urticaria or angioedema to remit on such a diet is presumptive evidence that some other cause is operative. Similar but somewhat less rigid diets than this can also be utilized (Sheldon *et al.*, 1967). In some patients, sensitivity to food dyes, natural salicylates, and/or benzoic acid derivatives may be subtle causes of chronic urticaria (Lockey, 1971; Juhlin *et al.*, 1972; Michaelsson and Juhlin, 1973) and diets specifically eliminating these materials are sometimes useful (Noid *et al.*, 1974; Warin and Champion, 1974). Approximately 15% of aspirin-sensitive individuals (including those with asthma, rhinitis, or urticaria) have been found to be sensitive to tartrazine yellow #5 (Settipane *et al.*, 1975; Settipane and Pudupakkam, 1975). Interestingly, these aspirin-sensitive patients tended to segregate into two groups, one in whom bronchospasm was the predominant symptom and a second group in whom rhinitis, urticaria and angioedema predominated although there was considerable overlap. A recent American Academy of Allergy investigation of the incidence of well-documented tartrazine sensitivity in patients with chronic intractable urticaria reported a value of 8% (Settipane and Padupakkam, 1975).

Urticaria and angioedema can also be the presenting symptom or an associated symptom of an underlying systemic illness (Braverman, 1967). Therefore, all patients should be screened for the presence of collagen vascular diseases such as systemic lupus erythematosus as well as for evidence of carcinoma. Recently systemic vasculitides have been found to be associated with lesions that are visually indistinguishable from urticaria. Included in this group were patients with Sjogren's syndrome, rheumatoid arthritis, and systemic lupus erythematosus either with or without cryoglobulinemia (Soter *et al.*, 1974a). Skin biopsy of these cutaneous lesions revealed true vasculitis with necrosis of the vessel wall, a polymorphonuclear leukocyte infiltrate, and, when cryoglobulinemia was present, deposition of immunoglobulin and complement. The complement activation profile reflected the particular class of immunoglobulin involved. Thus IgM and IgG cryoglobulins activated the classical pathway while IgA cryoglobulins spared C1, C4, and C2, suggesting alternate pathway activation.

Undetected infections have long been considered a cause of chronic urticaria; however, the incidence is probably quite small. Urticaria has been well documented during the prodrome of viral infections such as infectious hepatitis (Ljunggren and Moller, 1971; Koehn and Thorne, 1972; Lockshin and Hurley, 1972) and infectious mononucleosis (Aoyama *et al.*, 1970), and a large number of helminthic parasites are clearly associated with urticaria including ascaris, ancyclostoma, strongyloides, filaria, echinococcus, schistosoma, trichinella, toxocara, and fasciola (Warin and Champion, 1974). These parasitic infections are usually associated with a prominent eosinophilia. Although urticaria has been reported in association with various bacterial and fungal infections, in most cases it is not clear whether the two processes were related, occurred simultaneously by chance, or were influenced by medications taken. Cases have been reported in which removal of a dental abscess (Unger, 1960; Shelley, 1969) or gangrenous gallbladder (Chester *et al.*, 1959) led to prompt resolution of chronic urticaria while larger surveys have generally found no association between infections present in patients with urticaria and the clinical course of their hives (Rorsman, 1962). Similarly the association of tinea or monilia infections and urticaria is, in most cases, coincidental. In general, a thorough history and physical examination should provide the information needed to determine whether further workup in search of an underlying infection is warranted. Certainly any symptom or sign of such infection should be pursued and, if found, treatment instituted. However, doing routine gallbladder series, intravenous pyelograms, or even dental X-rays in search of the cause of chronic urticaria or angioedema is usually unwarranted. Table 2 summarizes an initial evaluation that all chronic urticaria or angioedema patients should receive. Then as specific diagnoses are considered, special tests, as outlined in Table 3, should be obtained.

Urticaria has also been observed as a manifestation of carcinoma of the colon (Sheldon *et al.*, 1954), rectum, or lung and may have an increased incidence in hyperthyroidism (Champion *et al.*, 1969; Isaacs and Ertel, 1971). However, these too account for only a very small proportion of patients with urticaria. Women with urticaria commonly complain that it exacerbates at the time menses begins, and, in some, cyclic urticaria is seen in association with menses (Champion *et al.*, 1969). Although immunological reactions to endogenous hormones have been proposed, there is little evidence to support such a mechanism. However, it is clear that hormones can play a role in modulating the severity of symptoms and in rare cases may play a role in the etiology (Farah and Shbaklu, 1971). Certainly the emotional status of the individual also affects the course of urticaria and angioedema as it does allergic rhinitis, atopic dermatitis, or asthma. Thus the resolution of conflicts and the easing of frustrations and daily stresses of living can be of considerable assistance in successfully managing patients with urticaria and an-

TABLE 2. Routine Evaluation of Chronic Urticaria and Angioedema

1. History
2. Physical examination
3. Chest X-ray
4. Blood tests
   a. Complete blood count and differential
   b. Sedementation rate
   c. Serology
   d. L.E. Prep, antinuclear factor, rheumatoid factor
   e. Protein electrophoresis
5. Stool for ova and parasites
6. Skin biopsy

gioedema (Levine, 1975). Numerous investigations of patients with chronic urticaria or angioedema have suggested that psychogenic factors were *responsible* for the illness in many patients. This contention remains a viable possibility since an alternative etiology cannot be identified in approximately 75% of cases. However, patients with hereditary angioneurotic edema fulfill all the criteria utilized to implicate psychogenic factors as being etiological in their disease, but this notion has been abandoned since an abnormal blood protein has been identified as the underlying defect. Possibly this disease dramatizes the temptation to implicate the patient's psyche as the cause of symptoms rather than as a modifying influence when the etiology is unknown and we are forced to acknowledge our own ignorance.

4. Physical Urticarias and Angioedema

The physical urticarias and angioedema share the common property of being reproducibly induced by environmental factors such as a change in temperature, or by direct stimulation of the skin by pressure, stroking, or vibration.

4.1. Cold Urticaria

Cold urticaria is a disorder characterized by the rapid onset of pruritis, erythema, and swelling after exposure to a cold stimulus. The location of the swelling is confined to those portions of the body that have contacted the cold, although the symptoms are often maximal after the exposed area is warmed. Patients typically experience symptoms while outside on cold, windy days, but holding cold objects can cause hand swelling and eating cold foods may cause lip swelling. Swelling of the tongue and pharynx is less common while laryngeal

TABLE 3. Tests Used in the Diagnosis of Urticaria and Angioedema

Food and drug reactions: Elimination of offending agent: challenge with suspected foods, lamb and rice diet, special diets eliminating natural salicylates and food additives
Inhalent allergens: Skin tests, *in vitro* histamine release from human basophils
Collagen vascular diseases and cutaneous vasculitis: Skin biopsy, CH50, C4, C3, factor B, immunofluorescence of tissue
Malignancy with angioedema: CH50, C1, C$\bar{1}$ INH determinations
Cold urticaria: Ice cube test
Cholinergic urticaria: Mecholyl skin test, exercise challenge
Solar urticaria: Exposure to defined wavelengths of light, red cell protoporphyrin, fecal protoporphyrin, and coproporphyrin
Dermographism: Stroking with narrow object, e.g., tongue blade, fingernail
Pressure urticaria: Application of pressure for defined time and intensity
Vibratory angioedema: Vibration with laboratory vortex for 4 min
Aquagenic urticaria: Challenge with tap water at various temperatures
Urticaria pigmentosa: Skin biopsy, test for dermographism
Hereditary angioedema: C4, C2, C$\bar{1}$ INH by protein and function
Familial cold urticaria: Challenge by cold exposure and measurement of temperature, WBC, and sedimentation rate; skin biopsy
C3b inactivator deficiency: C3, factor B, C3b inactivator determinations
Idiopathic: Skin biopsy, immunofluorescence

edema or abdominal complaints are rarely, if ever, seen. Total body exposure such as while swimming can cause massive mediator release, resulting in hypotension. Since fatalities by drowning have been reported secondary to the cold exposure presumably caused by the hypotension (Horton *et al.*, 1936), patients should be warned that swimming is contraindicated.

This disease can begin in any age group and has no obvious sex predilection. When the diagnosis is suspected, a simple test that can confirm the initial impression is to place an ice cube on the patient's forearm for 4 min and observe the area for 10 min afterward. If the patient has cold urticaria, the area will become pruritic about 2 min after removal of the ice cube, and by 10 min a large hive the shape of the ice cube will form as shown in Figure 3. Cold urticaria has been reported in association with a variety of diseases characterized by abnormal immunoglobulins which have some cold-dependent property. Thus it is seen in cryoglobulinemia, cold agglutinin disease, cryofibrinogenemia, and paroxysmal cold hemoglobinuria (the Donath–Landsteiner antibody associated with secondary syphilis) (Moroz and Rose, 1971). The mechanism of production of urticaria in these diseases is unknown; however, in some studies (Costanzi and Coltman, 1967; Costanzi *et al.*, 1969) isolated cryoglobulins have been shown to be capable of transferring the disease. These proteins can fix complement when aggregated by cryoprecipitation; thus it is possible that histamine release may occur via the C3a and C5a anaphylatoxins.

In most patients, however, an abnormal circulating protein is not evident. We have studied mediator release in 12 such patients by placing one hand in ice water for 4 min and serially determining the plasma histamine level in the brachial vein draining that hand (Figure 4). In all patients a peak of histamine release was observed between 4 and 8 min after the hand had been removed from the ice

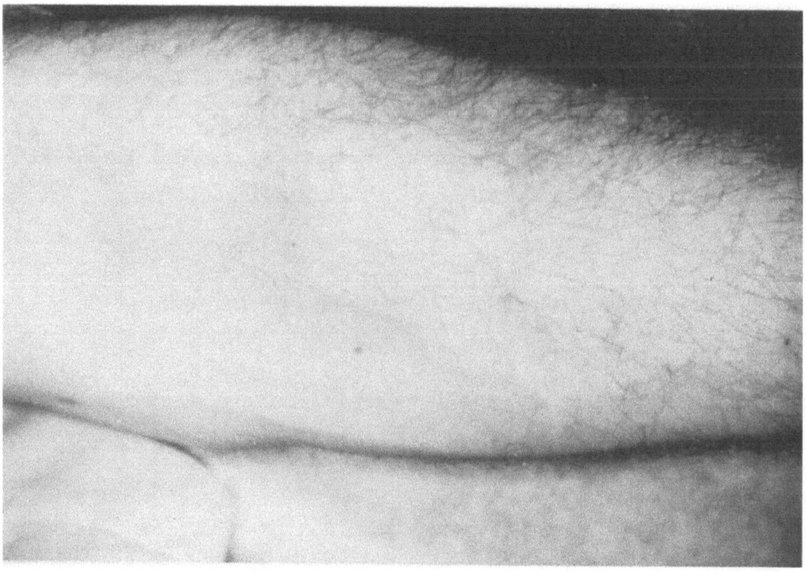

Figure 3. Positive ice cube test in a patient with cold urticaria.

water (Kaplan *et al.*, 1975; Kaplan and Beaven, 1976) while assays of the same samples for serotonin and bradykinin were negative. These results have been confirmed, and simultaneous release of the eosinophilotactic tetrapeptides (ECF-A) (Soter *et al.*, 1976b) as well as a chemotactic factor specific for neutrophils was observed (Wasserman *et al.*, 1977). In a patient with a history of repeated episodes of hypotension on wading in the ocean, a 50-point drop in diastolic blood pressure was observed coincident with the peak histamine level; thus it is likely that histamine contributes to both the urticaria and the hypotension characteristic of this disorder. In two of these 12 patients the cold urticaria could be passively transferred to normals and was shown to be mediated by IgE; however, the mechanism by which temperature changes lead to IgE-dependent histamine release is unknown. IgE-mediated cold urticaria has also been reported in another series of such patients (Houser *et al.*, 1970) while two patients have been described having IgM-dependent cold urticaria (Wanderer *et al.*, 1971). Although this disease generally responds to antihistamines, cyproheptadine (periactin) appears to be particularly effective (Wanderer and Ellis, 1971). We have found that 12–32 mg of cyproheptadine daily, in divided doses, will turn the ice cube test negative in most patients and affords considerable objective relief of their symptoms when exposed to cold. Although cold "desensitization" can apparently be achieved by gradual increasing exposure of patients (Bentley-Phillips *et al.*, 1976), we view this approach as less practical and potentially dangerous. A single family with delayed urticaria in response to cold appears to represent a different disorder, and extensive

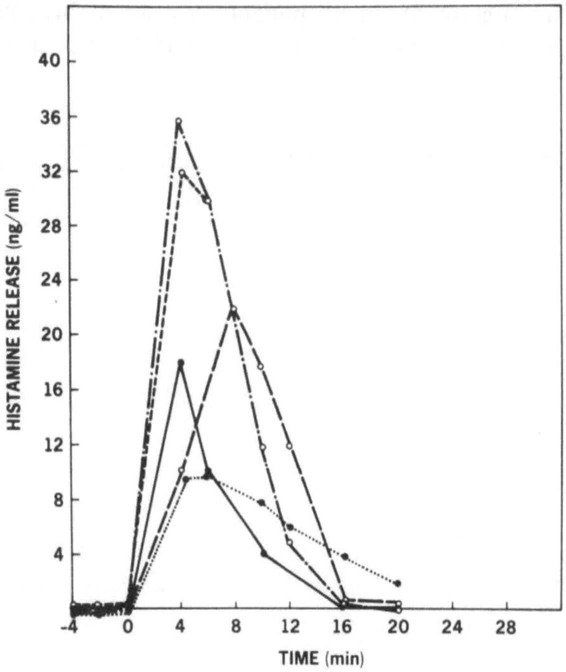

Figure 4. Histamine release obtained after challenge of six cold urticaria patients by placing one hand in ice water for 4 min. The "zero" time is when the hand was removed from the ice bath.

studies of mediator release, complement, and immunoglobulins failed to reveal an abnormality (Soter *et al.*, 1977).

4.2. Cholinergic Urticaria

Cholinergic or heat urticaria can occur in a local or generalized form. The local form is observed when a warm stimulus is in contact with the skin and when suspected can be tested for by using a test tube of warm water (Baer and Hauber, 1971). This is an extremely rare disorder (the local form), and there are no reported investigations of its pathogenesis. Generalized cholinergic urticaria is characterized by the onset of small punctate wheals surrounded by a prominent erythematous flare associated with exercise, hot showers, sweating, and anxiety (Grant *et al.*, 1935). It tends to appear first over the upper thorax and neck but can spread distally to involve virtually the entire body. In some patients these hives can become confluent and resemble angioedema while other patients may have symptoms characteristic of cholinergic stimulation such as lacrimation, salivation, and diarrhea. These various stimuli have the common feature of being mediated by cholinergic nerve fibers which innervate the musculature via parasympathetic neurons and innervate the sweat glands by cholinergic fibers that travel with the sympathetic nerves (Herxheimer, 1956) (Figure 5). The characteristic lesion of cholinergic urticaria can be reproduced by an intradermal injection of 0.01 mg mecholyl in 0.1 ml saline, and a localized hive surrounded by smaller satellite lesions is diagnostic (Baer and Hauber, 1971). These patients therefore demonstrate a "hypersensitivity" to cholinergic mediators, but they have no evidence of an immunoglobulin-mediated allergy to acetylcholine. It is possible that this disease involves an intrinsic cellular abnormality which leads to mediator release in the

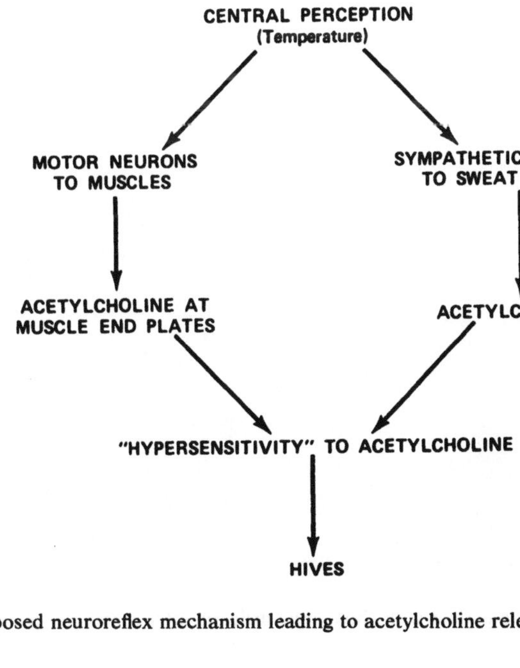

Figure 5. Proposed neuroreflex mechanism leading to acetylcholine release in cholinergic urticaria.

presence of cholinergic agents. Evidence that a neurogenic reflex is involved is provided by the observation that placing a patient's hand in warm water with a tourniquet tied proximal to that arm does not cause localized hives while removal of the tourniquet can lead to a generalized eruption. Thus a central perception of the temperature change appears to be followed by an efferent reflex leading to the urticaria. Such a reflex could also account for the association of hives with anxiety, although it should be emphasized that in these instances the emotional reaction itself may be normal. A photograph of typical cholinergic urticaria is shown in Figure 6, in which lesions were induced by having the patient run in place for 10 min. Histamine release associated with cholinergic urticaria has been reported (Kaplan *et al.*, 1975) but was demonstrable only in a small number of patients whose symptoms were particularly severe. The drug of choice for the management of cholinergic urticaria is hydroxazine (Atarax), and most patients respond to a dose between 100 and 200 mg/day (Moore-Robinson and Warin, 1908). It is considerably more effective than conventional antihistamines, suggesting that it has some additional action; it might, for example, interrupt the neurogenic reflex which leads to the urticaria.

4.3. Dermographism

The ability to "write on skin," termed "dermographism," can occur as an isolated disorder which often presents as traumatically induced urticaria. It can be diagnosed by observing the skin after stroking it with a tongue blade or fingernail. In these patients the white line secondary to reflex vasoconstriction is followed by pruritis, erythema, and linear swelling as in a classical wheal-and-flare reaction. In approximately 50% of patients passive transfer studies have suggested an IgE-mediated reaction (Aoyama *et al.*, 1970; Newcomb and Nelson, 1973), but the

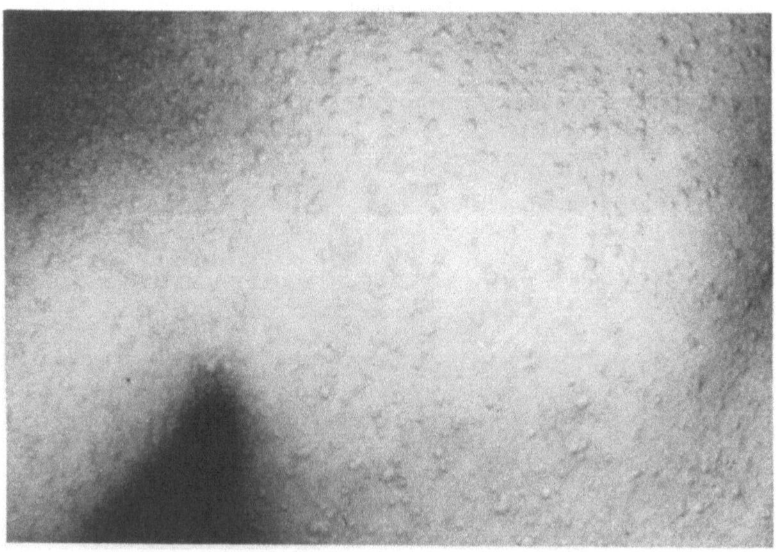

Figure 6. Hives induced in a patient with cholinergic urticaria after running in place for 10 min.

antigen has not been identified. The drug of choice for this disease is diphenhydramine (Benadryl), although different patients may prefer different antihistamines depending on their relative efficacy as opposed to adverse side effects. Dermographism of a milder degree may be seen in patients with chronic urticaria caused by a variety of different etiologies, as will be discussed subsequently. Severe dermographism is seen associated with urticaria pigmentosa or systemic mastocytosis, and in the systemic disease the wheals may last for many hours. Large doses of antihistamines are required to relieve the symptoms, and evidence of histamine release in urticaria pigmentosa as well as in idiopathic dermographism has been reported (Greaves and Sondergaard, 1970).

4.4. Pressure Urticaria (Angioedema)

The gradual onset of hives or swelling after pressure has been applied to the skin is called "pressure urticaria" or "pressure-induced angioedema." The urticaria may be associated with tight garments such as the elastic on socks, tight wristbands, belts, and brassierre straps or with sustained pressure such as buttock swelling after being seated for long periods of time. The time of induction of symptoms is quite variable, ranging from a few minutes after the stimulus to delayed reactions occurring as long as 24 hr later; a time interval of 4–6 hr is typical. Although the lesions are caused by direct pressure to the skin, these patients are not dermographic. Thus far there are no reports of mediator release in pressure urticaria or angioedema. It is usually unresponsive to antihistamines, and, for severe cases, low doses of systemic steroids are necessary.

4.5. Solar Urticaria

Solar urticaria is a rare disorder in which brief exposure to light causes the development of urticaria within 1–3 min. Typically pruritis occurs first, at about 30 sec, followed by erythema and edema confined to the light-exposed area and surrounded by a prominent erythematous zone caused by an axon reflex. The lesions then usually disappear within 1–3 hr. When large areas of the body are exposed, systemic symptoms may occur including hypotension and asthma. Although most patients reported have been in the third or fourth decade, solar urticaria can occur in any age group and has no association with other allergic disorders.

Solar urticaria has been classified into six types, depending on the wavelength of light which induces lesions and the ability or inability to passively transfer the disorder with serum (Harber *et al.*, 1963; Sams *et al.*, 1969; Baer and Hauber, 1971). Types I and IV can be passively transferred and may therefore be antibody (? IgE) mediated and are associated with wavelengths of 2800–3200 Å and 4000–5000 Å, respectively. The antigen has not been identified. Type IV, activated at 4000 Å, is clearly a metabolic disorder in which protoporphyrin IX acts as a photosensitizer and is synonymous with erythropoietic protoporphyria. In contrast to other forms of porphyria, the urinary porphyrin excretion is normal; however, red cell protoporphyrin is elevated and fecal protoporphyrin and coproporphyrin levels are elevated. It responds to oral β-carotene, which absorbs light at the same wavelength as protoporphyrin IX (Moshell and Bjornson, 1977). The mechanism producing light urticaria in types II, III, and V is unknown, but these are induced by inciting wavelengths of 3200–4000 Å, and 2800–5000 Å, respectively, and cannot be passively transferred with serum. As a simple screen, fluorescent tubes which emit a broad, continuous spectrum can be used to test the patient, and filters can then be used to define the spectrum which causes urticaria. Ordinary windowglass of 3 mm thickness will absorb most ultraviolet radiation below 3200 Å and will thereby protect patients with type I solar urticaria. Therapy of this disease requires avoidance of sunlight, use of protective garments to cover the skin, and use of topical preparations to absorb or reflect light. A 5% solution of *p*-aminobenzoic acid in ethanol, as in sunscreen lotions, can be helpful in the 2800–3200 Å range; however, it is more difficult to screen out the visible spectrum. The most effective agents for this purpose contain titanium oxide and/or zinc oxide. The efficacy of antihistaminics, antimalarials, and corticostroids in these disorders is not clear and needs to be evaluated for each type.

4.6. Aquagenic Urticaria

A few cases have been reported of patients who developed small wheals after contact with water, regardless of its temperature, which were distinguishable from cold urticaria or cholinergic urticaria. This entity has been termed "aquagenic urticaria" (Tromovitch, 1967; Chalamidas and Charles, 1971) and can be tested for by direct application of a compress of tap water or distilled water to the skin. The diagnosis should be reserved for those rare cases which give a positive test to water and in which tests for all other forms of physical urticaria are negative.

5. Hereditary Forms of Urticaria and Angioedema

5.1. Familial Cold Urticaria

Familial cold urticaria is a rare form of cold intolerance which is inherited as an autosomal dominant and histologically is not truly urticaria. Approximately 30 min after exposure to cold, a systemic reaction occurs consisting of burning papular skin lesions accompanied by fever, chills, arthralgias, myalgias, headache, and leukocytosis. Biopsy of the skin lesions reveals edema and an intense inflammatory infiltrate consisting almost entirely of polymorphonuclear leukocytes with eosinophils prominent about dilated capillaries (Tindall *et al.*, 1969; Douglas and Bleumink, 1974).

5.2. Hereditary Vibratory Angioedema

Hereditary vibratory angioedema has been described in a single family in whom it was inherited in an autosomal dominant pattern. It is properly viewed as a physically induced angioedema (Table 1) since patients complain of intense pruritis and swelling within minutes after vibratory stimuli (Patterson *et al.*, 1972). The patients are not dermographic and do not have pressure urticaria. The lesions can be reproduced by gently stimulating the patient's forearm with a laboratory vortex for 4 min. Rapid swelling of the entire forearm and a portion of the upper arm ensues, and histamine has recently been shown to be released secondary to such a vibratory stimulus (Metzger *et al.*, 1976). With care, patients can avoid vibratory stimuli and their symptoms can otherwise be partially relieved with diphenhydramine (Benadryl). We have observed a milder form of vibration-induced swelling in some patients with cholinergic urticaria (Kaplan *et al.*, 1972), suggesting that there may be some pathogenic relationship between those diseases although they are distinct clinical entities.

5.3. C3b Inactivator Deficiency

Two patients have been reported who are deficient in the C3b inactivator (Alper *et al.*, 1972; Thompson and Lachmann, 1977). The complement profile in these patients suggests "spontaneous" activation of the alternate complement pathway consisting of depletion of factor B, markedly depressed C3 levels, and a circulating inactive C3 by-product without evidence of further degradation to C3c or C3d (Alper *et al.*, 1972). The mechanism by which this pathway is activated as a consequence of the absent inactivator is unknown; however, intravenous replacement with C3b inactivator leads to elevation of the patients' C3. Of particular interest is that one patient had histaminuria and one of his presenting symptoms was urticaria. This may reflect rapid degradation of C3 with liberation of C3a anaphylatoxin. Family members had half-normal levels of the C3b inactivator, suggesting an autosomal recessive inheritance.

5.4. Urticaria and Amyloidosis

Familial urticaria has also been seen in conjunction with the combination of amyloidosis, nerve deafness, and limb pain (Muckle and Wells, 1962; Kennedy *et al.*, 1966). It appears to be inherited as an autosomal dominant (Anderson *et al.*, 1967; Black, 1969) in which the urticaria has been described having features of cholinergic urticaria, angioedema, or classical hives. The rash is associated with limb pain and seems to be intensified by cold weather.

5.5. Hereditary Angioedema

Hereditary angioedema is an autosomal dominant disorder caused by absence of the $C\bar{1}$ inactivator ($C\bar{1}$ INH) (Donaldson and Evans, 1963) in which patients may have attacks of swelling involving almost any portion of the body. A traumatic episode may initiate an attack; however, such a triggering event may not be evident and the swelling appears to occur "spontaneously." It is *not* associated with urticaria, and patients with both urticaria and angioedema without a family history invariably have a normal $C\bar{1}$ INH. In addition to the family history, the presence of visceral involvement suggests the hereditary disorder. The most severe complication is laryngeal edema, which has been a major cause of death in this disease. Patients can also have abdominal attacks (Donaldson and Rosen, 1966) lasting 1–2 days consisting of vomiting, severe abdominal pain, and guarding in the absence of fever, leukocytosis, or abdominal rigidity. This can, at times, be difficult to distinguish from an acute abdomen; however, the attacks are self-limited and have been shown to be caused by edema of the bowel wall (Pearson *et al.*, 1972).

Patients with hereditary angioedema have measurable levels of the *activated* first component of complement (C$\bar{1}$), although this protein usually circulates as an unactivated enzyme. The serum level of C4 is diminished even when the patient is free of symptoms and is usually undetectable during an attack (Ruddy *et al.*, 1968). A C4 determination is therefore the simplest test to diagnose hereditary angioedema. C2, the other substrate of C$\bar{1}$, is usually within normal limits when the patient is as symptomatic, but it also is diminished during an attack (Austen and Sheffer, 1965). When a diminished C4 level is obtained, a direct assay of protein C$\bar{1}$ INH level should be performed. A diminished or absent level of C$\bar{1}$ INH confirms the diagnosis; however, approximately 20% of patients have a normal or elevated C$\bar{1}$ INH protein (Rosen *et al.*, 1971). In these cases the protein is not functional and often has an abnormal electrophoretic mobility. Thus a functional C$\bar{1}$ INH assay is then necessary to determine whether the diagnosis is really hereditary angioedema.

The pathogenesis of the swelling appears to involve both the complement pathway and the plasma kinin-forming pathway as depicted in Figures 7 and 8. Intracutaneous injection of C$\bar{1}$ into normals causes the formation of a small wheal while injection into a patient with hereditary angioedema yields localized angioedema (Klemperer *et al.*, 1968). A kinin-like peptide has been isolated from these patients, and its formation appears to be inhibited in C2-deficient plasma (Donaldson *et al.*, 1969). However, direct demonstration of such a kinin-like peptide on interaction of C$\bar{1}$ with C4 and C2 or C2 alone is lacking. Twenty-four-hour urine histamine excretion is also increased during attacks of angioedema, suggesting that C3a and/or C5a is being generated. Although the plasma levels of C3 and C5 are normal in this disorder, C3 turnover is enhanced (Carpenter *et al.*, 1969). The lesions, however, are not pruritic and antihistamines have no effect on the clinical course of the disease.

C$\bar{1}$ INH also inhibits activated Hageman factor (Schreiber *et al.*, 1973), kallikrein (Gigli *et al.*, 1970), and plasmin (Schreiber *et al.*, 1973); thus it is also an important modulator of bradykinin generation. Patients appear to be hyperresponsive to injections of kallikrein (Juhlin and Michaelsson, 1969) as they are to C$\bar{1}$, and elevated levels of plasma bradykinin have been observed during attacks (Talamo *et al.*, 1969). There is also evidence that the C$\bar{1}$ activation observed in

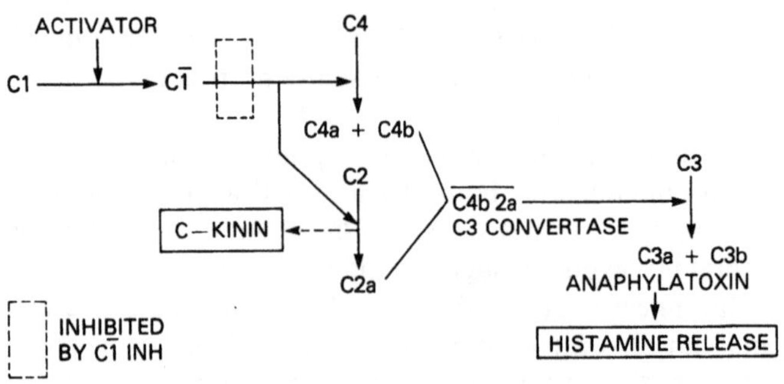

Figure 7. Interaction of C$\bar{1}$ with C4 and C2 indicating the position of inhibition by C$\bar{1}$ INH and the liberation of a putative C2-kinin. The formation of C3 convertase (C4b 2a) and cleavage of C3 to yield C3a anaphylatoxin are also shown.

hereditary angioedema may be Hageman factor dependent (Donaldson, 1968; Eisen and Loveday, 1972). Thus some Hageman-factor-dependent enzyme may be initiating the classical complement cascade. Plasmin has been shown to be capable of activating C$\bar{1}$s (Ratnoff and Naff, 1967) and may represent one such enzyme.

The ultrastructural lesion seen in tissues of patients with hereditary angioneurotic edema consists of gaps in the postcapillary venule endothelial cells with edema and virtually no cellular infiltrate (Sheffer *et al.*, 1971). Similar lesions are induced by injection of C$\bar{1}$ esterase (C$\bar{1}$) or the purified kinin-like polypeptide isolated from hereditary angioedema plasma (Willms *et al.*, 1975).

The treatment for attacks of hereditary angioedema often involves intermittent administration of subcutaneous epinephrine. However, there are no studies to support its efficacy since attacks usually abate in 3–4 days even if no medication is given. A tracheostomy is indicated if laryngeal edema occurs, and mild analgesics may be utilized to relieve the discomfort of severe swelling and/or abdominal pain. Intravenous fluids may be necessary if the patient is unable to eat or drink. Successful prevention of attacks has been reported (Davis *et al.*, 1974) utilizing large doses of an antifibrinolytic agent such as ϵ-aminocaproic acid (Lundh *et al.*, 1968; Frank *et al.*, 1972) or tranexamic acid (Sheffer *et al.*, 1972). The precise mechanism of action of these agents is unknown; however, they not only inhibit plasmin, which may activate C1 as well as Hageman factor (Kaplan and Austen, 1971), but also inhibit the activation of C$\bar{1}$ by immune complexes, suggesting a direct effect on the C1 molecule (Soter *et al.*, 1975). In Figure 8 is shown a proposed model for the pathogenesis of hereditary angioedema indicating the reactions inhibited by C$\bar{1}$ INH. At the present time, the drugs of choice appear to be androgen derivatives, which have been shown to prevent attacks of swelling in patients with hereditary angioedema (Spalding, 1960; Davis *et al.*, 1974). Danazole, a nonvirilizing androgen, prevents attacks of hereditary angioedema (Gelfand *et al.*, 1976; Rosse *et al.*, 1976), and the patients synthesize normal C$\bar{1}$ INH and their

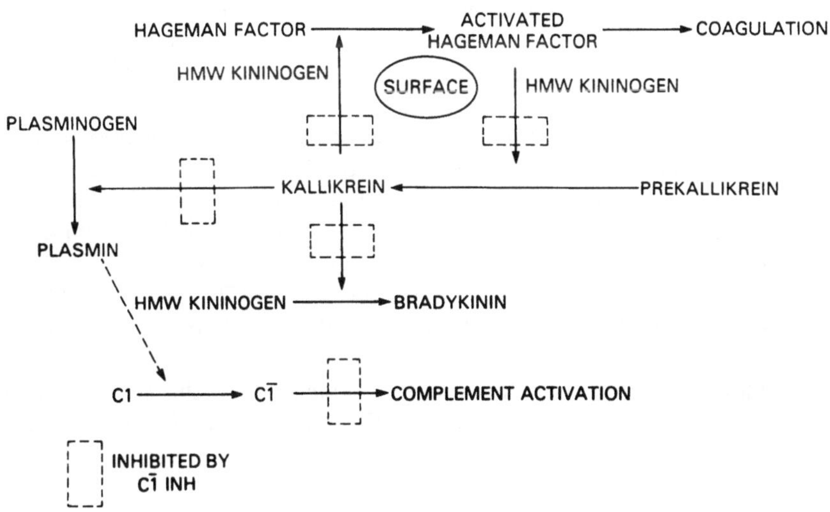

Figure 8. Hageman-factor-dependent pathways and early steps of the classical complement pathway indicating their possible interrelationships and the reactions inhibited by C$\bar{1}$ INH.

C4 level returns to normal. Thus patients with this disease are probably heterozygotes, possessing one normal gene whose function has been suppressed. Evidence of diminished hepatic synthesis of $C\bar{1}$ INH in patients with this disorder has been reported (Johnson *et al.*, 1971). Administration of the androgen leads to synthesis of the normal gene product.

A secondary form of this disease has been described in patients with lymphoma who have circulating low-molecular-weight IgM and depressed $C\bar{1}$ INH levels. This entity has an unusual complement utilization profile in that C1 depletion is more prominent than C4, C2, or C3 depletion, thus distinguishing it from the hereditary disorder (Caldwell *et al.*, 1972). The depressed $C\bar{1}$ INH level is assumed to be depletion secondary to binding and inactivation of the $C\bar{1}$.

6. Vasculitis and Urticaria

It has become clear that patients with immune complex disease such as serum sickness (Arbesman and Reisman, 1971; Warin and Champion, 1974) or systemic lupus erythematosus (Paver, 1971) can have urticaria as a manifestation of the underlying disease. Biopsy of such lesions shows evidence of a necrotizing vasculitis involving small venules (hypersensitivity angiitis) (Copeman and Ryan, 1970; Braverman and Yen, 1975), and immunofluorescent studies demonstrate deposition of immunoglobulins and complement. In patients with serum sickness, IgE-dependent histamine release as well as histamine release secondary to complement activation may contribute to the urticaria seen. Patients presenting with urticaria secondary to cutaneous vasculitis have been described (Soter *et al.*, 1974b) who could not be readily classified as having an underlying collagen-vascular disease. An elevated sedimentation rate, arthralgias, and myalgias as well as fever and leucocytosis were the main associated abnormalities. Like patients with palpable purpura associated with a variety of diseases, patients could be divided into a group with serum hypercomplementemia and a second group in whom the serum complement was normal (Soter *et al.*, 1976a). The group with hypocomplementemia had lesions characterized by infiltration with neutrophils, fibrin deposition, and prominent nuclear debris. The normocomplementemic group had lesions in which lymphocytes predominated and there was prominent perivenular fibrin deposition. In each, there was evidence of mast cell degranulation and true vessel wall necrosis. Other isolated cases of chronic urticaria also have been reported to involve cutaneous vasculitis and hypocomplementemia (McDuffie *et al.*, 1973; Marder *et al.*, 1976). The pathogenic mechanism in the normocomplementemic group is unknown. Hypocomplementemia in chronic urticaria was also found in 10 to 72 patients reported by Mathison *et al.* (1977), and each of these 10 patients had detectable circulating immune complexes, cutaneous vasculitis, and immunoglobulin and complement deposition at the dermal–epidermal junction as well as in blood vessel walls. Thus there is evidence that the subpopulation of patients with chronic urticaria and hypocomplementemia may have an underlying immune complex disease.

7. Chronic Idiopathic Urticaria and Idiopathic Angioedema

Reports of the incidence of identification of the etiological agent in chronic urticaria and angioedema range from 10% to as high as 80%. However, a successful diagnosis in most studies is probably not greater than 20%. Of course, different physicians, clinics, or allergy centers see different populations of patients, and this may in part account for the wide variance reported. We have studied over 100 patients with chronic urticaria for whom no etiological agent could be identified after evaluation by competent allergists in the community. Our incidence of successful subsequent identification of a causal factor is 5%. These patients appear to have a disorder that is "idiopathic." As a group they are not atopic individuals, i.e., they do not have an increased incidence of eczema, allergic rhinitis, or extrinsic asthma compared to the incidence of these disorders in the absence of chronic urticaria. Their IgE levels, as a group, are within normal limits. Some patients are dermographic, although this is usually of milder degree than is seen with the IgE-dependent dermographism described earlier, and curiously the dermographism may wax and wane just as the urticaria may vary from severe to mild or may intermittently subside. These patients have a normal white blood count and sedimentation rate and have no evidence of systemic disease. When patients with this type of urticaria are biopsied, the lesion appears as shown in Figure 9. There is perivascular cuffing consisting predominantly of lymphocytes, as well as monocytes and mast cells. In some patients a prominent eosinophilic infiltrate is also present. This is not a true vasculitis since there is no necrosis of the vessel wall, nuclear dust is not seen, neutrophils are not prominent, and immunofluorescent studies for the deposition of immunoglobulins and complement have thus far been negative. It is of interest that in a recent textbook of dermatopathology (Lever and Schaumburg-Lever, 1975) there is no lesion identified as chronic

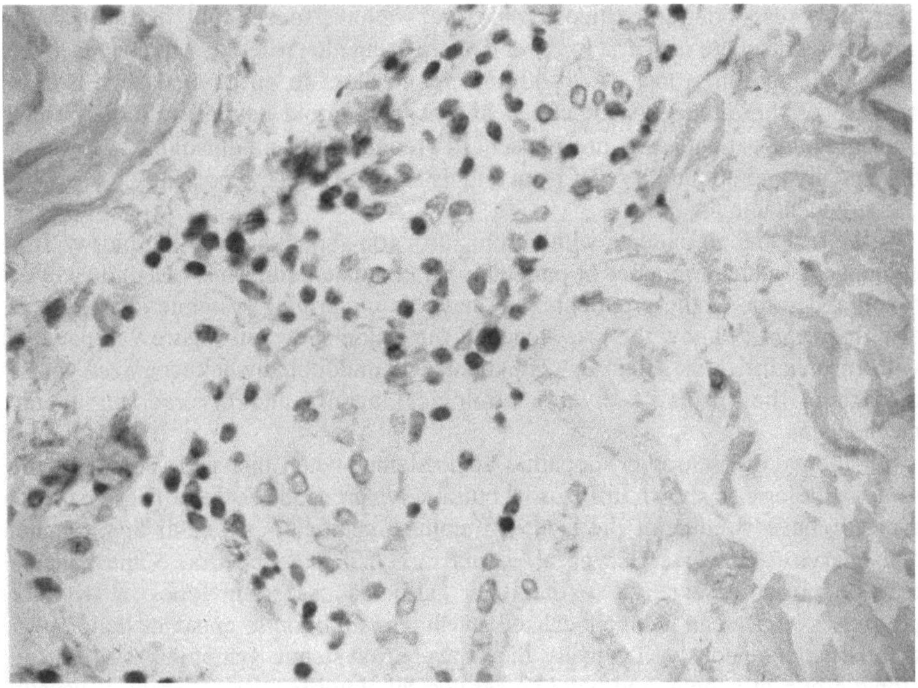

Figure 9. Hematoxylin- and eosin-stained skin biopsy specimen from a patient with chronic idiopathic urticaria.

urticaria, but the observed pathology closely resembles a form of erythema multiforme without bullae formation (type II erythemia multiforme). Some of our patients do have target lesions which, on routine biopsy, are indistinguishable from nontargeted urticarial lesions. The biopsy data do, in fact, suggest a lesion that is not typical of acute urticaria since this should classically consist of edema formation with a small number of eosinophils. Such lesions may be seen in mild early delayed hypersensitivity reactions and have been described as late consequences of IgE-mediated reactions when the antigen dose is high (Dolovich *et al.*, 1973). A single study reported diminished *in vitro* release of histamine from basophils of patients with chronic urticaria when challenged with anti-IgE, suggesting that their cells have in some fashion been deactivated (Kern and Lichtenstein, 1976). The only study of mediator release in chronic idiopathic urticaria has resulted from the use of suction blisters (Kaplan *et al.*, 1978). The results demonstrated that blister fluid histamine levels were markedly elevated in this patient population; however, patients also had elevated blister fluid histamine levels over normal-appearing skin. In these patients, one could not distinguish whether the histamine had been released into the tissue prior to the procedure, although urticaria was not seen, or whether the procedure caused local histamine release that is not seen in normal controls. Nevertheless, all patients had a significant elevation of blister fluid histamine levels taken over a lesion and were clearly distinguishable from normal controls.

Therapy generally consists of supportive measures using antihistamines such as hydroxazine (Atarax), cyproheptadine (Periactin), and diphenhydramine (Benadryl) for relief of pruritis. However, these agents relieve the pruritis but often have no effect on the appearance of the lesions. In our series, approximately 90% of patients responded to corticosteroids, and we have successfully managed many patients with severe urticaria for over 4 years using alternate-day prednisone given in a single morning dose of 20–40 mg. We hesitate to go beyond such a dose because of the attendent side-effects of chronic steroid administration. A small percentage of patients are unresponsive to prednisone or prednisolone at doses of 60 mg daily and obtain no relief from antihistamines. There is presently no specific therapy available for them.

We feel that all patients with chronic urticaria should have a skin biopsy. It is evident that a small number of patients with bonafide cutaneous vasculitis will be found and some of these patients may have an underlying systemic disease. It is also important to know the prevalence of the lesion shown in Figure 9 in patients with chronic urticaria; subgroups of patients will undoubtedly be recognized whose disease is the result of diverse etiological agents and diverse pathogenic mechanisms.

Patients with chronic idiopathic angioedema, when biopsied, have had the same pathology as shown in Figure 9 but involving deeper vessels. These patients typically have swelling of the face, extremities, genitalia, as well as lips, tongue, and pharynx. However, laryngeal edema rarely, if ever, occurs. Some patients may be pressure sensitive so that tight garments or certain types of work or physical exercise can induce localized swelling in addition to episodes that appear to arise spontaneously. Typically they have no systemic symptoms, are not an atopic group of people, and have no serological abnormalities. Therapy is usually attempted with high doses of antihistamines such as diphenhydramine (Benadryl) and corticosteroids as outlined for chronic urticaria if the frequency and severity of attacks warrant it. A small number of patients have been described with complement abnormalities (Sissons *et al.*, 1974; Webb *et al.*, 1975; Ballow *et al.*, 1975), suggesting that chronic angioedema will also probably represent a heterogeneous group of diseases.

Much has been written describing the clinical presentation and therapy of chronic urticaria and angioedema. However, it is clear that in most cases the etiology and pathogenesis are unknown. Future studies should provide further insight into the nature of these diseases and lead to improved methods of therapy.

8. References

Alper, C. A., Rosen, F. S., and Lachmann, P. J., 1972, Inactivator of the third component of complement as an inhibitor of the properdin pathway, *Proc. Natl. Acad. Sci. USA* **69:**2910–2913.

Anderson, V., Buch, N. H., Jensen, M. K., and Killmann, S., 1967, Deafness, urticaria, and amyloidosis: A sporatic case with chromosomal aberration, *Am. J. Med.* **42:**449–456.

Aoyama, H., Katsumata, Y., and Olzawa, T., 1970, Dermographism-inducing principle of urticaria factitia, *Jpn. J. Dermatol.* **80:**122.

Arbesman, C. E., and Reisman, R. E., 1971, Serum sickness and human anaphylaxis, in: *Immunologic Diseases,* Vol. I (M. Samter, ed.), p. 495, Little, Brown, Boston.

Austen, K. F., and Sheffer, A. L., 1965, Detection of hereditary angioneurotic edema by demonstration of a reduction in the second component of human complement, *N. Engl. J. Med.* **272:**649–656.

Baer, R. L., and Hauber, L. C., 1971, Reactions to light, heat, and trauma, in: *Immunological Diseases* (M. Samter, ed.), p. 973, Little, Brown, Boston.

Ballow, M., Ward, G. W., Jr., Gershwin, M. E., and Day, N. K., 1975, Cl bypass complement-activation pathway in patients with chronic urticaria and angioedema, *Lancet* **2:**248–250.

Beall, G. N., 1964, Urticaria: A review of laboratory and clinical observations, *Medicine* **43:**131–151.

Bentley-Phillips, C. B., Black, A. K., and Greaves, M. W., 1976, Induced tolerance in cold urticaria caused by cold-evoked histamine release, *Lancet* **2:**63–66.

Benveniste, J., Henson, P. M., and Cochrane, C. G., 1972, Leukocyte-dependent histamine release from rabbit platelets. The role of IgE, basophils, and a platelet activating factor, *J. Exp. Med.* **136:**1356–1377.

Benveniste, J., Kamoun, P., and Polonsky, J., 1975, Aggregation of human platelets by purified platelet activating factor from human and rabbit basophils, *Fed. Proc.* **34:**985 (abstr.).

Black, J. T., 1969, Amyloidosis, deafness, urticaria, and limb pains: A hereditary syndrome, *Ann. Intern. Med.* **70:**989–994.

Bokisch, V. A., Müller-Eberhard, H. J., and Cochrane, C. G., 1969, Isolation of a fragment (C3a) of the third component of human complement containing anaphylatoxin and chemotactic activity and description of an anaphylatoxin inactivator of human plasma, *J. Exp. Med.* **129:**1109–1130.

Boswell, R. N., Austen, K. F., and Goetzl. E. J., 1978, Intermediate molecular weight eosinophil chemotactic factors in rat peritoneal mast cells: Immunologic release, granule association, and demonstration of structural heterogeneity, *J. Immunol.* **120:**15–20.

Braverman, I. M., 1967, Urticaria as a sign of internal disease, *Postgrad. Med.* **41:**450–454.

Braverman, I. M., and Yen, A., 1975, Demonstration of immune complexes in spontaneous and histamine-induced lesions and normal skin of patients with leucocytoclastic angiitis, *J. Invest. Dermatol.* **64:**105–112.

Caldwell, J. R., Ruddy, S., Schur, P., and Austen, K. F., 1972, Acquired $C\bar{1}$ inhibitor deficiency in lymphosarcoma, *Clin. Immunol. Immunopathol 1:39–52.*

Carpenter, C. B., Ruddy, S., Shehadeh, I. H., Muller-Eberhard, H. J., Merrill, J. P., and Austen, K. F., 1969, Complement metabolism in man: Hypercatabolism of the fourth (C4) and third (C3) components in patients with renal allograft rejection and hereditary angioedema, *J. Clin. Invest.* **48:**1495–1505.

Chalamidas, S. L., and Charles, C. R., 1971, Aquagenic urticaria, *Arch. Dermatol.* **104:**541–546.

Champion, R. H., Roberts, S. O. B., Carpenter, R. G., and Roger, J. H., 1969, Urticaria and angioedema, *Br. J. Dermatol.* **81:**588–597.

Chester, A., Liebowitz, H., and Marklow, H., 1959, Causes of chronic urticaria including infection, *N. Y. State J. Med.* **59:**1786.

Clark, R. A. F., Gallin, J. I., and Kaplan, A. P., 1975, The selective eosinophilic chemotactic activity of histamine, *J. Exp. Med.* **142:**1462–1476.

Clark, R. A. F., Gallin, J. I., and Kaplan, A. P., 1976, Mediator release from basophil granulocytes in chronic myelogenous leukemia: Demonstration of the eosinophil chemotactic activity of histamine, *J. Allergy Clin. Immunol.* **58:**623–634.

Clark, R. A. F., Sandler, J. A., Gallin, J. I., and Kaplan, A. P., 1977, Histamine modulation of eosinophil migration, *J. Immunol.* **118:**137–145.

Cochrane, C. G., and Müller-Eberhard, H. J., 1968, The derivation of two distinct anaphylatoxin activities from the third and fifth components of human complement, *J. Exp. Med.* **127:**371–386.

Cochrane, C. G., Revak, S. D., Aiken, B. S., and Wuepper, K. D., 1972, The structural characteristics and activation of Hageman factor, in: *Inflammation: Mechanism and Control* (I. Lepow and P. Ward, eds.), pp. 119–129, Academic, New York.

Cochrane, C. G., Revak, S. D., and Wuepper, K. D., 1973, Activation of Hageman factor in solid and fluid phases: A critical role of kallikrein, *J. Exp. Med.* **138:**1564–1583.

Colman, R. W., Bagdasarian, A., Talamo, R. C., Scott, C. F., Seavey, M., Guimaraes, J. A., Pierce, J. V., and Kaplan, A. P., 1975, Williams trait: Human kininogen deficiency with diminished levels of plasminogen proactivator and prekallikrein associated with abnormalities of the Hageman factor dependent pathways, *J. Clin. Invest.* **56:**1650–1662.

Copeman, P. W. M., and Ryan, J. J., 1970, The problems of classification of cutaneous angiitis with reference to histopathology and pathogenesis, *Br. J. Dermatol.* **82(5):**2.

Costanzi, J. J., and Coltman, J. C., Jr., 1967, Kappa chain precipitable immunoglobulin G (IgG) associated with cold urticaria. I. Clinical observations, *Clin. Exp. Immunol.* **2:**167–178.

Costanzi, J. J., Coltman, C. A., Jr., and Donaldson, V. H., 1969, Activation of complement by a monoclonal cryoglobulin associated with cold urticaria, *J. Lab. Clin. Med.* **74:**902–910.

Cowdry, S. C., and Reynolds, J. S., 1969, Acute urticaria in infectious mononucleosis, *Ann. Allergy* **27:**182–187.

Daha, M. R., Fearon, D. T., and Austen, K. F., 1976a, C3 nephritic factor (C3 Nef): Stabilization of fluid phase and cell bound alternative pathway convertase, *J. Immunol.* **116:**1–7.

Daha, M. R., Fearon, D. T., and Austen, K. F., 1976b, Isolation of alternative pathway C3 convertase containing uncleaved B and formed in the presence of C3 nephritic factor (C3 Nef), *J. Immunol.* **116:**568–570.

Davis, A. E., Arnaout, M. A., Alper, C. A., and Rosen, F. S., 1977, Transfer of C3 nephritic factor from mother to fetus: Is C3 nephritic factor IgG, *N. Engl. J. Med.* **297:**144–146.

Davis, P. J., Davis, F. B., and Charache, P., 1974, Long term therapy of hereditary angioedema (HAE): Preventive management with fluoxymesterone and oxymetholone in severely affected males and females, *Johns Hopkins Med. J.* **135:**391–398.

DeWeck, A. L., 1971, Immunological effects of aspirin anhydride, a contaminant of commercial acetylsalicylic acid preparations, *Int. Arch. Allergy Appl. Immunol.* **41:**393–418.

Dolovich, J., Hargreave, F. E., Chalmers, R., Shier, K. J., Gauldie, J., and Bienenstock, J., 1973, Late cutaneous allergic responses on isolated IgE-dependent reactions, *J. Allergy Clin. Immunol.* **52:**38–46.

Donaldson, V. H., 1968, Mechanisms of activation of C1 esterase in hereditary angioneurotic edema plasma *in vitro:* The role of Hageman factor, a clot-promoting agent, *J. Exp. Med.* **127:**411–429.

Donaldson, V. H., and Evans, R. R., 1963, A biochemical abnormality in hereditary angioneurotic edema, *Am. J. Med.* **35:**37–44.

Donaldson, V. H., and Rosen, F. S., 1966, Hereditary angioneurotic edema: A clinical survey, *Pediatrics* **37:**1017–1027.

Donaldson, V. H., Ratnoff, O. D., DaSilva, W. D., and Rosen, F. S., 1969, Permeability-increasing activity in hereditary angioneurotic edema plasma. II. Mechanism of formation and partial characterization, *J. Clin. Invest.* **48:**642–653.

Douglas, H. M. G., and Bleumink, E., 1974, Familial cold urticaria. *Arch. Dermatol.* **110:**382–388.

Eisen, V., and Loveday, C., 1972, Activation of arginine and tyrosine esterase in serum from patients with hereditary angioedema, *Br. J. Pharm.* **46:**157–166.

Farah, F. S., and Shbaklu, Z., 1971, Autoimmune progesterone urticaria, *J. Allergy Clin. Immunol.* **48**:257–261.

Fearon, D. T., and Austen, K. F., 1975a, Initiation of C3 cleavage in the alternative complement pathway, *J. Immunol.* **115**:1357–1361.

Fearon, D. T., and Austen, K. F., 1975b, Properdin: Initiation of alternative complement pathway, *Proc. Natl. Acad. Sci. USA* **72**:3220–3224.

Fearon, D. T., and Austen, K. F., 1975c, Properdin: Binding to C3b and stabilization of the C3b-dependent C3 convertase, *J. Exp. Med.* **142**:856–863.

Fearon, D. T., Austen, K. F., and Ruddy, S., 1974, Properdin factor D: Characterization of its active site and isolation of the precursor form, *J. Exp. Med.* **139**:355–366.

Fernandez, H. N., Henson, P. M., Otani, A., and Hugli, T. E., 1978, Chemotactic response to human C3a and C5a anaphylatoxins. I. Evalution of C3a and C5a leukotaxis *in vitro* and under simulated *in vivo* conditions, *J. Immunol.* **120**:109.

Frank, M. M., Sergent, J. S., Kane, M. A., and Alling, D. W., 1972, Epsilon aminocaproic and therapy of hereditary angioneurotic edema: A double blind study, *New Engl. J. Med.* **286**:808–812.

Gallin, J. I., and Kaplan, A. P., 1974, Mononuclear cell chemotactic activity of kallikrein and plasminogen activator and its inhibition by $C\bar{1}$ INH and alpha-2 macroglobulin, *J. Immunol.* **113**:1928–1934.

Gelfand, J. A., Sherins, R. J., Alling, D. W., and Frank, M. M,, 1976, Treatment of hereditary angioedema with danazol: Reversal of clinical and biochemical abnormalities, *N. Engl. J. Med.* **275**:1444–1448.

Gewerz, H., Shin, H. S., and Mergenhagen, S. E., 1968, Interactions of the complement system with endotoxic lipopolysaccharide: Consumption of each of the six terminal complement components, *J. Exp. Med.* **128**:1049–1057.

Gigli, I., Mason, J. W., Colman, R. W., and Austen, K. F., 1970, Interaction of plasma kallikrein with the $C\bar{1}$ inhibitor, *J. Immunol.* **104**:574–581.

Goetzl, E. J., and Austen, K. F., 1975, Purification and synthesis of eosinophil tetrapeptides of human lung tissue: Identification as eosinophil chemotactic factor of anaphylaxis, *Proc. Natl. Acad. Sci. USA* **72**:4123–4127.

Goetzl, E. J., Wasserman, S. I., and Austen, K. F., 1974, Modulation of the eosinophil chemotactic response in immediate hypersensitivity, in: *Progress in Immunology II*, Vol. 4 (L. Brent and J. Holborow, eds.), pp. 41–50, North-Holland, Amsterdam.

Golbert, T. M., Patterson, R., and Pruzansky, J. J., 1969, Systemic allergic reactions to ingested antigens, *J. Allergy* **44**:96.

Götze, O., and Müller-Eberhard, H. J., 1971, The C3-activator system: An alternative pathway of complement activation, *J. Exp. Med.* **134**:905.

Götze, O., and Müller-Eberhard, H. J., 1974, The role of properdin in the alternate pathway of complement activation, *J. Exp. Med.* **139**:44–57.

Grant, J. A., Dupree, E., Goldman, A. S., Schultz, D. R., and Jackson, A. L., 1975, Complement-mediated release of histamine from human leukocytes, *J. Immunol.* **114**:1101–1106.

Grant, R. T., Pearson, R. S. B., and Corneau, W. J., 1935, Observations on urticaria provoked by emotion, by exercise and by warming the body, *Clin. Sci.* **2**:253–272.

Greaves, M. W., and Sondergaard, J., 1970, Urticaria pigmentosa and factitious urticaria: Direct evidence for release of histamine and other smooth muscle-contracting agents in dermographic skin, *Arch. Dermatol.* **101**:418–425.

Griffin, J. H., and Cochrane, C. G., 1976, Mechanisms for the involvement of high molecular weight kininogen in surface-dependent reactions of Hageman factor, *Proc. Natl. Acad. Sci. USA* **73**:2554–2558.

Griffin, J. H., Harper, E., and Cochrane, C. G., 1975, Studies on the activation of human blood coagulation factor XII (Hageman factor) by soluble collagen, *Fed. Proc.* **34**:860.

Harber, L. C., Holloway, R. M., Sheatley, V. R., and Baer, R. L., 1963, Immunologic and biophysical studies in solar urticaria, *J. Invest. Dermatol.* **41**:439–443.

Hathaway, W. E., and Alsever, J., 1970, The relation of "Fletcher factor" to factors XI and XII, *Br. J. Haematol.* **18**:161–169.

Hathaway, W. E., Belhausen, L. P., and Hathaway, H. S., 1965, Evidence of a new plasma thromboplastin factor, I. Case report, coagulation studies and physicochemical properties, *Br. J. Haematol.* **26**:521–532.

Herxheimer, A., 1956, The nervous pathway mediating cholinergic urticaria, *Clin. Sci.* **15**:195–204.

Horton, B. T., Brown, G. E., and Roth, G. M., 1936, Hypersensitivities to cold with local and systemic manifestations of a histamine-like character: Its amenability to treatment, *J. Am. Med. Assoc.* **107**:1263–1269.

Houser, D. D., Arbesman, C. E., Ito, K., and Wicher, K., 1970, Cold urticaria: Immunologic studies, *Am. J. Med.* **49**:23–33.

Isaacs, N. J., and Ertel, N. H., 1971, Urticaria and pruritis: Uncommon manifestations of hyperthyroidism, *J. Allergy Clin. Immunol.* **48**:73–81.

Ishizaka, K., DeBernardo, R., Tomioka, H., Lichtenstein, L., and Ishizaka, T., 1972, Identification of basophil granulocytes as a site of allergic histamine release, *J. Immunol.* **108**:1000–1008.

Johnson, A. M., Alper, C. A., Rosen, F. S., and Crain, J. M., 1971, C1 inhibitor: Evidence for decreased hepatic synthesis in hereditary angioneurotic edema, *Science* **173**:553–554.

Juhlin, L., and Michaelsson, G., 1969, Vascular reactions in hereditary angioedema, *Acta Derm. Venereol.* **49**:20–25.

Juhlin, L., Michaelsson, G., and Zetterstrom, O., 1972, Urticaria and asthma induced by food and drug additives in patients with aspirin sensitivity, *J. Allergy Clin. Immunol.* **50**:92–98.

Kaplan, A. P., 1977, Mediators of urticaria and angioedema, *J. Allergy Clin. Immunol.* **60**:324–332.

Kaplan, A. P., and Austen, K. F., 1970, A prealbumin activator of prekallikrein, *J. Immunol.* **105**:802–811.

Kaplan, A. P., and Austen, K. F., 1971, A prealbumin activator of prekallikrein. II. Derivation of activators of prekallikrein from active Hageman factor by digestion with plasmin, *J. Exp. Med.* **133**:696–712.

Kaplan, A. P., and Austen, K. F., 1972, The fibrinolytic pathway of human plasma: Isolation and characterization of the plasminogen proactivator, *J. Exp. Med.* **136**:1378–1393.

Kaplan, A. P., and Beaven, M. A., 1976, *In vivo* studies of the pathogenesis of cold urticaria, cholinergic urticaria, and vibration-induced swelling, *J. Invest. Dermatol.* **67**:327–332.

Kaplan, A. P., Kay, A. B., and Austen, K. F., 1972, A prealbumin activator of prekallikrein. III. Appearance of chemotactic activity for human neutrophils by the conversion of human prekallikrein to kallikrein, *J. Exp. Med.* **135**:81–97.

Kaplan, A. P., Goetzl, E. J., and Austen, K. F., 1973, The fibrinolytic pathway of human plasma. II. Generation of chemotactic activity by activation of plasminogen proactivator, *J. Clin. Invest.* **52**:2591–2597.

Kaplan, A. P., Meier, H. L., Yecies, L. D., and Heck, L. W., 1974, Hageman factor and its substrates: The role of factor XI (PTA), prekallikrein, and plasminogen proactivator in coagulation, fibrinolysis, and kiningeneration, in: *The Kallikrein System in Health and Disease: Fogarty International Center Proceedings, No. 27* (J. I., Pisano and K. F. Austen, ed.), pp. 237–254, U.S. Government Printing Office, Washington, D.C.

Kaplan, A. P., Gray, L., Shaff, R. E., Horakova, Z., and Beaven, M. A., 1975, *In vivo* studies of mediator release in cold urticaria and cholinergic urticaria, *J. Allergy Clin. Immunol.* **55**:394–402.

Kaplan, A. P., Horakova, Z., and Katz, S. I., 1978, Assessment of tissue fluid histamine levels in patients with urticaria, *J. Allergy Clin. Immunol.* **61**:350–354.

Kater, L. A., Austen, K. F., and Goetzl, E. J., 1975, Identification and partial purification of a platelet activating factor (PAF) from rat, *Fed. Proc.* **34**:985 (abstr.).

Kay, A. B., and Austen, K. F., 1971, The IgE-mediated release of an eosinophil leukocyte chemotactic factor from human lung, *J. Immunol.* **107**:889–902.

Kay, A. B., Stechschulte, D. J., and Austen, K. F., 1971, An eosinophil leukocyte chemotactic factor of anaphylaxis, *J. Exp. Med.* **133**:602–619.

Kellermeyer, R. W., and Breckenridge, R. T., 1965, The inflammatory process in acute gouty arthritis. I. Activation of Hageman factor by sodium urate crystals, *J. Lab. Clin. Med.* **65**:307–315.

Kennedy, D. D., Rosenthal, F. D., and Sneddon, I. B., 1966, Amyloidosis presenting as urticaria, *Br. Med. J.* **1**:31–32.

Kern, F., and Lichtenstein, L. M., 1976, Defective histamine release in chronic urticaria, *J. Clin. Invest.* **57**:1369–1377.

Klemperer, M. R., Donaldson, V. H., and Rosen, F. S., 1968, The vasopermeability response in man to purified C1 esterase, *J. Clin. Invest.* **47**:604 (abstr.).

Koehn, G. G., and Thorne, E. G., 1972, Urticaria and viral hepatitis, *Arch. Dermatol.* **106**:422.

Kohler, P. F., 1973, Clinical immune complex disease: Manifestations in systemic lupus erythematosus and hepatitis B virus infection, *Medicine* **52:**419–429.

Lever, W. F., and Schaumburg-Lever, G., 1975, *Histopathology of the Skin,* p. 133, Lippincott, Philadelphia.

Levine, B. B., 1966, Immunochemical mechanisms of penicillin allergy, *N. Engl. J. Med.* **275:**1115–1125.

Levine, M. I., 1975, Chronic urticaria, *J. Allergy Clin. Immunol.* **55:**276–283.

Lewis, T., 1927, *The Blood Vessels of the Human Skin and Their Responses,*Shaw and Sons, London.

Ljunggren, B., and Moller, H., 1971, Hepatitis presenting as transient urticaria, *Acta Derm. Venereol.* **51:**295–297.

Lockey, S. D., 1971, Reactions to hidden agents in foods, beverages, and drugs, *Ann. Allergy* **29:**461–466.

Lockshin, N. A., and Hurley, H., 1972, Urticaria as a sign of viral hepatitis, *Arch. Dermatol.* **105:**570–571.

Lundh, B., Laurell, A., Wetterqvist, H., White, T., and Granerus, G., 1968, A case of hereditary angioneurotic edema successfully treated with eaminocaproic acid, *Clin. Exp. Immunol.* **3:**733–745.

Mandle Jr., R. J., and Kaplan, A. P., 1977, Hageman factor substrates. II. Human plasma prekallikrein. Mechanism of activation by Hageman factor and participation in Hageman factor dependent fibrinolysis, *J. Biol. Chem.* **252:**6097–6104.

Mandle, R. J., Jr., Colman, R. W., and Kaplan, A. P., 1976, Identification of prekallikrein and HMW kininogen as a circulating complex in human plasma, *Proc. Natl. Acad. Sci. USA* **73:**4179.

Marder, R. J., Rent, R., and Enoi, E. Y. C., 1976, C1q deficiency associated with urticarial-like lesions and cutaneous vasculitis, *Am. J. Med.* **61:**560–565.

Mathison, D. A., Arroyave, L. M., Bhat, K. N., Hurewitz, D. S., and Marnell, D. J., 1977, Hypocomplementemia in chronic urticaria, *Ann. Intern. Med.* **86:**534–538.

McDuffie, F. C., Sams Jr., W. M., Maldonado, J. E., Andreini, P. H., Conn, D. L., and Samayoa, E. A., 1973, Hypocomplementemia with cutaneous vasculitis and arthritis, *Mayo Clin. Proc.* **48:**340.

McKee, W. D., 1966, The incidence and familial occurrence of allergy, *J. Allergy* **38:**226–235.

McMillan, C. R., Saito, H., Ratnoff, O. D., and Walton, A. D., 1974, The secondary structure of human Hageman factor (factor XII), *J. Clin. Invest.* **54:**1312–1322.

Meier, H. L., Pierce, J. V,, Colman, R. W., and Kaplan, A. P., 1977, Activation and function of human Hageman factor: The role of high molecular weight kininogen and prekallikrein, *J. Clin. Invest.* **60:**18–31.

Metzger, W. J., Kaplan, A. P., Beaven, M. A., Irons, J., and Patterson, R., 1976, Hereditary vibratory angioedema: Confirmation of histamine release in a type of physical hypersensitivity, *J. Allergy Clin. Immunol.* **57:**605–608.

Michaelsson, G., and Juhlin, L., 1973, Urticaria induced by preservatives and dye additives in food and drugs, *Br. J. Dermatol.* **88:**525–532.

Moore-Robinson, M., and Warin, K. P., 1908, Some clinical aspects of cholinergic urticaria, *Br. J. Dermatol.* **80:**794–799.

Moroz, L. A., and Rose, B., 1971, The cryopathies, in: *Immunological Diseases* (M. Samter, ed.), p. 459, Little, Brown, Boston.

Morrison, D. C., and Cochrane, C. G., 1974, Direct evidence for Hageman factor (factor XII) activation by bacterial lipopolysaccharides (endotoxins), *J. Exp. Med.* **140:**787–811.

Moshell, A. N., and Bjornson, L., 1977, Photoprotection in erythropoietic protoporphyria: Mechanism of protection by beta carotene, *J. Invest. Dermatol.* **68:**157–160.

Moskowitz, A. N., Schwartz, H. J., Michel, B., Ratnoff, O. D., and Astrup, T., 1970, Generation of kinin-like agents by chondroitin sulfate, heparin, chitin sulfate, and human articular cartilage: Possible pathophysiologic implications, *J. Lab. Clin. Med.* **76:**790–798.

Muckle, T. J., and Wells, M., 1962, Urticaria, deafness, and amyloidosis: A new heredo-familial syndrome, *Q. J. Med.* **31:**235–248.

Müller-Eberhard, H. J., and Gotze, O., C3 proactivator convertase and its mode of action, *J. Exp. Med.* **135:**1003–1008.

Müller-Eberhard, H. J., Polley, M. J., and Calcott, M. A., 1967, Formation and functional significance of a molecular complex derived from the second and the fourth component of human complement, *J. Exp. Med.* **125**:359–380.

Naff, G. B., Pensky, J., and Lepow, I. H., 1964, The macromolecular nature of the first component of human complement, *J. Exp. Med.* **119**:593–613.

Newcomb, R. W., and Nelson, H,, 1973, Dermographia mediated by immunoglobulin E, *Am. J. Med.* **54**:174–180.

Niewiarowski, S., Bankowski, E., and Rogowicka, I., 1965, Studies on the adsorption and activation of the Hageman factor (factor XII) by collagen and elastin, *Thromb. Diath. Haemorr.* **14**:387–400.

Noid, H. E., Schulze, T. W., and Winkelman, R. K., 1974, Diet plan for patients with salicylate-induced urticaria, *Arch. Dermatol.* **109**:886–889.

Orange, R. P., and Austen, K. F., 1972, Immunologic and pharmacologic receptor control of the release of chemical mediators from human lung, in: *The Biological Role of the Immunoglobulin E System* (K. Ishizaka and D. H. Dayton, Jr., eds.), p. 151, National Institutes of Health, Bethesda, Md.

Orange, R. P., Murphy, R. C., Karnovsky, M. L., and Austen, K. F., 1973, The physicochemical characteristics and purification of slow reacting substance of anaphylaxis, *J. Immunol.* **110**:760–770.

Orfunos, C. E., Schaumburg-Lever, G., and Lever, W. F., 1974, Dermal and epidermal types of erythema multiforme, *Arch. Dermatol.* **109**:682–688.

Patterson, R., Mellies, C. J., Blankenship, M. L., and Pruzansky, J. J., 1972, Vibratory angioedema: A hereditary type of physical hypersensitivity, *J. Allergy Clin. Immunol.* **50**:174–182.

Paver, W. K., 1971, Discoid and subacute systemic lupus erythematosus associated with urticaria, *Aust. J. Dermatol.* **12**:113.

Pearson, K. D., Buchignani, J. S., Shimkin, P. M., and Frank, M. M., 1972, Hereditary angioneurotic edema of the gastrointestinal tract, *Am. J. Roentgenol. Radium Ther. Nucl. Med.* **116**:256–261.

Pillemer, L., Blum, L., Lepow, I. H., Ross, O. A., Todd, E. W., and Wardlaw, A. C., 1954, The properdin system and immunity. I. Demonstration and isolation of a new serum protein, properdin, and its role in immune phenomena, *Science* **120**:279–285.

Ratnoff, O. D., and Naff, G. B., 1967, The conversion of C′1S to C′1 esterase by plasmin and trypsin, *J. Exp. Med.* **125**:337–358.

Ratnoff, O. D., Davie, E. W., and Mallet, D. L., 1961, Studies on the action of Hageman factor: Evidence that activated Hageman factor in turn activates plasma thromboplastin antecedent, *J. Clin. Invest.* **10**:803–819.

Rocklin, R. E., and David, J. R., 1971, Detection of *in vitro* cellular hypersensitivity to drugs, *J. Allergy Clin. Immunol.* **48**:276–282.

Rorsman, H., 1962, Studies on basophil leukocytes with special reference to urticaria and anaphylaxis, *Acta Derm. Venereol.* **42**:1–20 (Suppl. 48).

Rosen, F. S., Alper, C. A., Pensky, J., Klemperer, M. R., and Donaldson, V. H., 1971, Genetic heterogeneity of the C1 esterase inhibitor in patients with hereditary angioneurotic edema, *J. Clin. Invest.* **50**:2143–2149.

Rosse, W. F., Logue, G. L., and Silberman, H. R., 1976, The effect of synthetic androgens on the clinical course and C1 esterase ($C\bar{1}$ INH) levels in hereditary angioneurotic edema (HANE), *Clin. Res.* **24**:428A.

Roth, G. J., Stanford, N., and Majerus, P. W., 1975, Acetylation of prostaglandin synthase by aspirin, *Proc. Natl. Acad. Sci. USA* **72**:3073–3076.

Ruddy, S., Gigli, I., Sheffer, A. L., and Austen, K. F., 1968, The laboratory diagnosis of hereditary angioedema, in: *Allergology, Proceedings of the Sixth International Congress of Allergology* (Rose, Richter, Sehon, and Frankland, eds.), pp. 351–359, Excerpta Medica, Amsterdam.

Sams, W. M., Jr., Epstein, J. H., and Winkelmann, R. K., 1969, Solar urticaria: Investigation of pathogenic mechanisms, *Arch. Dermatol.* **99**:390–397.

Samter, M., and Beers, Jr., R. F., 1967, Concerning the nature of intolerance to aspirin, *J. Allergy* **40**:281–293.

Schreiber, A. D., Kaplan, A. P., and Austen, K. F., 1973, Inhibition by $C\bar{1}$ INH of Hageman factor fragment activation of coagulation, fibrinolysis, and kinin generation, *J. Clin. Invest.* **52**:1402–1409.

Schreiber, R. D., Medicus, R. G., Gotze, O., and Müller-Eberhard, H. J., 1975, Properdin and nephritic factor-dependent C3 convertases: Requirement of native C3 for enzyme formation and the function of bound C3b as properdin receptor, *J. Exp. Med.* **142**:760–772.

Settipane, G. A., and Pudupakkam, R. K., 1975, Aspirin intolerance. III. Subtypes, familial occurrence, and cross-reactivity with tartrazine, *J. Allergy Clin. Immunol.* **56**:215–221.

Settipane, G. A., Chafee, F. H., Postman, I. M., Levine, M. I., Saker, J. H., Barrick, R. H., Nicholas, S. S., Schwartz, M. D., Honsinger, R. N., and Klein, D. E., 1975, Significance of tartrazine sensitivity in chronic urticaria of unknown etiology, *J. Allergy Clin. Immunol.* **57**:541–546.

Sheffer, A. L., Craig, J. M., Willms-Kretschmer, K., Austen, K. F., and Rosen, F. S., 1971, Histopathological and ultrastructural observations on tissues from patients with hereditary angioneurotic edema, *J. Allergy* **47**:292–297.

Sheffer, A. L., Austen, K. F., and Rosen, F. S., 1972, Tranexamic acid therapy in hereditary angioneurotic edema, *N. Engl. J. Med.* **287**:452–454.

Sheldon, J. M., Mathews, K. P., and Lovell, R. G., 1954, The vexing urticaria problem: Present concepts of etiology and management, *J. Allergy* **25**:525–560.

Sheldon, J. M., Lovell, R. G., and Mathews, K. P., 1967, *A Manual of Clinical Allergy,* 2nd ed. p. 196, Saunders, Philadelphia.

Shelley, W. B., 1969, Urticaria of nine years duration cleared following dental extraction, *Arch. Dermatol.* **100**:324–325.

Sissons, J. G. F., Williams, D. G., Peters, D. K., and Boulton-Jones, J. M., 1974, Skin lesions, angioedema, and hypocomplementemia, *Lancet* (Dec.) **7**:1350–1352.

Soter, N. A., Austen, K. F., and Gigli, I., 1974a, The complement system in necrotizing angiitis of the skin: Analysis of complement component activities in serum of patients with concomitant collagen-vascular diseases, *J. Invest. Dermatol.* **63**:219–226.

Soter, N. A., Austen, K. F., and Gigli, I., 1974b, Urticaria and arthralgias as manifestation of necrotizing angiitis, *J. Invest. Dermatol.* **63**:485–490.

Soter, N. A., Austen, K. F., and Gigli, I., 1975, Inhibition by e-aminocaproic acid of the activation of the first component of the complement system, *J. Immunol.* **114**:928–932.

Soter, N. A., Mihm Jr., M. C., Gigli, I., Dvorak, H. F., and Austen, K. F., 1976a, Two distinct cellular patterns in cutaneous necrotizing angiitis, *J. Invest. Dermatol.* **66**:334–350.

Soter, N. A., Wasserman, S. I., and Austen, K. F., 1976b, Cold urticaria: Release into the circulation of histamine and eosinophil chemotactic factor of anaphylaxis during cold challenge, *N. Engl. J. Med.* **294**:687–690.

Soter, N. A., Joshi, N. P., Twarog, F. J., Zeiger, R. S., Rothman, P. M., and Colton, H. R., 1977, Delayed cold-induced urticaria: A dominantly inherited disorder, *J. Allergy Clin. Immunol.* **59**:294–297.

Spaulding, W. B., 1960, Methyl testosterone therapy for hereditary episodic edema (hereditary angioneurotic edema), *Ann. Intern. Med.* **53**:739–745.

Swinny, B., 1941, The atopic factor in urticaria, *South. Med. J.* **34**:855–858.

Szczeklik, A., Oryglewski, R. J., and Czerniawska-Mysik, 1975, Relationship of inhibition of prostaglandin biosynthesis by analgesics to asthma attacks in aspirin-sensitive patients, *Br. Med. J.* **1**:67.

Talamo, R. C., Haber, E., and Austen, K. F., 1969, A radioimmunoassay for bradykinin in plasma and synovial fluid, *J. Lab. Clin. Med.* **74**:816–827.

Thompson, R. A., 1972, C3 inactivating factor in the serum of a patient with chronic hypocomplementemia proliferative glomerulonephritis, *Immunology* **22**:147–158.

Thompson, R. A., and Lachmann, P. J., 1977, A second case of human C3b inhibitor (KAF) deficiency, *Clin. Exp. Immunol.* **27**:23–29.

Thompson, R. E., Mandle, R. J., Jr., and Kaplan, A. P., 1977, Association of factor XI and high molecular weight kininogen in human plasma, *J. Clin. Invest.* **60**:1376–1480.

Tindall, J. P., Beeker, S. K., and Rosse, N. F., 1969, Familial cold urticaria, *Arch. Intern. Med.* **124**:129–134.

Tomioka, H., and Ishizaka, K., 1971, Mechanisms of passive sensitization. II. Presence of receptors for IgE in monkey mast cells, *J. Immunol.* **107**:971–978.

Tromovitch, T. A., 1967, Urticaria from contact with water, *Calif. Med.* **106**:400–401.

Unger, A. H., 1960, Chronic urticaria. II. Association with dental infections, *South. Med. J.* **53**:178–181.

Vallota, E. H., and Müller-Eberhard, H. J., 1973, Formation of C3a and C5a anaphylatoxins in whole human serum after inhibition of the anaphylatoxin inactivatior, *J. Exp. Med.* **137:**1109–1123.

Vallota, E. H., Gotze, O. Spiegelberg, H. L., Forristal, J., West, C. D., and Müller-Eberhard, H. J., 1974, A serum factor in chronic hypocomplementemic nephritis distinct from immunoglobulins and activating the alternative pathway of complement, *J. Exp. Med.* **139:**1249–1261.

Vane, J. R., 1971, Inhibition of prostaglandin synthesis as a mechanism of action for aspirin-like drugs, *Nature (London) New Biol.* **231:**232–235.

Waldbott, G. L., and Merkle, K., 1952, Urticaria due to pollen, *Ann. Allergy* **10:**30–35.

Wanderer, A. A., and Ellis, E. F., 1971, Treatment of cold urticaria with cyproheptadine, *J. Allergy Clin. Immunol.* **48:**366–371.

Wanderer, A. A., Maselli, R., Ellis, R. F., and Ishizaka, K., 1971, Immunologic characterization of serum factors responsible for cold urticaria, *J. Allergy Clin. Immunol.* **48:**13–22.

Warin, R. P., and Champion, R. H., 1974, *Urticaria,* p. 33, Saunders, London.

Wasserman, S. I., Soter, N. A., Center, D. M., and Austen, K. F., 1977, Cold urticaria: Recognition and characterization of a neutrophil chemotactic factor which appears in serum during experimental cold challenge, *J. Clin. Invest.* **60;**189–196.

Webb, D. R., Pearsall, H. R., and Sumida, S. E., 1975, Depression of third component of complement (C3) in chronic angioedema, *J. Allergy Clin. Immunol.* **55:**106 (abstr.).

Weiss, A. S., Gallin, J. I., and Kaplan, A. P., 1973, Fletcher factor deficiency: Abnormalities of coagulation, fibrinolysis, chemotactic activity, and kinin generation attributable to absence of prekallikrein, *J. Clin. Invest.* **53:**622–633.

Willms, K., Rosen, F. S., and Donaldson, V. H., 1975, Observations in the ultrastructure of lesions induced in human and guinea pig skin by C1 esterase and polypeptide from hereditary angioneurotic edema (HANE) plasma, *Clin. Immunol. Immunopathol.* **4:**174–188.

Wilner, G. D., Nossel, H. L., and Leroy, E. C., 1968, Activation of Hageman factor by collagen, *J. Clin. Invest.* **47:**2608–2615.

Wuepper, K. D., 1973, Prekallikrein deficiency in man, *J. Exp. Med.* **138:**1345–1355.

Wuepper, K. D., Bokisch, V. A., Müller-Eberhard, H. J., and Stoughton, R. B., 1972, Cutaneous responses to human C3a anaphylatoxin in man, *Clin. Exp. Immunol.* **11:**13–20.

Wuepper, K. D., Miller, D. R., and LaCombe, M. J., 1975, Flaujeac trait: Deficiency of human plasma kininogen, *J. Clin. Invest.* **56:**2663–1672.

Yurchak, A. M., Wicher, K., and Arbesman, C. E., 1970, Immunologic studies on aspirin, *J. Allergy* **46:**245–253.

9

Food Hypersensitivity

CHARLES D. MAY

1. Introduction

In prehistoric times when man sought to satisfy hunger by eating unfamiliar or contaminated foodstuffs, erroneous incrimination of an item in the diet as a cause of symptoms was surely common—and it still is. Once spoilage was a ready explanation and the concept of "ptomaine" poisoning was popular; nowadays "allergy" is a favorite explanation for a supposed relation between symptoms and a food. Volumes could be filled with the array of unfounded beliefs about the relation of food to well-being.

Considering that nutrition is as essential for survival of the individual as reproduction is for the species, little wonder man is preoccupied with food and sex and for both strives to cover ignorance by fantasies and superstitions. Feelings about food easily become embroiled in neurotic complaints, and so naturally confusion becomes widespread about the place of food in the causation of symptoms.

The task of modern scientific medicine is to develop objective dependable means for making accurate associations between foods and explicit disorders and to ascertain the underlying mechanisms. There may be many undiscovered ways whereby substances in food could cause symptoms, but first unequivocal associations between foods and symptoms must be made rather than thoughtless use of "allergy" as an explanation.

In scientific circles allergy generally implies an immunological mechanism, but in connection with food the term has lost precision through careless usage. In this discussion "hypersensitivity" is used instead to denote an immunological basis for an adverse reaction to food.

The importance of knowledge of true immunological reactions to food is not based on fear of maiming or killing. Popular beliefs about "allergy" to food are a menace to health. Unjustified dietary restrictions threaten optimal nutrition.

CHARLES D. MAY • Department of Pediatrics, National Jewish Hospital and Research Center, and Department of Pediatrics, University of Colorado Medical School, Denver, Colorado 80206.

Mistaken assignment of symptoms to food may delay proper medical search for serious disease. Dissemination of unrestrained, unscientific, and unsubstantiated assertions through the mass media that processed foods cause widespread vague complaints makes it difficult for physicians to practice rational medicine and places unwarranted burdens on the food industry and government regulatory agencies. A solution to this problem can come only from sound knowledge of adverse reactions to foods, particularly immunological reactions.

2. Plan of Presentation

This review provides a summation rather than an exhaustive presentation of the current knowledge about food hypersensitivity, along with some concepts that may aid in comprehension or stimulate additions through research. One goal is to reveal that food hypersensitivity now deserves a respectable place in clinical immunology; another is to give the background for a practical approach to diagnosis and management, sorely needed for rational care of persons with genuine hypersensitivity reactions to food.

The material is arranged to foster a sound educational approach to the subject by an orderly progression from basic immunology and clinical immunology through clinical manifestations as a preparation for dealing intelligently with clinical applications. Practitioners are urged to follow this plan rather than skipping to the end in the vain hope of learning without labor.

3. Basic Immunology

In attempts to portray the immunological system in the intestine, data obtained from studies of animals are often freely intermingled with findings in humans without taking fully into account that the former findings may have little or no relevance to the latter. Experiments with animals are of great value as preliminary studies and in development of techniques, but ultimately clinical relevance must be determined by direct investigations in human beings. In this review information obtained from humans will be used exclusively.

All the details of the components of the immunological system of the intestine will not be given, only sufficient information to serve as a basis for considering mechanisms of immunological reactions to antigenic substances of food in humans. Although the mucosa extending from the nose and mouth to the anus can participate in immunological reactions, in this section only the local system in the intestinal mucosa and correlated generalized immunological processes will be discussed.

3.1. Local Components

Antigen which penetrates the epithelium of the intestinal mucosa reaches plasma or lymphoid cells in the lamina propria capable of producing immunoglobulins A, E, G, and M and probably others (Tomasi, 1972; Lamm, 1976; Crabbé and Heremans, 1966; Bull *et al.*, 1971; Tada and Ishizaka, 1970; Brown *et al.*, 1975; Savilahti, 1972a,b; Ogra and Karzon, 1969). These immunoglobulins are primarily secreted into the lumen of the gut but sometimes may pass into the circulation. IgA and IgM acquire an additional component during secretion through the epithelium, a secretory piece, which endows them with resistance to digestion and an affinity for attachment to the mucosal surface. Secretory IgA is normally the preponderant immunoglobulin in the intestinal juice, but IgE, IgG, and IgM are present normally and in varying amounts in pathological circumstances. These immunoglobulins in intestinal secretions comprise antibodies specific for the antigen which stimulated their production and may bind food antigens and so influence the absorption of undigested antigenic substances from the gut. The concept that a major function of secretory IgA is to curb the absorption of antigenic materials from the gut was set forth years ago (Tomasi, 1972; Good and Rodey, 1970) and is being taken up eagerly at present to explain the pathogenesis of allergic disorders (Soothill *et al.*, 1976).

The activities of this local system of specific antibody production may not necessarily be reflected in titers of antibodies in the blood. However, when the production becomes sufficiently active the flood of antibodies escapes via the lymphatics into the circulation as well as by secretion through the epithelium to the lumen of the intestine.

Lymphocytes are found in lymphoid follicles (Peyer's patches) in the lamina propria and interspersed between the epithelial cells of the villi of the intestinal mucosa. T cells among these have the potential of participating in cell-mediated immunity (Ferguson *et al.*, 1976). On antigenic stimulation, blast transformation and lymphokine secretion could occur.

3.2. Systemic Components

Intact antigenic substances may pass through the intestinal mucosa into the circulation. Consequently, antibody-producing cells throughout the body may be exposed to the stimulus of food antigens. The specific antibodies to food proteins in the serum are believed to be largely derived from cells in the peripheral lymph nodes, spleen, and circulating lymphocytes, but IgA antibodies come primarily from the local production in the intestinal mucosa. Likewise, T lymphocytes throughout the body could be exposed to food antigen and cell-mediated immunity could ensue.

3.3. Developmental Features

Substantial synthesis of antibodies begins after birth in the human on exposure to environmental antigens. Prematurely born infants of 35–36 weeks' gestation can produce specific antibodies to bovine serum albumin (Rieger and Rothberg, 1975). IgA production is slow at first, so that IgA is absent or barely detectable in the serum until 1–2 weeks after birth. This results in an apparent relative deficiency in the neonatal period, then serum levels rise gradually but are not maximal until puberty (Haworth and Dilling, 1966).

Normally antibody response to food proteins introduced in the first months of life leads to maximum levels of specific antibody in the serum in about 6 months (Kletter *et al.*, 1971a,b). The serum titers of specific food antibodies then slowly decline until virtually absent in normal adults, which may be associated with acquisition of a state of immunological tolerance or unresponsiveness (Korenblat *et al.*, 1968). Immune responses to the first ingestion of food antigens may be less as age advances, but the general pattern of response to new foods may be similar in later life. Only in persons genetically prone to producing IgE antibody do the serum levels of specific IgE to food antigen become appreciable (Kletter *et al.*, 1971c; Björkstén and Johansson, 1975).

There is a possibility of intrauterine sensitization of the human fetus because, as mentioned, antibody production can be stimulated by 35 weeks' gestation. There have been a few reports of allergic reactions to foods on the first introduction into the diet soon after birth, but the manner of sensitization is not settled. In some cases the infant may have become sensitized by antigen secreted in the breast milk, in others by passive sensitization with reagin from the mother's serum because of an exceptional leakage through the placenta, ordinarily impervious to reagin. Another possibility is penetration of antigen to a fetus genetically destined to produce IgE readily, in case the pregnant woman ingests large amounts of an antigenic food like milk, eggs, or wheat (Ratner, 1928; Donnally, 1930; Kaufman, 1971).

3.4. Genetic Factors

There are obviously many opportunities for genetic characteristics to influence the occurrence and nature of hypersensitivity reactions to food. The subject is beyond the scope of this chapter, but the most pertinent examples are the various genetically determined defects in the immune system, the deficiencies of enzymes involved in digestion and assimilation of nutrients, and the cytotoxic effects of food substances peculiar to persons who develop gluten-sensitive enteropathy. These will receive further attention in the sections on clinical matters.

3.5. Components of Immunological Reactions

In addition to sensitization through humoral antibodies and possibly through the mechanisms of cell-mediated immunity, hypersensitivity reactions to food depend on other essential components and systems, e.g., cells (neutrophils, mast cells, etc.), the complement system, mediators (histamine, etc.), end organs (capillaries, smooth muscle, mucus glands), digestive processes, and physiological systems that transport undigested antigenic food substances across the intestinal mucosa. Unless the crucial roles of these are kept in mind, preoccupation with the evidence of immunological sensitization may leave one mystified by clinical events.

3.6. Types of Immunological Reactions

In the preceding discussion of sensitization of humans by antigens from food, it is evident that any of the known types of immunological reaction can be expected following ingestion of the responsible foods. The terms "immediate" and "delayed" should be viewed as more appropriate to the chronology of clinical events and may be somewhat misleading if transposed to immunological mechanisms. Surely when antigen encounters specific antibodies or sensitized cells the reaction is immediate whatever the time required for the ensuing chain of events that may or may not lead to clinically observable manifestations. One could use the well-known grouping of immunological reactions into types I–IV. Considering the present limitations in our ability to identify which mechanism is involved in hypersensitivity reactions to food, it may be enough to speak of reactions as "reagin mediated" and "not reagin mediated," as follows.

3.6.1. Reagin Mediated

Reagin-mediated reactions are based on attachment of IgE (and possibly other reagins) to mast cells and basophils and consequent release of mediators on interaction with antigen. The mediators act on capillaries, smooth muscle, and mucus glands to give the characteristic pathology and clinical manifestations.

3.6.2. Not Reagin Mediated

Antibodies of IgG and IgM and perhaps other classes and sensitized cells may react with antigen to (1) form complexes with or without biological activity, (2) activate the complement system with a potential for pathologic consequences, or (3) stimulate proliferation of lymphocytes and lymphokine production. The subsequent pathology may or may not result in clinically observable manifestations due to mediators, inflammation, cytopathic, or proliferative disturbances.

3.6.3. Mixed Reactions

An individual could be sensitized both by reagins and by the other types of sensitization and therefore exhibit reactions containing elements of reaginic and nonreaginic mechanisms, or one mechanism may prepare the way for another.

4. Clinical Immunology

Application of the facts of basic immunology to clinical diagnosis and treatment, along with consideration of factors which influence the immune reactions, forms the content of the clinical immunology of hypersensitivity reactions to food.

4.1. The Mucosal Barrier and the Immune System

The mucosa of the gastrointestinal and the respiratory tracts may be considered to have evolved to allow the body to sustain its structure and carry on its functions through exchanges with the air and by extraction of nutrients from foods, while excluding pathogenic organisms and noxious materials. In essence, as conceived by Claude Bernard, a discriminating barrier is interposed between the external and internal environments. The mucosa excites admiration for its role in the highly successful survival of the human race under ordinary environmental circumstances. However, the barrier may be overwhelmed by excessive or unnatural demands or fail because of disruption by pathological disturbances or genetic imperfections.

The effectiveness of the barrier in the gastrointestinal tract depends on many elements, of which the following are of special relevance to comprehension of hypersensitivity reactions to foods:

1. The physiological processes for transport of macromolecular substances through the cells lining the gastrointestinal tract
2. The role of the immune system
3. Immunodeficiency disorders

Hypersensitivity reactions to food in humans direct our attention to the manner by which antigenic substances in food reach immunocompetent cells, to the immune responses, and to the immunopathology of reactions that ensue when the sensitized individual ingests specific antigens contained in food.

The discrimination of the barrier of the gastrointestinal tract did not evolve to perfection and so the immune system seems to provide a second line of defense in prevention of excessive invasion of the body by antigenic material, analogous to the bodily mechanisms which serve to detoxify noxious materials that manage to penetrate the barrier. Indeed, unless some antigen could have penetrated or crossed the barrier to reach immunocompetent cells, the immune system would probably not have come to play an important role in protection of the internal environment from pathogenic organisms in the external environment.

For all but a relative few, the barrier and the immune system are normally able to exclude antigens from food to a degree and in a fashion that prevents any ill effects from the minimal amounts of intact antigens which do penetrate the barrier and from the consequent immune reactions in sensitized persons.

4.1.1. Antigenic Penetration of the Mucosal Barrier

Penetration of the barrier by antigenic material and some of the immunological responses in the normal human were demonstrated early in the history of immunology in a series of clearly conceived and carefully executed studies by Schloss and Walzer and their associates (Anderson *et al.,* 1925; DuBois *et al.,* 1925; Lippard *et al.,* 1936; Lippard, 1939; Walzer, 1927; Brunner and Walzer, 1928; Wilson and Walzer, 1935; Sherman *et al.,* 1937; Gray and Walzer, 1938a,b, 1940; Gray *et al.,* 1940). Important aspects of our present understanding of food hypersensitivity are based on the observations of these clinical investigators. Walzer (1927) developed a procedure based on the finding of Prausnitz and Küstner that antibodies in sera from persons exhibiting reagin-mediated allergic reactions may be fixed in the skin of nonallergic subjects. Walzer and associates found that when a food was administered intranasally, orally, intraduodenally, or rectally to a nonallergic subject in whom 24 hr previously a skin site had been prepared with intracutaneous injection of serum from a person allergic to the corresponding food, a characteristic wheal-and-flare reaction occurred in the prepared site (Brunner and Walzer, 1928; Wilson and Walzer, 1935; Sherman *et al.,* 1937; Gray and Walzer, 1938a,b, 1940; Gray *et al.,* 1940). The local reaction appeared 10–15 min after the food was eaten, indicating that intact antigenic material had been quickly absorbed into the circulation.

By means of this type of experiment, various factors increasing intestinal absorption of antigen were identified; namely, amount of antigen ingested, administration alone into an empty stomach vs. mixture with benign foods, cooking, reduction of gastric acidity, and smaller amounts of food could evoke positive reactions during gastrointestinal disturbances. The intestinal tracts of normal persons were found to be permeable to intact antigen from infancy throughout adulthood. Estimates indicated that only minute amounts of intact antigen were able to penetrate the mucosa, but the content in sera was sufficient to specifically sensitize animals injected with sera obtained after ingestion of antigenic foods, and also to induce systemic allergic reactions when injected intravenously into a subject sensitive to a particular food (Gray *et al.*, 1940).

Walzer's group also showed that exposed mucosa of the gastrointestinal tract (ileum, rectum) of nonallergic subjects could be sensitized by intramucosal injection of sera from persons allergic to foods (Gray and Walzer, 1938a; Gray *et al.*, 1940). When the nonallergic subjects ingested the corresponding foods, characteristic reactions occurred in the prepared sites (remote from contact with the food) consisting of vasodilation, edema, and mucus secretion. This showed that the intestinal mucosa contained elements capable of fixing antibodies and exhibiting the immunopathological consequences of the reagin-mediated type of reaction.

Schloss and associates detected absorption of antigen and traced the course of antibody to cow milk and egg proteins which appeared in the serum when these foods were first introduced into the diets of infants (Anderson *et al.*, 1925; DuBois *et al.*, 1925; Lippard *et al.*, 1936; Lippard, 1939). They made serial observations with intracutaneous skin tests, the Prausnitz–Küstner procedure, and complement-fixation tests for antigen and antibody in serum. Antigenic materials from the foods were found to appear in the blood on ingestion of the foods, later followed by specific antibodies. In normal persons relatively large amounts of food protein were required to produce absorption of antigen and production of specific antibody, and intracutaneous tests were positive transitorily, but positive P-K tests with sera were not observed. Nor did the infants develop symptoms from the foods. In contrast, among eczematous infants some were found whose sera also persistently yielded positive P-K tests and exacerbations of eczema were seen (Lippard, 1939). In infants with gastrointestinal disturbances, relatively small amounts of cow milk or egg resulted in detectable specific antigen in the serum and antibody persisted in the serum for months. In normals the antigen disappeared from the serum as the antibody titer increased. Even if ingestion of the food continued, the serum antibody titer declined to low levels in children and until no longer detectable in adults. The positive skin tests unaccompanied by positive P-K tests also soon disappeared. Positive skin tests associated with positive P-K tests persisted. The same sequence of events was observed at any period of infancy when the foods were introduced for the first time, not just in the early months after birth (Lippard *et al.*, 1936).

Schloss and Walzer and their coworkers considered absorption of minute amounts of food antigens and the characteristic antibody responses in the serum and skin to be physiological or clinically insignificant in normal persons but viewed the consequences in some abnormal (eczematous, allergy-prone individuals) to be important in the etiology and pathogenesis of clinical reactions to foods. They showed that the same phenomena were observed with the first ingestion of a variety of foods, e.g., cow milk, egg, fish, almonds, and peanuts. Perhaps the same would occur with any food protein newly introduced into the diet.

Of special importance is the direct bearing of the findings of these early investigators on clinical medicine because the observations were made with humans. Furthermore, the concepts of stimulus–response relationships and symptomatic vs. asymptomatic hypersensitivity to food, so essential to the clinical understanding, are clearly evident in their studies. Recent studies with humans using modern technology have confirmed and refined some of the observations of Schloss and Walzer and co-workers (Gruskay and Cooke, 1955; Rothberg, 1969). Nothing fundamental has been added to their evidence of antigen penetration of the intestinal mucosa in humans or to their description of the general nature of the response in serum antibodies. Further details have been learned of production and responses in specific antibodies of the various classes of immunoglobulins.

The recent findings in animals regarding the processes which permit and modulate antigen penetration of the mucosa are of interest but are not yet shown to hold for humans (Walker and Isselbacher, 1974).

4.1.2. Immunodeficiency Disorders

Considering the prominent place of SIgA in establishing a barrier to penetration of antigens through the mucosa, the frequency of diarrhea and malabsorption in the syndrome of selective IgA deficiency is not surprising (Crabbé and Heremans, 1966). Likewise, in any of the immunodeficiency disorders which lower host resistance to overgrowth of microorganisms and parasites, the mucosal barrier may be overwhelmed. The frequent occurence of gastrointestinal disease in immunodeficiency disorders is fully documented in a recent comprehensive review (Ament, 1975). Food antigens also may penetrate the mucosa and lead to specific antibodies in the serum more readily in selective IgA deficiency (Buckley and Dees, 1969; Tomasi and Katz, 1971; Huntley *et al.*, 1971). Cunningham-Rundles *et al.* (1978) reported that 59% of patients with selective IgA deficiency had circulating immune complexes, 50% had milk precipitins, 23% had precipitins to bovine serum, and 13% had precipitins to fetal calf serum.

4.2. Detection of Reaginic Sensitization

4.2.1. Skin Tests

Introduction of pollen antigen into the skin as a means of detecting sensitization was first described in 1873 (Blackley, 1873), but the technique was not employed in studies of sensitivity to food antigen until 1912 (Schloss, 1912). Ever since, the use of skin tests with food antigen has had a strange history of conflicting unscientific opinions regarding their usefulness. The confusion has been sustained by lack of verification of the antigenic performance of extracts of food substances used in skin tests and failure to determine objectively the relation between the results of the skin tests and occurrence of symptoms after ingestion of corresponding foods.

Verification of a reagent (extract or constituent of food) for use in detection of sensitization requires demonstration that the amount used does not elicit nonspecific or irritant reactions in nonallergic subjects but will identify by significant wheal reactions all those persons who will develop symptoms on ingestion of the food, preferably using a double-blind procedure for the challenge. Not until 1966 was such verification undertaken, when exemplary studies showed that a purified antigen from codfish was able to detect 100% of children exhibiting clinical reaction to cod (Aas, 1966a,b).

Proper use of skin tests with food substances or extracts for detection of reaginic sensitization entails

1. Verification of the reagent or extract by determining the amount and technique which will evoke significant wheal reactions in hypersensitive persons and not in normals. A wheal reaction 10–15 min after introduction of antigen into the skin indicates sensitization with specific reagin-type antibody, the prototype being IgE. The reaction is due to release of histamine from mast cells.
2. Ascertainment of the degree or size of reaction which identifies all persons who will manifest symptoms in a double-blind food challenge, i.e., who are sensitive to a degree likely to be associated with symptoms when the food is consumed in ordinary amounts in the usual varied diet.

Where these requirements are met, food skin tests are useful for the detection of reaginic sensitization to food antigens and for identification of those persons who should be subjected to double-blind food challenge to establish whether the diagnosis should be clinically significant (symptomatic) hypersensitivity to the food under consideration or clinically insignificant (asymptomatic) hypersensitivity. In either case, the individual is shown by a designated response in the skin test to be sensitized by reaginic antibody to the food antigen (Bock *et al.*, 1977, 1978b).

The foregoing statements are contrary to widely held opinion, based on untested assumptions, that skin tests with food substances are worthless and misleading. Actually the same considerations and interpretations apply to skin tests with inhalants as with ingestants, and the reliability is dependent on proper use whichever antigenic material is employed.

An IgG antibody termed "heat-stable, short-term sensitizing" has been demonstrated in sera from three children who developed symptoms 12–36 hr after ingesting milk (Parish, 1970, 1971). A wheal reaction appeared within minutes in skin tests with milk proteins, but there were differences from the reaginic IgE antibody; human mast cells could not be passively sensitized to give antigenic histamine release, and its activity was not destroyed at 56°C and appeared to be complement dependent. Further studies on the role of this type of IgG antibody in food hypersensitivity will be of interest. The transitory positive skin tests to food antigens described many years ago (Lippard, 1939) in normal infants receiving foods for the first time who did not develop symptoms of food hypersensitivity may be explained by this type of IgG antibody; systematic search by serial studies for this type of skin reactivity and this IgG antibody among normal infants fed cow milk may be rewarding.

4.2.2. P-K Test

The Prausnitz–Küstner procedure was a useful method for demonstration of reaginic antibodies in serum but has now been abandoned for general use because of the risk of transmitting hepatitis from the donor of the serum to the recipient.

4.2.3. RAST

A newborn infant may be so lovable because the inevitable flaws are not yet evident. So it may be with new diagnostic tests. The RAST (radioallergosorbent test) was widely embraced in its infancy, but the limitations are now coming to be realized. In those studies where objective oral challenge with food is compared with results of skin test and RAST with the corresponding antigen, RAST has not proved superior to the skin test in detecting reaginic sensitization to food antigens or in correlation with clinical reactions to foods (Aas and Lundkvist, 1973; Aas, 1978). Comparisons of skin tests and RAST with inhalant antigens have also failed to find RAST superior to properly performed skin tests (Norman *et al.*, 1973).

RAST is a measurement of specific IgE in the circulation (where it has a relatively short stay), and therefore the serum content depends on the current rate of production and disposal. The skin test detects IgE fixed in the skin and provides a less variable index of the state of sensitization. Only by studies comparing skin tests and RAST with the results of objective food challenges can their relative worth be determined for identification of the degree of sensitivity likely to be correlated with clinically significant hypersensitivity to food; properly performed skin tests have been superior to RAST (Aas, 1978; Lee and May, unpublished data).

Skin tests are inexpensive and the results are available at once for interpretation by the physician. RAST is impractical for the practitioners' office, and determinations by commercial laboratories are expensive and there is an inevitable delay in obtaining the results.

4.2.4. Quality of Reagents

Skin tests and RAST are equally dependent on the quality of the antigens available. At present only a few food proteins have been isolated and partially purified. Commercial extracts of foods provided as antigenic material are not prepared in a uniform manner and are not standardized for content of antigenic material or stability. Therefore, the extracts employed must be subjected to verification of their performance as sources of antigen just as should be done with extracts of inhalants. This would seem a proper function of the conscience of commercial vendors or of a government regulatory agency. If the antigenic content of relatively crude extracts can be verified, isolation of pure antigens of foods may not be necessary for clinical practice, although desirable for certain research.

4.2.5. Other Tests

Cellular responses discernable by the skin window technique, degranulation of basophils, and *in vitro* release of histamine from leukocytes all may be used to detect responses to antigen in reaginic sensitization; while they offer no advantages in clinical practice, they are useful in research.

4.3. Detection of Nonreaginic Sensitization

4.3.1. Humoral Antibodies

Nonreaginic antibodies to food proteins have usually been measured in the serum by methods involving spontaneous precipitation with antigen or diffusion in gel, passive hemagglutination, or induced precipitation of antibody bound to radioactively labeled antigen (Williams and Chase, 1977). Relatively high concentration of antibody is required for detection by spontaneous precipitation or diffusion in gel methods. The binding of isotopically labeled antigen is the most sensitive and readily quantitated (Minden *et al.*, 1966).

As already discussed, in normal persons food antigens can penetrate the intestinal barrier and reach immunocompetent cells, so, as might be anticipated, a heterogeneous antibody response is stimulated. Specific antibodies to food antigens are found regularly in IgG, IgM, and IgA classes of immunoglobulins in the serum when a food is first introduced into the diet; normally the titers reach a peak in a few months and then decline as time passes even though the food continues to be consumed (Lippard *et al.*, 1936; Lippard, 1939; Kletter *et al.*, 1971a,b,c; Korenblat *et al.*, 1968).

Obviously the mere detection of antibody to a food antigen in the serum by a sensitive method will not serve for clinical distinction between normal and abnormal persons. Therefore, considerations which must be kept in mind are (1) whether there are unusual *amounts* or *kinds* of antibody, (2) if there is *persistence* of elevated levels beyond the usual duration, and (3) whether the intestinal barrier may be disrupted as in selective IgA immunodeficiency and gastrointestinal disorders (Wilson *et al.*, 1974; May *et al.*, 1977).

4.3.2. Cell-Mediated Immunity

Proliferation of lymphocytes has been observed in the intestinal mucosa in gastrointestinal disorders (Ferguson *et al.*, 1976). On addition of food antigen to cultures of peripheral lymphocytes, significant stimulation may occur. The degree of stimulation is usually much less than seen in unequivocal cell-mediated immunity, such as tuberculin sensitivity, and occurs as frequently in normals as in individuals hypersensitive to food. Simultaneous skin tests with the same food antigens have not produced characteristic delayed reactions, but perhaps injection of a larger amount of antigen would give a different result (Amache *et al.*, 1969; Scheinmann *et al.*, 1976; May and Alberto, 1972a,b).

The magnitude of antigenic lymphocyte stimulation is greatest when the humoral antibody titer in the serum is high (May and Alberto, 1972a). Active lymphocyte proliferation has been observed (without addition of antigen) in cultures of peripheral lymphocytes obtained after food challenge of persons hypersensitive to food (May and Alberto, 1972b); this spontaneous lymphocyte proliferation may have resulted from adsorbed antigen acting on antigen-reactive cells in the circulation committed to humoral antibody production rather than because of cell-mediated immunity.

4.3.3. Complement and Antigen–Antibody Complexes

Activation of complement could be an indication of involvement of humoral antibodies or antigen–antibody complexes in hypersensitivity reactions to food. One report (Matthews and Soothill, 1970) of reduction of serum content of C3 after challenge of individuals hypersensitive to cow milk was not confirmed in later studies (Savilahti, 1973).

Penetration of antigen through the mucosa to encounter antibody in the tissues and the circulation affords an opportunity for formation of antigen–antibody complexes. The possibility of circulating complexes of food antigen and antibody was examined in a study of lupus erythematosus (Carr *et al.*, 1972). Findings with respect to complement fixation and antigen–antibody complexes in mucosal lesions in celiac disease and food intolerance will be presented in the next section.

4.3.4. Immunopathology of the Mucosa

After years of arduous investigations with human subjects, characteristic pathological changes in the mucosa of the gastrointestinal tract have been associated with certain adverse reactions to foods in infants and with celiac sprue due to gluten sensitivity. The etiological role of foods in production of this mucosal lesion has been well documented in so-called intolerance of infants to cow milk (Savilahti, 1973; Kuitunen *et al.*, 1973; Shiner *et al.*, 1975b; Fontaine and Navarro, 1975) and soy proteins (Ament and Rubin, 1972) and in gluten-sensitive enteropathy in children and adults (Katz and Falchuk, 1975), but the mucosal lesion is also found in other conditions (Perara *et al.*, 1975). The pathogenesis of the lesion in gluten sensitivity has been considerably clarified by recent studies (Katz and Falchuk, 1975; Strober *et al.*, 1975; Hekkens and Pena, 1974) which implicate immunological mechanisms acting in conjunction with cellular interactions with gluten.

As identical pathological changes in the mucosa appear to occur in this type of reaction to various foods, and examination of biopsy of the jejunal mucosa is recognized as a definitive diagnostic procedure, the general features and the participation of immunological mechanisms will be outlined.

For the purpose of the present discussion the normal mucosa of the jejunum may be considered to consist of villi covered with columnar epithelium which is renewed by proliferation of epithelial cells at the base. In the course of maturation the epithelial cells acquire a brush border containing disaccharidases and other enzymes. Occasional lymphocytes are interspersed among the epithelial cells of the villi. Underneath the villi is the lamina propria, containing mostly lymphocytes and immunoglobulin-producing plasma cells but also some mast cells and eosinophils. These are elements of a dynamic system which may respond to pathological insult rapidly or recover in a period of hours.

The pathological changes in the jejunal mucosa observed in food intolerance and gluten sensitivity consist of destruction of the mature epithelium at the tip of the villi, with loss of brush border and constituent enzymes, and acceleration in production of replacement cells at the base. There is an increase in cells in the lamina propria; lymphocytes or plasma cells may predominate according to the stimulus. As a result, the villus becomes flattened and the cellularity at the base is conspicuously increased. The histology of the normal mucosa and the pathology of this lesion are amply illustrated elsewhere (Perara *et al.*, 1975).

Another type of pathology is found in the gastric and the intestinal mucosa in a condition called "allergic gastroenteropathy," probably the result of a different immunological mechanism, in which eosinophilic infiltration predominates with or without destruction of gastric glandular or intestinal villous epithelium and shortening of these structures (Waldmann *et al.*, 1967; Katz *et al.*, 1977).

Functional derangements, such as secondary intestinal disaccharidase deficiency, are to be expected from such damage to the mucosa, and complications such as leakage of blood and serum would not be surprising.

The cellular elements of the mucosa provide the potential for sensitization and immunological reactions of all types between antigen and humoral antibodies or by cell-mediated response. By means of immunofluorescent staining of biopsy specimens obtained before and after food challenge in cases of intolerance or gluten sensitivity, the reaction in the lamina propria was found to consist of variable preponderance of antibody-forming cells of IgA, IgM, or IgE classes, and deposits of immune complexes and C3 have been identified (Savilahti, 1973; Shiner *et al.*, 1975a; Savilahti, 1972a,b; Shiner and Ballard, 1972). The finding of an increase in the number of interepithelial lymphocytes in mucosal biopsies has opened speculation about a contribution of cell-mediated immunity to the pathology (Ferguson *et al.*, 1976).

Mucosal biopsy specimens can now be maintained in good functional condition *in vitro*. This has permitted more refined studies of responses of normal and sensitized mucosa to exposure to antigen and other manipulations (Katz and Falchuk, 1975; Strober *et al.*, 1975). Findings with this *in vitro* model have been profoundly illuminating and indicate that the pathogenesis of the mucosal lesion characteristic of celiac sprue and food intolerances may be the result of conjoint action of a binding capacity of the incriminated food substances for mucosal epithelial cells in some persons and ensuing activation of immunological reactions. The elements in the process appear to be genetically determined in keeping with the familial incidence of the clinical disorders.

5. Clinical Manifestations

The first step in a rational approach to hypersensitivity reactions to foods is to make certain that what appears to be a definite association of a food with symptoms is actually a correct observation. One's confidence in his ability to make a correct association is likely to be greatly inflated until punctured by some objective means of testing his assumptions concerning relations between foods and symptoms. Adherents to scientific medicine realize that the most valid clinical observations depend on elimination of the preconceptions of physician and patient: in this case, resort to an arrangement in which neither the observer nor the observed knows whether a suspected food is being ingested. Only in this way can sound knowledge be obtained as to whether symptoms ascribed to ingestion of foods are based on bodily disturbances or stem from the imaginations of patients, parents, or physicians, as has been learned by blind food challenges (May, 1976; Bock *et al.*, 1978a). This procedure is described in Section 6.

5.1. Adverse Reactions to Foods

Even if symptoms are shown objectively and unequivocally to be associated with ingestion of a food, all that can be said is that an adverse reaction has been witnessed. There are many causes of adverse reactions to food, the major categories being deficiency of intestinal enzymes (disaccharidases), noxious natural constituents (poisons), contaminants (microorganisms, parasites, toxins, chemicals), psychological factors, and immunological reactions.

Many of the symptoms of adverse reactions are shared by the various categories; the differential diagnosis is considered in Section 6. One must not leap from confirmation that a food is associated with an adverse reaction to an assumption the cause is hypersensitivity on an immunological basis.

5.2. Unproven "Syndromes"

The emotional stress of life often appears in the guise of physical disturbances, especially subjective complaints such as headache, fatigue, and nervous manifestations like altered mood or activity. Currently, unsubstantiated claims have been widely promulgated, particularly in the mass media, that ill-defined syndromes termed "hyperkinesis" and "tension-fatigue" are caused by "allergic" reactions to food and additives for preservation, coloring, or flavoring of food. Scientific studies have not yielded substantial support for these notions, least of all that an immunological mechanism could be involved (Spring and Sandoval, 1976; Wender, 1977).

5.3. Immunological Reactions to Foods

5.3.1. Classification

Traditionally, hypersensitivity reactions have been classified as immediate or delayed according to the interval between ingestion and symptoms. This has been unsatisfactory and misleading because this interval is influenced by various secondary factors apart from the type of immune mechanism, such as amount of food, degree of sensitivity, and nature of the pathological response. As already proposed for the immunological mechanisms in Section 4, it now also seems opportune to strive to classify reactions clinically as reagin mediated or not reagin mediated, thereby focusing attention on the fundamental immunopathological processes rather than the timing of superficial events.

5.3.2. Symptomatic vs. Asymptomatic

An important concept to bear in mind as one seeks to comprehend clinical manifestations is the quantitative requirements in stimulus–response relationships.

When a sensitized person ingests the responsible food, a complex sequence of events must happen before symptoms can occur (Figure 1). Each event from penetration of the mucosal barrier by antigen through interaction among antigen, antibodies, and cells, to final stimulus and response of an end organ is governed by the dependence of response on the magnitude of the stimulus. This means that for a *symptomatic* clinical reaction to appear, enough antigen must reach and combine with a sufficient amount of an appropriate antibody to react with susceptible cells to a degree that will produce a response in end organs of a magnitude detectable by clinical observations. If the quantitive requirements of the stimulus–response relationship are not met sufficiently at each step, the reaction will be unrecognizable clinically or be *asymptomatic*.

5.3.3. Prevalence

The prevalence of immunological adverse reactions to food cannot be stated precisely because diagnosis has probably been grossly inaccurate; widely divergent estimates reflect the opinions of enthusiasts and skeptics. A conservative opinion is that genuine symptomatic hypersensitivity to food is most often encountered in infants (five cases in 1000 infants) and less frequently with advancing age, being uncommon in adults.

5.4. Reagin-Mediated Reactions

5.4.1. Manifestations

Reagin-mediated hypersensitivity reactions to food, confirmed by food challenges, appear in minutes to less than 2 hr after ingestion of a food with the following manifestations (May, 1976; Bock *et al.*, 1978a):

Anaphylaxis	Angioedema	Rhinitis
Abdominal pain	Rash	Vomiting
Urticaria	Diarrhea	Allergic dermatitis
Asthma		

These are the familiar overt symptoms of allergy and although easily recognized are often erroneously ascribed to foods. In fact, only about one-third of clinical histories of adverse reactions to food were confirmed by blind food challenges. Subjective complaints (headache or altered behavior, activity, or mood) were not confirmed (May, 1976; Bock *et al.*, 1978a).

Overt symptoms of reagin-mediated reactions to food may be seen at any age, including neonates, but gastrointestinal and cutaneous manifestations are preponderant in infancy and childhood.

Many disorders may involve one or more manifestations that resemble reagin-mediated hypersensitivity to foods, among which gastrointestinal disorders are most troublesome in practical differential diagnosis. Easily mistaken for hypersensitivity reactions are gastrointestinal symptoms due to deficiencies of intestinal enzymes which may be congenital or acquired, secondary to mucosal damage from any cause. Disaccharidase deficiencies are revealed by acidic stools and increased content of reducing substances, often leading to irritations and erythema of the buttocks (Ament, 1972). Otherwise distinguishing features of the various disorders should steer the informed clinician away from erroneous diagnoses.

5.4.2. Detection of Reaginic Sensitization

The general principles of detection of reagin-mediated reactions to food have been presented in Section 4. Reaginic antibody may be fixed in the skin from birth onward (Kuhns, 1965). With different lots of food extracts from one source (Greer Laboratories, Lenoir, North Carolina) which were verified for usefulness in skin tests, reaginic sensitization has been dependably detected in reagin-mediated food hypersensitivity (Bock *et al.*, 1977, 1978b). Skin tests were performed by the puncture technique using 1:20 w/v concentration of extracts; a net wheal reaction of 3 mm diameter or greater in 10–15 min identified all the subjects among whom were to be found those exhibiting clinical reactions of reaginic hypersensitivity in blind food challenges. Reference is made again to the comments on immediate wheal reactions in the skin due to an IgG antibody in the discussion of skin tests in Section 4; appearance of symptoms in infants exhibiting this type of sensitization may not occur immediately, but instead 12–36 hr after ingestion of a food (Parish, 1970, 1971).

As already discussed, RAST and other tests for reaginic activity are not superior to properly utilized skin tests with verified extracts.

5.4.3. Foods Causing Reactions

Among 20 foods commonly believed to be responsible for hypersensitivity reactions to food, in studies of over 100 infants and children (Bock *et al.*, 1977, 1978b) only the following were actually found to cause clinical reactions: peanuts and other nuts, cow milk, hen egg, and soy bean. Reaginic sensitization to other

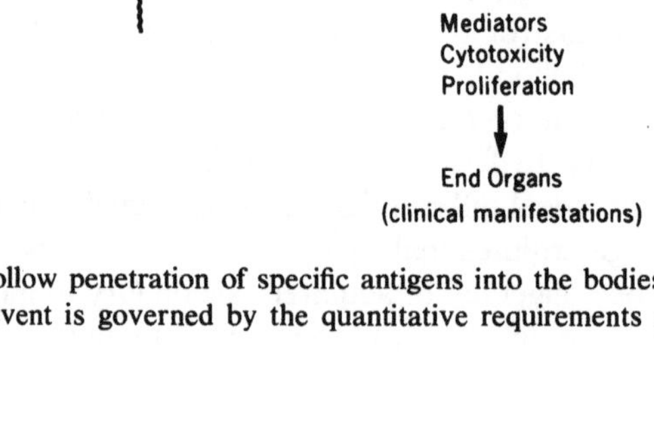

Figure 1. Events that follow penetration of specific antigens into the bodies of sensitized persons. The outcome of each event is governed by the quantitative requirements of a stimulus–response relationship.

foods, but too weak to be associated with clinically significant or symptomatic reactions, was frequent in allergic subjects but indicative only of asymptomatic sensitization. Relatively few foods may be responsible for confirmable, clinically significant hypersensitivity reaction to foods ingested in ordinary amounts.

5.5. Reactions Not Reagin Mediated

5.5.1. General Characteristics

Under the heading of reactions not reagin mediated are grouped disorders where the evidence of foods being etiological is convincing and a basic role for an immunologic mechanism is certain or probable but the delineation of the pathogenesis may be incomplete. Because of limitations in information in the past, some of the adverse reactions to food in this category were appropriately referred to as food "intolerance." Knowledge of the clinical and immunological features has now reached a state where it seems feasible to attempt to picture this group of adverse reactions to food as an orderly array of hypersensitivity reactions to food, even though the blemishes in the depiction will be evident.

To say that this group of reactions is not reagin mediated is meant to convey the idea that other immune mechanisms are exclusively or principally involved—more explicitly, the manifestations are associated with interactions between food antigens and IgA, IgG, and IgM classes of antibody and cells in the ways described in Sections 3 and 4. This does not exclude the possibility of a reagin-mediated mechanism being a prerequisite or a partner in clinical and pathological manifestations through preliminary or concomitant effects of the mediators released.

The limited variety of manifestations of hypersensitivity reactions to food not mediated by reagin are

Pneumonitis	Enteropathies	Urticaria
Asthma	Occult or gross bleeding (anemia)	Allergic dermatitis
Vomiting	Protein losing (edema)	Contact dermatitis
Diarrhea	Malabsorption (steatorrhea)	
Subnormal growth		

The end organs can respond in correspondingly few ways. The impression of a vast assortment of clinical symptoms arises from the ramifications induced by age, sites of the major pathological impact, chronicity, and complications or secondary effects, and by mixtures of underlying circumstances and mechanisms. The somewhat simplistic grouping of clinical disorders to be presented at least affords an orderly approach to diagnosis and management.

An outstanding clinical feature is the time interval between ingestion of an offending food and the appearance of symptoms, in general being a matter of several hours or days in contrast to minutes or less than 2 hr as is the case with reagin-mediated reactions. This delay in appearance of symptoms reflects the time required for progression of the immunopathology to a clinically recognizable stage rather than any latency in onset of the immune response, which begins immediately on contact of antigen with antibody or sensitized cell.

5.5.2. Acute Gastroenteropathy

Diarrhea in infants, sometimes accompanied by vomiting, which develops 12–36 hr after ingestion of particular foods, especially cow milk, and which quickly subsides if the food is withdrawn from the diet is the prime feature of the reactions now generally referred to as food "intolerance" (Savilahti, 1973; Kuitunen *et al.*, 1975; Shiner *et al.*, 1975b; Fontaine and Navarro, 1975; Ament and Rubin, 1972). Over the years clinical descriptions of what were probably examples of this sort of reaction to foods have used various terms, such as "cow's milk idiosyncracy" (Vendel, 1948), "milk allergy," and "intractable" or "protracted" diarrhrea (Lloyd-Still *et al.*, 1973).

This type of reaction occurs in the early months of infancy and is usually transient so that by the age of 2–3 years the guilty foods can be eaten without provoking symptoms. Unless the responsible food is identified and eliminated, the diarrhrea will persist and may become life threatenting (Lloyd-Still *et al.*, 1973; Shwachman *et al.*, 1973), or chronic enteropathy may develop (Fällström *et al.*, 1965); acute dehydration and metabolic and nutritional deficits supervene.

A variety of enteropathy caused by gluten sensitivity is not transient but may begin in infancy as acute diarrhea. Differentiation from transient acute gastroenteropathy can ultimately be made only when it is found that intolerance to wheat and other gluten-containing foods is permanent. This variety is discussed later in Section 5.5.4.

The more regularly biopsy of the jejunal mucosa is obtained in acute gastroenteropathy not found to be reagin mediated, the more a characteristic lesion is shown to be present (Kuitunen *et al.*, 1973; Walker-Smith *et al.*, 1978); the immunopathology of this lesion is described in Section 4. The resemblance to the mucosal lesion in the chronic malabsorptive condition gluten-sensitive enteropathy is so close or identical that the pathogenesis may well be similar.

Evidence is mounting that this form of acute gastroenteropathy is at least in part due to a hypersensitivity reaction to food. The characteristic changes in jejunal mucosa may even be present when clinical symptoms are not provoked by a single challenge with a suspected food; that is, it may be subclinical or asymptomatic evidence of sensitization. Immunofluorescent staining of biopsy specimens demonstrated that IgG and IgM antibodies are most conspicuously involved, but sometimes IgE antibodies may play a part (Shiner *et al.*, 1975a). However, skin tests rarely evoke wheal reactions, and typical manifestations of reagin-mediated reactions seldom accompany the diarrhea. Further elucidation of the pathogenesis of acute gastroenteropathy as a hypersensitivity reaction to food will surely come from *in vitro* studies with biopsy specimens, as has been the case with gluten-sensitive enteropathy.

Acute gastroenteropathy occurs in the early months of infancy, or soon after breast feeding is replaced or supplemented with other foods, which is also the period when IgG and IgM antibodies to cow milk proteins and other foods in the diet are regularly detected in the sera from normal infants (Rothberg and Farr, 1965; Kletter *et al.*, 1971a,b; May *et al.*, 1977), whereas IgE antibodies to milk proteins are detected in the sera only in genetically predisposed, sensitized infants (Kletter *et al.*, 1971c). The prevalence of acute gastroenteropathy and these serum antibodies in the period of infancy may not be merely fortuitous; if attention is paid to the amount and kind of antibody and not just the presence, the significance of increase in specific food antibodies of the IgG and IgM classes in the mucosal lesion may seem more relevant (May *et al.*, 1977). The stage may be set for the sort of interplay of genetic and immunological factors found in the pathogenesis of gluten-sensitive enteropathy. Absence or minimal levels of serum antibodies to a suspected food have not proved to be compatible with gastroenteropathy on an immunological basis (May, unpublished). Also suggestive is the fact that the prevalence of acute gastroenteropathy declines after infancy as do serum levels of food antibodies, except in persons with persistent reaginic hypersensitivity to food (May *et al.*, 1977).

5.5.3. Chronic Gastroenteropathy

In the 1960s reports appeared of groups of infants and a few children who at first seemed to be suffering from different chronic entities, the major presenting feature being either hypochromic anemia unresponsive to iron or edema and hypoproteinemia (Wilson *et al.*, 1962; Waldmann *et al.*, 1967). Underlying occult blood loss and excessive protein loss from the gut were found to account for the clinical features. Diarrhea was mild and intermittent, and, although chronicity was a feature, steatorrhea was not. Growth failure was common. In some patients manifestations characteristic of reagin-mediated hypersensitivity were seen, namely, urticaria, eczema, rhinitis, or asthma. Cow milk was discovered to frequently be the cause, the cure was effected by its elimination from the diet, but usually milk could be tolerated in later months or years. Ultimately the various supposed entities were seen to be manifestations of transient chronic gastroenteropathy (Wilson *et al.*, 1974).

The clinical differences between acute and chronic gastroenteropathy may depend on (1) whether the offending food is identified and completely eliminated promptly and long enough for recovery to occur; or (2) how old the patient is, as the gut of the infant may be more easily provoked into acute diarrhea; or (3) the immunopathogenesis of the acute and chronic forms may not be identical.

Biopsies of the jejunal mucosa in some of the patients with chronic enteropathy revealed marked infiltration of the lamina propria by cosinophils as the only abnormality; flattening of the villi was not observed, in contrast to the pathological findings in gluten-sensitive enteropathy (Waldmann *et al.*, 1967). Eosinophilia was also frequent in the peripheral blood, and the term "eosinophilic gastroenteropathy" is favored by some. Precipitins to milk proteins were demonstrated in abnormally high titers in the sera of the majority of the patients, but comprehensive search for a specific immune mechanism was not undertaken.

Thus this chronic although transient form of gastroenteropathy was shown to be an adverse reaction to food (milk) protein, probably a hypersensitivity reaction of unknown immune mechanism, analogous to transient acute gastroenteropathy, but with different pathological changes in the jejunal mucosa insofar as the few studies to date can be judged. Special notice should be taken of the greater prevalence of reported cases in infancy and childhood and the transient nature. Food antigens have not been identified as etiological in all cases of chronic gastroenteropathy (Wilson *et al.*, 1974; Katz *et al.*, 1977). Biopsy of gastric mucosa may be preferable for diagnosis because characteristic lesions were more prominent and more regularly found than in jejunal mucosa (Katz *et al.*, 1977). Reaginic sensitization has been demonstrated in some cases (Katz *et al.*, 1978), and, as mentioned, there may be a combination of immune mechanisms.

Clarification of the immunological basis would surely come from studies of specimens of mucosa by immunofluorescence techniques and with the *in vitro* organ culture system used so fruitfully in research on the pathogenesis of gluten-sensitive enteropathy.

5.5.4. Gluten-Sensitive Enteropathy

In contrast to the preceding transient enteropathies the celiac-sprue malabsorption syndrome, which may be more precisely designated "gluten-sensitive enteropathy," is not transient, but the basic defect is hereditary and irreversible; sensitivity to gluten persists throughout life (Hekkens and Pena, 1974).

The clinical features of the fully developed condition are almost unmistakable, but many unusual presenting manifestations have been described (Ament, 1972; Katz and Falchuk, 1975; Strober *et al.*, 1975). Classically, a miserable, wasted individual with distended abdomen passes voluminous, foul, fatty stools. By means of oral tests for absorption of fat or carbohydrate or determination of fat in the feces, the absorptive defect can be confirmed.

Definitive diagnosis depends on biopsy of the jejunal mucosa where the characteristic lesion is found. This lesion is not unique to gluten-sensitive enteropathy but, as already mentioned, occurs in acute gastroenteropathy in infants caused by cow milk, soy protein, and possibly other food proteins; this is the most confusing condition to be distinguished in differential diagnosis in infancy. Other disorders in which the mucosal lesion may be found are listed elsewhere (Perara *et al.*, 1975).

The mucosal lesion and the immunopathology are described in Section 4. The immunological component of the pathogenesis is now sufficiently established as an essential part to justify inclusion of gluten-sensitive enteropathy among hypersensitivity reactions to food. Complete clarification of the resemblances and differences in the pathogenesis of the mucosal lesions in gluten-sensitive enteropathy and in the other gastroenteropathies caused by hypersensitivity to foods will probably bring surprises.

5.5.5. Chronic Pneumonitis

A relatively few infants and children, compared to the number with acute and chronic gastroenteropathy, have been described with chronic pulmonary infiltrations associated with ingestion of cow milk (Heiner *et al.*, 1962; Holland *et al.*, 1962; Anderson *et al.*, 1974; Boat *et al.*, 1975). These reactions may represent a variant of nonreaginic hypersensitivity reactions to milk—gastrointestinal manifestations being prominent in some and pulmonary involvement conspicuous in others. Avoidance of milk is curative in many patients in either group, and high titers of serum antibodies to milk are frequent in both.

This form of pneumonitis ordinarily begins within the first 6 months of life. Vomiting, choking, coughing, and dysphagia are frequent complaints while diarrhea is mild and intermittent. Eosinophilia and severe hypochromic anemia are usually present. Roentgenograms of the lungs reveal patchy infiltration. In some patients pulmonary hemosiderosis was diagnosed by hemoptysis and the finding of iron-laden macrophages in gastric and bronchial aspirates.

Intradermal skin tests with milk proteins were often found to evoke wheal reactions within 15 min. Total serum IgE was often elevated, but negative Prausnitz–Küstner tests with patients' sera and milk proteins were not present. At the time, the skin-sensitizing IgG antibody was not known, and therefore sera were not tested for it, but the immediate reaction in the skin tests may have been due to this type of antibody (Parish, 1970, 1971).

As was found in chronic gastroenteropathy, not only did the sera of patients with this type of chronic pneumonitis exhibit abnormally high titers of precipitins, using a gel diffusion technique, but also precipitins to seven or more protein constituents of milk were found. Sera of normal infants contained detectable milk precipitins much less frequently and in low titer, and precipitins were not obtained to more than three milk proteins.

In the two latest reports of this chronic pneumonitis the general features and the immunological responses to milk proteins were confirmed and extended to suggest an Arthus-type reaction involving IgG milk antibodies. RAST tests for specific IgE antibodies to milk proteins showed none to be present in the sera (Anderson *et al.*, 1974; Boat *et al.*, 1975).

In view of the frequency of symptoms compatible with aspiration of milk into the lungs, the suggestion that this may be responsible for the pneumonitis is rational (Anderson *et al.*, 1974). Other conditions in which aspiration of food is common also lead to a similar chronic pneumonitis but without associated signs of gastroenteropathy (Nelson, 1964; Kletter *et al.*, 1972).

The point to be emphasized here is that the titers and variety of milk antibodies in the sera from patients with chronic pneumonitis and gastroenteropathy are much greater than found in normal infants and children. When milk is avoided, the abnormalities of milk antibodies from the serum disappear simultaneous with improvement in the pneumonitis, as is true for the gastroenteropathies.

The available evidence indicates that the acute and chronic gastroenteropathies and the chronic pneumonitis described result from similar nonreaginic immune mechanisms involving interactions of food (milk) antigens, IgG and other antibodies, and cells in the mucosa or alveoli, and that these are examples of hypersensitivity reactions to food. Reaginic sensitization probably plays a role in some cases (Katz *et al.*, 1978).

There could be a genetic predisposition in the affected persons which accounts for susceptibility to immunopathology. However, the transient nature of these conditions, leading to spontaneous recovery in later infancy or early childhood, is compatible with maturation of some related process such as penetrability of the intestinal barrier or cellular modulation of antibody production.

5.5.6. Concluding Comments

Separation of distinctive syndromes due to hypersensitivity reactions to food for clinical convenience endangers a dynamic view of sensitization to food antigens and the potential for hypersensitivity reactions. Returning to the concept of the immune system as a second line of defense reinforcing the barrier of the intestinal mucosa against invasion of the body by foreign proteins, the list of disorders which may lead to abnormal penetration of the barrier or breakdown of the secondary defense seems almost interminable. Consider the many pathological disturbances of the gastrointestinal system and the complex assortment of disorders of the immune system and the genetic control and developmental defects to which both systems are liable. It is striking that so few foods are involved in nonreaginic hypersensitivity reactions; cow milk, soybean, and wheat account for almost all reported cases.

Sensitization to food antigens will frequently occur, and specific antibodies and sensitized cells will be identified by the various immunological methods. The properly oriented clinician will be alert to the circumstances that may result in sensitization to a food antigen, but he will remember that clinically significant, symptomatic hypersensitivity reactions to the food depend on the quantitative stimulus–response relationship which governs every step in the immune response (Figure 1). Enough response must take place all along the way to give clinically recognizable manifestations at the end. Otherwise, the sensitization has no clinical consequence at the time, although the potential for pathological significance remains.

Because all the components of the various immune responses may be present in sensitization to food antigen, further demonstration can be anticipated of involvement of hypersensitivity reactions to food in immune complex diseases and other immunological disorders. This awaits better methods for quantitative detection of specific components of immune complexes.

Better to bear in mind the dynamics of sensitization and hypersensitivity reactions to food than to memorize syndromes and tests, unless one prefers perpetual confusion and mystery.

6. Clinical Applications

What follows is derived from the foregoing account of the processes underlying the clinical manifestations of reactions to food based on immunological mechanisms, i.e., genuine hypersensitivity to antigens in food. The approach to diagnosis is for those who strive to practice rational scientific medicine. The struggle is not easy amid demands for relief from symptoms by quick and simple means. Practical and simple are not the same—to be truly practical clinically is to follow the correct procedures to reach definitive solutions to patients' problems, simple or not. Where knowledge is incomplete the way may be blocked, but irrational groping will not hasten progress toward sensible clinical management of food hypersensitivity.

The greatest obstacle to a comfortable, confident, practical approach to food hypersensitivity is the traditional, unfounded attitude that knowledge of the subject is too limited to allow rational clinical analysis. No longer can this slender reed be used to support confusion or gullibility.

The purpose of this section is to give the general approach to clinical application of present knowledge of hypersensitivity reactions to food without trying to cover the details.

Orderly approach to diagnosis of hypersensitivity reactions to foods requires

1. Thoughtful history and careful physical examination

2. Objective confirmation of the history of an adverse reaction by double-blind food challenge
3. Differentiation of hypersensitivity from other adverse reactions to foods
4. Evidence of specific immunological sensitization
   a. Reaginic: skin tests
   b. Nonreaginic: serum antibodies, biopsy of mucosa of the gastrointestinal tract
5. Elimination diet

6.1. History and Physical Examination

A full, freely given history and careful physical examination will go far toward settling the foremost questions: Are the manifestations actually compatible with food hypersensitivity caused by an immune mechanism, and which foods may be guilty? Skepticism is indicated, but the physician should listen sympathetically with an open mind. Aside from the manifestations of food hypersensitivity, he should be alert to clues of other categories of adverse reactions to food.

6.2. Confirmation of Reported Adverse Reaction to Food

In our experience even the most trustworthy patients and parents as well as the most sincere physicians are not exempt from erroneous association of symptoms with foods. Therefore, confirmation of suspicions by double-blind food challenge is strongly recommended.

Obviously, life-threatening anaphylactic reactions to food will not be doubtful, and victims must not be subjected to the hazard of intentional challenge.

Sound observations of reactions to foods cannot be made unless the patient is free of symptoms or brought to a steady state at the time of challenge. To this end, for as long as necessary before challenging, all suspected foods are eliminated from the diet, or when the symptoms are suggestive but no particular food can be incriminated the diet listed in Table 1, composed of items rarely causing sensitization, should be utilized.

Capsules are filled by someone other than the observers with a dry form of the food product to be tested. The commonest offenders can be obtained at a grocery in the dry state (for example, cow milk, soybean flour, whole wheat flour, whole egg, peanuts, and other nuts). Other wet foods of real concern can be freeze-dried and powdered. Opaque, dye-free, size #1 capsules* will hold 200–500 mg of dry food. Subjects 5–6 years of age and older will swallow 20 capsules in a few minutes with gentle persuasion.

With subjects under 6 years of age, the dry or wet food will have to be masked in some other item in the diet, which is completely satisfactory under 3 years and relatively so in the 3–6 year range. The amount of dry food administered as a test dose is governed by the apparent degree of the suspected hypersensitivity, ranging from 10 mg to 2 g for the initial dose.

The subject should be under continuous surveillance during food challenge, preferably in an office or hospital setting, to secure definitive observations.

*Obtainable from Tutag Pharmaceuticals, 2599 West Midway Blvd., Broomfield, CO 80020.

TABLE 1. Elimination Diet

Foods allowed at mealtime		
Rice		Asparagus
Puffed rice		Beets
Rice cakes (Chico San, Inc.)		Carrots
Rice Krispies		Lettuce
		Sweet potatoes
Pineapple	Canned fruit, juices, and nectars of these	White vinegar
Apricots		Olive oil
Cranberrie		
Peaches		
Pears		
Apples		Honey, 2 oz a day
Lamb		Cane or beet sugar
Chicken		Salt
		Oleomargarine, milk free
Tapioca		Crisco, Spry
Snacks		
1 box rice cereal midmorning and midafternoon		
Avoid		
Any food not on this list (check labels)		

Capsules are given by someone blind to the contents and under close supervision to make certain all are swallowed without exploration of the contents. The capsules are given just before a meal of the restricted diet (preferably before breakfast), and the restricted diet is continued throughout the period of observations. When a test dose must be masked in an item from the restricted diet, it is fed with a meal of the restricted diet by someone blind to what is being masked.

Any symptoms which occur are recorded by observers unaware of what food is being tested. To detect reactions reported by history to have occurred within 24 hr, the subject must be examined every 15 min for 2 hr for immediate reactions and then at least hourly for 8–12 hr and at 24 hr for later reactions.

If no reaction is evoked by the initial dose, the challenge should be repeated with increasingly large doses on successive separate occasions (about two- to tenfold increments) until an unequivocal reaction is witnessed or no symptoms are provoked by 8 g of dry food. If 8 g is tolerated blindly, the food in its natural form can be added to the diet visibly after the subject is told that no reaction was induced by it. The water content of the foods naturally varies widely; for cow milk, 8 g of dry product is equivalent to 62 g (2 oz) in the liquid state.

Unequivocal reagin-mediated reactions will occur within 2 hr of ingestion of the test dose. Reactions not mediated by reagin usually begin within 4–25 hr of the test dose. No other foods should be added to the diet until the food under test has been consumed in a customary portion at least once daily for a week, while any symptoms continue to be reported. Preferably challenges with each food should be separated by 2-week intervals to avoid overlap of symptoms.

If no symptoms occur, a placebo control is not necessary, but in case of doubt, especially with unimpressive vomiting or subjective complaints, double-blind administration of glucose in capsules or in the same item used to mask the test food will clarify matters.

A single unequivocal positive reaction to a food tested in a double-blind food challenge, conducted as described, may be considered definitive evidence of an adverse reaction to a food. Confirmation of the role of gluten sensitivity in a patient with chronic malabsorption is a separate consideration to be dealt with later.

A commonly expressed dictum is that occurrence of symptoms after open administration of a food on three successive trials may be considered proof of an allergic reaction. Actually, other adverse reactions would be exhibited in the same way, e.g., disaccharidase deficiency and especially psychological reactions. It seems more human and judicious to evoke symptoms once in a definitive blind food challenge than to inflict discomfort three times in open challenges in an effort to make up for the shortcomings of the open procedures. There is no substitute for double-blind challenge.

6.3. Differential Diagnosis

Once an adverse reaction has been objectively and unequivocally shown to result from ingestion of a food, a hypersensitivity reaction must be differentiated from other adverse reactions. Then the search for an association with immunological sensitization can begin.

Fortunately certain considerations simplify the task of the practitioner. Reagin-mediated reactions manifest relatively distinctive features in infants, children, and adults, and identification of reaginic sensitization is straightforward. Reactions not reagin mediated are most common in infancy and childhood, except for malabsorption in adults caused by gluten-sensitive enteropathy. Only a few foods have been shown to be etiological in nonreaginic reactions. With the aid of a careful history and physical examination, the experienced, capable physician will not often find the differential diagnosis complicated if the manifestations are viewed in their entirety; most conditions have some distinctive features which separate them from disorders arising from food hypersensitivity. The most flagrant examples of the gastroenteropathies and the pneumonitis previously associated with food hypersensitivity are seldom seen now in the United States, conceivably because an excessive zeal in eliminating cow milk from the diet of infants is developing.

Serum levels of immunoglobulins A, E, G, and M are useful in identification of immunodeficiency disorders. Blood content of hemoglobin and serum proteins, test for occult blood in feces, and roentgenograms of the lungs may disclose characteristic features of gastroenteropathies or pneumonitis caused by food hypersensitivity.

Other investigations will be dictated by the findings in the history and physical examination, for example, chloride in sweat when cystic fibrosis is suspected. Appropriate examinations for infectious agents may be indicated. Further radiological studies are needed when anatomical or inflammatory lesions of the gastrointestinal or urinary tracts are suspected. Protracted diarrhea with irritation of the buttocks calls for testing the feces for pH below 6 and excessive content of reducing substances. If indicated, tolerance tests with specific disaccharide or monosaccharide can be performed with customary procedures (Ament, 1972).

6.4. Evidence of Specific Immunological Sensitization

The nature and detection of the immune processes in hypersensitivity reactions to food have received extensive consideration in Sections 3 and 4. Comprehension of the contents of those sections is assumed, and here only the practical application will be emphasized.

6.5. Reactions Reagin Mediated

Skin tests with extracts of foods is the most useful, practical, and economic procedure for clinical identification of reaginic sensitization. The adequacy of the extracts in specific antigen content and freedom from irritants must be verified as was done by us for one commercial source (Bock *et al.,* 1977, 1978b); with those extracts a net wheal of 3 mm or greater diameter evoked by a 1:20 weight/volume concentration administered by the puncture technique served to identify the degree of hypersensitivity likely to be associated with a reagin-mediated hypersensitivity reaction to ingestion of a food.

In addition to usefulness in making an association between an adverse reaction to a food and reaginic hypersensitivity, skin tests properly performed and interpreted can serve as screening tests to identify the relatively few persons with whom food challenges may evoke a hypersensitivity reaction (Bock *et al.,* 1977, 1978b).

In infants and children most reagin-mediated hypersensitivity reactions have been found in our experience to be caused by a few foods (cow milk, egg, soybean, and nuts) out of a panel of 20 foods commonly incriminated (Bock *et al.,* 1977, 1978b). In some regions other foods may be more common offenders, depending on dietary habits (Aas, 1966a). Although some individuals may give histories of reactions to many other foods, these are not often confirmed by blind food challenge, and therefore routine skin testing with a large number of food extracts will not be advantageous. Use of unverified extracts is apt to be misleading.

The level of reagin in the serum measured by the radioallergosorbent (RAST) method correlates well with the degree of sensitization detected by skin test. Verification of the adequacy of the food antigen employed is essential for both tests. RAST has not been found superior to the skin test for reliable detection of reaginic sensitization to foods in our experience. The RAST test has no advantages in clinical practice. There is great need for improvement in quality of the commercially produced antigenic material required for both tests.

Several other procedures are available for detection of reaginic sensitization, namely microscopic examination for basophil degranulation or for cellular responses in the skin window technique and *in vitro* determination of antigenic histamine release. None of these is superior to the skin test or has any advantages for clinical purposes.

Widespread eczema presents a problem for skin tests, and RAST may give spurious reactions in eczema (Lee and May, unpublished data), so that food challenge must be depended on at present.

When characteristic symptoms and evidence of reaginic sensitzation are not found, the search for an immunological basis of an adverse reaction to food must be extended to nonreaginic mechanisms.

6.6. Reactions Not Reagin Mediated

6.6.1. Serum Antibodies

Because food antigens penetrate the intestinal barrier in everyone, an antibody response may be evoked in any normal immunocompetent person. Therefore, the mere presence of antibodies to food in the serum cannot meet diagnostic needs, but their detection does mean that a state of immunological sensitization exists. However, if the distinction between mere presence and the amount and kind of antibodies to food proteins in sera receives more attention, the role of these antibodies in the pathogenesis of hypersensitivity reactions to food and their diagnostic usefulness may be more clearly perceived.

Antibodies in the serum have been measured by various methods—precipitins, precipitation of antibody-bound antigen, and hemagglutination (Williams and Chase, 1971/1977)—all of which may reflect the total heterogeneous antibody population but predominantly IgG and IgM classes. The titer of serum antibodies to foods introduced in infancy declines steadily after infancy and may become undetectable in normal adults. In individuals hypersensitive to food this decline may not take place and the titers remain up at the infantile level (May *et al.*, 1977). The titer and variety of serum antibodies are greatly increased in some cases of gastroenteropathy and chronic pneumonitis associated with hypersensitivity to food antigens (Wilson *et al.*, 1962, 1974; Heiner *et al.*, 1962; Holland *et al.*, 1962). Therefore, the finding of exceptionally high titers of serum antibodies to foods at any age, or persistence of the levels found normally in infancy into and beyond childhood, should enhance suspicion that an associated adverse reaction to a food may be a hypersensitivity disorder.

Bear in mind that the amounts and variety of antibodies in serum ordinarily detected by these methods in normal persons vary according to age and probably have no pathological significance. Beware of attempts to arouse concern over the mere presence of serum antibodies to each food antigen that happens to be studied, for example, soybean. We have been through this with cow milk.

The methods for measurement of these serum antibodies are not suitable for occasional use in the practitioner's office, but should be available in laboratories where serious, comprehensive evaluation of hypersensitivity reactions to food is to be undertaken.

6.6.2. Biopsy of Mucosa of the Gastrointestinal Tract

Definitive diagnosis of the food-induced transient gastroenteropathies and the persistent gluten-sensitive enteropathy depends on finding characteristic lesions in biopsy specimens of jejunal or gastric mucosa. The lesions are not exclusively associated with these conditions but are regularly present. The differential diagnosis, pathogenesis, and microscopic characteristics of the lesions are described briefly in Sections 4 and 5, and comprehensive discussions are available in the literature (Strober *et al.*, 1975; Perara *et al.*, 1975).

Mucosal biopsy requires special skills in procurement, examination, and interpretation. But without the information obtainable through this procedure, investigation of adverse reactions to food will be incomplete, and a diagnosis of a hypersensitivity reaction not mediated by reagin cannot be firmly established.

6.6.3. Cell-Mediated Immunity

There is insufficient evidence of a clinically significant contribution of cell-mediated immune reactions to call for a search for this type of response in nonreaginic hypersensitivity reactions to food. The meager antigenic stimulation of lymphocytes in culture reported in some cases (Amache *et al.*, 1969; Scheinmann *et al.*, 1976; May and Alberto, 1972a,b) cannot be taken as conclusive evidence of a cell-mediated immune response on the basis of food hypersensitivity.

6.6.4. Elimination Diet

The elimination diet recommended for use in the procedure for food challenge may have to serve a diagnostic purpose when other methods are lacking or fail to give adequate support for a diagnosis of hypersensitivity reactions to foods. One must be alert to the deceptiveness of offering a suspected food visibly in the diet, and accept only overt manifestations and not subjective complaints in evaluation of the response. Especially in chronic gastroenteropathies in infancy, the implication of gluten may require a period of elimination from the diet.

6.7. Management

6.7.1. Diet

If the procedures set forth are used to establish a diagnosis of food hypersensitivity, foods will not be removed from the diet excessively on inadequate grounds to the detriment of nutrition. Avoidance of single foods of little nutritional worth should not be a hardship. Even when a major food like cow milk must be kept from an infant's diet, optimal nutrition can still be achieved with substitutes such as soybean or protein-free preparations. Exclusion of wheat requires some ingenuity in construction of an appetizing wholesome diet and careful reading of labels, but is not really formidable. Not often do properly conducted studies lead to exclusion of more than one major foodstuff, because a limited variety of foods cause most reactions. In fact, we have not encountered an individual, even in infancy, who could not be given a diet which took into account all his genuine, confirmed hypersensitivity reactions to foods and also achieved optimal nutrition. This is not the place to offer extensive dietetic information; besides, what is needed more is adherence to rational diagnostic procedures, thereby limiting the need for elaborate dietary arrangements to preserve optimal nutrition and the contentment of the patient.

6.7.2. Cromolyn

After correct diagnosis of true hypersensitivity reactions to the relatively few foods involved and the simple requirement for avoidance of guilty foods have been observed, there will be little need for drug treatment of reagin-mediated reactions. The rationale for use of cromolyn (disodium cromoglycate) would presumably be to inhibit reagin-mediated reactions, where a drug seems least needed. Trials of the drug now in progress may suffer from inadequacies in diagnostic procedures. Scanty reports to date do not present a compelling case for common usage of cromolyn in food hypersensitivity (Freier and Berger, 1973; Dannaeus *et al.*, 1977).

A bothersome thought is that suppression of symptoms of reagin-mediated reactions may encourage continued ingestion of foods capable of evoking other immune responses in the affected individuals. Should production of antibodies other than reagins be stimulated, there is the possibility that reactions not mediated by reagin would develop from continued ingestion of food antigen, e.g., immune complex disorders.

No doubt if cromolyn is approved for general use for reagin-mediated hypersensitivity reactions to foods, there will be wholesale prescription for all manner of vague symptoms loosely ascribed to food "allergy."

6.7.3. Corticosteroids

Individuals severely afflicted with gluten-sensitive enteropathy may benefit from treatment with corticosteroids for a period, as may those who do not seem to respond to exclusion of gluten from the diet (Katz and Falchuk, 1975; Ament, 1972), and some patients with eosinophilic gastroenteropathy (Katz *et al.*, 1978).

6.7.4. Hyposensitization

Allergists have deep faith in injection therapy for hyposensitization in pollen sensitivity, but this feeling has not spread to food sensitivity. This is all the more strange because successful hyposensitization of a food-sensitive person was reported about the same time that attempts at hyposensitization in hay fever became popular (Schloss, 1912). Since then there have been only a few anecdotal reports of success. The reasons hyposensitization with foods was not generally accepted are not known. The natural history of decline with age in clinical symptoms caused by food hypersensitivity could easily be mistaken as successful desensitization. It does not seem prudent to embark on programs of oral or injection hyposensitization in the transient forms of immunological hypersensitivity to food.

However, oral administration of graded doses of protein is not without rationale insofar as stimulation of secretion of specific SIgA antibodies in the gut is concerned, which conceivably could strengthen the intestinal mucosal barrier against penetration by specific antigen (Hanson *et al.*, 1977). In addition, there is the possibility of hastening acquisition of immunological unresponsiveness to food proteins, which appears to happen in later life (Korenblat *et al.*, 1968; Thomas and Parrott, 1974). Exploration of these possibilities is for future research. At present there are no substantial, relevant data to support use of food proteins for oral or parenteral attempts at hyposensitization in immunological hypersensitivity to foods. Injection of food proteins also may stimulate production of humoral antibodies involved in nonreaginic hypersensitivity and immune complex disease.

6.7.5. Prophylaxis

There are many uncertainties about the rationale and the success of prevention of hypersensitivity to foods by delaying introduction of common offenders into the diet until late infancy. Even if convincing evidence were on hand that hypersensitivity to a food could be prevented in this manner, and not simply delayed until exposure to the food did occur, selection of the infants and the foods to be subjected to this management would be guesswork at present. To lengthen this review with a sound critique of the literature on this subject seems unwarranted. The curious reader can begin his search with Matthews and Soothill (1970), Savilahti (1973), and Halpern *et al.* (1973).

7. Envoi

From looking back on this survey of the literature on food hypersensitivity the gaps in our knowledge are easily discerned. The scene as a whole gives the impression that sophisticated research in many aspects of immunological reactions to food substances is finally under way. The challenges presented by the ramifications of the many fundamental processes involved in the immunology of the gastrointestinal tract and adverse reactions to foodstuffs are as exciting as any in the field of science. This review has been a modest effort to convey some of the findings and the prospect of a new era to academicians and practitioners alike, for they do not differ in the need for understanding.

ACKNOWLEDGMENTS

While the author bears full responsibility for this review, he was greatly aided by his associates, Dr. S. Allan Bock, Dr. Wai-Ying Lee, and Ms. Linda Remigio. Their intellectual stimulation and skillful effort during our clinical and laboratory studies was essential to this undertaking.

8. References

Aas, K., 1966a, Studies of hypersensitivity to fish—A clinical study, *Int. Arch. Allergy* **29:**346.

Aas, K., 1966b, Studies of hypersensitivity to fish—Allergological and serological differentiation between various species of fish, *Int. Arch. Allergy* **30:**257.

Aas, K., 1978, The diagnosis of hypersensitivity to ingested foods: Reliability of skin prick testing and radioallergosorbent test with different materials, *Clin. Allergy* **8:**39.

Aas, K., and Lundkvist, U., 1973, The radioallergosorbent test with a purified allergen from codfish, *Clin. Allergy* **3:**255.

Amache, N., Ky, N. T., and Hazard, J., 1969, La culture des lymphocytes dans l'allergie alimentaire, *Rev. Fr. Allerg.* **8:**215.

Ament, M. E., 1972, Malabsorption syndromes in infancy and childhood I, II, *J. Pediatr.* **81:**685, 867.

Ament, M. E., 1975, Immunodeficiency syndromes and gastrointestinal disease, *Pediatr. Clin. N. Am.* **22:**807.

Ament, M. E., and Rubin, C. E., 1972, Soy protein—another cause of the flat intestinal lesion, *Gastroenterology* **62:**227.

Anderson, A. F., Schloss, O. M., and Myers, C., 1925, The intestinal absorption of antigenic protein by normal infants, *Proc. Soc. Biol. Med.* **23:**180.

Anderson, J. A., Weiss, L., Rebuck, J. W., Cabal, L. A., and Sweet, L. C., 1974, Hyperreactivity to cow's milk in an infant with LE and tart cell phenomenon, *J. Pediatr.* **84:**59.

Björkstén, F., and Johansson, S. G. O., 1975, *In vitro* diagnosis of atopic allergy: The occurrence and clustering of positive RAST results as a function of age and total IgE concentration, *Clin. Allergy* **5**:363.

Blackley, C. H., 1873, *Experimental Researches on the Causes and Nature of Catarrhus Aestivis*, p. 84, London.

Boat, T. F., Polmar, S. H., Whitman, V., Kleinerman, J. I., Stern, R. C., and Doershuk, C. F., 1975, Hyperreactivity to cow milk in young children with pulmonary hemosiderosis and cor pulmonale secondary to nasopharyngeal obstruction. *J. Pediatr.* **87**:23.

Bock, S. A., Buckley, J., Holst, A., and May, C. D., 1977, Proper use of skin tests with food extracts in diagnosis of hypersensitivity to food in children, *Clin. Allergy* **7**:375.

Bock, S. A., Lee, W.-Y., Remigio, L., and May, C. D., 1978a, Studies of hypersensitivity reactions to foods in infants and children, *J. Allergy Clin. Immunol.* **62**:327.

Bock, S. A., Lee, W.-Y., Remigio, L., Holst, A., and May, C. D., 1978b, Appraisal of skin tests with food extracts for diagnosis of food hypersensitivity, *Clin. Allergy* **8**:559.

Brown, W. R., Borthistle, B. K., and Chen, S.-T., 1975, Immunoglobulin E (IgE) and IgE-containing cells in human gastrointestinal fluids and tissues, *Clin. Exp. Immunol.* **20**:227.

Brunner, M., and Walzer, M., 1928, Absorption of undigested proteins in human beings—The absorption of unaltered fish proteins in adults, *Arch. Intern. Med.* **42**:173.

Buckley, R. H., and Dees, S. C., 1969, Correlation of milk precipitins with IgA deficiency, *N. Engl. J. Med.* **281**:465.

Bull, D. M., Bienenstock, J., and Tomasi Jr., T. B., 1971, Studies on human intestinal immunoglobulin A, *Gastroenterology* **60**:370.

Carr, R. I., Wold, R. T., and Farr, R. S., 1972, Antibodies of bovine gamma globulin (BGG) and the occurrence of a BGG-like substance in systemic lupus erythematosus sera, *J. Allergy Clin. Immunol.* **50**:18.

Crabbé, P. A., and Heremans, J. F., 1966, The distribution of immunoglobulin-containing cells along the human gastrointestinal tract, *Gastroenterology* **51**:305.

Cunningham-Rundles, C., Brandeis, W. E., Good, R. A., and Day, N. K., 1978, Milk precipitins, circulating immune complexes, and IgA deficiency, *Proc. Natl. Acad. Sci. (USA)* **75**:3387.

Dannaeus, A., Foucard, T., and Johansson, S. G. O., 1977, The effect of orally administered sodium cromoglycate on symptoms of food allergy, *Clin. Allergy* **7**:109.

Donnally, H. H., 1930, The question of the elimination of foreign protein (egg-white) in woman's milk, *J. Immunol.* **19**:15.

DuBois, R. O., Schloss, O. M., and Anderson, A. F., 1925, The development of cutaneous hypersensitiveness following the intestinal absorption of antigenic protein, *Proc. Soc. Exp. Biol. Med.* **23**:176.

Fällström, S. P., Winberg, J., and Andersen, H. J., 1965, Cow's milk induced malabsorption as a precursor of gluten intolerance, *Acta Paediatr. Scand.* **54**:101.

Ferguson, A., McClure, J. P., and Townley, R. R. W., 1976, Intraepithelial lymphocyte counts in small intestinal biopsies from children with diarrhea, *Acta. Pediatr. Scand.* **65**:541.

Fontaine, J. L., and Navarro, J., 1975, Small intestinal biopsy in cow's milk protein allergy in infancy, *Arch. Dis. Child.* **50**:357.

Freier, S., and Berger, H., 1973, Disodium cromoglycate in gastrointestinal protein intolerance, *Lancet* **1**:913.

Good, R. A., and Rodey, 1970, IgA deficiency, antigenic barriers, and autoimmunity, editorial, *Cell. Immunol.* **1**:147.

Gray, I., and Walzer, M., 1938a, Studies in mucous membrane hypersensitiveness. III. The allergic reaction of the passively sensitized rectal mucous membrane, *Am. J. Dig. Dis. Nutr.* **4**:710.

Gray, I., and Walzer, M., 1938b, Studies in absorption of undigested protein in human beings. VII. Absorption of protein introduced by tube into the duodenum, *Am. J. Dig. Dis. Nutr.* **5**:345.

Gray, I., and Walzer, M., 1940, Studies in absorption of undigested protein in human beings. VIII. Absorption from the rectum and a comparative study of absorption following oral, duodenal, and rectal administrations, *J. Allergy* **11**:245.

Gray, I., Harten, M., and Walzer, M., 1940, Studies in mucous membrane hypersensitiveness IV. The allergic reactions in the passively sensitized mucous membranes of the ileum and colon in humans, *Ann. Intern. Med.* **13**:2050.

Gruskay, F. L., and Cooke, R., 1955, The gastrointestinal absorption of unaltered protein in normal infants and in infants recovering from diarrhea, *Pediatrics* **16**:763.

Halpern, S. R., Sellars, W. A., Johnson, R. B., Anderson, D. W., Saperstein, S., and Reisch, J. S.,

1973, Development of childhood allergy in infants fed breast, soy, or cow milk, *J. Allergy Clin. Immunol.* **51**:139.

Hanson, L. A., Ahlstedt, S., Carlsson, B., and Fallstrom, S. P. 1977, Secretory IgA antibodies against cow's milk proteins in human milk and their possible effect in mixed feeding, *Int. Arch. Allergy* **54**:457.

Haworth, J. C., and Dilling, L., 1966, Concentration of γA-globulin in serum saliva, and nasopharyngeal secretions of infants and children, *J. Lab. Clin. Med.* **67**:922.

Heiner, D. C., Sears, J. W., and Kniker, W. T., 1962, Multiple precipitins to cow's milk in chronic respiratory disease, *Am. J. Dis. Child.* **103**:634.

Hekkens, W. Th. J. M., and Pena, A. S. (eds.), 1974, *Coeliac Disease* (Proceedings of the Second International Coeliac Symposium), Leiden.

Holland, N. H., Hong, R., Davis, N. C., and West, C. D., 1962, Significance of precipitating antibodies to milk proteins in the serum of infants and children, *J. Pediatr.* **61**:181.

Huntley, C. C., Robbins, J. B., Lyerly, A. D., and Buckley, R. H., 1971, Characterization of precipitating antibodies to ruminant serum and milk proteins in humans with selective IgA deficiency, *N. Engl. J. Med.* **1**:7.

Katz, A. J., and Falchuk, Z. M., 1975, Current concepts in gluten sensitive enteropathy (celiac sprue), *Pediat. Clin. North Am.* **22**:767.

Katz, A. J., Goldman, H., and Grand, R., 1977, Gastric mucosal biopsy in eosinophilic (allergic) gastroenteritis, *Gastroenterology* **73**:705.

Katz, A. J., Falchuk, Z. M., Garovoy, M., Zeiger, R. S., and Twarog, F. J., 1978, Eosinophilic gastroenteritis in childhood: Basis for allergic etiology (abstr.), *J. Allergy Clin. Immunol.* **61**:157.

Kaufman, H. S., 1971, Allergy in the newborn: Skin test reactions confirmed by the Prausnitz–Küstner test at birth, *Clin. Allergy* **1**:363.

Kletter, B., Gery, I., Freier, S., and Davies, A. M., 1971a, Immune responses of normal infants to cow milk. I. Antibody type and kinetics of production, *Int. Arch. Allergy* **40**:656.

Kletter, B., Gery, I., Freier, S., and Davies, A. M., 1971b, Immune responses of normal infants to cow milk. II. Decreased immune reactions in initially breast-fed infants, *Int. Arch. Allergy* **40**:667.

Kletter, B., Gery, I., Freier, S., Noah, Z., and Davies, M. A., 1971c, Immunoglobulin E antibodies to milk proteins, *Clin. Allergy* **1**:249.

Kletter, B., Noach, Z., Rotem, Y., Moses, S., and Freier, S., 1972, The significance of food antibodies in familial dysautonomia, *Clin. Allergy* **2**:373.

Korenblat, P. E., Rothberg, R. M., Minden, P., and Farr, R. S., 1968, Immune responses of human adults after oral and parenteral exposure to bovine serum albumin, *J. Allergy* **41**:226.

Kuhns, W. J., 1965, Studies of immediate wheal reactions of reaginic antibodies in pregnancy and in the newborn infant, *Proc. Soc. Exp. Biol. Med.* **118**:377.

Kuitunen, P., Rapola, J., Savilahti, E., and Visakorpi, J. D., 1973, Response of the jejunal mucosa to cow's milk in the malabsorption syndrome with cow's milk intolerance, *Acta. Paediatr. Scand.* **62**:585.

Kuitunen, P., Visakorpi, J. D., Savilahti, E., and Pelkonen, P., 1975, Malabsorption syndrome with cow's milk intolerance, *Arch. Dis. Child.* **50**:351.

Lamm, M. E., 1976, Cellular aspects of immunoglobulin A, *Adv. Immunol.* **22**:223.

Lippard, V. W., 1939, Immunologic response to ingestion of foods by normal and by eczematous infants, *Am. J. Dis. Child.* **57**:524.

Lippard, V. W., Schloss, O. M., and Johnson, P. A., 1936, Immune reactions induced in infants by intestinal absorption of incompletely digested cow's milk protein, *Am. J. Dis. Child.* **51**:562.

Lloyd-Still, J. D., Shwachman, H., and Filler, R. M., 1973, Protracted diarrhea of infancy treated by intravenous alimentation. I. Clinical studies of 16 infants, *Am. J. Dis. Child.* **125**:358.

Matthews, T. S., and Soothill, J. F., 1970, Complement activation after milk feeding in children with cow's milk allergy. *Lancet* **2**:893.

May, C. D., 1976, Objective clinical and laboratory studies of immediate hypersensitivity reactions to foods in asthmatic children. *J. Allergy Clin. Immunol.* **58**:500.

May, C. D., and Alberto, R., 1972a, *In vitro* responses of leucocytes to food proteins in allergic and normal children: Lymphocyte stimulation and histamine release, *Clin. Allergy* **2**:335.

May, C. D., and Alberto, R., 1972b, *In vivo* stimulation of peripheral lymphocytes to proliferation after oral challenge of children allergic to foods, *Int. Arch. Allergy* **43**:525.

May, C. D., Remigio, L., Feldman, J., Bock. S. A., and Carr, R. I., 1977, A study of serum antibodies to isolated milk proteins and ovalbumin in infants and children. *Clin. Allergy* **7**:583.

Minden, P., Reid, R. T., and Farr, R. S., 1966, A comparison of some commonly used methods for detecting antibodies to bovine albumin in human serum, *J. Immunol.* **96**:180.

Nelson, T. L., 1964, Spontaneously occurring milk antibodies in mongoloids, *Am. J. Dis. Child.* **108**:494.

Norman, P. S., Lichtenstein, L. M., and Ishizaka, K., 1973, Diagnostic tests in hay fever, *J. Allergy Clin. Immunol.* **52**:210.

Ogra, P. L., and Karzon, D. T., 1969, Distribution of poliovirus antibody in serum, nasopharynx and alimentary tract following segmental immunization of lower alimentary tract with poliovaccine. *J. Immunol.* **102**:1423.

Parish, W. E., 1970, Short-term anaphylactic IgG antibodies in human sera, *Lancet* **2**:591.

Parish, W. E., 1971, Detection of reaginic and short-term sensitizing anaphylactic or anaphylactoid antibodies to milk in sera of allergic and normal persons, *Clin. Allergy* **1**:369.

Perara, D., Weinstein, W., and Rubin, C. E., 1975, Small intestinal biopsy, *Hum. Pathol.* **6**:157.

Ratner, B., 1928, A possible causal factor of food allergy in certain infants, *Am. J. Dis. Child.* **36**:277.

Rieger, C. H. L., and Rothberg, R. M., 1975, Development of the capacity to produce specific antibody to an ingested food antigen in the premature infant, *J. Pediatr.* **87**:515.

Rothberg, R. M., 1969, Immunoglobulin and specific antibody synthesis during the first weeks of life of premature infants, *J. Pediatr.* **75**:391.

Rothberg, R. M., and Farr, R. S., 1965, Anti-bovine serum albumin and anti-alpha lactalbumin in the serum of children and adults, *Pediatrics* **35**:571.

Savilahti, E., 1972a, Immunoglobulin-containing cells in the intestinal mucosa and immunoglobulins in the intestinal juice in children, *Clin. Exp. Immunol.* **11**:415.

Savilahti, E., 1972b, Intestinal immunoglobulins in children with coeliac disease, *Gut* **13**:958.

Savilahti, E., 1973, Immunochemical study of the malabsorption syndrome with cow's milk intolerance, *Gut* **14**:491.

Scheinmann, P., Gendrel, D., Charlas, J., and Paupe, J., 1976, Value of lymphoblast transformation test in cow's milk protein intestinal intolerance, *Clin. Allergy* **6**:515.

Schloss, O. M., 1912, A case of allergy to common foods, *Am. J. Dis. Child.* **3**:342.

Sherman, H., Kaplan, C., and Walzer, M., 1937, Studies in mucous membrane hypersensitiveness. II. Passive local sensitization of the nasal mucous membrane, *J. Allergy* **9**:1.

Shiner, M., and Ballard, J., 1972, Antigen–antibody reactions in jejunal mucosa in childhood coeliac disease after gluten challenge, *Lancet* **1**:1202.

Shiner, M., Ballard, J., Brook, C. G. D., and Herman, S., 1975a, Intestinal biopsy in the diagnosis of cow's milk protein intolerance without acute symptoms, *Lancet* **2**:1060.

Shiner, M., Ballard, J., and Smith, M. E., 1975b, The small-intestinal mucosa in cow's milk allergy, *Lancet* **1**:136.

Shwachman, L., Lloyd-Still, J. D., Khaw, T., and Antonowicz, I., 1973, Protracted diarrhea of infancy treated by intravenous alimentation. II. Studies of small intestinal biopsy results. *Am. J. Dis. Child.* **125**:365.

Soothill, J. F., Stokes, C. R., Turner, M. W., Norman, A. P., and Taylor, B., 1976, Predisposing factors and the development of reaginic allergy in infancy, *Clin. Allergy* **6**:305.

Spring, C., and Sandoval, J., 1976, Food additives and hyperkinesis: A critical evaluation of the evidence, *J. Learning Disabil.* **9**:560.

Strober, W., Falchuk, Z. M., Rogentine, G. M., Nelson, D. L., and Klaeveman, H. L., 1975, The pathogenesis of gluten-sensitive enteropathy, *Ann. Intern. Med.* **83**:242.

Tada, T., and Ishizaka, K., 1970, Distribution of IgE-forming cells in lymphoid tissues of the human and monkey, *J. Immunol.* **104**:377.

Thomas, H. D., and Parrott, M. V., 1974, The induction of tolerance to a soluble protein antigen by oral administration, *Immunology* **27**:631.

Tomasi, T. B., Jr., 1972, Secretory immunoglobulins, *N. Engl. J. Med.* **287**:500.

Tomasi, T. B., and Katz, L., 1971, Human antibodies against bovine immunoglobulin M in IgA deficient sera, *Clin. Exp. Immunol.* **9**:3.

Vendel, S., 1948, Cow's milk idiosyncrasy in infants, *Acta Paediatr.* **35**:Suppl. V.

Waldmann, T. A., Wochner, R. D., Laster, L., and Gordon, R. S., Jr., 1967, Allergic gastroenteropathy—A cause of excessive gastrointestinal protein loss, *N. Engl. J. Med.* **276**:761.

Walker, W. A., and Isselbacher, K. J., 1974, Uptake and transport of macromolecules by the intestine—Possible role in clinical disorders, *Gastroenterology* **67**:531.

Walker-Smith, J., Harrison, M., Kilby, A., Phillips, A., and France, N., 1978, Cow's milk-sensitive enteropathy, *Arch. Dis. Child.* **53**:375.

Walzer, M., 1927, Studies in absorption of undigested proteins in human beings. I. A simple direct method of studying the absorption of undigested protein, *J. Immunol.* **14**:143.

Wender, E., 1977, Food additives and hyperkinesis, *Am. J. Dis. Child.* **131**:1204.

Williams, C. A., and Chase, M. W., (eds.), 1971/1977, *Methods in Immunology and Immunochemistry,* Academic, New York. Vol. III, 1971, Chapter 13, Precipitation reaction; Chapter 14, Precipitation analysis by diffusion in gels, Vol. IV, 1977, Chapter 16, Agglutination and Flocculation.

Wilson, J. F., Heiner, D. C., and Lahey, M. E., 1962, Evidence of gastrointestinal dysfunction in infants with iron deficiency anemia: A preliminary report, *J. Pediatr.* **60**:787.

Wilson, J. F., Lahey, M. E., and Heiner, D. C., 1974, Further observations on cow's milk-induced gastrointestinal bleeding in infants with iron-deficiency anemia, *J. Pediatr.* **84**:335.

Wilson, S. J., and Walzer, M., 1935, Absorption of undigested proteins in human beings. IV. Absorption of unaltered egg protein in infants, *Am. J. Dis. Child.* **50**:49.

10

Drug Allergy

A. L. DE WECK

1. Introduction

The development of chemotherapy and the steadily increasing number of available drugs make it almost impossible to comprehensively review allergic reactions to drugs. Therefore, this chapter represents only a brief general outline of the mechanisms of such reactions and of their main clinical aspects.

The true incidence of allergic reactions to drugs is difficult to evaluate because systems of reporting and objective diagnostic tests for drug allergy are frequently unsatisfactory. Nevertheless, on the basis of drug-monitoring studies in hospitals in various parts of the world, it has been estimated that as many as 5% of hospital admissions are due to some untoward reaction to a drug and that about 10% of hospitalized patients experience at least one adverse drug reaction (Parker, 1975; Thoburn *et al.*, 1966). Since 30–40% of all adverse drug reactions appear to be of allergic nature, it leaves us with an overall incidence of about 5% of allergic reactions to drugs. This is probably a low estimate. Therapeutic habits change rapidly. For that reason some drugs which were responsible for a majority of drug reactions in the past (e.g., organic arsenicals, gold salts) have become of mere historical interest. However, clinical and experimental studies performed while these drugs were still in wide use have contributed to our understanding of the basic mechanisms of allergic reactions to drugs. Readers are referred to a number of reviews and monographs (Ackroyd and Rook, 1964; de Warte, 1972; de Weck, 1971a; Gillette *et al.*, 1974; Levine, 1965; Meyler and Herxheimer, 1975; Parker, 1975).

Terms used for the classification of untoward drug reactions have varied widely. It is therefore necessary to define the most commonly used terms:

a. *Overdosage:* The untoward effects are directly related to the administered amount of drug (absolute overdosage, e.g., barbiturate suicide) or to its unexpected accumulation due to some excretory or metabolic abnormality in the patient (e.g., kidney or liver failure).

A. L. DE WECK • Institute of Clinical Immunology, Inselspital, 3010 Bern, Switzerland. This work was supported in part by the Swiss National Science Foundation (Grant No. 3.468.75).

b. *Intolerance:* The untoward effect represents a qualitatively normal pharmacological effect of the drug which, however, is quantitatively increased (e.g., cinchonism after low doses of quinine).
c. *Idiosyncrasy:* The reaction to the drug is qualitatively abnormal and does not correspond to the drug's usual pharmacological action. Such reactions do not, however, depend on an immunological mechanism. (e.g., hemolytic anemia to primaquine in 6GPD-deficient individuals).
d. *Side effects:* This term should be restricted to the undesirable but unavoidable pharmacological actions of the drug (e.g., sedative effects of antihistaminic drugs).
e. *Secondary effects:* These are indirect but not inevitable consequences of the primary action of the drug (e.g., disturbances of the normal bacteriological flora in patients receiving longterm antibiotic therapy).
f. *Allergic reactions:* Hypersensitivity or allergic reactions are the result of an immune response of the organisms leading to the formation of specific antibodies or of sensitized lymphocytes, or both.

This chapter will deal exclusively with adverse reactions to drugs which are due to immunological mechanisms. Ideally, an objective diagnosis of drug allergy should always rest on the demonstration of specific antibodies and/or of sensitized lymphocytes to the offending drug. Unfortunately, this is still difficult to achieve in most drug allergies. The diagnosis of drug allergy is more often established at the bedside than in the laboratory.

2. Clinical Manifestations of Drug Allergy

2.1. Anaphylactic Shock

Aside from injections of foreign serum or stinging insects, some drugs appear to be frequent cause of anaphylactic reactions in man. These reactions are characterized by an acute cardiovascular collapse and hypotension. Typically the reaction develops rapidly and reaches a maximum within 5–30 min. Accompanying symptoms may include nausea and vomiting, urticaria, pruritus and diffuse erythema, bronchospasm, laryngeal edema, cardiac arrhythmia, and hyperperistalsis. Often the anaphylactic symptoms are limited to malaise and vertigo, but in other cases the outcome may be fatal in a few minutes. Anaphylactic reactions may apparently also be the cause of myocardial infarction and sudden cardiac arrest (Levine, 1976). The most common cause of anaphylactic reactions in man is still penicillin therapy. In the early 1960s fatalities from anaphylactic shock to penicillins were estimated at about 300 per year in the United States, but it is difficult to obtain precise informations on the true incidence (Idsøe *et al.,* 1968). Among other less frequent causes of anaphylactic shock or of shock resembling anaphylaxis are the radiopaque organic iodides, local anesthetics, vitamin B_{12}, streptomycin, dextrans, bromsulfalein, fluorescein, tetracycline, cephalosporins, organic mercurials, opiates (heroin), and sodium dehydrocholate.

Accidental intravascular injection of some drugs also elicits shock on a nonimmunological basis. Some acute reactions immediately following penicillin injection may be due to the toxic-embolic effect of procaine on the central nervous system or to microemboli of penicillin crystals (Hoigné and Schoch, 1959). Shock reactions to roentgenological contrast media have been attributed to nonimmunological histamine liberation effects (Brasch *et al.*, 1970), although patients with previous reactions to contrast media appear to develop anaphylactic reactions more readily on renewed administration than the general population (Schatz *et al.*, 1975).

2.2. Serum Sickness Syndrome

A syndrome clinically indistinguishable from true serum sickness is produced by a variety of nonprotein drugs, among which penicillins, streptomycin, sulfonamides, diphenylhydantoin, thiouracils, and some cholecystographic media have been described as offenders. The serum sickness syndrome usually develops 5–14 days after the first administration of the drug and is characterized by a generalized urticarial skin rash, fever, joint swelling, and lymphadenopathy. Brief episodes of glomerulonephritis and involvement of other organs are not rare. In serum sickness syndrome due to penicillins, skin-sensitizing antibodies (IgE) are usually present. However, it is common to find positive skin tests only after all symptoms have subsided (de Weck and Blum, 1965). Other types of antibodies might therefore account for some of the other symptoms such as fever and swelling of joints.

2.3. Cutaneous Manifestations

Cutaneous manifestations due to immunological mechanisms occur in most patients with drug allergies, but they are not characteristic for a particular drug and identical lesions may sometimes be caused by nonimmunological mechanisms (Fellner and Baer, 1965b; Fellner and Harris, 1972). They include pruritus, urticaria which may persist for several weeks or months after withdrawal of the drug, morbilliform exanthemas ("rash"), erythemas, exfoliative dermatitis, erythema multiforme and bullous eruptions, fixed drug eruptions (Welsh, 1961), purpura with and without thrombocytopenia (Peterson and Manick, 1967), and eczema and photosensitization (Mayer, 1950).

2.4. Hematological Manifestations

2.4.1. Thrombocytopenia

Short-lived thrombocytopenia is common in acute allergic reactions, including those due to protein and environmental antigens. Drug-induced thrombocytopenia is currently most often caused by quinidine and quinine, sulfonamides and sulfonamide derivatives, chloramphenicol, chlorothiazide, thiouracils, meprobamate, and phenylbutazone. Sedormid (allylisopropylacetylcarbamide), the classic offender with which Ackroyd (1958) so convincingly established the immunological basis of drug-induced thrombocytopenia, is no longer in use.

The clinical manifestations are primarily hemorrhage and petechial skin lesions, but associated symptoms such as fever and arthralgia may also be present.

After withdrawal, bleeding usually subsides within a week. Thrombocytopenia often recurs at various intervals on readministration of the drug. A transient and clinically silent drop of the thrombocyte level appears to be associated with a large number of drug reactions. The fall in thrombocyte level on exposure to a minimal drug dose has even been proposed as a diagnostic criterion. In drug-induced thrombocytopenic purpura it is often possible to demonstrate an antiplatelet factor which causes agglutination of the patient's platelets as well as of compatible normal platelets *in vitro* in the presence of the drug. Platelets alone are not agglutinated by such antibodies, except in the presence of the drug. The antigenic determinant seems therefore formed by union of the drug with the platelet membrane. Soluble drug–antibody complexes as such may, however, also be toxic for the platelet membrane.

2.4.2. Agranulocytosis

A number of drugs have been associated with agranulocytosis, most commonly aminopyrine and pyrazolone derivatives, thiouracils, sulfonamides, anticonvulsants, tolbutamide, chloramphenicol, and phenothiazines (Huguley, 1964; Meyler and Herxheimer, 1975). Following cessation of drug therapy, improvement may be expected in 1–2 weeks, provided that death due to infection has not supervened. Readministration of minute amounts of the offending drug will again lead to an abrupt fall in leukocyte levels. It is not clear whether the changes observed in the bone marrow morphology (Moeschlin, 1958) reflect an exhaustive stimulation of the marrow following rapid leukocyte destruction or whether the interaction of drug and specific antibodies may also have some toxic effect on granulocyte precursors. There are some well-documented instances in which immunological mechanisms have been demonstrated (Moeschlin and Wagner 1952; Thierfelder *et al.*, 1967).

2.4.3. Aplastic Anemia

Chloramphenicol is the best known cause of aplastic anemia following administration of a drug. A number of other drugs including sulfonamides, phenylbutazone, anticonvulsants, and organic solvents such as benzene cause aplastic anemia, but immunological mechanisms have not been clearly demonstrated in all instances.

2.4.4. Hemolytic Anemia

Hemolytic anemia due to drug allergy must be distinguished from the drug-induced hemolytic anemia due to an inherited defect of glucose-6-phosphate dehydrogenase in red blood cells. In this latter group of patients, anemia can be induced by primaquine and other antimalarial substances, sulfonamides, antipyretic drugs, sulfones, and nitrofurans. On the other hand, hemolytic anemias based on immunological mechanisms have been well documented with mesantoin, quinine, and quinidine (Freedman *et al.*, 1956), acetophenetidin (Dausset and Contu, 1964), paraaminosalicylic acid, dipyrone, antazoline, penicillins (Bird *et al.*, 1975; Petz and Fudenberg, 1966; Swanson *et al.*, 1966), and methyldopa (Worrledge *et al.*, 1966).

2.5. Vasculitis and Connective Tissue Damage

Vascular changes are often demonstrated in subjects with serum sickness, drug fever, and drug-induced syndromes in which the damage is primarily localized in a single organ. The lesions tend to occur in small vessels and range from mild cellular infiltration to acute necrosis (Symmers, 1962). In severe forms, vessels in many organs may be involved, including those in the skin and kidneys. Aside from petechial skin lesions, proteinuria and manifestations of renal failure, symptoms often include fever, dermatitis, arthralgia, and edema and less frequently myositis, coronary arteritis, pneumonitis, and gastrointestinal bleeding. The drugs most frequently implicated in severe vasculitis are the penicillins, pyrazolone derivatives, sulfonamides, pronazines, tetracyclines, thiazides, quinidine, busulfan, iproniazid, allopurinol, iodides, metamphetamine, and the thiouracils. A clinical syndrome resembling rheumatoid arthritis and systemic lupus erythematosus with or without LE cell phenomenon has been described following prolonged hydralazine therapy and less frequently following therapy with other drugs, such as procainamide (Hahn *et al.*, 1972; Tan, 1974). A pseudolupus syndrome has also been attributed to pyrazolone derivatives in preparations used for the treatment of thrombophlebitis (Müller *et al.*, 1975). Several other reports attribute chronic inflammatory changes in the connective tissue to drugs (Meyler and Herxheimer, 1975). Frequently, the precise immunological mechanism of these lesions has not been established.

2.6. Hepatic Damage

Chloroform and carbon tetrachloride are potent liver poisons and when given in sufficiently large doses invariably cause hepatic damage. Chlorpromazine, thiouracil, sulfonamides, and paraaminosalicylic acid, on the other hand, cause liver damage in only a small proportion of the patients treated. The liver damage may consist of two types: (1) intrahepatic biliary obstruction may dominate the picture, while (2) in other cases hepatocellular damage and necrosis are more prominent. The clinical picture closely resembles that of infective hepatitis, and it is quite possible that some of the early reports of allergic liver damage were in fact cases of viral hepatitis (Lunel *et al.*, 1966). The cholestatic form is most frequently caused by chlorpromazine but has been reported following administration of methyltestosterone, thiouracil, and propylthiouracil. Hepatocellular damage frequently accompanied by fever, skin rash, lymphadenopathy, blood eosinophilia, and infiltration of the liver with eosinophils, lymphocytes, or plasmacytes has been reported in connection with sulfonamides, paraaminosalicylic acid, indandione derivatives, halothane, methoxyflurane, phenylbutazone, nitrofurantoins, indomethacin, isoniazid, chlorpropamide, erythromycin estolate, and α-methyldopa (Davies and Holmes, 1972; Zimmermann, 1972).

2.7. Fever

Fever is a common manifestation of drug allergy (Cluff and Johnson, 1964). It is usually associated with other symptoms but may also occur alone. Among the more prominent causes of drug fever are quinidine, sulfonamides, iodine, thiouracils, procainamide, streptomycin, penicillins, anticonvulsants, antithyroid drugs, paraaminosalicylic acid, and mercurial diuretics. Little work has been done up to now on the molecular mechanisms causing drug fever. Attempts to detect a pyrogenic factor in the blood of patients sensitive to streptomycin has been unsuccessful (Snell, 1961). Fever may sometimes be the only clinical manifestation of drug hypersensitivity. It might be assumed that drug fever could be a manifestation of a generalized delayed-type reaction involving the release of pyrogenic factors on contact of sensitized lymphocytes with the allergen, but this has not yet been substantiated in man.

2.8. Nephropathy

Glomerulonephritis is commonly observed in the serum sickness syndrome and in drug-induced acute vasculitis. A less common form of renal damage due to drug allergy is acute interstitial nephritis (Baker and Williams, 1963). Acute tubular necrosis has also been reported following prolonged hypotension in acute anaphylactic reactions, but this represents rather a secondary complication. Tubular necrosis following bouts of hemolytic anemia may also be observed. A few cases of interstitial nephritis with deposits of penicillin-specific antigen–antibody complexes and development of autoantibodies against tubular basement membranes have been reported (Baldwin *et al.*, 1968; Border *et al.*, 1974). The possible role of hypersensitivity in the development of chronic interstitial nephritis following long-term intake of phenacetin or salicylates is not yet clear (Prescott, 1966).

2.9. Pulmonary Manifestations

Bronchial asthma after ingestion or injection of drugs is occasionally observed alone but is frequently associated with urticaria. The patient may have a history of asthma and of nasal polyps, in which case aspirin, indomethacin, and some foodstuff dyes (e.g., tartrazine) appear to be the most common causes. However, the nature of aspirin-induced asthma is unlikely to be immunological in most cases (Samter and Beers, 1967). Bronchial asthma is also observed in hypersensitive patients on inhalation of penicillins and related compounds (Davies *et al.*, 1974). Pulmonary infiltrations with eosinophilia, fever, hilar adenopathy, and so-called allergic pneumonitis are less well characterized. They have been reported to response to nitrofurantoins (Pearsall *et al.*, 1974), sulfonamides, aminosalicylic acid, penicillins, disodium cromoglycate, mephenasin, and azathioprine (Sharma, 1973).

2.10. Miscellaneous

Lymphadenopathy is frequently observed with serum sickness. Prolonged treatment with hydantoin and oxazlidine derivatives has been reported to cause clinical and pathological changes suggestive of malignant lymphoma (Hyman and Sommers, 1966). In a member of cases of immunoblastic lymphadenopathy (Lukes and Tindle, 1975), the disease has taken a fatal course. Hypersensitivity reactions to penicillin or griseofulvin have been reported as preceding the development of the disease. The association of myocarditis, coronary arteritis, and pericarditis has also occasionally been reported with drug hypersensitivity (Meyler and Herxheimer, 1975). However, convincing evidence that such lesions rest on immunological mechanisms has been lacking.

3. Immunochemistry and Immunopathology of Drug Reactions

3.1. Chemical Properties Involved in the Allergenic Potential of Drugs

Most of our understanding on the immunochemical mechanisms involved in drug allergy is based on experimental studies with low-molecular-weight simple chemical compounds (or haptens). The use of haptens as antigenic determinants in experimental animals has provided an efficient method of investigating the structural basis of immunological specificity (Eisen, 1959; Landsteiner, 1945). From these studies, a certain number of rules have emerged which appear to be valid also in allergy to low-molecular-weight chemotherapeutic agents. These rules are as follows:

a. The *formation of an immunogenic conjugate* between a simple chemical (or hapten) and a carrier molecule is an *absolute requirement* for the induction of an immune response to the hapten. Sensitization to the hapten *in vivo* occurs on conjugation with autologous carriers. Although proteins are usually the most efficient carriers, oligopeptides and polysaccharides have also been considered as potentially immunogenic carriers. In recent years, however, direct conjugation of simple chemicals to structural elements of cell membranes (especially of monocytes and macrophages) has been thought to play an important role in the induction of sensitization (de Weck, 1975). The type of binding between the antigenic determinants and its carriers is also of importance. On the basis of numerous experimental studies, it has been assumed that only conjugates formed by covalent binding are immunogenic. Experiments using methylated albumins or electrostatically charged oligopeptides as carriers indicate, however, that molecules strongly attached to such carriers by noncovalent bonds may also behave as immunogens (Green *et al.*, 1966). Obviously, a minimal stability in binding strength is required.

b. The *ability of a simple chemical to induce an immune response in vivo rests on its ability to conjugate in vitro*. Simple chemicals which are potent sensitizers are also highly reactive and can be readily shown to form conjugates with proteins *in vivo* (Gell *et al.*, 1948). Those chemicals unable to form covalent bonds with proteins *in vitro* show no or only a very low incidence of sensitization. The extent to which a simple chemical is reversibly bound to serum proteins such as albumin has no apparent influence on its ability to sensitize. Among the members of a family of simple chemicals with different chemical reactivity, there is a distinct correlation between the rate of conjugation with proteins as measured *in vitro* and the incidence of sensitization *in vivo* (Eisen, 1969). Furthermore, in several instances, the antibodies formed on sensitization with a simple chemical *in vivo* are specific not for the original compound injected but for the modified haptenic structure formed on covalent binding to a protein carrier (de Weck, 1962). The protein carrier or cell membrane structures of the host may contribute to the specificity of the response (partial autoimmunity).

c. Whenever an *in vivo* immune response has occurred following injection of chemicals which are nonreactive with proteins *in vitro,* further investigations invariably show that the immunological activity is due to some *antigenic contaminants* or to the *metabolic degradation* of the administered compound to some *reactive intermediate*. The only known exception may be the strong adsorption of low-molecular-weight compounds to cell membranes, as appears to be the case with some metal salts (e.g., nickel, beryllium, and chromium salts) (Hutchinson *et al.,* 1975). In most cases the immunogen appears to require a minimal size: it is therefore very unlikely that low-molecular-weight nonconjugating drugs could induce an immune response as such.

d. *Elicitation of allergic reactions of the immediate type due to antibodies require multivalent antigens acting as a passive link between antibody-combining sites.* In the case of anaphylactic reactions due to the interaction of antigen with homocytotropic antibodies (reagins, IgE) bound to the mast cell membrane, bridging of adjacent immunoglobulin molecules by antigens which must be at least bivalent (i.e., two antigenic determinants per molecule) appears to be required (de Weck *et al.,* 1973; Levine, 1965; Parker *et al.,* 1962a). It has been shown convincingly in the penicillin system that antigens carrying three to six penicilloyl determinants per molecule at some suitable distance from each other are optimal elicitors (de Weck and Schneider, 1969; Levine and Redmond, 1968). Elicitation of anaphylactic reactions by univalent haptens, on the other hand, has remained an exception (Frick *et al.,* 1968; de Weck *et al.,* 1973). Reactions to univalent haptens are probably the result of nonspecific aggregation of the hapten *in vivo* or of binding to cell membranes yielding multivalent antigens.

Drugs which elicit clinical anaphylactic reactions *in vivo* in sensitized individuals may do so only if they possess a relatively high degree of protein reactivity and form multivalent hapten–carrier conjugates within a short time. A higher degree of chemical reactivity is required to elicit an anaphylactic reaction than to sensitize, since anaphylaxis requires significant amounts of multivalent conjugates. Even if this requirement is met, which is rarely the case, some unconjugated drug will often still be present in large excess and will compete for available antibody-combining sites (''built-in inhibition''), provided that the sensitizing antigenic determinant formed on conjugation and the unconjugated drugs have sufficient structural similarities to permit cross-reactivity. Therefore, immediate-type skin tests with unconjugated chemicals or drugs are frequently negative even in sensitized animals or individuals who readily react to preformed multivalent conjugates. In some cases, eliciting antigens may be formed directly without conjugation to protein carriers if the drug is able to dimerize or polymerize, yielding thereby multivalent antigenic determinants. Such *polymers* may be non-immunogenic since their potential conjugating capacity has been exhausted by the formation of the polymer. Accumulation of dimers and polymers in penicillin solutions is probably responsible for the bulk of anaphylactic reactions to penicillin (de Weck *et al.,* 1968; Dewdney, 1977). Of significance may also be the presence of *macromolecular contaminants* (e.g., protein impurities or macromolecular additives capable of functioning as carriers (Batchelor *et al.,* 1967; Stewart, 1967; Kristofferson, *et al.,* 1977; de Weck *et al.,* 1969).

While bivalent antigens may suffice to induce anaphylactic reactions, the induction of Arthus reactions and activation of complement require the formation of a tridimensional multimolecular antigen–antibody lattice. Accordingly, Arthus reactions may be elicited only by trivalent antigens and are rarely observed in drug allergy.

e. *Delayed-type allergic reactions* occur when *T lymphocytes* have been sensitized to simple chemicals, forming conjugates *in vivo*. Conjugates eliciting delayed-type reactions must have a chemical structure (hapten *and* carrier) very similar if not identical to that responsible for sensitization (Gell and Benacerraf, 1961). Experimental evidence suggests that the mononuclear infiltration characteristics of delayed-type reactions is due to synthesis and release of inflammatory mediators (lymphokines) from specific T lymphocytes on renewed contact with the sensitizing simple chemical. Although the molecular mechanism which triggers these events is not yet elucidated, indirect evidence suggests that it is basically different from the mere bridging of adjacent immunoglobulin receptors by multivalent antigens, as observed for mast cells in anaphylaxis. Experiments on the stimulation of penicillin-sensitive T lymphocytes *in vitro* suggest that their activity may be triggered only by antigenic determinants actively presented on the membrane of other living cells, preferentially monocytes (de Weck, 1975). Whether B lymphocytes may, like mast cells, also be activated by passive bridging of immunoglobulin receptors through multivalent antigens has not been conclusively established. *In vitro* at least, the presence of monocytes or macrophages (acting as antigen-presenting cells) appears to be necessary to stimulate sensitized T and/or B lymphocytes with soluble hapten–protein conjugates. Nonconjugated haptens or monovalent hapten–amino acid conjugates are definitely unable to stimulate sensitized lymphocytes to proliferate or to produce lymphokines (Spengler *et al.*, 1974). In delayed-type reactions initiated by lymphokines, secondary antibody response *in situ* by infiltrating B lymphocytes as well as antibody-dependent reactions involving cytophilic antibodies on monocytes and infiltrating mast cells probably contribute to the inflammatory events in later stages of the reaction (Askenaze, 1977).

3.2. Induction of Immune Responses to Drugs: Main Factors Involved

The induction of the immune response to drugs appears to be governed by the same rules and factors that play a role in experimental sensitization to simple chemical compounds. Some factors are inherent to the sensitizing drug, whereas others involve the host.

3.2.1. Chemical Factors Involving the Sensitizing Drug

a. Chemical Structure and Reactivity. Most drugs in clinical use are not such highly reactive chemicals as to readily form stable conjugates when incubated with proteins *in vitro*. Furthermore, the incidence of clinical allergic reactions to drugs is generally low, and correlation between chemical reactivity and sensitization index is usually difficult to establish. However, highly reactive chemicals such as dinitrochlorobenzene and chloramine T have a high sensitization index in man. Furthermore, when the incidence of the immune response is evaluated not from the incidence of overt clinical reactions but by objective immunological procedures, good correlations may be demonstrated between chemical reactivity and sensitizing capacity (e.g., penicillins). The involvement of enzymatic and metabolic processes in the coupling of drugs to proteins *in vivo* is increasingly recognized (Remmer and Schüppel, 1972), even though in many instances the reactive derivatives responsible for drug allergy have not been identified.

b. Cross-Sensitization. Cross-sensitization occurs when allergic reactions induced by one compound are subsequently elicited by one or more related compounds. The range of cross-sensitization to drugs is extremely variable. Among the clinically frequent causes of cross-reactions, substances of the so-called para group (i.e., possessing a free amino group in the para position of a benzene ring) such as benzocaine, paraaminobenzoic acid, paraphenylenediamine, procaine, and sulfonamides, compounds with the phenothiazine structure, and those possessing the penicillin nucleus (penicillins and cephalosporins) should be emphasized. The range of cross-sensitization may vary with time and repeated exposure, as observed also in experimental sensitization to haptens (Steiner and Eisen, 1966). Immunochemical studies have shown wide individual variations in range of cross-sensitization to penicillins with various side chains and have also demonstrated heterogeneity in the affinity of antibodies formed in individual patients.

c. Dose, Duration, and Number of Courses of Therapy. There is a general feeling that the higher the dose and the longer the period of administration, the greater the probability of sensitization, but it is very difficult to collect reliable data in this regard. With penicillin or insulin, courses of therapy with moderate doses repeated at various intervals seem to lead more frequently to sensitization than prolonged treatment without free intervals. On the other hand, minute doses are certainly capable of inducing sensitization in some genetically predisposed individuals.

d. Mode of Administration. Except for contact dermatitis, the route of administration appears to be of little importance in determining the type of hypersensitivity and clinical symptoms produced. Application of allergenic drugs to the skin is usually associated with a high incidence of sensitization (favorable conditions for the formation of conjugates?), whereas the oral route appears to be less likely to foster sensitization. Some drugs, such as chlorprothixene, which on topical application frequently cause contact dermatitis, have an extremely low sensitization index when given orally. To what extent this phenomenon may be related to the fact that feeding with haptens may induce immunological tolerance (Chase, 1946) is not clear. Oral administration of drugs such as penicillin and sulfonamides to sensitive patients can also induce severe allergic reactions such as anaphylactic shock (Spark, 1971). The oral route therefore is by no means entirely "safe." Additives and solvents, of which oils, carboxymethylcellulose, and emulsifiers may be examples, may have an adjuvant effect by favoring retention of antigen and by causing local inflammation. The depot forms of insulin, for example, induce an immune response more readily than rapidly resorbed preparations (Frankhauser, 1969).

3.2.2. Factors Involving the Patient

In general, it can be said that the patient rather than the drug determines the incidence of sensitization. Allergic reactions occur in a comparatively small number of patients who take drugs, since drugs with an unusually high allergic potential (e.g., phenylethylhydantoin) are either kept from distribution or soon withdrawn.

a. Age and Sex. Allergic reactions to drugs appear to be less frequent in children than in adults (Berkowitz *et al.*, 1953). This may represent the effect of accumulated exposure rather than an intrinsic difference between children and adults in the capacity to respond. Severe allergic reactions may also be observed in very small infants; death from anaphylactic shock to penicillin may occur even in babies (passive sensitization from maternal blood or milk). Aged people seem somewhat less prone to become sensitized. There is no definite evidence, with some exceptions, that the incidence of drug reactions on similar exposure would be higher in females than in males.

b. Genetic Factors. Genetic factors play an important role in the development of hypersensitivity to drugs. It has been claimed that patients with an atopic constitution are predisposed to develop immediate-type hypersensitivity to drugs, especially penicillin (Miller, 1967; Rajka and Skog, 1965), but this statement does not appear to hold true (Green and Rosenblum, 1971). Immediate-type allergy to *injected* allergens such as penicillin, insect venoms, and insulin (in contrast to inhaled or ingested allergens) does not appear to be more common in atopic than in nonatopic patients. Anaphylactic sensitivity to penicillin frequently develops in nonatopic individuals, and many patients with allergy to drugs have no allergic background. Genetic factors probably also condition an individual specifically for sensitization to a given drug or chemical. In experimental sensitization to various chemicals, it has become evident that the immune response is specifically under the influence of genetic factors, among which the so-called immune response genes (Ir genes) which are linked to major histocompatibility complex genes have attracted the most attention (Benacerraf and Germain, 1978). Genetic differences in the sensitivity of guinea pigs to various drugs such as phenetidin, aspirin, hydralazine, and penicillin have been established (Ellmann *et al.*, 1971; Geczy and de Weck, 1975). The rapidly evolving field of pharmacogenetics also provides evidence that a number of individual variations in the metabolism of drugs are genetically determined. Genetic factors could therefore intervene at several levels in the biochemical pathways leading to sensitization, such as the formation of reactive metabolites or the selectively inherited ability to form antibodies specific for a given chemical structure. Typing for histocompatibility antigens of the HLA system in patients allergic to penicillins, however, has not yet revealed any clear-cut association with any allele of the HLA *A* or *B* locus (Spengler and de Weck, 1977).

c. Underlying Diseases. The incidence of drug allergy may be influenced by disease affecting the metabolism and excretion of the drug, such as chronic hepatic or renal disease, although these have probably a more direct influence on toxic effects. Theoretically, drug reactions should occur less frequently in patients whose immunological responsiveness is impaired. However, hypogammaglobulinemic patients are still capable of developing exanthematous eruptions to drugs (Good *et al.*, 1962). Patients with sarcoidosis and viral diseases with impaired cellular hypersensitivity seem less prone to develop contact dermatitis and drug exanthemas, but they still manifest urticarial and anaphylactic reactions (Chase, 1966).

d. Variations in Immunological Response to Drugs. Studies of the immune response to penicillins have shown that the incidence of an immune response after administration of a drug may be considerably higher than would be expected from the mere incidence of overt clinical allergic reactions. For example, a large percentage of patients receiving penicillin develop IgM antibodies. According to the sensitivity of the hemagglutination technique used, the percentage reported has varied between 20% and 100%. It is now certain that an immune response to a drug may not be evident clinically. Caution should therefore be exercised in the interpretation of clinical data not based on immunochemical investigations and the use of suitable techniques for antibody detection. The clinical manifestations of the hypersensitivity state may be governed not only by the types of antibodies formed but also by the relative proportion of the various immunoglobulins present at various times. For example, in most cases, the presence of IgM antibodies to penicillin does not lead to clinical symptoms and the presence of IgG antibodies sometimes appears to be protective. In patients developing IgE antibodies and anaphylactic reactivity, high titers of IgG antibody may be sufficient to compete for antigens and prevent anaphylactic reactions. In penicillin urticaria and in the serum sickness syndrome, the disappearance of skin lesions often coincides with a marked rise of the antipenicilloyl IgG level in the serum. A summary of the immunoglobulins formed on administration of penicillin and of their biological and pathological properties is given in Table 1.

There is an increasing awareness of the role of delayed-type hypersensitivity in clinical drug reactions (Redmond and Levine, 1968). Drug fever and especially the typical maculopapular exanthemas common to several drug reactions might be the expression of delayed-type hypersensitivity. The development of suitable test reagents and of methods of investigation for sensitized lymphocytes *in vitro* has revealed that specific sensitized T lymphocytes are frequently present in the peripheral blood of patients allergic to drugs.

4. Principal Allergenic Drugs

It is obviously impossible to give in this chapter a complete list of drugs capable of functioning as allergens. The reader is referred to several comprehensive sources (Meyler and Herxheimer, 1975; Rosenheim and Moulton, 1958; Dash and Jones, 1972).

4.1. Penicillins and Cephalosporins

The following penicillin derivatives may act as sensitizers:

a. Penicillin itself, which may react through its β-lactam ring to yield penicilloyl radicals with carrier molecules possessing free amino or hydroxyl groups (Schneider and de Weck, 1965, 1967) (Figure 1).
b. Reactive metabolites or degradation products such as penicillenic acids, penicilloic acids and penicillamine, which possess reactive groups and are therefore capable of forming stable conjugates with suitable antigenic carriers *in vitro* and *in vivo*.
c. Antigenic contaminants which, according to their structure, may or

TABLE 1. Clinical Forms of Allergic Reactions to Penicillins: Immunological Parameters

Clinical reaction	Interval between penicillin administration and symptoms	Main symptoms	Antibodies involved	Specificity
No reaction	Undetermined	None	IgM or IgG	BPO[a]
Anaphylactoid reaction	1–5 min after i.v. injection	Neurological and sensorial	None	None
Anaphylactic shock	5–120 min	Cardiovascular collapse	IgE	BPO and minor determinants
Immediate urticaria	2–24 hr	Urticaria	IgE	BPO
Serum-sickness-like disease	1–3 weeks	Urticaria, fever arthralgias, adenopathies	IgE and IgG	BPO and minor determinants
Chronic urticaria	Variable	Urticaria and pressure urticaria	IgE	Minor determinants and BPO
Exanthema	5–10 days	Morbilliform exanthema, rash	Sensitized lymphocytes	BPO and minor determinants
Hemolytic anemia	Variable	Anemia with positive Coombs test	IgG and IgM	BPO

[a] BPO, benzylpenicilloyl, major determinant.

may not have some degree of cross-reactivity with the drug itself or its degradation products. In the case of penicillin prepared by microbiological methods, antigenic contaminants may be proteins of the culture medium or of the *Penicillium* mold extracted together with penicillin (Batchelor *et al.*, 1967).

Reactions to penicillins are an example of the complexity of the mechanisms which lead to drug allergy. The steps followed in the study of such mechanisms should include (1) chemical study of the drug's reactivity and of its eventual metabolites and derivatives with various types of potential carrier molecules *in vitro;* (2) immunization of animals either with the drug itself or with suitable drug–protein conjugates prepared *in vitro;* (3) detection of antibodies and cellular hypersensitivity to the drug in experimental animals using various techniques (skin tests, hemagglutination, radioimmunoassays, lymphocyte cultures) and suitable drug–carrier conjugates for the elicitation of immunological reactions; (4) detection of antibodies and sensitized lymphocytes in patients spontaneously sensitized to the drug. On the basis of such studies, the following conclusion regarding the mechanisms of penicillin allergy have been drawn: (1) The bulk of antibodies formed on sensitization to penicillin are of penicilloyl specificity (major determinant). For various reasons however, the presence of penicilloyl-specific antibodies, especially when they are not of the skin-sensitizing type, may remain clinically silent; (2) a number of other haptenic antigenic determinants (minor determinants)

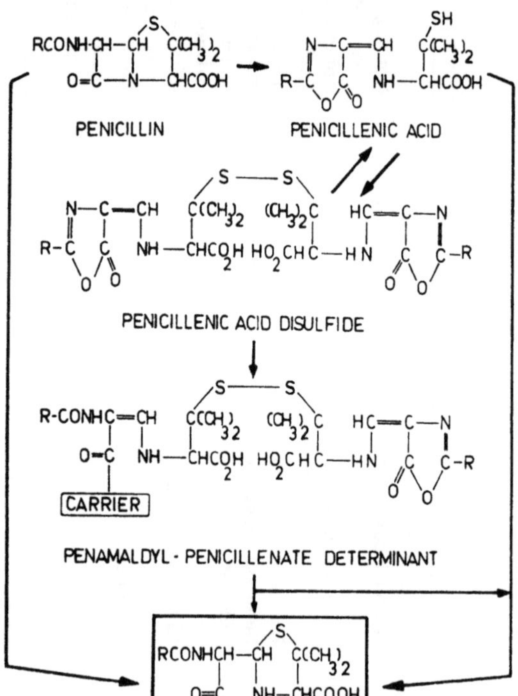

Figure 1. Chemical pathways leading to the formation of the benzylpenicilloyl (BPO) determinant.

arise from penicillin and may play a variable role in clinical penicillin allergy. Some have not yet been identified. Skin tests, passive transfer, and inhibition experiments indicate that at least three determinants (penicilloyl, a penicillin derivative, and a penicilloic acid derivative) play a significant role in clinical allergic reactions to penicillin. (3) Most available commercial penicillin preparations contain very small amounts of antigenic contaminants (Kristofferson *et al.*, 1977), and it is still debated whether these contaminants play an important role in the induction of penicillin in allergy and in the elicitation of allergic reactions.

Penicillin allergy is still the most common of all drug allergies and the most frequent cause of anaphylactic shock in man. The incidence of allergic reactions among various semisynthetic penicillins appears to vary somewhat. Because of special chemical features such as the presence of an additional side-chain amino group, ampicillin seems to be a frequent sensitizer, but the clinical reaction more often takes the form of an exanthema than that of urticaria or anaphylaxis. The facts that exanthemata occur after ampicillin treatment in the large majority of patients with infectious mononucleosis (Bierman *et al.*, 1972) or hyperuricemia (Boston, 1972) and that ampicillin therapy may often be pursued despite exanthemata have led several authors to doubt the immunological nature of this manifestation.

In principle, all penicillins are capable of showing cross-reactivity, including cephalosporins, although to a quite variable extent (Batchelor *et al.*, 1967; Dewdney, 1977).

4.2. Other Antibiotics

Allergic reactions to tetracyclines are relatively uncommon, although a few instances have been reported (Fellner and Baer, 1965a). Phototoxic skin reactions to tetracycline, especially with demethyltetracycline, are well known. Chloramphenicol, besides inducing aplastic anemia, can also cause skin allergy of the delayed type as well as urticarial and anaphylactic reactions. Allergic reactions to streptomycin are usually of the delayed type, although immediate reactions including anaphylactic shock have been reported. In practically all instances, the precise immunochemical mechanisms have not been uncovered.

4.3. Sulfonamides

Sulfonamides cause a large number of allergic reactions, usually involving the skin and frequently accompanied by fever. Several cases of epidermal necrolysis have been reported (Meyer and Herxheimer, 1975). The immunochemical mechanisms of the various reactions to sulfonamides have not been extensively investigated. Experiments in animals indicate that oxidation products may be responsible for conjugation (Schwarz and Schwarz-Speck, 1960) and for those manifestations of sulfonamide hypersensitivity which involve light as a pathogenetic factor.

4.4. Aspirin

In several reports, aspirin is ranked second only to penicillin as the most frequent cause of allergic reactions to drugs; in other statistics it is third, closely following sulfonamides. Despite several attempts, immunochemical causes of reactions to aspirin have not been satisfactorily established. Samter and Beers (1967) have proposed that the apparent allergic effects of aspirin are not due to an immunological mechanism but to an abnormal reactivity of peripheral chemoreceptors. However, some manifestations of aspirin intolerance also appear to be associated with immunological responses. We have shown that most commercial aspirin preparations contain highly reactive and immunogenic contaminants such as aspirin anhydride and acetylsalicyl salicylic acid (de Weck, 1971b; Bundgaard and de Weck 1975). Some patients developing urticaria after aspirin ingestion seem to be sensitized to these determinants, as shown by positive skin test with aspirylpolylysine, serological detection of antiaspiryl antibodies (Phills and Perelmutter, 1974), and positive lymphocyte stimulation tests (de Weck, 1974). However, the majority of patients intolerant to aspirin and other drugs (e.g., indomethacin) or azo dyes (tartrazine) appear to develop symptoms (esentially asthma, rhinitis, and nasal polyposis) through nonimmunological mechanisms possibly related to interference with prostaglandin synthesis (Szczerlik *et al.*, 1975). Familial occurrence of this abnormality, which may also be detected in children, has been reported (Lockey *et al.*, 1973).

4.5. Antipyretic and Analgesic Drugs

Systemic and cutaneous allergic reactions as well as blood dyscrasias due to the administration of pyrazolone derivatives, such as aminopyrine, phenylbutazon, and phenacetin, are well known. A number of these manifestations may be due to nonimmunological mechanisms. However, we have recently shown that allergy to phenacetin is due to its metabolites hydroxyphenetidine and *p*-hydroxyphenetidine (Ruegger *et al.*, 1973). Sensitization to these metabolites can be readily demonstrated by classic immunological techniques in patients allergic to phenacetin, provided that the metabolites and not phenacetin itself are used to prepare the test reagents.

5. Diagnosis of Drug Allergy

5.1. Case History

Every practicing physician should be familiar with the large variety of clinical syndromes due to drug hypersensitivity. The diagnosis of drug allergy is, with few exceptions, still made on the basis of history alone. Some clinical criteria may help in the diagnosis of an allergic drug reaction. The reactions should (1) not resemble the pharmacological action of the drug; (2) be elicited by a minute amount of the drug; (3) occur only after an induction period of at least 5–7 days following primary exposure to the drug; (4) include symptoms classic for allergic reactions to natural macromolecular antigens (anaphylaxis, urticaria, serum sickness syndrome, asthma); (5) reappear promptly on readministration of the drug in small amounts; (6) be reproduced by drugs possessing similar cross-reacting chemical structures. Even when these criteria are all fulfilled, it may not be possible to establish the immunological nature of the reaction. Manifestations of an immunological reaction may sometimes be limited to a single organ or organ system;

classic symptoms of allergic reactions such as urticaria or asthma may not be present. On the other hand, symptoms suggestive of allergy may be due to the direct release of pharmacological mediators (e.g., histamine release by codein) or to pharmacological effects on cellular receptors (e.g., asthma due to aspirin). The late appearance of a reaction after initial administration of the drug in contrast to a prompt reappearance of symptoms on readministration is also no absolute demonstration of the allergic nature. For example, a latent period of one to several weeks before appearance of symptoms might also be required for the development of cumulative drug toxicity. On the other hand, when readministration of the drug occurs only after a long absence, allergic symptoms may not reappear immediately but may require again a "booster" interval of several days. Allergic reactions can also occur immediately on the first apparent exposure to drug if this drug cross-reacts with some other compounds to which the patient has previously been sensitized. Consequently, clinical criteria alone are often inadequate to establish the diagnosis of allergic reaction to a drug. A large number of alleged reactions to penicillin can be attributed to other causes. Often, so many drugs have been given at the time of the allergic reaction that a diagnosis based on history alone amounts to little more than a guess. Efforts should be made to establish objectively the presence of specific immunological agents, i.e., antibodies or sensitized lymphocytes.

5.2. Skin Tests

Scratch, prick, or intradermal tests with drug solutions are supposed to detect skin-sensitizing antibodies and reactivity of the immediate type, whereas epicutaneous or "patch" tests may reveal contact sensitization and hypersensitivity of the delayed type. The frequent failure of immediate-type skin tests with drugs can be readily explained by the previously described molecular requirements for anaphylactic reactions. On the other hand, positive skin reactions of diagnostic value may certainly be elicited by penicillins or other reactive chemical compounds such as chloramine T.

A frequent difficulty in intradermal testing is the poor solubility of many drugs in water and the difficulty in preparing test solutions which are not primarily irritating to the skin. While skin tests may remain negative even in clear-cut cases of drug hypersensitivity, they are occasionally helpful. In particular, epicutaneous testing with drugs may prove rewarding (Felix and Comaish, 1974), even in cases in which the clinical manifestation has been systemic rather than localized contact dermatitis. Positive patch tests with drugs may often be observed in hypersensitive individuals, provided that the right allergen is used (e.g., phenetidin in phenacetin allergy) and provided that the drug is applied in a solvent facilitating its penetration through the epidermis (e.g., dimethylsulfoxide). Under controlled conditions, positive reactions represent an objective demonstration of hypersensitivity, but the final interpretation depends on the history. Some objections to the use of skin tests in diagnosis of drug allergy must be kept in mind, such as the risk of sensitizing patients and the more serious risk of producing systemic reactions in highly sensitive individuals. Fatalities due to skin testing with drugs are extremely rare but have been reported (Idsøe *et al.*, 1968).

Progress in the diagnosis of drug allergy would be considerably advanced if suitable skin test reagents became generally available. In these, the antigenic determinants formed by the drug on conjugation *in vivo* would be represented on a multivalent conjugate, using a nonimmunogenic oligopeptide as carrier. This principle has been used successfully for the preparation of penicilloylpolylysine, a reagent which has proved to be very useful for the detection of some forms of penicillin allergy (Parker *et al.*, 1962a). Similar improvements in diagnosis of allergy to other drugs could be achieved, if the antigenic determinants were identified and the corresponding conjugates prepared.

5.3. *In Vitro* Tests

5.3.1. Detection of Antibodies by Serological Tests

When the drug is able to bind covalently to erythrocytes on incubation *in vitro*, as is the case with penicillin, hemagglutinating antibodies are readily detected (de Weck, 1964; Thiel *et al.*, 1964). They are in general of the IgG or IgM type, but their concentration is often too low to permit detection, In penicillin allergy, the presence of hemagglutinating antibodies may be coincidental unless confirmed by history and skin tests. Little of diagnostic value is to be expected from classic immunological methods, such as immunodiffusion and immunoelectrophoresis. Drugs functioning as univalent haptens do not cause precipitation. Methods involving study of the primary binding of a labeled drug to immunoglobulins could be more promising but would be of no value unless the antigenic determinants involved in allergy, i.e., the result of the *in vivo* conjugation of the drug, cross-reacted with the labeled compound. Differential assays such as the radioallergosorbent test (RAST) for detection of IgE antibodies are of greater diagnostic significance. In penicillin allergy, a good correlation among skin tests, history of penicillin allergy, and antipenicilloyl IgE antibodies has been established (Wide and Juhlin, 1971; Kraft *et al.*, 1977). However, these correlations become less reliable about 6 months after an alleged clinical allergic reaction, since antibody titers in serum decline rather rapidly in most patients without further contact with the allergenic drug.

The use of passive cutaneous anaphylaxis in rabbits or guinea pigs with sera from hypersensitive patients has been reported, but the technique is not very reliable and detects immunoglobulin classes which are probably of secondary clinical interest. Passive transfer of serum from hypersensitive patients to man or monkeys has the advantage of circumventing the risk of direct skin tests but is less reliable than direct skin testing. Sophisticated methods such as polarization fluorescence (Dandliker *et al.*, 1965) and inactivation of hapten-coated bacteriophages (Haimovich *et al.*, 1967) have not gained general acceptance.

5.3.2. Histamine Release

Blood basophils appear to release histamine on contact with allergens *in vitro*, but this test, first proposed by Shelley (1963), has long been considered as too insensitive and unreliable for the detection of allergy to drugs. It has been claimed that rat mast cells may detect human IgE and that a corresponding assay for clinical diagnosis of drug allergy can be developed (Korotzer and Haddad, 1970; Phills and Perelmutter, 1974). Histamine release from basophils can be detected by morphological or biochemical means. Recently, detection of penicillin hpersensitivity by histamine release using actively or passively sensitized human leukocytes has become possible.

5.3.3. Lymphocyte Reactivity

The wide application of lymphocyte cultures for immunological studies has persuaded a number of workers to use this technique as a diagnostic test in drug allergy. Specific lymphocyte transformation detected by various means (morphology, autoradiography, incorporation of labeled DNA precursors) may occur when an allergenic drug is placed in contact *in vitro* with the lymphocytes of hypersensitive individuals. Reports about the reproducibility and reliability of this procedure, however, are rather conflicting. Some authors claim an almost 100% correlation with the clinical history (Halpern *et al.*, 1967), but others are more cautious. Nevertheless, the lymphocyte transformation test (LTT) has lately become one of the most frequently used diagnostic tests in drug allergy. It seems to be a useful procedure provided that technical pitfalls are avoided. One of its main advantages is that, in contrast to drug-specific antibodies, drug-sensitive lymphocytes persist in the peripheral blood of allergic individuals even several years after the last known contact with the sensitizing drug. Most lymphocytes stimulated by drugs are T lymphocytes, but experiments in immediate-type allergies to penicillin (e.g., urticaria) have implicated B lymphocytes as well (de Weck, 1975). Another manifestation of specific lymphocyte reactivity, the macrophage migration inhibition test, has also been recommended (Rocklin and David, 1971). In penicillin allergy at least, the phenomenon of macrophage migration inhibition may be caused also by antigen–antibody complexes and appears to be rather unreliable. In any case, it is obvious that cellular tests *in vitro* merely indicate the presence of specific memory cells for a given antigen and cannot have predictive value.

5.4. Provocation Tests

Provocation tests in drug allergy should be undertaken rarely, if at all, and only with utmost caution. They are absolutely contraindicated in patients who have experienced a clinically severe reaction and with drugs known to be capable of inducing fatal reactions. Provocation tests must be restricted to very special circumstances, e.g., when the suspected drug must be given for lifesaving purposes. The doses suggested in several textbooks for so-called provocation tests, as for detecting sensitivity to contrast media in radiological procedures or before therapeutic use of antisera, are often so large that they are likely to kill any highly sensitive patient! Provocation tests must be carried out with allergen doses in the nanogram and microgram range, and then carefully and progressively increased only when reactions are initially negative.

6. Therapy

Treatment of clinical drug reactions is dealt with in handbooks of therapeutics, but some points concerning prophylaxis and hyposensitization could be made here.

6.1. Prophylaxis

Drugs known to have a high allergenic potential, such as penicillins, should be given only for serious clinical indications. Although this may seem obvious, the huge increase in drug consumption shows that this principle is not always adequately observed. Patients should always be asked whether they have experienced previous reactions to the prescribed drug. It seems reasonable and essential indeed that they be informed of the nature of the drug being prescribed. When an allergic reaction has occurred, presumably following the administration of a drug, every attempt should be made to secure an objective diagnosis and to inform the patient, so that similar reactions may be avoided in the future. In the case of penicillin allergy, skin tests and serological investigations, best performed 1–3 months after the clinical reaction, will make the patient quite aware of his hypersensitivity. A confirmed hypersensitivity to a drug usually represents an absolute contraindication to its renewed administration. The duration of drug hypersensitivity, however, seems to vary widely from patient to patient. In some individuals allergic to penicillin, high levels of skin-sensitizing antibodies are still detected 12–15 years after the last known clinical reaction. In others, the hypersensitivity may no longer be detectable after a few months. In such patients, readministration of the drug may be tolerated at the onset but will promptly cause an anamnestic response which may be quite dangerous.

6.2. Hyposensitization

In drug allergy, desensitization is seldom required except when the drug is considered lifesaving and no substitutes are available. In such cases, a so-called rush hyposensitization may be attempted. Success has been reported, especially in penicillin allergy (Reisman *et al.*, 1962; Zolov *et al.*, 1967), but the procedure is not without danger and should be carried out only on hospitalized patients under adequate cover of antihistamines, corticosteroids, and readily available emergency outfit.

Since univalent haptens are blocking antibody-combining sites and preventing the reaction of immunoglobulins with multivalent antigens, the principle of hapten inhibition has been applied to the prevention of allergic reactions to penicillin in hpersensitive patients. It has been demonstrated that the addition of an univalent penicillin derivative (penicillinoylformyllysine) permits the administration of penicillin without untoward clinical reactions even in patients with high-grade penicillin hypersensitivity of the immediate type (de Weck *et al.*, 1975). However, in a relatively low percentage of allergic patients, highly sensitive to the so-called minor determinants, the univalent hapten itself (probably through some secondary conjugation) is eliciting allergic reactions. The principle of hapten inhibition could therefore not be used blindly in all penicillin allergic patients, but those reacting directly to the hapten must first be screened out by a skin test.

7. References

Ackroyd, J. F., 1958, Thrombocytopenic purpura due to drug hypersensitivity, in: *Sensitivity Reactions to Drugs* (Rosenheim and Moulton, eds.), pp. 28–62, Blackwell, Oxford.

Ackroyd, J. F., and Rook, A. J., 1964, Drug reactions, in: *Clinical Aspects of Immunology* (P. G. H. Gell and R. R. A. Coombs, eds.), pp. 448–496, Davis, New York.

Askenaze, P. W., 1977, Role of basophils, mast cells and vasoamines in hypersensitivity reactions with a delayed time course, *Progr. Allergy* **23:**199–320.

Baker, S. B., and Williams, R. T., 1963, Acute interstitial nephritis due to drug sensitivity, *Br. Med. J.* **1:**1655–1658.

Baldwin, D. S., Levine, B. B., McCluskey, R. T., and Gallo, G. R., 1968, Renal failure and interstitial nephritis due to penicillin and methicillin, *N. Engl. J. Med.* **279:**1245–1252.

Batchelor, F. R., Dewdney, J. M., Weston, R. D., and Wheeler, A. W., 1966, The immunogenicity of cephalosporin derivatives and their cross-reaction with penicillin, *Immunology* **10:**21–33.

Batchelor, F. R., Dewdney, J. M., Feinberg, J. G., and Weston, R. D., 1967, A penicilloylated protein impurity as a source of allergy to benzylpenicillin and 6-aminopenicillanic acid, *Lancet* **1:**1175–1177.

Banacerraf, B., and Germain, R. N., 1978, The immune response genes of the major histocompatibility complex, *Immunol. Rev.* **38:**70–119.

Banacerraf, B., and McDevitt, H. O., 1972, Histocompatibility-linked immune response genes, *Science* **175:**273–279.

Berkowitz, M., Glaser, J., and Johnstone, D. E., 1953, The incidence of allergy to drugs in pediatric practice, *Ann. Allergy* **11:**561–566.

Bierman, C. W., Pierson, W. E., Zeitz, S. J., Goffman, L. S., and Van Arsdel, P. P., Jr., 1972, Reactions associate with ampicillin therapy, *J. Am. Med. Assoc.* **220:**1098–1100.

Bird, G. W. G., Wingham, J., Gunstone, R. F., and Smith, A. J., 1975, Acute haemolytic anemia due to IgM and IgA penicillin antibody, *Lancet* **2:**462.

Border, W. A., Lehman, D. H., and Egan, J. D., 1974, Antitubular basement-membrane antibodies in methicillin-associated interstitial nephritis, *N. Engl. J. Med.* **291:**381–384.

Boston Collaborative Drug Surveillance Program, 1972, Excess of ampicillin rashes associated with allopurinol or hyperuricemia, *N. Engl. J. Med.* **286:**505–507.

Brasch, R. C., Rockoff, S. D., Kuhn, C., and Chraplyvy, M., 1970, Contrast media as histamine liberators. II. Histamine release into venous plasma during intravenous urography in man, *Invest. Radiol.* **5:**510–513.

Bundgaard, H., and de Weck, A. L., 1975, The role af amino-reactive impurities in acetylsalicylic acid allergy, *Int. Arch. Allergy Appl. Immunol.* **49:**119–124.

Chase, M. W., 1946, Inhibition of experimental drug allergy by prior feeding of the sensitizing agent, *Proc. Soc. Exp. Biol. Med.* **61:**257–259.

Chase, M. W., 1966, Delayed-type hypersensitivity and the immunology of Hodgkin's disease, with a parallel examination of sarcoidosis, *Cancer Res.* **26:**1097–1120.

Cluff, L. E., and Johnson, J. E., 1964, Drug fever, *Prog. Allergy* **8:**149.

Dandliker, W. B., Halbert, S. P., Florin, M. C., Alonso, R., and Schapiro, H. C., 1965, Study of penicillin antibodies by fluorescence polarization and immunodiffusion, *J. Exp. Med.* **122:**1029–1048.

Dash, C. H., and Jones, H. E. H., 1972, *Mechanisms in Drug Allergy,* Churchill Livingstone, London.

Dausset, J., and Contu, L. A., 1964, A case of haemolytic anemia due to phenacetin allergy, *Vox. Sang.* **9:**599–607.

Davies, G. E., and Holmes, J. E., 1972, Drug induced immunological effects on the liver, *Br. J. Anaesthesiol.* **44:**941–945.

Davies, R. J., Hendrick, D. J., and Pepys, J., 1974, Asthma due to inhaled chemical agents: Ampicillin, benzylpenicillin, 6-aminopenicillanic acid and related substances, *Clin. Allergy* **4:**227–247.

de Warte, R. D., 1972, Drug allergy, in: *Allergic Diseases: Diagnosis and Management* (R. Patterson, ed.), p. 393, Lippincott, Philadelphia.

Dewdney, J., 1977, Immunology of the antibiotics, in: *The Antigens,* Vol. 4 (M. Sela, ed.), pp. 74–245, Academic, New York.

de Weck, A. L., 1962, Studies on penicillin hypersensitivity. I. The specificity of rabbit "antipenicillin" antibodies, *Int. Arch. Allergy Appl. Immunol.* **21:**20–37.

de Weck, A. L., 1964, Penicillin allergy: Its detection by an improved hemagglutination technique, *Nature (London)* **202:**975–977.

de Weck, A. L., 1968, Comparison of the antigen's molecular properties required for elicitation of various types of allergic tissue damage, in: *Immunopathology* (P. Graber and P. A. Miescher, eds.), pp. 295–309, Schwabe, Basel.

de Weck, A. L., 1971a, Drug reactions, in: *Immunological Diseases* (M. Samter, ed.), pp. 415–440, Little, Brown, Boston.

de Weck, A. L., 1971b, Immunological effects of aspirin anhydride, a contaminant of commercial acetylsalicylic acid preparations, *Int. Arch. Allergy Appl. Immunol.* **41**:393–418.

de Weck, A. L., 1974, Immunological and nonimmunological mechanisms of intolerance reactions to aspirin, in: *Selected Therapeutic Problems in Rheumatoid Arthritis* (G. H. Fallet and T. L. Fischer, eds.), pp. 31–35, Urban & Schwarzenberg, Munich.

de Weck, A. L., 1975, Molecular mechanisms of T and B lymphocyte triggering, *Int. Arch. Allergy Appl. Immunol.* **49**:247–254.

de Weck, A. L., and Blum, G., 1965, Recent clinical and immunological aspects of penicillin allergy, *Int. Arch. Allergy Appl. Immunol.* **27**:21–256.

de Weck, A. L., and Schneider, C. H., 1969, Molecular and stereochemical properties required of antigens for the elicitation of allergic reactions, in: *Problems of Immunological Diseases* (O. Westphal, H. E. Bock, and E. Grundmann, eds.), pp. 32–46, Springer, Heidelberg.

de Weck, A. L., Schneider, C. H., and Gutersohn, J., 1968, The role of penicilloylated protein impurities, penicillin polymers and dimers in penicillin allergy, *Int. Arch. Allergy Appl. Immunol.* **33**:535–567.

de Weck, A. L., Schneider, C. H., and Leemann, W., 1969, Hypersensitivity to carboxymethylcellulose as a cause of anaphylactic reactions in cattle, *Nature (London)* **223**:621–623.

de Weck, A. L., Schneider, C. H., Spengler, H., Toffler, O., and Lazary, S., 1973, Inhibition of allergic reactions by monovalent haptens, in: *Mechanisms of Reaginic Allergy* (A. Sehon, ed.), pp. 323–337, Dekker, New York.

de Weck, A. L., Jeunet, F., Schulz, K. H., Louis, P., Girard, J. P., Grilliat, J. P., Moneret-Vautrin, D., Storck, H., Wüthrich, B., Spengler, H., Juhlin, L., Scheiffarth, F., Warnatz, H., Wortmann, F., and Vigary, S., 1975, Clinical trial of Ro 6–0787: A monovalent specific hapten inhibitor of penicillin allergy, *Z. Immunitaetsforsch.* **150**:138–160.

Eisen, H. N., 1959, Hypersensitivity to simple chemicals, in: *Cellular and Humoral Aspects of the Hypersensitive States* (H. S. Lawrence, ed.), pp. 89–122, Hoeber, New York.

Ellmann, L., Inman, J., and Green, I., 1971, Strain difference in the immune response to hydralazine in inbred guinea pigs, *Clin. Exp. Immunol.* **9**:927–937.

Fankhauser, S., 1969, Neuere Aspekte der Insulintherapie, *Schweiz. Med. Wochenschr.* **99**:414–420.

Felix, R. H., and Comaish, J. S., 1974, The value of patch and other skin tests in drug eruptions, *Lancet* **1**:1017–1019.

Fellner, M. J., and Baer, R. L., 1965a, Anaphylactic reaction to tetracycline in a penicillin-allergic patient, *J. Am. Med. Assoc.* **192**:997–998.

Fellner, M. J., and Baer, R. L., 1965b, Cutaneous reaction to drugs, *Med. Clin. North Am.* **49**:709–724.

Fellner, M. J., and Harris, H., 1972, Adverse cutaneous reactions to drugs, in: *Drug Induced Diseases,* Vol. 4 (L. Meyer and H. M. Peck, eds.), pp. 382–402, Excerpta Medica, North-Holland, Amsterdam.

Freedman, A. L., Barr, P. S., and Brody, E. A., 1956, Hemolytic anemia due to quinidine: Observations on its mechanism, *Am. J. Med.* **20**:806–816.

Frick, O. L., Nye, W., and Raffel, S., 1968, Anaphylactic reactions to univalent haptens, *Immunology* **14**:563–568.

Geczy, A. F., and de Weck, A. L., 1975, Genetic control of sensitization to structurally unrelated antigens and its relationship to histocompatibility antigens in guinea pigs, *Immunology* **28**:331–342.

Gell, P. G. H., and Benacerraf, B., 1961, Delayed hypersensitivity to simple protein antigens, *Adv. Immunol.* **1**:319–343.

Gell, P. G. H., Harrington, C. R., and Michel, R., 1948, Antigenic function of simple chemical compounds: Correlation of antigenicity with chemical reactivity, *Br. J. Exp. Pathol.* **29**:578–589.

Gillette, J. R., Mitchell, J. R., and Brodie, B. B., 1974, Biochemical mechanisms of drug toxicity, *Ann. Rev. Pharmacol.* **14**:271–288.

Good, R. A., Kelley, W. D., Rötstein, J., and Varco, R. L., 1962, Immunological deficiency diseases, *Progr. Allergy* **6**:187–319.

Green, G. R., and Rosenblum, A., 1971, Report of the penicillin study group: American Academy of Allergy, *J. Allergy Clin. Immunol.* **48**:331–343.

Green, I., Paul, W. E., and Benacerraf, B., 1966, The behavior of hapten-poly-L-lysine conjugates as complete antigens in genetic responders and as haptens in nonresponder guinea pigs, *J. Exp. Med.* **123**:859–879.

Hahn, B. H., Sharp, G. C., Irvin, W. S., Kantor, O. W., Gardner, C. A., Bagby, M. K., Perry, H. M., Jr., and Osterland, C. K., 1972, Immune responses to hydralazine and nuclear antigens in hydralazine-induced lupus erythematosus, *Ann. Intern. Med.* **76**:365–374.

Haimovich, J., Sela, M., Dewdney, J. M., and Batchelor, F. R., 1967, Anti-penicilloyl antibodies: Detection with penicilloylated bacteriphage and isolation with a specific immunoadsorbent, *Nature (London)* **214**:1369–1370.

Halpern, B., Ky, N. T., and Amache, N., 1967, Diagnosis of drug allergy *in vitro* with the lymphocyte transformation test. *J. Allergy Clin. Immunol.* **40**:168–181.

Hoigné, R., and Schoch, K., 1959, Anaphylaktischer Schock und akute nicht allergische Reaktionen nach Procain-Penicillin, *Schweiz. Med. Wochenschr.* **89**:1350–1356.

Huguley, C. M., 1964, Drug-induced blood dyscrasias. II. Agranulocytosis, *J. Am. Med. Assoc.* **188**:817–818.

Hutchinson, F., MacLeod, T. M., and Raffle, E. J., 1975, Nickel hypersensitivity, *Br. J. Dermatol.* **93**:557–561.

Hyman, G., and Sommers, S. C., 1966, The development of Hodgkin's disease and lymphoma during anticonvulsant therapy, *Blood* **28**:416–427.

Idsøe, O., Guthe, T., Willcox, R. R., and de Weck, A. L., 1968, Nature and extent of penicillin side reactions with particular references to 151 fatalities from anaphylactic shock, *Bull. WHO* **38**:159–188.

Korotzer, J., and Haddad, Z. H., 1970, *In vitro* detection of human IgE-mediated immediate hypersensitivity reactions to pollens and penicillin(s) by a modified rat mast cell degranulation technique, *J. Allergy Clin. Immunol.* **45**:126.

Kraft, D., Roth, A., Mischer, P., Pichler, H., and Ebner, H., 1977, Specific and total serum IgE measurements in the diagnosis of penicillin allergy: A long term follow-up study, *Clin. Allergy* **7**:21–28.

Kristofferson, A., Ahlstedt, S., Pettersson, E., and Svärd, P. O., 1977, Antigens in penicillin allergy. I. A radioimmunoassay for detection of penicilloylated protein contaminants in penicillin preparations, *Int. Arch. Allergy Appl. Immunol.* **55**:13–27.

Landsteiner, K., 1945, *The Specificity of Serological Reactions*, Harvard University Press, Cambridge, Mass.

Levine, B. B., 1965, The nature of the antigen-antibody complexes which initiate anaphylactic reactions. I, *J. Immunol.* **94**:111–131.

Levine, B. B., and Redmond, A. P., 1968, The nature of the antigen-antibody complexes initiating the specific wheal-and-flare reactions in sensitized man, *J. Clin. Invest.* **47**:566–567.

Levine, H. D., 1976, Acute myocardial infarction following wasp sting, *Am. Heart J.* **91**:365–374.

Lo Buglio, A. F., and Jandl, J. H., 1967, The nature of the alpha-methyl-dopa red-cell antibody, *N. Engl. J. Med.* **276**:658–665.

Lockey, R. F., Rucknagel, D. L., and Vanselow, N. A., 1973, Familiar occurrence of asthma, nasal polyps and aspirin intolerance, *Ann. Intern. Med.* **78**:57–63.

Lukes, R. J., and Tindle, B. H., Immunoblastic lymphadenopathy, 1975, *N. Engl. J. Med.* **292**:1–4.

Lunel, J., Albot, G., and Pagniez, R., 1966, Etude critique des ictères à la chlorpromazine, *Sem. Hop. Paris* **42**:1791–1807.

Mayer, R. L., 1950, Compounds of quinone structure as allergens and cancerogenic agents, *Experientia* **6**:241–250.

Meyler, L., and Herxheimer, A., 1975, *Side Effects of Drugs*, Vol. 8, Excerpta Medica Foundation, Amsterdam.

Miller, F. F., 1967, History of drug sensitivity in atopic persons, *J. Allergy Clin. Immunol.* **40**:46–49.

Moeschlin, S., 1958, Agranulocytosis due to sensitivity to drugs, in: *Sensitivity Reactions to Drugs* (M. L. Rosenheim and R. Moulton eds.) pp. 77–89, Blackwell, Oxford.

Moeschlin, S., and Wagner, K., 1952, Agranulocytosis due to the occurrence of leukocyte-agglutinins, *Acta Haematol.* **8**:29–41.

Müller, J. W., Grob, P. J., Joller, H. I., and Guggisberg, H. E., 1975, Pseudolupus: Eine schwere Nebenwirkung eines Venenpräparates? *Schweiz. Med. Wochenschr.* **105**:665–668.

Parker, C. W., 1975, Drug allergy, *N. Engl. J. Med.* **292:**511–514, 732–736, 957–960.

Parker, C. W., de Weck. A. L., Kern, M., and Eisen, H. N., 1062a, The preparation and some properties of penicillenic acid derivatives relevant to penicillin hypersensitivity, *J. Exp. Med.* **115:**803–819.

Parker, C. W., Kern, M., and Eisen, H. N., 1962b, Polyfunctional dinitrophenyl haptens as reagents for elicitation of immediate-type allergic skin responses, *J. Exp. Med.* **115:**789–801.

Pearsall, H. R., Ewalt, J., Tsoi, M. S., Sumida, S., Backus, D., Winterbauer, R. H., Webb, D. R., and Jones, H., 1974, Nitrofurantoin lung sensitivity: Report of a case with prolonged nitrofurantoin lymphocyte sensitivity and interaction of nitrofurantoin-stimulated lymphocytes with alveolar cells, *J. Lab. Clin. Med.* **83:**728–737.

Peterson, W. C., and Manick, K. P., 1967, Purpuric eruptions associated with use of carbromal and meprobamate, *Arch. Dermatol.* **95:**40–42.

Petz, L. D., and Fudenberg, H. H., 1966, Coombs-positive hemolytic anemia caused by penicillin administration, *N. Engl. J. Med.* **274:**171–178.

Phills, J. A., and Perelmutter, L., 1974, IgE-mediated and non IgE-mediated allergic-type reactions to aspirin, *Acta Allergol.* **29:**474–490.

Prescott, L. F., 1966, The nephrotoxicity of analgesics, *J. Pharm. Pharmacol.* **18:**331–353.

Rajka, G., and Skog, E., 1965, On the relation between drug allergy and atopy, *Acta Allergol.* **20:**387–394.

Redmond, A. P., and Levine, B. B., 1968, Delayed skin reactions to benzylpenicillin in man, *Int. Arch. Allergy Appl. Immunol.* **33:**193–206.

Reisman, R. E ., Rose, N. R., Witebsky, E., and Arbesman, C., 1962, Penicillin allergy and desensitization, *J. Allergy Clin. Immunol.* **33:**178–187.

Remmer, H., and Schüppel, R., 1972, The formation of antigenic determinants, in: *International Encyclopedia of Pharmacology and Therapeutics,* Vol. 1 (M. Samter and C. W. Parker, eds.), pp. 67–89, Pergamon, Oxford.

Rocklin, R. E., and David, J. R., 1971, Detection *in vitro* of cellular hypersensitivity to drugs, *J. Allergy Clin. Immunol.* **48:**276–282.

Rosenheim, M. L., and Moulton, R. (eds.), 1958, *Sensitivity Reactions to Drugs,* Blackwell, Oxford.

Ruegger, R., Spengler, H., de Weck, A. L., and Dubach, U. C., 1973, Immunologische Aspekte der Sensibilisierung auf Phenacetin, *Dtsch. Med. Wochenschr.* **98:**762–764.

Samter, M., and Beers, R. F., 1967, Concerning the nature of intolerance to aspirin, *J. Allergy Clin. Immunol.* **40:**281–293.

Schatz, M., Patterson, R., O'Rourke, J., Mickelsen, J., and Northup, C., 1975, The administration of radiographic contrast media to patients with a history of a previous reaction, *J. Allergy Clin.Immunol.* **55:**358–366.

Schneider, C. H., and de Weck, A. L., 1965, A new chemical aspect of penicillin allergy: The direct reaction of penicillin with ϵ-amino groups, *Nature (London)* **208:**57–59.

Schneider, C. H., and de Weck, A. L., 1967, The reaction of benzylpenicillin with carbohydrates at neutral pH with a note on the immunogenicity of hapten–polysaccharide conjugates, *Immunochemistry* **4:**331–343.

Schwarz, K., and Schwarz-Speck, M., 1960, Experimentally induced photoallergy to sulfonilamide, *Acta Allergol.* **7:**224–231.

Sharma, O. P., 1973, Drug induced pulmonary disease, *Ann. Intern. Med.* **78:**616.

Shelley, W. B., 1963, Indirect basophil degranulation test for allergy to penicillin and other drugs, *J. Am. Med. Assoc.* **184:**171–178.

Snell, E. S., 1961, An examination of the blood of febrile subjects for pyrogenic properties, *Clin. Sci.* **21:**115–124.

Spark, R. P., 1971, Fatal anaphylaxis due to oral penicillin, *J. Clin. Pathol.* **56:**407–411.

Spengler, H., and de Weck, A. L., 1977, Evaluation of genetic control of the immune response to penicillin in man, *Monogr. Allergy* **11:**116–123.

Spengler, H., de Weck, A. L., and Geczy, A. F., 1974, Studies on the molecular mechanisms of lymphocyte stimulation by penicillin and penicillin derivatives, in: *Proceedings of the Eighth Leucocyte Conference,* pp. 501–507, Academic, New York.

Steiner, L. A., and Eisen, H. N., 1966, Variations in the immune response to a simple determinant, *Bacteriol. Rev.* **30:**383–396.

Stewart, G. T., 1967, Allergenic residues in penicillins, *Lancet* **1:**1177–1183.

Swanson, M. A., Chanmougan, D., and Schwartz, R. S., 1966, Immunohemolytic anemia due to antipenicillin antibodies, *N. Eng. J. Med.* **274:**178–181.

Symmers, W. S. C., 1962, The occurrence of angiitis and of other generalized diseases of connective tissues as a consequence of the administration of drugs (with a note on drug allergy as a cause of thrombotic purpura), *Proc. R. Soc. Med.* **55:**20–28.

Szczerlik, A., Gryglewski, R. J., and Czerniawska-Mysik, G., 1975, Relationship of inhibition of prostaglandin biosynthesis by analgesics to asthma attacks in aspirin-sensitive patients, *Br. Med. J.* **1:**67–69.

Tan, E. M., 1974, Drug-induced autoimmune disease, *Fed. Proc.* **33:**1894–1897.

Thiel, J. A., Mitchell, S., and Parker, C. W., 1964, The specificity of hemagglutination reactions in human and experimental penicillin hypersensitivity, *J. Allergy Clin. Immunol.* **35:**399–424.

Thierfelder, S., Eulitz, M., and Karl, M. L., 1967, Immunologische Studien an einem Pyramidon-Leukozytenantikörper, *Klin. Wochenschr.* **45:**78–83.

Thoburn, R., Johnson, J. E., and Cluff, L. E., 1966, Studies on the epidemiology of cephalothin and penicillin allergy. *J. Am. Med. Assoc.* **198:**345–348.

Wegmann, A., and Renker, H., 1976, Das Elektrokardiogramm im anaphylaktischen Schock des Menschen, *Klin. Wochenschr.* **54:**453–459.

Welsh, A. L., 1961, *The Fixed Eruption,* Thomas, Springfield, Ill.

Wide, L., and Juhlin, L., 1971, Detection of penicillin allergy of the immediate-type by radioimmunoassay of reagins (IgE) to penicilloyl conjugates, *Clin. Allergy* **1:**171–177.

Worrledge, S. M., Carstairs, K. C., and Dacie, J. V., 1966, Autoimmune hemolytic anemia associated with α-methyldopa, *Lancet* **2:**135–139.

Zimmermann, H. J., 1972, Drug induced hepatic injury, in: *International Encyclopedia of Pharmacology and Therapeutics,* Vol. 1 (M. Samter and C. W. Parker, eds.), pp. 299–365, Pergamon, Oxford.

Zolov, D., Redmond, A. P., and Levine, B. B., 1967, Immunological studies of desensitization in penicillin allergy, *J. Allergy Clin. Immunol.* **39:**107.

11

Insect Allergy: Stinging and Biting Insects

ROBERT E. REISMAN

1. Introduction

Allergic reactions due to the common stinging insects bee, wasp, yellow jacket, and hornet will be the primary emphasis of this chapter. In addition, reactions due to fire ants, which are nonwinged hymenoptera, and biting insects will be briefly considered.

2. Stinging Insects: "Winged" Hymenoptera

Stinging insect allergy has been recognized for many years. Today it is a significant problem. Documented fatalities occur yearly as a result of insect stings (Barnard, 1973), and the morbidity is much greater. In recent years new information regarding the pathogenesis of allergy and immunity to stinging insects has been forthcoming. The implications of this information are quite important for a number of reasons. First, reliable guidelines are being developed for the first time for the diagnosis and treatment of stinging insect allergy. Second, these concepts have important implications relevant to other types of allergic reactions such as pollen and drug allergy. Third, the traditional approaches to diagnosis and treatment of stinging insect allergy, in which there still is a great deal of faith, may be entirely without validation.

2.1. Clinical Aspects

2.1.1. Causative Agents

The four major stinging insects are the bee, wasp *(Polistes)*, yellow jacket, and hornet. All belong to the order Hymenoptera of the class Insecta. The

ROBERT E. REISMAN • Departments of Medicine and Pediatrics, State University of New York, Buffalo, New York 14203.

honeybee and bumblebee are members of the superfamily Apoidea. Both bees tend to sting only when provoked. The bumblebee is a rare offender. Because of the common use of the honeybee for production of honey and in plant fertilization, exposure to this insect is quite common. Multiple stings from honeybees are quite common, particularly if their hive is endangered. The honeybee is the only stinging insect which loses its stinging mechanism in the stinging process, thereby suffering self-evisceration and death.

The wasp, yellow jacket, and hornet belong to the superfamily Vespoidea. The wasp usually builds a honeycomb nest under eaves and in rafters. Wasps are relatively few in number in such nests. The hornet constructs a large *papier mache* type nest hanging from trees or shrubs. The yellow jacket builds its hive in the ground or under logs and is the most common cause of insect sting reactions. The yellow jacket is the insect most often inadvertently disturbed in the course of common activities such as gardening, lawnmowing, and picnicking.

2.1.2. Prevalence of Reactions

Anaphylactic reactions cause at least 40 reported deaths per year in this country according to information obtained from vital statistic registries (Barnard, 1973). It is most likely that other deaths go unrecognized. In several retrospective large population studies, the incidence of a past history of an allergic reaction of a nonfatal type from an insect sting was about 0.4% (Chafee, 1970; Settipane and Boyd, 1970). The reaction rates may vary a great deal depending on location and degree of exposure.

2.1.3. Clinical Features

Allergic reactions due to stinging insects may occur at any age. The majority of reactions have occurred in individuals under the age of 20. There is a 2:1 male-to-female ratio. These factors may be a reflection of exposure rather than any specific age or sex predilection. Population studies have suggested that approximately 33–40% of individuals suffering systemic reactions have had a personal history of atopic disease (Brown and Bernton, 1970; Frazier, 1964; Mueller, 1959; Mueller *et al.*, 1975; Schwartz and Kahn, 1970).

The yellow jacket has been incriminated as the most common cause for allergic reactions followed by the bee, wasp, and hornet (Barr, 1974; Brown and Bernton, 1970; Frazier, 1964). This will vary considerably depending on immediate environmental conditions. As insect identification is often very difficult, usually only the bee, which leaves its stinger in place, can be reliably identified.

Stings occurring around the head and neck most commonly cause allergic reactions (Brown and Bernton, 1970; Frazier, 1964). It must be emphasized, however, that reactions may occur from stings occurring on any area of the body.

2.1.4. Types of Reactions

A variety of reactions have been described from insect stings, ranging from acute anaphylaxis to unusual reactions such as serum sickness and neuritis. They may be summarized as follows:

Normal: transient swelling, erythema, pain.
Large local: peak 48–72 hr; may last up to 1 week.
Anaphylaxis.
Neurological and vascular reactions.
Toxic.
None.

a. Anaphylaxis. The most serious reaction following an insect sting is acute anaphylaxis. The symptoms which occur are those typical of anaphylaxis from any cause. The majority of reactions begin within several to 15 min after the sting, although there have been rare reports of reactions developing at later periods of time. It has been suggested that the sooner the reaction occurs the more severe it might be. The clinical symptomatology which occurs in anaphylaxis is variable from patient to patient. Reactions include generalized urticaria, flushing, angioedema, upper airway edema, bronchospasm, circulatory collapse with shock and hypotension, gastrointestinal symptoms manifested by bowel spasm and diarrhea, and uterine contractions. A chief cause of death has been upper airway edema involving the pharynx, epiglottis, and trachea. Significant amounts of secretions have been associated with the edema. Circulatory involvement was thought to be responsible for fatalities in other patients, and several individuals have been described in whom autopsy findings were essentially normal. The symptom complex which occurred following insect stings was the same in a large series of individuals who had fatal and nonfatal results (Barnard, 1970, 1973; Jensen, 1962; O'Connor *et al.*, 1964; Schenken *et al.*, 1953).

The majority of individuals who die as a result of an insect sting are adults (Barnard, 1973; Jensen, 1962, O'Connor *et al.*, 1964). This conflicts somewhat with the incidence prevalence of the under age 20 group. Although the reason for the increased mortality in adulthood is not clear, one might speculate that it is due to the presence of cardiovascular disease or other pathological changes associated with age. The adults may have less tolerance for the profound biochemical and physiological changes which accompany anaphylaxis.

Most individuals had no previous warning of the development of stinging insect allergy. In two studies only 18% and 47% of patients who developed fatal reactions had a history of any prior insect sting problems (Barnard, 1973; O'Connor *et al.*, 1964). Large local reactions from preceding insect stings have been described in 10–40% of individuals who subsequently had generalized systemic reactions (Brown and Bernton, 1970; Insect Allergy Committee Report, 1972). There seems to be little relationship between the time interval leading to the systemic reaction and the previous innocuous sting. Furthermore, numerous individuals have reported a reaction occurring with the first sting.

b. Local Reactions. The usual reaction from an insect sting is mild transitory pain, erythema, and swelling about the sting site. On occasion, moderate to severe local reactions occur. Swelling extends from the sting site over an extensive area and may last for several days. For example, swelling from a sting on the finger may extend to the elbow. The pathogenesis of this type of reaction will be discussed below.

c. Neurological and Vascular Complications. There have been a number of individual case reports of unusual reactions occurring in a temporal relationship to an insect sting (Ashworth, 1964; Burke and Jellinek, 1954; Day, 1962; Fogel *et al.*, 1967; Goldstein *et al.*, 1965; Means, 1973; Ross, 1939; Rytand, 1955; Sheehan, 1965; Venters*et al.*, 1961). These reactions usually involve the vascular or neurological system and include such reactions as vasculitis, nephrosis, serum sickness, neuritis, and encephalitis. In some instances these reactions are also associated with the occurrence of the more typical acute anaphylactic symptoms. Neurological and vascular symptoms have occurred from several days to a week following the sting and have been progressive over long periods of time. The etiology of these reactions is still unknown, although there are suggestions that immunological responses may play some role.

d. Toxic. Toxic reactions may occur as a result of multiple stings. Insect venom contains a number of potent pharmacological agents. As a result of the pharmacological properties of these substances, one may develop vascular collapse, shock, hypotension, and even death.

e. "None." There are some individuals, primarily beekeepers, who develop negligible reactions at the site of bee stings. These reactions are less than "normal." From a clinical viewpoint these individuals represent the antithesis of the allergic individual and have provided a source for study of the mechanisms of immunity.

2.2. Immunopathogenesis

2.2.1. Nature of Antigen

a. Venom and Body Protein. Extracts prepared by mashing or grinding whole insect bodies have been used for over 40 years for the diagnosis and treatment of insect-allergic individuals. The origins of these extracts date back to observations made by Benson (Benson and Semenov, 1930; Benson, 1939b), who believed that the allergen responsible for anaphylaxis was present throughout the whole body of the bee as well as in the venom. In these early observations, Benson studied several beekeepers who became anaphylactically sensitive to bee stings. These individuals also may have been sensitive to body proteins encountered during exposure to bee dust and unfortunately do not represent the typical anaphylactically sensitive patient.

In more recent years the question of potency of whole body extracts has been assessed. In the early 1960s Shulman and colleagues examined the immunochemical and antigenic relationships of various stinging insects and their parts (Shulman, 1968). They described the presence of a "tissue"-specific antigen present in bee venom and not present in the rest of the bee body. These observations led to clinical studies designed to reexamine the diagnostic and therapeutic effectiveness of whole body extracts and particularly to compare results to the use of pure venoms.

The usefulness of whole body extracts as diagnostic agents was reexamined in several reports. In a well-controlled study, Schwartz (1965) found that skin test reactions with whole body insect extracts were the same in allergic patients as in individuals who had never had any type of reaction from a stinging insect and concluded that whole body extract testing did not differentiate allergic from nonallergic individuals. Pioneer studies by Loveless and Fackler (1956) suggested that the venom might be a better diagnostic test antigen, although there was some overlap in test results with control groups. Subsequently other studies seemed to confirm this observation. Hunt *et al.* (1975) found venom skin tests to be reliable and correlate with results of histamine release studies.

Further *in vitro* studies have been done to measure the binding of IgE-specific antibodies with venom and whole body insect extracts. Using the histamine release system, Sobotka *et al.* (1974b) found venom to be quite effective in releasing histamine from cells of allergic individuals. Poor release was found with whole body extracts. In the only study showing some activity of whole body extracts, Yocum *et al.* (1973) did find substantial release of histamine. Apparently in these studies a number of whole body extracts were screened before a potent one could be found. Unfortunately, venom was not used for comparison in this latter study.

In our laboratory using the RAST procedure and comparing whole body extracts and bee venom as coupling antigens, the majority of insect-sensitive sera reacted to both antigens but to a greater degree to bee venom (Light *et al.*, 1976b).

To summarize the results of these diagnostic studies performed in more recent years, it would appear that venom contains the allergen responsible for sensitivity. Whole body extracts apparently contain very little potent allergen. Preliminary studies have also suggested that there is considerable variation in the potency of different whole body extracts (Arbesman *et al.*, 1975) Whether a potent whole body extract can be prepared is still an open question.

b. Venom Fractions. Bee venom has been fractionated into at least eight distinct components with a likelihood that there are at least several others. The major identifiable components are phospholipase A, hyaluronidase, melittin, apamin, and a more recently described high-molecular-weight protein (Hoffman *et al.*, 1977; Shepherd *et al.*, 1974). Phospholipase A appears to be a major allergen in bee venom (Light *et al.*, 1976a; Sobotka *et al.*, 1974a). Phospholipase A specific IgE antibodies have been identified by RAST and histamine release techniques. In addition, it now appears that other allergens may be important, particularly the high-molecular-weight components and hyaluronidase. Whether there is any clinical significance in differentiating the active allergenic component of bee venom has yet to be determined.

The contents of other insect venoms vary from bee venom (Table 1). Histamine, 5-hydroxytryptamine, and kinins have been identified in wasp venom (Bhoola *et al.*, 1961; Jacques and Schachter, 1954; Neumann and Habermann, 1954). Hornet venom contains these substances as well as acetylcholine. As yet there have not been sufficient quantities of these venoms available for appropriate fractionation studies.

c. Single Insect and Multiple Insect Sensitivity. As noted above, honeybees are classified in the superfamily Apoidea, and the other stinging insects, wasps, hornets, and yellow jackets are in the superfamily Vespoidea. This entomological difference also has significance in terms of allergenic specificity.

Observations in the past regarding single insect sensitivity have been quite common. For example, beekeepers quite immune to the sting of the bee have had acute allergic reactions resulting from the stings of yellow jackets or wasps. Sensitive individuals have occasionally been able to identify the specific insect causing their reaction while tolerating other insect stings with no difficulty.

More recent studies using *in vitro* procedures such as histamine release and RAST have addressed this problem fairly directly. The results of the studies with one large group of sera taken from insect-sensitive individuals is shown are Figure 1 (Light and Reisman, 1976). Clearly there are sera reacting with one or multiple venoms. Thus bee or yellow jacket or hornet sensitivity may be quite specific. In studies of *Polistes* (wasp) anaphylaxis, sensitivity as measured by leukocyte histamine release was confined to wasp venom. No release was found with honeybee venom (Findlay *et al.*, 1977).

2.2.2. Nature of Antibody

As acute systemic reactions following insect stings occur immediately and have the cardinal signs of typical anaphylaxis, an IgE immunopathogenesis is certainly likely. Results of skin tests and *in vitro* tests have suggested that most if not all anaphylactic reactions are mediated by IgE antibodies. In one study of a large number of patients who had had sting anaphylaxis and were selected at random there were some who failed to have detectable IgE antibodies (Table 2) (Reisman *et al.*, 1975). It was possible that the appropriate venom was not used for testing or that the IgE antibodies may have disappeared in a short period of time. Most recent observations from our own laboratory have indicated that there are a small number of patients seen shortly after an acute anaphylactic reaction in whom an IgE pathogenesis for the reaction could not be determined either by skin testing or by *in vitro* testing. Until this problem is resolved there is still a possibility of a non-IgE pathogenesis for these reactions. The unusual reactions such as nephrosis or neurological disease which have been reported following insect stings

TABLE 1. Pharmacologically and Biochemically Active Constituents of Various Insect Venoms

Bee	Wasp	Hornet
	Biogenic amines	
Histamine	Histamine	Histamine
Dopamine, norepinephrine	Serotonin	Serotonin
	Dopamine, norepinephrine	Acetylcholine
	Protein and polypeptide toxins (nonenzymatic)	
Mellitin	Wasp kinin	Hornet kinin
Apamin		
MCD-peptide		
Minimine		
	Enzymes	
Phospholipase A	Phospholipase A	Phospholipase A
Phospholipase B	Phospholipase B	Phospholipase B
Hyaluronidase	Hyaluronidase	Hyaluronidase
Acid phosphatase		Acid phosphatase

do not have an identifiable immunological pathogenesis (Light *et al.*, 1977). In some patients serum antibodies have been found, but it is not clear that these are part of the pathogenesis of the reaction.

In considering the pathogenesis of allergic reactions to stinging insects it is also appropriate to discuss the question of immunity. As already noted, beekeepers may well represent the antithesis of the allergic individual. Analysis of sera obtained from beekeepers revealed high levels of bee venom specific IgG (Light *et al.*, 1975). These antibodies are capable of blocking bee venom induced histamine release from cells of allergic individuals. On occasion beekeepers also have elevated levels of specific IgE antibodies. Studies suggest that when these IgE antibodies are also accompanied by high levels of IgG antibodies immunity rather than allergy is the response.

Following an acute allergic reaction IgE antibodies are stimulated and rise to peak titers in 2–3 weeks. This response is quite similar to that seen in ragweed-sensitive patients who develop an anamnestic response as a result of ragweed pollen exposure. In addition to this IgE antibody response some patients mount an IgG antibody response following this one sting reaction.

2.3. Diagnosis

The diagnosis of an acute allergic reaction due to a stinging insect is usually self-evident. The major problem is usually the identification of the insect responsible for the reaction. Most individuals are unable to differentiate the various types of stinging insects. Only the honeybee is readily identifiable because it leaves its stinger in place.

As mentioned above, skin testing or *in vitro* testing with extracts prepared from whole insect bodies has been used as a means of documenting and perhaps quantitating sensitivity for many years. Objective data now suggest that this is quite unreliable. Even in the past, experienced practitioners often have either omitted testing or discounted the results. It has been suggested that perhaps the only real value in such testing has been the identification of the rare individual who is highly sensitive to whole body extracts and would require minimal initial therapeutic doses.

Diagnostic testing with venom is in its early stages. It would appear that

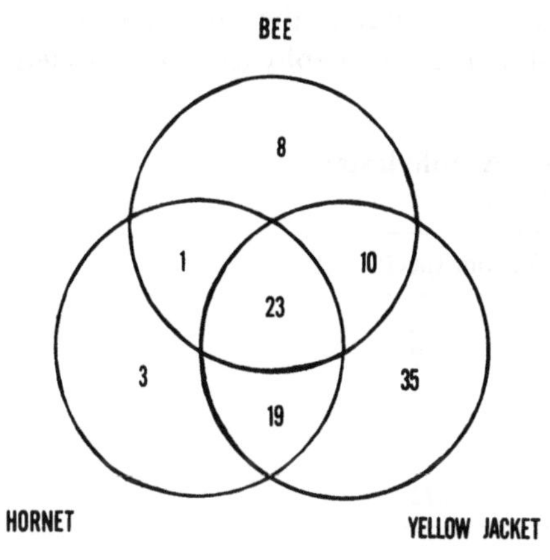

Figure 1. Venn diagram summarizing the presence of IgE antibodies reacting with bee, yellow jacket, and hornet venoms in the sera of 99 insect-sensitive patients. As can be noted, antibodies may be present reacting with one, two, or all three venoms.

venom testing is a highly reliable method of diagnosing the presence of insect sensitivity. Potential problems may occur because venom in higher concentrations does cause reactions in nonallergic individuals, presumably as a result of direct pharmacological action of its contents. As with skin testing, *in vitro* tests such as histamine release and RAST are also highly reliable for measuring the presence of specific IgE antibodies reacting with venom. Collection of sufficient quantities of honeybee venom for both testing and therapy should present no problem. Using the simple method of electrical stimulation designed by Benton *et al.* (1963), bee venom can be obtained in large quantities. Collection of venoms from other types of stinging insects may well be a problem and may require sufficient time, effort, and funding.

One of the more interesting problems currently under investigation is duration of insect sensitivity. Preliminary studies suggest that there is a great individual difference in the persistence of sensitivity in the absence of any type of treatment or resting. A number of individuals have been seen who have had acute allergic reactions with high levels of specific IgE antibodies. These antibody titers may fall off rapidly to the point where a year later they are undetectable. In contrast, of specific IgE. These observations are quite analogous to those made in individuals with other sensitivities such as penicillin.

2.4. Therapy

2.4.1. Principles of Avoidance

Simple precautions may decrease the risk of insect stings. Individuals at risk should be careful about outside activities. Foods and odors readily attract insects. Outdoor cooking and eating should be done with care. Garbage should be well wrapped and covered. Lawnmowing, hedge clipping, and gardening should be done with a great deal of caution. Shoes should be worn when walking in grass or fields. Cosmetics, perfumes, hair sprays, and bright colors may attract insects and should be avoided when outside by people at risk. Insecticides may be of some help.

2.4.2. Medical Therapy

Acute allergic reactions due to insect stings are treated in the same manner as anaphylaxis from any cause. The principles and therapy of anaphylaxis are outlined

TABLE 2. Stinging Insect Anaphylaxis: Analysis of 109 Sera

	Venom-specific IgE
Bee	46
Yellow jacket	57
Hornet	36
Total number of sera with antibodies	72

in Chapter 18. The drug of choice for immediate treatment of anaphylactic reactions is epinephrine hydrochloride administered in a dose ranging from 0.2 to 0.5 ml. On rare occasions intravenous injections may be necessary. Individuals at risk are taught to self-administer epinephrine and to keep epinephrine available at all times. Antihistamines such as diphenhydramine hydrochloride, 50 mg, may be given orally or parenterally depending on specific symptomatology. Other medications which may be needed include aminophylline, vasopressors, and oxygen. Careful attention must be given to the maintenance of the airway as upper airway edema has been identified as a common cause for fatality. Acute allergic reactions usually occur within a matter of minutes following an insect sting. If untreated and not fatal, symptomatology may be self-limited and disappear within several hours. Rarely the reaction may continue for a long period of time. In those circumstances steroids may be necessary.

Treatment of local reactions generally consists of the application of cold and the use of oral antihistamines and analgesics. When the reactions are extremely large and painful, steroids are quite beneficial in reducing the swelling. As the pathogenesis of the unusual neurological and vascular complications which occur in the temporal relationship to the insect sting is really unknown, specific therapy is not clear. In some situations steroid therapy has been used and appeared to be beneficial.

2.4.3. Immunotherapy

The results of immunotherapy will be addressed from two viewpoints: clinical and immunological. Current studies have also made it possible to relate these two parameters.

a. Clinical Studies. Numerous clinical studies have suggested that traditional whole body insect therapy is effective. These studies are well summarized in the literature and are reviewed by Barr (1971). The most complete study was done by the Insect Committee of the American Academy of Allergy (1972). In this study over 2500 patients who had acute allergic reactions were followed for periods up to 10 years. Five hundred and sixty-nine patients on therapy were restung. Over 95% had less reaction when restung. In contrast, about 65% of 345 patients who did not receive specific whole body immunotherapy had less reaction when restung. These figures have been used to suggest the efficacy of whole body extract therapy. The major deficiencies in this study are the lack of identification of the insect responsible for the initial and subsequent sting, the failure to point out any emergency medication taken by patients at the time of the resting, and the lack of knowledge of the present state of sensitivity at the time of resting. While these factors all may equate in the two groups of patients, it is necessary to point out that they are the important factors relevant to the anticipated reaction following an insect sting. There are comparable reports of other large numbers of patients receiving specific injection therapy and subsequently restung with lower reaction rates (Barr, 1974; Frazier, 1964; Mueller, 1959; Mueller *et al.*, 1975). Similar criticisms apply to these studies.

In recent years treatment failures with whole body extracts have been reported with increased frequency. Subsequently two patients who continued to have reactions despite apparently adequate whole body extract therapy were successfully treated with pure venom. The success of bee venom therapy was documented by the lack of reaction to subsequent stings as well as corroborative immunological studies (Busse *et al.*, 1975; Lichtenstein *et al.*, 1974).

In a more recent blind study comparing the effects of bee venom, whole bee body extract, and placebo in groups of documented sensitive individuals, bee venom was found to be highly successful in protecting the individuals at risk. Whole body extract and placebo were equally ineffective in providing success (Hunt *et al.*, 1978b). Thus in these short-term studies whole body insect extracts were ineffective therapeutic agents. Further studies of venom therapy in large numbers of patients and for longer periods of time suggest that it is highly effective (Amodio *et al.*, 1978; Loveless and Fackler, 1956; Reisman *et al.*, 1978).

b. Immunological Studies. Measurement of venom-specific IgE and venom-specific IgG provide the immunological parameters to evaluate the response to immunotherapy. These antibodies appeared to be a reflection of the "state of allergy" and the "state of immunity."

Sequential serum samples from bee and yellow jacket sensitive individuals have been analyzed for the levels of venom-specific IgE. In the initial study patients were examined who received injection treatment with whole body extracts and compared to an untreated group. Venom-specific IgE decreased in almost all individuals regardless of whether or not injection therapy was administered (Reisman *et al.*, 1976). Subsequent studies have been done analyzing the levels of IgE antibodies in patients receiving venom immunotherapy.

In some patients shortly after initiation of venom immunotherapy there is stimulation of venom-specific IgE. This is quite similar to findings with ragweed immunotherapy. Thus it may be theoretically possible to actually increase the sensitivity early in the course of therapy. With continued and prolonged venom injections, most patients have a declining titer of venom-specific IgE (Reisman *et al.*, 1978; Sobotka *et al.*, 1978). Both the treated and untreated patients show considerable individual variation in the rate of this decrease of IgE antibodies which appears unrelated to the initial antibody titer or to the amount of therapy administered.

As noted previously, following an insect sting and acute allergic reaction individuals occasionally do have elevated levels of bee venom specific IgG (Figure 2). Beekeepers frequently stung and without reaction also have high levels of specific IgG antibodies. Evidence has been accumulated to suggest that these antibodies are related to clinical immunity to insect stings. Following whole body extract therapy there is no stimulation of IgG antibodies reacting with bee venom (Reisman *et al.*, 1976). Thus whole body extracts appear to be immunologically ineffective as measured by this important parameter. In contrast, venom does stimulate the production of specific IgG antibodies. Antibodies appear to be stimulated when doses of venom greater than 1μ are administered. In successfully treated patients in whom a subsequent resting fails to cause an allergic reaction detectable levels of serum venom-specific IgG are present. These IgG antibodies do appear to be the immunological corollary to clinical immunity (Reisman *et al.*, 1978; Sobotka *et al.*, 1978). Thus both clinical and immunological studies indicate that venom is an appropriate agent for the specific immunotherapy. Venoms have recently become available for general use.

Large local reactions due to insect stings also present an unsettled problem. About half the patients have an IgE pathogenesis for these reactions and therefore would be considered possibly at risk for future stings. A small percentage of patients who have had large local reactions do progress and develop systemic reactions. It is our feeling that patients who have had these reactions and have documented specific IgE antibodies are candidates for immunotherapy.

One controversial question remaining today is the use of whole body extracts as therapeutic agents. It is this author's personal opinion that current clinical and immunological evidence cannot support the use of presently available whole body extracts.

3. Fire Ant

The fire ant is in the Hymenoptera order and belongs to the superfamily Formicedae and family Myrmicimae. Two species of imported fire ants, *Solenopsis richteri* and *Solenopsis invicta*, are responsible for the majority of allergic reactions. The fire ant is found in 13 southern states, particularly in the Gulf Coast area, and is responsible for extensive crop damage each year.

In recent years systemic reactions due to the stings of the fire ant have been reported with increased frequency (James *et al.*, 1976); Lockey, 1974; Rhoades *et al.*, 1975; Triplett, 1973). The fire ant attaches itself to its victim by biting with its jaws and then pivots around about the head, stinging in multiple sites in a circular pattern with its stinger located on the abdomen. Within 24 hr of the sting a sterile pustule develops which is diagnostic of the fire ant's sting. Allergic symptoms which occur following such stings are typical of acute anaphylaxis. Symptoms occur within minutes and may involve any of the organ systems.

Skin tests with extracts prepared from whole bodies of fire ants appear to be very reliable in identifying the allergic individuals, with very few false-positive reactions in nonallergic controls (James *et al.*, 1976). Venom of the fire ant has also been used as a diagnostic agent. These results suggest that the antigens

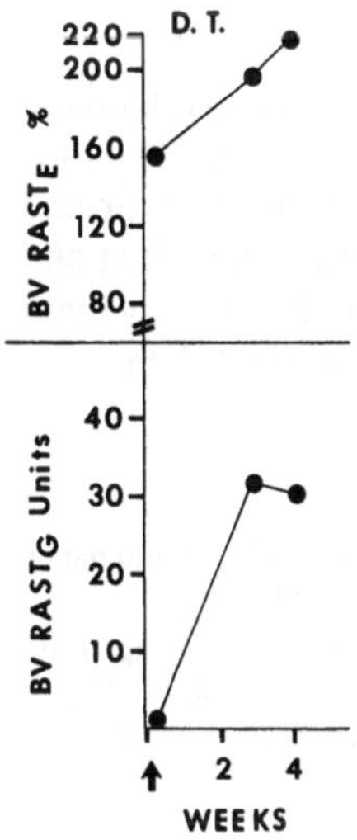

Figure 2. Effect of a sting, causing an anaphylactic reaction, on bee venom specific IgE and IgG. Production of both antibodies was stimulated by this antigenic stimulus. The arrow indicates the sting, and time is measured in weeks. Bee venom specific IgE is measured in RAST % and bee venom specific IgG in units.

responsible for the allergic reaction are either common to the venom and body constituents or possibly unique to the venom and preserved in the body in the preparation of whole body extract.

Fire ant venom has been well studied and does differ considerably from other Hymenoptera venoms. Recent studies (Baer *et al.*, 1977) have shown three allergenic fractions in fire ant venom.

Immunotherapy with whole body fire ant extracts appears to be quite effective. Numerous restings have occurred in treated patients with excellent results. As the whole body fire ant extract is a good diagnostic agent, this therapeutic response might be anticipated. It is important to point out, however, that controlled clinical observations of the response to subsequent stings in allergic individuals not receiving immunotherapy have not been reported. In addition, serological studies defining the nature of immunity to fire ant stings have not been conducted.

Recently anaphylaxis from the sting of the harvester ant *(Pogonomyrmex maricopa, Pogonomyrmex rugosus)*, another kind of nonwinged Hymenoptera, has been described (Pinnas *et al.*, 1977). Specific IgE antibodies were detected by direct skin tests and leukocyte histamine release using harvester ant venom.

4. Biting Insects

A large number of biting insects including the mosquito, flea, black fly, chigger, louse, bed bug, sand fly, and deer fly have been described as the cause of allergic reactions, usually of the local type, both immediate and delayed (Arean and Fox, 1955; Bowen, 1944; Gudgel and Brauer, 1970; Mease, 1943). The mosquito and flea have been most extensively studied (Benson, 1939a; Feingold and Benjamini, 1961; Rockwell and Johnson, 1952). Although immediate skin test reactions have been reported with these insect extracts, demonstration of serum insect specific IgE antibodies has been very difficult. Thus there is poor documentation for an IgE pathogenesis for these biting insect reactions. Delayed skin test reactions with flea extract have correlated with clinical delayed reactions from the actual bites.

Anaphylaxis due to kissing bug and bed bug bites has been described with good documentation (Churchill, 1930; Nichols, 1963; Parson, 1955).

Immunotherapy has been attempted with biting insect extracts, with mixed results. In several studies of flea immunotherapy there were divergent opinions concerning effectiveness (Feingold and Bejamini, 1961; Hatoff, 1946; McIvor and Cherney, 1941). Good therapeutic results have been reported with kissing bug and mosquito extracts. Overall, carefully controlled clinical studies of the effectiveness of biting insect extracts are lacking, as are confirmatory immunological data.

5. References

Amodio, F., Markley, L., Valentine, M. D., Sobotka, A., and Lichtenstein, L. M., 1978, Maintenance immunotherapy for Hymenoptera sensitivity, *J. Allergy Clin. Immunol.*, **61:**134.

Arbesman, C. E., Wypych, J. I., and Reisman, R. E., 1975, Standardization of stinging insect extracts: International WHO-IABS symposium on Standardization and Control of Allergy Administered to Man, Geneva 1974, in: *Development of Biological Standardization*, Vol. 29, pp. 249–257, Karger, Basel.

Arean, V. M., and Fox, I., 1955, Dermal alteration in severe reactions to the bite of the sandfly, *Culicoides furens*, *Am. J. Clin. Pathol.* **25:**1359.

Ashworth, B., 1964, Encephalopathy following a sting, *J. Neurol. Neurosurg. Psychiat.* **27:**542.

Baer, H., Liu, D. T., Hooton, M., Blum, M., James, F., and Schmid, W. H., 1977, Fire ant allergy: Isolation of three allergenic proteins from whole venom, Abstracts of scientific papers of the program of the American Congress of Allergy and Immunology, presented March 26–30, 1977, New York City.

Barnard, J. H., 1970, Nonfatal results in third degree anaphylaxis from Hymenoptera stings, *J. Allergy* **45:**92.

Barnard, J. H., 1973, Studies of 400 Hymenoptera sting deaths in the United States, *J. Allergy Clin. Immunol.* **52:**259.

Barr, S. E., 1971, Allergy to Hymenoptera stings—Review of the world literature 1953–1970, *Ann. Allergy* **29:**49.

Barr, S. E., 1974, Allergy to Hymenoptera stings, *J. Am. Med. Assoc.* **228:**718.

Benson, R. L., 1939a, Diagnosis and treatment of sensitization to mosquitos, *J. Allergy* **8:**47.

Benson, R. L., 1939b, Diagnosis of hypersensitiveness to the bee and to the mosquito, *Arch. Intern. Med.* **64:**1306.

Benson, R. L., and Semenov, H., 1930, Allergy in its relation to bee sting, *J. Allergy* **1:**105.

Benton, A. W., Morse, R. A., and Stuart, J. D., 1963, Venom collection from honeybee, *Science* **142:**228.

Bhoola, K. D., Calle, J. D., and Schachter, M., 1961, Identification of acetylcholine, 5-hydroxytryptamine, histamine and a new kinin in hornet venom *(V. crabro)*, *J. Physiol.* **159:**167.

Bowen, R., 1944, Insects and allergic problems, *South. Med. J.* **44:**836.

Brown, H., and Bernton, H. S., 1970, Allergy to the Hymenoptera, *Arch. Intern. Med.* **125:**665.

Burke, D. M., and Jellinek, H. L., 1954, Nearly fatal case of Schoenlein-Henoch syndrome following insect bites, *Am. J. Dis. Child.* **88:**772.

Busse, W. W., Reed, C. E., Lichtenstein, L. M., and Reisman, R. E., 1975, Immunotherapy in bee-sting anaphylaxis: Use of honeybee venom, *J. Am. Med. Assoc.* **231:**1154.

Chafee, F. H., 1970, The prevalence of bee sting allergy in an allergic population, *Acta Allergol.* **25:**292.

Churchill, T. P., 1930, Urticaria due to bedbug bite, *J. Am. Med. Assoc.* **95:**1975.

Day, J. M., 1962, Death due to cerebral infarction after wasp stings, *Arch. Neurol.* **7:**184.

Feingold, B. F., and Benjamini, E., 1961, Allergy to flea bites: Clinical and experimental observations, *Ann. Allergy* **19:**1275.

Figley, K. D., 1940, May fly (Ephemerida) hypersensitivity, *J. Allergy* **11:**376.

Findley, S. R., Weiner, L. S., Gillaspy, J. E., and Grant, J. A., 1977, Polistes anaphylaxis, Abstracts of scientific papers of the program of the American Congress of Allergy and Immunology, presented March 26–30, 1977, New York City.

Fogel, B. J., Weinberg, T., and Markowitz, M., 1967, A fatal connective tissue disease following a wasp sting, *Am. J. Dis. Child.* **114:**325.

Frazier, C. A., 1964, Allergic reactions to insect stings: A review of 180 cases, *South. Med. J.* **57:**1028.

Goldstein, N. P., Rucker, C. W., and Klass, D. W., 1965, Encephalopathy and papilledema after bee sting, *J. Am. Med. Assoc.* **193:**155.

Gudgel, E. F., and Brauer, F. H., 1970, Acute and chronic reactions to black fly bites (simulium fly), *Arch. Dermatol.* **70:609.**

Hatoff, A., 1946, Desensitization to insect bites, *J. Am. Med. Assoc.* **130:**856.

Hoffman, D. R., Shipman, W. H., and Babin, D., 1977, Allergens in bee venom, II. Two new high molecular weight allergenic specificities, *J. Allergy Clin. Immunol.* **59:**147.

Hunt, K. J., Sobotka, A. K., Valentine, M. D., Zeleznick, L. D., and Lichtenstein, L. M., 1975, Diagnosis of Hymenoptera hypersensitivity by skin testing with Hymenoptera venoms, *J. Allergy Clin. Immunol.* **55:**74.

Hunt, K. J., Sobotka, A. K., Valentine, M. D., Zeleznick, L. D., and Lichtenstein, L. M., 1978a, Sensitization following Hymenoptera whole body extract therapy, *J. Allergy Clin. Immunol.* **61:**48.

Hunt, K. J., Valentine, M. D., Sobotka, A. K., Benton, A. W., Amodio, F. J., and Lichtenstein, L.

M., 1978b, A controlled trial of immunotherapy in insect hypersensitivity, *N. Engl. J. Med.* **249:**157.

Insect Allergy Committee Report, 1972, American Academy of Allergy, unpublished.

Jacques, R., and Schachter, M., 1954, The presence of histamine, 5-hydroxytryptamine and a potent slow contracting substance in wasp venom, *Biol. J. Pharmacol.* **9:**53.

James, F. K., Pence, H. L., Driggers, D. P., Jacobs, R. L., and Horton, D. E., 1976, Imported fire ant hypersensitivity: Studies of human reactions to fire ant venom, *J. Allergy Clin. Immunol.* **58:**110.

Jensen, O. M., 1962, Sudden death due to stings from bees and wasps, *Acta Pathol. Microbiol. Scand.* **54:**9.

Lichtenstein, L. M., Valentine, M. D., and Sobotka, A. K., 1974, A case for venom treatment in anaphylactic sensitivity to hymenoptera sting, *N. Engl. J. Med.* **290:**1223.

Light, W. C., and Reisman, R. E., 1976, Stinging insect allergy: Changing concepts, *Postgrad. Med.* **59:**153.

Light, W. C., Reisman, R. E., Wypych, J. I., and Arbesman, C. E., 1975, Clinical and immunological studies of beekeepers, *Clin. Allergy* **5:**389.

Light, W. C., Reisman, R. E., Ilea, V. S., Wypych, J. I., Okazaki, T., and Arbesman, C. E., 1976a, Studies of the antigenicity and allergenicity of phospholipase A_2 of bee venom, *J. ALlergy Clin. Immunol.* **58:**322.

Light, W. C., Reisman, R. E., Rosario, N. A., and Arbesman, C. E., 1976b, Comparison of the allergenic properties of bee venom and whole bee body extract, *Clin. Allergy* **6:**293.

Light, W. C., Reisman, R. W., Shimizu, M., and Arbesman, C. E., 1977, Unusual reactions following insect stings: Clinical features and immunologic analysis, *J. Allergy Clin. Immunol.* **59:**391.

Lockey, R. F., 1974, Systemic reactions to stinging ants, *J. Allergy Clin. Immunol.* **54:**132.

Loveless, M. H., and Fackler, W. R., 1956, Wasp venom allergy and immunity, *Ann. Allergy* **14:**347.

Markley, L., Amodio, F., Sobotka, A. K., Valentine, M. D., and Lichtenstein, L. M., Immunotherapy with commercial venom preparations. *J. Allergy Clin. Immun.* **61:**134.

McIvor, B. C., and Cherney, L. S., 1941, Studies in insect bite desensitization, *Am. J. Tropical Med.* **21:**493.

Means, E. D., 1973, Nervous system lesions after sting by yellow jacket, *Neurology* **23:**881.

Mease, J. A., 1943, Deer fly desensitization, *J. Am. Med. Assoc.* **122:**227.

Mueller, H. L., 1959, Further experiences with severe allergic reactions to insect stings, *N. Engl. J. Med.* **261:**374.

Mueller, H. L., Schmid, W. H., and Rubinsztain, R., 1975, Stinging insect hypersensitivity: A 20 year study of immunologic treatment, *Pediatrics* **55:**530.

Neumann, W., and Habermann, E., 1954, Beiträge zur Charakterisierung der Wirkstoffe des Bienengiftes. *Arch. Exp. Pathol. Pharmakol.* **222:**367.

Nichols, N., 1963, Allergic reactions to "kissing bug" bites, *Calif. Med.* **98:**267.

O'Connor, R., Stier, R. A., Rosenbrook, W., Jr., and Erickson, R. W., 1964, Death from "wasp" sting, *Ann. Allergy* **22:**385.

Parson, D. J., 1955, Bedbug bite anaphylaxis misinterpreted as coronary occlusion, *Ohio Med. J.* **51:**669.

Pinnas, J. L., Strunk, R. C., Wang, T. M., and Thompson, H. C., 1977, Harvester ant sensitivity: *In vitro* and *in vivo* studies using whole body extracts and venom, *J. Allergy Clin. Immunol.* **59:**10.

Reisman, R. E., Wypych, J. I., and Arbesman, C. E., 1975, Stinging insect allergy: Detection and clinical significance of venom IgE antibodies, *J. Allergy Clin. Immunol.* **56:**443.

Reisman, R. E., Light, W. C., Wypych, J. I., and Arbesman, C. E., 1976, Immunological studies of the effect of whole body insect extracts in the treatment of stinging insect allergy, *J. Allergy Clin. Immunol.* **57:**547.

Reisman, R. E., Arbesman, C. E., and Lazell, M., 1978, Venom immunotherapy, *J. Allergy clin. Immunol.* **61:**135.

Rhoades, R. B., Schafer, W. L., Schmid, W. H., Wubbena, P. F., Dozier, R. M., Townes, A. W., and Wittig, H. L., 1975, Hypersensitivity to the imported fire ant, *J. Allergy Clin. Immunol.* **56:**84.

Rockwell, E. M., and Johnson, P., 1952, The insect bite reactions. II. Evaluation of the allergic reaction, *J. Invest. Dermatol.* **19:**137.

Ross, A. T., 1939, Peripheral neuritis: Allergy to honeybee stings, *J. Allergy* **10:**382.

Rytand, D. A., 1955, Onset of the nephrotic syndrome during a reaction to bee sting, *Stanford Med. Bull.* **13:**224.

Schenken, J. R., Tamisiea, J., and Winter, F. D., 1953, Hypersensitivity to bee sting, *Am. J. Clin. Pathol.* **23:**1216.

Schwartz, H. J., 1965, Skin sensitivity in insect allergy, *J. Am. Med. Assoc.* **194:**113.

Schwartz, H. J., and Kahn, B., 1970, Hymenoptera sensitivity, II. The role of atopy in the development of clinical hypersensitivity, *J. Allergy* **45:**87.

Settipane, G. A., and Boyd, G. K., 1970, Prevalence of bee sting allergy in 4,992 Boy Scouts, *Acta Allergol.* **25:**286.

Sheehan, R. K., 1965, Serum sickness and recurrent angioedema after bee sting, *J. Am. Med. Assoc.* **193:**155.

Shepherd, G. W., Elliott, W. B., and Arbesman, C. E., 1974, Fractionation of bee venom. I. Preparation and characterization of four antigenic components, *Prep. Biochem.* **4:**71.

Shulman, S., 1968, Insect allergy: Biochemical and immunological analysis of the allergens, in: *Progress in Allergy,* Vol. 12 (P. Kallos and B. H. Waksman, eds.), pp. 246–317, Karger, New York.

Sobotka, A. K., Franklin, R., Valentine, M. D., Adkinson, N. F., and Lichtenstein, L. M., 1974a, Honeybee venom: Phospholipase A as the major allergen, *J. Allergy Clin. Immunol.* **53:**103.

Sobotka, A. K., Valentine, M. D., Benton, A. W., and Lichtenstein, L. M., 1974b, Allergy to insect stings. I. Diagnosis of IgE-mediated Hymenoptera sensitivity to venom-induced histamine release, *J. Allergy Clin. Immunol.* **53:**170.

Sobotka, A. K., Valentine, M. D., and Lichtenstein, L. M., 1978, The immune response to hymenoptera venoms, *J. Allergy Clin. Immunol.* **61:**136.

Triplett, R. F., 1973, Sensitivity to the imported fire ant: Successful treatment with immunotherapy, *South. Med. J.* **66:**477.

Venters, H. D., Vernier, R. L., Worthen, H. G., and Good, R. A., 1961, Bee sting nephrosis: A study of the immunopathologic mechanisms, *Am. J. Dis. Child.* **102:**688.

Yocum, M. W., Johnstone, D. E., and Condemi, J. J., 1973, Leukocyte histamine release in Hymenoptera allergic patients, *J. Allergy Clin. Immunol.* **52:**265.

12

Nasal Hypersensitivity

JOHN T. CONNELL

1. Introduction

The nose weeps and obstructs for a variety of reasons, some physiological and some pathological. An understanding of these reasons is necessary to diagnose and treat patients, but our current concepts of why the nose weeps and obstructs are fragmentary.

"Nasal hypersensitivity" is a phrase used to indicate hyperreactive response of the nasal mucosa. Rhinorrhea, a normal reaction, may be increased and incite nose blowing, sneezing, and postnasal drip. Congestion may occur with or without rhinorrhea. In addition, pathological symptoms such as itching and anosmia may be present. Pain is relatively infrequent and is usually associated with pathology of the sinuses. Classically, one almost always thought of an IgE-mediated allergic rhinitis as the underlying pathology, whether or not an offending antigen could be identified. More recent information, derived from studies of cell biology, immunology, chemistry, and histology, indicates that diseases other than allergic rhinitis may be the cause of some of these symptoms. The purpose of this chapter is to review nasal disease by clinical syndromes and then to explore other explanations for nasal symptoms. In so doing, some speculation will be employed where definitive knowledge is lacking.

How and why may nasal hypersensitivity occur? The nasal mucosa is exposed to a variety of stimuli; it is exposed to environmental air, has a complex nervous system, and has a rich vascular supply. Normal functions of the nose include preparation of inspired air for the lower respiratory tract and olfaction. During every 24 hr the nasal mucosa removes particles greater than 5 μm and noxious gases from as much as 20 m^3 of inspired air; a liter of fluid is added to humidify the air; and up to 10% of body heat may be expended to warm the air. The ambient air usually contains a number of contaminants such as pollen and various dusts and chemicals in the form of solids or gases. Removal of the contaminants from

JOHN T. CONNELL • Nasal Diseases Study Center, Holy Name Hospital, Teaneck, New Jersey 07666.

the airstream onto the mucosa may incite symptoms through allergic, immune, pharmacological, or physical mechanisms. The rich vascular supply of the nose exposes it to a myriad of ingested and digested allergens and chemicals and products or by-products of systemic activities such as mediators and hormones. The neurogenic system of the nose, through parasympathetic and sympathetic pathways, may be the source of abnormal or excessive stimuli which could cause symptoms.

2. Common Syndromes of Nasal Disease

When many cases of rhinitis are associated with a number of similar features, the similarities tend to suggest that a unique clinical entity is present. Over the years a number of syndromes evolved which were based primarily on clinical observations and laboratory findings. Where substantial evidence exists, the syndrome is recognized as a disease, such as with allergic rhinitis. On the other hand, other syndromes, such as vasomotor rhinitis, are more tenuous and may actually represent one or more unique diseases.

In the following section the syndromes associated with rhinitis are presented, recognizing that substantial differences of opinion may exist among different physicians as to their authenticity.

2.1. Seasonal Allergic Rhinitis

Symptoms of seasonal allergic rhinitis are rhinorrhea associated with sneezing and nose blowing, varying degrees of congestion, and nasal itching. Lacrimation and itching of the eyes, indicating allergic conjunctivitis, and itching of the ears and throat often accompany the nasal symptoms. The symptoms occur at specific times of the year, coinciding with the presence of pollens or mold spores in the environment. For example, ragweed pollen is in the air during the last 2 weeks of August and most of the month of September, at which times patients sensitive to the pollen have symptoms. This diagnosis is confirmed by positive skin tests or other methods for demonstrating IgE-specific antibody. Eosinophils are found in the nasal smears of about 70% of patients. The findings of an allergic factor clearly associated with the symptoms described at a specific time of the year are highly suggestive of disease associated with immunological perturbations. Little difficulty is encountered in making the diagnosis in typical cases. In fact, the patients themselves often make the correct diagnosis.

2.2. Perennial Allergic Rhinitis

Some patients with a nonseasonal and chronic pattern of symptoms found in seasonal allergic rhinitis are thought to have a perennial form of the disease. Again, the diagnosis is confirmed when antigen-specific antibody can be identified in the sera from these patients and the patients have exacerbations of symptoms when exposed to the specific antigen. The antigens commonly associated with perennial symptoms are dust, feather pillows, and animal dander, but may be almost any airborne particle in the environment capable of sensitizing an individual. Dust, the substance most frequently incriminated, may cause allergic symptoms due to allergens in the dust. In addition, physical irritation or nonallergic chemical contents of the dust can incite rhinorrhea via nonimmune mechanisms. Difficulties may be encountered in making the diagnosis of perennial allergic rhinitis. Symptoms of some degree are often present continually, and recognition of those due to specific exposures to antigens is difficult or impossible. The association of exacerbations of symptoms to nonallergic stimuli such as weather changes, odors, and psychological factors, to name a few, may cloud the issue. Then, too, many patients have positive skin tests (Hagy and Settipane, 1976) or RAST (radioactive immunoadsorbent test) (Wide *et al.*, 1967) but for yet unknown reasons do not have symptoms. Thus the diagnosis of perennial allergic rhinitis is much more tenuous than that of seasonal rhinitis. There is a possibility that many of the symptoms in patients with chronic rhinitis are not IgE mediated but may evolve because of other mechanisms.

A further aid to the diagnosis of allergic rhinitis is a family history of allergy (Kallio *et al.*, 1966). This association has been recognized clinically for years. Only recently have genetic studies (Levine *et al.*, 1973; Marsh *et al.*, 1974) confirmed that genes play a role in determining the inheritance of the disease, although the exact nature of the transmission is unkown.

Laboratory tests are useful in confirming the diagnosis. The skin test and RAST have already been mentioned. An elevated total serum IgE level is suggestive of the allergic diathesis (Gleich *et al.*, 1971), although a few patients with elevated IgE may not have clinical symptoms while some with low IgE may have symptoms. Histamine release caused by exposure of peripheral basophils to specific antigen is an excellent indicator of hypersensitivity but is currently impractical as a routine clinical procedure. A provocative inhalation challenge of a patient with suspected allergy is a reasonable procedure, but it has many limitations and should be employed only with adequate controls. The major limitations are that only one antigen should be tested at a time since symptoms could occur immediately or their onset be delayed for some hours. Although a reaction might appear to be precipitated by a challenge, there is no proof that the reaction is immunologically mediated. Even though eosinophils are found in 70% of patients with uncomplicated allergic rhinitis, peripheral blood eosinophilia is usually less than 5%.

Physical examination of the nares is not diagnostic. In most cases the turbinates are edematous, although about 20% of patients do not have edema despite severe symptoms. Rhinorrhea is usually present; the nasal discharge is watery and clear. Almost every color has been used to describe the nasal mucosa, making this criterion of little value. The usual color in patients with ragweed hay fever is pale pink, but the membrane may have a different appearance in the chronic state.

The pathophysiology of allergic rhinitis is the genetic predisposition for the production of the IgE class of immunoglobulin, unknown conditions or stimuli which sensitize the IgE system to specific antigens, and attachment of the specific IgE molecules to the surface of mast cells. Subsequent exposure to the antigen results in binding of the antigen to the IgE molecules on sensitized mast cells, activating the mast cells to release histamine and possibly other vasoactive substances. The mediators secreted and released by the mast cells cause capillary dilatation and increase permeability, cholinergic stimulation causes glandular secretion of mucus, and stimulations of afferent nerve fibers cause itching.

Treatment of allergic rhinitis centers on the search for offending antigens. If these can be identified and eliminated, no other form of therapy is necessary. When antigen cannot be eliminated, hyposensitization therapy may reduce the severity of symptoms.

Nonspecific therapy includes a variety of drugs acting on different mechanisms. It should be noted that none of these prevents the union of antigen with the antigen-specific antibody on the mast cells; the drugs suppress mediator formation or release, compete with mediators at target cell receptor sites, reverse the effects of mediators on target tissues, or affect the cholinergic system.

Cromolyn sodium is thought to act on enzymatic systems within the mast cell, thereby preventing secretion of histamine (Cox, 1971; Lavin *et al.*, 1976). Corticosteroids may have an effect on the mast cell, but also act on target cells (Claman, 1975). Antihistamines compete with histamine released by the mast cell for H-1 receptor sites on target tissues. Antihistamines may have an additional role by blocking cholinergic stimuli and hence reducing rhinorrhea and associated symptoms. H-2 antihistamines have not been investigated thoroughly enough to determine whether or not they will be of significance in IgE-mediated disease. Atropine or atropinelike drugs inhibit the muscarinic effects of acetylcholine transmission. Decongestants reverse congestion by stimulating α-receptors on target cells, promoting vasoconstriction.

Even with the medications described above, symptoms are only partially and temporarily relieved. Many patients become refractory to their use. None of the drugs alters the basic course of the disease.

Complications in seasonal allergic rhinitis are rare. They may be more significant in perennial allergic rhinitis because of the prolonged duration of symptomatic episodes. Asthma is said to occur more frequently as a result of lack of hyposensitization (Sherman, 1968). However, the occurrence of asthma and hay fever simultaneously in the same individual may merely be coincidental and not related to hyposensitization. Nasal polyps sometimes occur but apparently in no greater incidence than that found in the nonatopic population. Younger patients have a higher incidence of middle ear problems, probably related to edema of the eustachian tubes. Sinus infections occur much more rarely than one might expect considering the severity of nasal obstruction.

2.3. Nonatopic or Infectious Rhinitis

"Nonatopic rhinitis," "infectious rhinitis," and "bacterial allergy" are terms used to signify that the disease process is not related to inhalant antigens but is in some manner thought to be caused by or associated with allergy to bacteria. The patients have a history of chronic nasal symptoms that is vaguely associated with episodes of suspected nasal infection. Exacerbation of symptoms coincides with or persists for a prolonged time after the infectious process subsides. Cooke (1947) postulated that the condition was related to bacteria or bacterial products. Efforts to elucidate offending bacterial antigens by immediate wheal and erythema skin tests have been, with rare exceptions, fruitful (Hampton *et al.*, 1963) but in most studies nonproductive (Swineford and Holman, 1949). One of the most compelling pieces of evidence supporting the hypothesis is that the symptoms may be reproduced in some patients by the injection of bacterial vaccines (Cooke, 1947). Interpretation of results of cultures of the nasopharynx is confusing since they may vary from time to time in the same patient. Even more tenuous is the assumption that the organism cultured is related to the disease process. Although allergic reactions to some bacteria or bacterial products (Cooke, 1947) are well recognized in other areas of medicine, little positive evidence exists to indicate that the mechanism is a frequent cause of chronic nasal disease.

The syndrome is vague, and that it actually exists is doubted by many physicians. On the other hand, there is such a preponderance of evidence associating bacteria to allergic and immune reactions that it is difficult not to believe a relationship to nasal disease exists, albeit the nature and incidence of the relationship are unclear. Since there are no well-defined diagnostic criteria, and there is doubt as to who may or may not have the disease, laboratory tests and characteristic physical findings are not defined.

Those who believe that the condition represents bacterial allergy employ a course of injection therapy with a mixed bacterial vaccine or a vaccine prepared from autogenous cultures of the nose and throat. Antihistamines and decongestants are relatively ineffective. Corticosteroids provide relief, but, since the disease is chronic, use of steroids is prolonged and potential side-effects must be considered. Surgery of the sinuses when abnormal was popular in the past but has now been abandoned.

2.4. Vasomotor Rhinitis

"Vasomotor rhinitis" is a term used to describe a syndrome of episodic chronic rhinitis characterized by acute onset of rhinorrhea and congestion. Nasal pruritis is absent or at least not prominent in most cases. Stimuli inciting attacks vary from patient to patient and for the same patient, and may include physical stimuli, inhalation of chemicals and gases, and psychological changes. Many patients do not recognize specific triggers of acute attacks. The physical findings usually described are a markedly edematous, pale membrane and a copious, clear discharge. Allergic stigmata and genetic predisposition are absent. IgE levels, if determined, are most often in the normal range. The nasal secretions are acellular except for epithelial cells. Unfortunately, diagnostic criteria vary from physician to physician, and the diagnois is frequently resorted to in lieu of positive findings. In essence, vasomotor rhinitis should be considered a syndrome and not a disease.

Nonspecific drug therapy as described for allergic rhinitis should be tried. In general, most patients are refractory to drug therapy and no effective treatment is known.

2.5. Rhinitis Medicamentosa

"Rhinitis medicamentosa" is a clinical condition brought on by excessive use of topical decongestants or systemic ingestion of some drugs. α-Adrenergic agonists are the prime topical offenders. Excessive use of these drugs causes "rebound phenomena," a condition in which use of the drug produces temporary decongestion which is rapidly followed by congestion more marked than that present ititially. The pharmacological mechanisms involved are not known. The drugs have no effect on the postganglionic nerve terminal or norepinephrine; the most likely site of action is on the target cell. The target cells, muscles of arterioles, theoretically could become depleted of metabolites through repeated and prolonged stimulation and dilate, leading to congestion.

Some antihypertensive agents may initiate nasal congestion through their action on norepinephrine storage in the postganglionic sympathetic nerves. Reserpine replaces and occupies the place of norepinephrine in storage areas (Norn and Shore, 1971). Guanethidine releases norepinephrine (Boura and Green, 1965) from the nerve terminal, producing a temporary adrenergic response. Continued use of guanethidine results in depletion of norepinephrine. Reduction of norepinephrine stores decreases the availability of the transmitter for the normal adrenergic stimulation of α-receptors on target cells. The result in some patients is vasodilatation and nasal congestion.

β-Stimulators are agents with the potential of causing nasal congestion through stimulation of β-receptors on target cells, leading to vasodilatation. β-Stimulators are not usually used in the nose, but we (Connell, 1973) have shown that a nasal spray of Salbutamol causes marked congestion. The possibility exists that systemic use of β-stimulators may bring on or aggravate congestion in some patients with chronic rhinitis.

Rhinitis and nasal congestion have been associated with a variety of conditions having to do with hormones in the female, such as the "rhinitis of pregnancy" and use of birth control pills. The hormones involved or the manner in which they cause symptoms is unknown.

When symptoms coincide with the use of oral medications, the diagnosis of rhinitis medicamentosa should be suspected. Frequently, a change in dose or formulation, or elimination of the medication, will be associated with a decrease in nasal symptoms. Only about one-third of patients in whom abuse of topical agents is suspected will improve with elimination of the drug. Those who do not improve most likely have underlying nasal disease for which the medication was first employed.

2.6. Anatomical Lesions as a Cause of Rhinitis

One frequent cause of rhinitis and nasal obstruction is an anatomical lesion, the most common being a deviated nasal septum. The reason for the obstruction is evident on physical examination, but an explanation for the rhinorrhea is unknown. Little attention has been given to the cycling of the nares in this regard. Normally, one nostril is more patent than the other, a condition persisting for 1–3 hr. There is less resistance to inspiration in the more patent nostril and consequently more air flows through it. It performs the work of filtering, humidifying, and heating inspired air. In time, the patent nostril becomes physiologically exhausted and congestion ensues. The contralateral naris simultaneously becomes decongested and assumes the work of breathing. The process described is analogous to the functional reserve observed in the kidney, lung, etc. When unilateral anatomical obstruction is present, the work of breathing is of necessity carried on by the unobstructed naris. Hypertrophy of the turbinate on the unobstructed side is a consequence, and rhinorrhea is frequently observed on this side. Surgical repair eliminates the obstruction and rhinorrhea eventually ceases, indicating that no other nasal disease exists. Anatomical obstruction or other disease which prohibits the congestion–decongestion reflexes from occurring normally may bring on nasal mucosal disease of an as yet undefined nature.

2.7. Neurogenic Rhinitis

The neurogenic supply to the nose supplying the vasculature and glands is by way of the sympathetic and parasympathetic systems. Hypothalamic tracts are involved in this pathway. Afferent fibers conducting the sensations of pain and itch are carried by the second division of the trigeminal nerve. The parasympathetic system primarily supplies the nasal glands. In normals, the parasympathetic supply has little effect on vasodilatation. It is possible that patients with nasal disease could react differently. The sympathetic system innervates arteries and arterioles and causes vasoconstriction through α-adrenergic receptors on target cells. One hypothesis explaining excessive rhinorrhea in neurogenic rhinitis is that the parasympathetic system or hypothalamic tracts are overreactive (Golding-Wood, 1970), causing overabundant secretions. Evidence to support such a hypothesis is for the most part derived from surgical or medical denervation of the parasympathetic system in patients with chronic rhinitis of the neurogenic type. Severing the vidian nerve, vidian neurectomy (Golding-Wood, 1970), produces almost immediate relief of the previously intractable rhinitis and suggests a cause-and-effect relationship. Relapse may occur in a year or so, a period of time compatible with nerve regeneration. If congestion is the major symptom, one possible explanation is an imbalance in α- and β-receptors opposite to that found in the lung (Szentivanyi and Fishel, 1965). We (Connell, 1973) have shown in man that Salbutomal, a β-agonist, causes nasal congestion, suggesting that β-stimulation of the nasal vasculature results in nasal congestion.

The neurogenic system plays a large role in the state of congestion through reflex arcs. A stream of air directed at one cornea causes contralateral nasal congestion (Solomon, 1967). Stimuli administered unilaterally, such as drugs or inhalation of pollen in an allergic individual, cause a unilateral change in congestion on the side stimulated and an opposite change in congestion on the contralateral side (Connell, 1968a).

Exercise causes marked decongestion of the nose. Whether this occurs through the neurogenic system or because of mediators via the blood is unknown. Clinicians have noted that in some individuals sexual excitement frequently leads to severe rhinorrhea, sneezing, and congestion. Both the nasal mucosa and the genitals have a rich parasympathetic supply. Hyperactivity of the parasympathetic system could stimulate both organs.

Indeed, if neurogenic rhinitis is caused by a defect in the parasympathetic supply to the nose and the defect is in the postganglionic neuron or target cell receptor site, the most conservative treatment is the use of local or systemic atropine. Injection of an anesthetic into parasympathetic ganglia is another approach, producing temporary parasympathetic blockade. If successful, an injection into the ganglia with a destructive compound such as alcohol can provide more permanent relief. Vidian neurectomy, which is a formidable surgical procedure, should be utilized only as a last resort and only in intractable rhinitis. Since nerves do not cross the midline, the procedure should be done bilaterally for best results.

2.8. Food Intolerance as a Cause of Rhinitis

Food intolerance may be of the immediate hypersensitivity type (IgE mediated)(May, 1976b) or of type(s) as yet undescribed. Some patients have nasal symptoms soon after ingesting specific food, and, in addition, have positive skin tests to that food. This condition, to a great extent, resembles allergic rhinitis with the exception that the antigen is ingested rather than inhaled. On the other hand, a significant number of patients have nasal symptoms at some time after ingesting a specific substance but do not have positive skin tests to that substance. An important example is rhinitis within minutes of ingesting alcohol, a relatively common finding in a significant number of patients with rhinitis. In these cases, the chemical may either be acting as a pharmacological agent or be partaking in a non-IgE-mediated immune reaction. If it is acting as a pharmacological agent, an additional requirement is a malfunction or abnormality of some other factor(s); otherwise, everyone would experience the symptom.

The treatment of choice in food idiosyncrasy is the identification and avoidance of offending foods.

2.9. Hormonal Rhinitis

The possible role of female hormones in producing rhinitis was previously mentioned under ''rhinitis medicamentosa.'' The manner in which these hormones cause rhinitis is unknown. It is significant that the vasculature of the genitalia and that of the nasal mucosa are of similar anatomical structure, being of the ''erectile'' type. A nasal smear of secretions from the nose of a premenstrual woman dries in a ''fern'' pattern, much as a vaginal smear would if obtained at the same time, illustrating an additional similarity between the two organs. Since progesterone increases vascularity and glandular secretion in the genitalia, it may also promote the same changes in the nose.

Some patients with hypothyroidism also have rhinitis and congestion. It is not clear whether this type of rhinitis is on a hormonal basis or is merely the result of thickening and edema of the subcutaneous tissues associated with hypothyroidism.

2.10. Atrophic Rhinitis

''Atrophic rhinitis'' is a condition in which the turbinates are small, the mucosa is thin, glandular secretion is scant, and dried crusts are frequently adherent to the mucosa. Subjectively, the patient complains of severe nasal congestion. The subjective sensation of congestion is at variance with the physiological state, for if airflow measurements are made objectively the nares are found to be excessively patent. Perhaps the most common cause of atrophic rhinitis, at least in its mildest form, is aging. Airway studies indicate a decreasing resistance to the flow of air with advancing years.

Other causes are extensive nasal surgery, Wegener's midline granulomatosis, and idiopathic atrophy in young people. Fortunately, these conditions are rare.

Atrophic rhinitis is said to be improved by surgical transplantation of bone or cartilage under the nasal mucosa (Togawa and Konno, 1976). In so doing, obstruction is increased, and, paradoxically, the patient loses the sensation of congestion. Estrogens have been tried with the hope that they will increase congestion of the turbinates.

2.11. Chemical Rhinitis

Some chemicals (soap powder) and gases (sulfur dioxide) have a proclivity for producing rhinitis. For the most part, the rhinorrhea is a physiological reaction, an attempt by the nose to clear irritating substances. The condition may be clinically significant in some individuals as an occupational or other hazard where continual exposure to such substances exists.

2.12. Rhinitis Associated with Nasal Polyps

Nasal polyps are grapelike structures which arise from the posterior nasal mucosa and most often from the mucosa of the sphenoid sinus. They extend into the nasal cavity where they are easily recognized by physical examination. They occlude the nares by varying degrees, often causing the patient to seek medical advice because he or she cannot breathe through the nose.

The etiology of nasal polyps is unknown. They occur no more frequently in patients with seasonal allergic rhinitis than in the general population (1% incidence in both groups) (Connell, 1974). They were commonly believed to be allergic in origin (Kern and Schenck, 1923), but this opinion is changing. Settipane and Chafee (1977) reported interesting statistics of nasal polyps in asthma and rhinitis in a total population of 4986. The frequency of nasal polyps was 4.2% in the total population, 6.7% in the asthmatic portion of the population, and 2.2% in that portion of the population having only rhinitis. Asthmatics with negative skin tests to allergens had significantly more polyps than asthmatics with positive skin tests (12.5% vs. 5.0%). The frequency of polyps increased with age. Of the total 211 cases of nasal polyps, 71% involved asthma and 29% involved rhinitis alone.

Histologically, polyps are relatively simple structures with a thin layer of epithelium, primitive basement membrane, and an unorganized system of meager connective tissue. The cellular contents of a polyp almost always include eosinophils, plasma cells, and lymphocytes. Mast cells are found in some polyps. These are cells intimately associated with the immune system, and it is not unexpected that the polyp contains most types of antibodies and other metabolites or mediators of the immune system. The cellular contents would strongly suggest that polyps have some relationship to immunity, but whether their formation is a purposeful one or totally disorganized remains to be determined. In any event, the polyp seems to be a small, localized "immunological factory." Patients with polyps almost always have rhinitis. The mucosa itself is grossly abnormal, appearing to be almost white or a very pale pink, and is frequently edematous.

The treatment of nasal polyps is empirical since their cause is unknown. If they occur in an atopic individual, hyposensitization therapy is tried, although there are no controlled studies to show that the therapy alters the course of nasal polyposis. Systemic or topical corticosteriods may provide temporary relief, and occasionally polyps may disappear with such therapy. That corticosteroids cause some polyps to shrink is expected since steroids cause a reduction in eosinophilia and lymphopenia. When polyps cause severe obstruction, as they often do, they should be surgically excised and an ethmoidectomy performed. Most discouraging to the patient and physician is that new polyps are frequently generated and additional polypectomies may be necessary.

2.13. Psychosomatic Rhinitis

Many patients and physicians consider rhinitis triggered by psychic stimuli as a clinical entity of psychosomatic origin. It cannot be denied that the symptoms of some patients are triggered by emotional stimuli. One interpretation of this finding is that the disease is psychosomatic, but this conclusion does not answer the question "why don't all people undergoing the same stress have the same nasal symptoms?" An alternative interpretation is that an organic pathological mechanism exists which is triggered by psychic stimuli. My own experience is that patients referred for psychosomatic rhinitis almost always have a histological lesion of the mucosa demonstrated by nasal biopsy, and, in reality, have organic disease.

3. Incidence of the Syndromes of Nasal Disease

The incidence of seasonal allergic rhinitis (Sherman, 1968) is about 5–10% of the population.

The incidence of chronic nasal disease is much more difficult to assess. No published figures are available describing its incidence. That it is prevalent is not disputed. For example, in a study of postnasal drip in an urban community (Connell, 1978), 150 individuals responded to a newspaper ad run only 3 days. All had chronic nasal symptoms for which they used over-the-counter preparations or home remedies or ignored because of previous therapeutic failures. Less than 2% were currently being treated by a physician. This example would suggest that chronic nasal disease is even more prevalent than allergy. An examination of physicians' records to determine the true incidence is fruitless, for the allergists' figures are slanted favoring allergic rhinitis and the rhinologists' records are skewed to the nonallergic diseases. Probably the most important factor distorting the incidence of specific nasal diseases is that the diagnostic criteria are inexact and the diagnoses arrived at, to a great extent, reflect the training and prejudices of the individual physician rather than the occurrence of the diseases.

An educated guess as to the occurrence of each disease entity is useful to illustrate our lack of knowledge in this area. Allergic rhinitis is the probable cause of symptoms in 15–30% of patients with chronic nasal disease. Anatomical lesions (primarily deviated septum) account for another 5–10%. Rhinitis medicamentosa is found in less than 3%, and, as stated, a chronic nasal disease underlies medicamentosa in most cases. Neurogenic, hormonal, atrophic, chemical, and polyp-associated rhinitis each account for less than 3%. The total incidence of the diseases enumerated thus far is less than 50%, indicating our lack of understanding of chronic nasal disease. As indicated in the text, the incidence of "nonatopic rhinitis" (or "infectious rhinitis" or "bacterial allergy"), "vasomotor rhinitis," and the rhinitis of food intolerance will vary tremendously with the individual physician's preference for a particular diagnosis. For some physicians inclusion of these last entities will ensure that they diagnose 100% of their cases. For other physicians, these entities will not be entirely acceptable and the cases will be classified as "etiology unknown."

4. Histological Classification of Nasal Disease

The foregoing description of the incidence of specific clinical entities of chronic nasal disease emphasizes the need for additional research. Of necessity, investigation by many disciplines of science will be required.

One approach to the problem is histological evaluation of the nasal mucosa. Considering the relative ease with which specimens of nasal tissue may be obtained, it is unfortunate that this approach has been so underutilized. In my own laboratory, we have studied biopsies from over 1300 patients in the last 10 years. The data obtained thus far reinforce some of the clinical syndromes described, introduce new diagnostic possibilities, and indicate more fruitful avenues of investigation. The following section describes these findings (Connell, 1977). An attempt is made to classify the histological findings by probable mechanisms. Since light microscopy is applicable only to certain types of pathology, the classification, as expected, falls short of solving the problem and raises additional questions which can only be answered by other disciplines.

Certain reservations should be made regarding the evaluation of histopathology. Histopathological features represent the state of a small piece of tissue at the time it was removed from the body. These features could vary from one time to another. Or the histological changes could be different in different parts of the mucosa. In practice, these criticisms are true for some cases, but in the majority of patients with chronic rhinitis pathological changes remain qualitatively, if not quantitatively, similar from time to time, judging by repeat biopsies, and from area to area when the specimen is large enough to make this judgment.

A very significant danger in attempting to classify diseases by histological findings is that some diseases may appear dissimilar at different times depending on exposure to antigen or other factors. The stages, which differ histologically, may, in error, be classified as two different diseases. Another important potential error is that two or more diseases may occur simultaneously and histological evidence for both be found in the same biopsy. These findings could be erroneously interpreted as a unique disease.

4.1. Normal Histology of the Nasal Membrane

The normal mucosa is briefly described for purposes of comparison with abnormal mucosa. The external lining of the nasal mucosa is ciliated columnar epithelium and goblet cells. The goblet cells secrete a mucous blanket which is propelled toward the posterior nares by the cilia. Fenestrated capillaries pierce the epithelium and emit a fluid less viscous than mucus which is required for humidification of inspired air (Cauna and Hinderer, 1969).

A basement membrane underlies the epithelial cells. Structurally, it appears as a thin, condensed outer layer and a less dense, but thicker inner layer. Both layers are acellular. The basement membrane is made up of complex glycoproteins and is probably a barrier to prevent solid or soluble products from penetrating the epithelium.

The tunica propria lies beneath the basement membrane and is composed of histiocytes, collagenous fibrils parallel to the basement membrane, vascular structures, and glands. Mast cells are scattered throughout the tunica and normally number 200–400/mm^3 of tissue. Eosinophils, lymphocytes, and plasma cells are rare in the normal mucosa.

4.2. Abnormal Histological Features Suggesting Nonimmunological Causes of Nasal Disease

4.2.1. Abnormalities of the Epithelium

Squamous cell epithelium is found in some cases of rhinitis. It rarely even has a cornified external layer. Squamous cells neither secrete mucous nor have cilia to propel the mucous blanket over the mucosal surface. Fenestrated capillaries, the probable source of fluid for humidification of inspired air, do not pierce the squamous cell epithelium as they do the columnar epithelium. Thus humidification, heating, and filtering functions of the nose are ablated by squamous epithelium. A squamous cell epithelium may coincide with the clinical diagnosis of atrophic rhinitis in some cases. The amount of secretion in the goblet cells, when they are present, is easily judged by special staining techniques. In the majority of cases, very little secretion is found in the goblet cells, but in a few cases the secretion is profuse. For example, in acute coryza, the goblet cells bulge with secretion. No clinical correlates have been made regarding the amount of or absence of secretion.

4.2.2. Basement Membrane Abnormalities

The basement membrane is postulated to be a barrier to penetration of foreign material. It appears to be thin or destroyed in patients who have had symptoms of IgE-mediated allergic rhinitis for some period of days.

A poorly developed basement membrane of the mucosa of the turbinates is almost always found in patients who have nasal polyps even though the turbinate mucosa is distinct and distant from the actual polyps. The explanation for this finding is not known, but patients with polyps have the same type of infiltrating cells as patients with allergic rhinitis. The similarity in infiltrating cells may be significant and in some way related to basement membrane destruction.

Basement membrane damage is occasionally seen in patients without apparent IgE disease or nasal polyps. Its meaning is unknown in these cases.

4.2.3. Absence of Cellular Infiltrates

In about 3% of patients biopsied, there is a complete absence of infiltrating cells of the immune system. The basement membrane is normal, as is the mast cell count. The only histological abnormality is severe edema.

The meager histological findings are surprising considering the severe symptoms and gross physical abnormalities found clinically. The mucosa is usually very pale, with markedly congested turbinates and copious, watery discharge. Symptoms are congestion and rhinorrhea, but nasal pruritis is usually absent. Eye symptoms do not accompany the condition.

The histological findings are compatible with a diagnosis of neurogenic rhinitis or hormonal rhinitis. Vasomotor rhinitis was described as a syndrome, and some clinical cases of the syndrome could well involve this type of pathology.

The absence of infiltrating cells is consistent with mechanisms described for neurogenic disease of the nose. Excessive parasympathetic stimulation would be expected to produce chemical abnormalities not detectable with light microscopy. One result of parasympathetic stimulation would be rhinorrhea. Similarly, hormonal influences would be expected to affect metabolic events, which again would not be visible. Infiltrates in the nasal mucosa would not be anticipated with hormonal disease.

The histological finding of edema in the absence of infiltrates could also be due to rhinitis medicamentosa. As described, rhinitis medicamentosa either is a biochemical disease of the postganglionic sympathetic neurons or is due to exhaustion of metabolites of the target cells. In either case, pathophysiological events cannot be detected with the microscope. In cases of rhinitis medicamentosa associated with a chronic nasal disease, cellular infiltrates would be expected, and would represent the pathology of the chronic nasal disease.

4.3. Abnormal Infiltrates Suggesting Nonimmunological Causes of Nasal Disease

4.3.1. Eosinophilic Infiltrates

An eosinophilic infiltrate not associated with any other abnormality is found in about 4% of nasal biopsies. Furthermore, in the patients who have these infiltrates, there is nothing in the history to suggest an IgE-mediated allergic rhinitis. IgE levels are normal. The patients complain of rhinorrhea but even more of congestion. Nasal pruritis is present in some cases but absent in most. Clinically, the mucosa varies from white to pale, or brownish-yellow, unlike that seen in allergic rhinitis.

Cases of this sort raise the question of whether or not the eosinophil can be present in a disease not associated with an immune reaction. For instance, mast cells may be capable of releasing ECF because of nonimmune stimuli. Infiltrates of eosinophils frequently seen in skin lesions of mastocytosis may represent nonimmune release of ECF. Or the spontaneous release of histamine from mast cells described by May (1976a) may be paralleled by spontaneous release of ECF. In another example, eosinophils infiltrate the myocardium beginning about 8–14 days after a myocardial infarction (Mallory *et al.*, 1939). The cause of the infiltrate is not known, but certainly an IgE-mediated reaction is not suspected. On the other hand, the lack of eosinophilic infiltrates in the 8–14 day period after infarction is reminiscent of the time required for a primary immune response to occur. Could it be that a primary immune response develops to some component of the infarcted tissue and only then are eosinophils found, or is this a nonimmune infiltrate? The question of whether or not the eosinophils play a role in nonimmune diseases cannot be answered with certainty at this time.

Another extremely important question regarding the role of the eosinophil is "can the eosinophil itself cause symptoms and disease?" The eosinophil contains arylsulfatase, a strongly basic chemical, various lysozymes, and main basic protein (Gleich, 1977). Arylsulfatase and lysozymes could be quite toxic if released in tissues. It is dangerous to overinterpret histological observations, but in cases of eosinophilic infiltrates it may be significant that many eosinophils appear to be ruptured, with granules spread into surrounding tissue. The findings do not appear to be artifacts and suggest the possibility that the eosinophil may be responsible for many of the symptoms observed. The mechanism(s) that might cause release of the contents of the eosinophil is not clearly understood.

The enigma of the role of the eosinophil in disease requires further clarification, and for the present this condition should be called "chronic nasal disease with eosinophilic infiltrates." The role of eosinophils in immunological phenomena is discussed in Chapter 2.

4.3.2. Polymorphonuclear (PMN) Infiltrates

Because most obvious cases of infection are diagnosed, treated, and not biopsied, it is rare to see PMN as the only infiltrating cell. However, this does occasionally occur, and the presumed diagnosis is an infectious process that is not apparent clinically. The patient will frequently give a history of questionable chronic sinusitis or other suspicious symptoms compatible with a smoldering infection. On physical examination the nasal mucosa will usually be bright or dark red. The PMN will be considered again as a factor in immune disease.

4.3.3. Mediator Cells

The mast cell as described by Selye (1965) is the body's "emergency kit" because it contains so many mediators for protection and repair. I would add that because of these mediators the mast cell is a microcellular "regulatory system." Mast cells are known to contain or synthesize a variety of potent chemicals (histamine, SRS-A, heparin, ECF) involved in normal as well as pathological processes. A variety of mechanisms have been described or postulated as stimuli for mediator release, including IgE-mediated allergic reactions, the complement system, neurogenic stimuli, physical changes, and drugs.

In approximately 25% of patients with chronic rhinitis the mast cell count is more than $2000/mm^3$ of tissue and has been observed as high as $40{,}000/mm^3$. The increase in mast cells may be the only pathological observation in a biopsy, or there may be other infiltrates. Eosinophilic infiltrates accompany mast cell increases in 30% of cases and may be explained by ECF released by mast cells. For unknown reasons, large numbers of plasma cells are seen in 30% of biopsies with increased mast cell counts.

The increase in mast cells has been called "nasal mastocytosis" (Connell, 1969b). It is clinically associated with chronic rhinorrhea and congestion but not nasal itching. Most patients do not have stigmata of IgE-mediated allergic rhinitis, and serum IgE is low or normal in the majority of cases. The color of the nasal mucosa is not unlike that found in the normal. About one in six patients has a history of migraine headache and one in five a history of asthma. Patients are usually refractory to antihistamines and oral decongestants; some may respond temporarily to intranasal or systemic corticosteroids. Based on their histories, many patients appear to have had mastocytosis for periods of 10–20 years without anything more than severe nasal symptoms.

The cause of the increase in mast cells is unknown. In a study of nasal mucosa obtained during 100 autopsies, 12% of subjects had increased numbers of mast cells (Connell, 1969c). Ten of the 12 had died of acute myocardial infarction or upper gastrointestinal disturbances and had nasal tubes (oxygen catheters or Levine tubes) in place for at least 24 hr before death. The tubes can disturb nasal physiology and irritate the mucosa and are presumed to cause the increase in mast cell counts. Other causes of nasal mastocytosis are unknown.

The proposed pathophysiology is that normal or abnormal stimuli of mediator secretion cause an excess amount of mediator to be released due to the increased number of mast cells.

4.4. Abnormal Infiltrates Suggesting Immunological Causes of Nasal Disease

4.4.1. Allergic Rhinitis (IgE Mediated)

Histological findings vary from time to time in patients with IgE-mediated allergic rhinitis. The variations in pathology are believed to exist because of duration of exposure to antigens to which the patient is sensitized. Histological findings are normal in patients with seasonal allergic rhinitis when they are not exposed to these antigens. After sufficient exposure (probably more than a week), basement membrane damage of varying degree is apparent (Rappaport *et al.*, 1953; Connell, 1968b). Healing of the basement membrane does not occur until exposure to antigen is eliminated for several weeks. Eosinophils are found in the tunica propria and infiltrate the epithelium. Information derived from histological examinations of skin test sites (Kline *et al.*, 1931) would suggest that the occurrence of the eosinophilic response parallels exposure; after nasal challenge eosinophils are found shortly after exposure begins and for 1 or 2 days after exposure ceases (Slavin *et al.*, 1964). A large amount of disorganized material which could be fragments of nuclei is frequently found. Eosinophilic granules are often seen in close approximation to these fragments, and hence the fragments are believed to represent degenerating eosinophils. Small numbers of lymphocytes and plasma cells may be found at various times in the tunica. Microscopic findings in allergic rhinitis vary with the degree and timing of exposure to antigen in relation to the time the mucosa is biopsied. The findings described are based on numerous biopsies from different patients and are a composite description rather than serial studies of the same patients.

The cause of damage to the basement membrane is not known. Presumably, it is not related to the antigen which is inhaled without effect by nonatopic individuals. At least some mediators of the mast cell are not involved because the basement membrane is normal in nasal mastocytosis (Connell, 1969b). Corticosteroids apparently do not protect the basement membrane (Rappaport *et al.*, 1953).

The occurrence of basement membrane damage is consistent with the clinical findings associated with "priming" (Connell, 1969a). Early seasonal exposure to relatively large amounts of inhaled antigen causes minimal or no symptoms. As exposure continues over days, smaller amounts of inhaled antigen may now produce severe symptoms. This situation is what has been called "priming." Late in the season or even after pollination ceases, patients may respond with severe symptoms to exposure to the antigen, or to other antigens to which they are sensitive by skin test but to which they rarely have symptoms when clinically exposed. The clinical observations and microscopic findings, when considered together, suggest that the basement membrane acts as a barrier which protects the structures in the tunica propria from antigen. When this membrane is damaged, antigenic substances can more readily enter the tunica and allergic reactions of greater intensity follow.

4.4.2. Immune Cell Infiltrates

An immune cell for these purposes is defined as a lymphocyte or plasma cell since these types are intimately involved in synthesis of antibodies. The eosinophil is included as an immune cell when present with lymphocytes or plasma cells because of its known association to many immune reactions. PMN leukocytes are frequently seen in conjuction with immune cell infiltrates. The function of the PMNs in these situations is not known. They are presumed to be part of the inflammatory reaction rather than a harbinger of infection.

A red mucosa is found on physical examination of patients who have infiltrates of lymphocytes and plasma cells. The appearance is not at all like that of the color of the membrane typically found in patients with IgE-mediated allergic rhinitis and is a point suggesting unique immunological diseases associated with lymphocyte and plasma cell infiltrates.

Immune cell infiltrates (usually of a mixed cell type) are found in approximately 60–75% of nasal biopsies. This high figure would suggest that an immune reaction is involved in the majority of patients with chronic nasal disease. Whether the immune reaction is a primary or secondary event in the disease process is not known. Twenty percent of this group have clinical evidence suggestive of an IgE-mediated perennial allergic rhinitis. If there is no evidence of IgE-mediated disease in the 40–55% with immune cell infiltrates, what is the significance of the infiltrates?

Type 2, 3, and 4 immune mechanisms have been inadequately investigated in the nasal mucosa. The studies which have been done are inconclusive but compatible with the hypothesis that type 2 and type 4 diseases could occur in the nose. In one study (Slavin *et al.*, 1964), nonatopic human subjects were immunized with emulsions of aqueous ragweed extract. Following a suitable interval, gauze soaked in aqueous ragweed extract was placed on the turbinates, after which biopsies were obtained. The mucosa became grossly reddened after this procedure, and histological examination revealed lymphocytic and monocytic infiltrates, suggesting a type 4 reaction. In another study (Zavala *et al.*, 1975) done in rabbits sensitized to bovine immunoglobulin G, bovine immunoglobulin G was placed on intact bronchial mucosa *in vivo*. Polymorphonuclears, lymphocytes, and mononuclear cells infiltrated the challenged mucosa. The reaction was dose dependent and proceeded to infarction and necrosis of the pulmonary tissues when excessive challenging doses were employed. The pathology suggested an Arthus reaction. The results of these studies indicate that the nasal mucosa could be involved in immune reactions other than type 1.

Is it reasonable to assume that such reactions might occur clinically? As previously mentioned, the nose removes particulate matter from a large volume of air each day. Elimination of particles from inspired air is accomplished by turbulence in the airstream which causes the particles to be deposited on the mucous blanket. Thus a variety of antigenic substances in varying amounts may be brought into intimate contact with the mucosa, and sensitization and rechallenge could occur under clinical conditions. Perhaps there is already clinical evidence of such an occurrence. Individuals who inhale the fumes of burning poison ivy or oak leaves develop a delayed and severe inflammation of the upper and lower respiratory tracts shortly after exposure, consistent with a type 4 reaction.

Clinicians are aware that many cases of chronic rhinitis are enigmas because the patients have no immediately recognizable exacerbation of symptoms on exposure to known antigenic substances but usually have a continuum of symptoms. Repeated and frequent contact to an antigen for which a type 2 or type 4 sensitivity was present could explain the chronicity of the disease and absence of acute exacerbations immediately after the exposure.

Another explanation of at least some of the cases of immune cell infiltrates may be related to the immunity associated with infection. Perhaps in these cases a persistent rhinitis is an immunological reaction to bacteria, even when clinical infection is not apparent or may not even exist (Cooke, 1947). Many cases of "intrinsic rhinitis" or "bacterial allergy" could fall into this category.

Only one cell type (either lymphocyte or plasma cell) is involved in about 10% of cases of immune cell infiltration. Possible explanations for such an occurrence when the lymphocyte is the infiltrating cell revolve around the specificity of the lymphocyte type. If, for instance, the lymphocytes were of a single family, i.e., T cells or B cells, certain inferences regarding relative immunodeficiency states might apply. Preponderance of one or another cell type has been described in atopic dermatitis (Corman, 1974). The finding of pure plasma cell infiltrates also raises intriguing theoretical and diagnostic possibilities.

The accuracy of these hypotheses regarding the meaning of lymphocytic and plasma cell infiltrates awaits further investigations.

4.4.3. PMN Infiltrates

PMN infiltrates were discussed in Section 4.3.2. They are included again as a possible immune cell infiltrate because of their relationship to immune reactions. For instance, the PMN is the earliest infiltrating cell in the immediate skin test (Kline *et al.*, 1931) and is the only infiltrating cell present when the wheal and erythema of the skin test is developing. The PMN is also the first infiltrating cell found in the mucosa of patients with immediate hypersensitivity to ragweed after nasal challenge with aqueous ragweed extract (Slavin *et al.*, 1964). PMNs are intimately associated with type 2 Arthus reactions and appear to play a role in complement-related diseases. Their role in noninfectious nasal diseases has not been elucidated, but they are found in significant numbers in some cases of chronic nasal disease where an infectious process is not apparent.

5. Summary

Nasal disease is more prevalent than even the medical profession realizes. Often, because our diagnoses are inadequate and therapy is ineffective, a significant number of patients will consult with several physicians in search of relief. Most learn to live with their diseases since at best they are not life threatening.

The current state of clinical knowledge and histological observations have been reviewed. There is a consistency between some clinical states and microscopic findings, but many histopathological conditions are yet to be explained.

6. References

Bourà, A. L. A., and Green, A. F., 1965, Adrenergic neurone blocking agents, *Annu. Rev. Pharmacol.* **5**:183–212.

Cauna, N., and Hinderer, K. H., 1969, Fine structure of blood vessels of the human nasal respiratory mucosa, *Ann. Otol. Rhinol. Laryngol.* **78**:865–879.

Claman, H. N., 1975, How corticosteroids work, *J. Allergy Clin. Immunol.* **55**:145–151.

Connell, J. T., 1968a, Reciprocal nasal congestion-decongestion reflex, *Trans. Am. Acad. Opthalmol. Otolaryngol.* **72**:422.

Connell, J. T., 1968b, The priming effect and its relationship to histopathologic changes in nasal biopsies, *J. Allergy* **41**:101.

Connell, J. T., 1969a, Quantitative pollen challenges. III. The priming effect in allergic rhinitis, *J. Allergy* **43**:33–44.

Connell, J. T., 1969b, Nasal mastocytosis, *J. Allergy* **43**:182.

Connell, J. T., 1969c, Incidence of nasal mastocytosis in 100 autopsied patients, unpublished data.

Connell, J. T., 1973, Effects of salbutamol on nasal congestion, unpublished data.

Connell, J. T., 1974, Incidence of nasal polyps in an unselected population, unpublished data.

Connell, J. T., 1977, Histological examinations of 1300 nasal biopsies from 1966–1977, unpublished data.

Connell, J. T., 1978, Causes of post-nasal drip, unpublished data.

Cooke, R. A., 1947, Bacterial allergy, in: *Allergy in Theory and Practice*, Saunders, Philadelphia.

Corman, R. H., 1974, B and T cells in dermatitis, *Mayo Clin. Proc.* **49**:531–536.

Cox, J. S. G., 1971, Disodium cromoglycate: Mode of action and its possible relevance to the clinical use of the drug, *Br. J. Dis. Chest* **65**:189–204.

Gleich, G. J., Averbeck, A. K., and Swedlund, H. A., 1971, Measurement of IgE in normal and allergic sera by radioimmunoassay, *J. Lab. Clin. Med.* **77**:690–698.

Gleich, G. J., 1977, The eosinophil: New aspects of structure and function, *J. Allergy Clin. Immunol.* **60**:73–82.

Golding-Wood, P. H., 1970, Vidian neurectomy and other transantral surgery, *Laryngology* **80**:1179–1189.

Hagy, W. H., and Settipane, G. A., 1976, Risk factors for developing asthma and allergic rhinitis, *J. Allergy Clin. Immunol.* **58**:330–336.

Hampton, S. F., Johnson, M. C., and Galakatos, E., 1963, Studies of bacterial hypersensitivity in asthma. I. The preparation of antigens of *Neisseria catarrhalis*, the induction of asthma by aerosols, the performance of skin and passive transfer tests, *J. Allergy* **34**:63–95.

Kallio, E. I. S., Bacal, H. L., Eisen, A., and Fraser, F. C., 1966, A familial tendency toward skin sensitivity to ragweed pollen. *J. Allergy* **38**:241–249.

Kern, R. A., and Schenck, H. P., 1923, Allergy, a constant factor in the etiology of so-called mucous nasal polyps, *J. Allergy* **4**:485–497.

Kline, B. S., Cohen, M. B., and Rudolph, J. A., 1931, Histological changes in allergic and non-allergic wheals. *J. Allergy* **3**:531.

Lavin, N., Rachelefsky, G. S., and Solomon, A. K., 1976, An action of disodium cromoglycate: Inhibition of cyclic 3',5'-AMP phosphodiesterase, *J. Allergy* **57**:80–88.

Levine, B. B., Stember, R. H., and Fotino, M., 1973, Ragweed hay fever: Genetic control and linkage to HL-A haplotypes, *Science* **178**:1201–1203.

Mallory, G. K., White, P. D., and Salcedo-Salgar, J., 1939, The speed of healing of myocardial infarction. A study of the pathologic anatomy of 72 cases, *Am. Heart J.* **18**:647–671.

Marsh, D. G., Bias, W. B., and Ishizaka, K., 1974, Genetic control of basal serum immunoglobulin E level and its effect on specific reaginic activity, *Proc. Natl. Acad. Sci. USA* **71(9)**:3588–3592.

May, C. D., 1976a, High spontaneous release of histamine *in vitro* from leukocytes of persons hypersensitive to food, *J. Allergy Clin. Immunol.* **58**:432–437.

May, C. D., 1976b, Objective and laboratory studies of immediate hypersensitivity reactions to foods in asthmatic children, *J. Allergy Clin. Immunol.* **58:**500–518.

Norn, S., and Shore, P. A., 1971, Failure to affect tissue reserpine concentrations by alteration of adrenergic nerve activity, *Biochem. Pharmacol.* **20:**2133–2135.

Rappaport, B. Z., Samter, M., Catchpole, H. R., and Schiller, F., 1953, The mucoproteins of the nasal mucosa of allergic patients before and after treatment with corticotropins, *J. Allergy* **24:**35–51.

Selye, H., 1965. *The Mast Cells*, p.6, Butterworth, Washington, D.C.

Settipane G. A., and Chafee F. H., 1977, Nasal polyps in asthma and rhinitis: A review of 6,037 patients, *J. Allergy Clin. Immunol.* **59:**17–21.

Sherman, W. B., 1968, *Hypersensitivity, Mechanisms and Management*, pp. 225 and 237, Saunders, Philadelphia.

Slavin, R. G., Fink, J. N., Becker, R. J., Tennenbaum, J. I., and Feinber, S. M., 1964, Delayed response to antigen challenge in induced delayed hyperreactivity, *J. Allergy* **35:**499–505.

Solomon, R. W., 1967, Ocular mechanisms producing reflex nasal obstruction, *J. Allergy Clin. Immunol.* **30:**109.

Swineford, O., Jr., and Homan, J., 1949, Studies in bacterial allergy. III. Results of 3860 skin tests with 34 crude polysaccharide and nucleoprotein fractions of 14 different bacteria, *J. Allergy* **20:**420–427.

Szentivanyi, A., and Fishel, C. W., 1965, Effect of bacterial products on responses to the allergic mediators, in: *Immunological Diseases* (M. Samter, ed.), Little, Brown, Boston.

Togawa, K., and Konno, A., 1976, Respiratory function in atrophic rhinitis, in: *Proceedings of the International Symposium on Infection and Allergy of the Nose and Paranasal Sinuses* (R. Takahaski, ed.), pp. 27–30, Scimed Publications, Tokyo.

Wide, L., Bennich, H., and Johansson, S. G. O., 1967, Diagnosis of allergy by an *in vitro* test for allergen antibodies, *Lancet* **2:**1105–1107.

Zavala, D. C., Rhodes, M. L., Richerson, H. B., and Oskvig, R., 1975, Light and immunofluorescent study of the Arthus reaction in the rabbit lung, *J. Allergy Clin. Immunol.* **56:**450–463.

13

Pathogenesis of Bronchial Asthma

MICHAEL H. GRIECO

1. Introduction

Bronchial asthma, a disease referred to in the Hippocratic writings, was vividly described by Aretaeus in the second century. Galen thought of asthma as the result of the accumulation of thick secretions coming down from the brain via conduits to the upper and lower respiratory tracts. The vagal nervous system and heredity were implicated as etiological factors by Eberle's treatise on the practice of medicine published in 1830 in Philadelphia. Thereafter numerous authors thought of spasmodic asthma as the result of perverted innervation of the vagi based on experimental demonstration that stimulation of the vagus nerve produced contraction of the bronchi. These reports and observations culminated in the hypothesis of Eppinger and Hess (1915) that asthma is due to functional imbalance of the autonomic nervous system resulting from vagotonia and excessive cholinergic activity and in the local "organ vagotonia" concept of Takino (1946).

Although thc symptoms of hay fever were described initially by Botallo in 1565, it was not until Bostock's report in 1819 that catarrhus aestivus, conjunctivitis, and asthma were recognized as associated clinical manifestations. In 1831 Elliotson presented the concept that hay fever was caused by emanation of pollen while Blackley in 1873 demonstrated, by scratch skin tests on the arm, that such patients were sensitive to the pollen. The role of immunological mechanisms in asthma was introduced by studies of anaphylaxis. In 1901 Richet conducted experiments with extracts of actinia from the sea anemone which led to a reaction, following a second injection into an experimental animal, termed "anaphylaxis," signifying loss of protection. Subsequently Von Pirquet in 1905 suggested that

MICHAEL H. GRIECO • R. A. Cooke Institute of Allergy and the Allergy, Clinical Immunology, and Infectious Disease Division, Medical Service, The Roosevelt Hospital, New York, New York 10019, and Department of Clinical Medicine, Columbia University College of Physicians and Surgeons, New York, New York 10032.

"anaphylaxis" be replaced by the term "allergy" to reflect altered reactivity rather than a loss of protection.

This chapter will reexamine these historical concepts of the pathogenesis of bronchial asthma in the light of our current understanding of the immunological and nonimmunological mechanisms involved.

2. Clinical Classification and Pathology

2.1. Classification

The essential feature of bronchial asthma is reversibility of obstruction. In contrast to "emphysema," which is defined by histological changes and chronic bronchitis by mucus production, the term "bronchial asthma" denotes a complex of symptoms characterized by paroxysmal wheezing and dyspnea due to bronchial obstruction resulting from bronchospasm, excessive mucoid production, and mucosal edema. A committee of the American Thoracic Society (1962) has placed emphasis on the host factors in defining asthma as "a disease characterized by an increased responsiveness of the trachea and bronchi to various stimuli and manifested by widespread narrowing of the airways that change in severity either spontaneously or as the result of treatment."

In 1918 Walker distinguished extrinsic and intrinsic factors involved in the causation of clinical symptoms. Today these terms are translated into "allergic" or "immunological" vs. "idiopathic" or "nonimmunological" asthma. Features characteristic of each are presented in Table 1. Allergic asthma is usually characterized by a family history of allergic diseases (eczema, rhinitis, or asthma) and provocation of symptoms by antigens believed to be acting by specific IgE-induced mast cell degranulation. A study (Stevenson *et al.*, 1975) of 234 patients revealed that most asthmatics had at least one major and one or more minor provoking factors. Reagin-mediated mechanisms constituted the major provoking factor in 25% of patients and were a minor factor in an additional 20%. Thus in only 45% were reaginic mechanisms responsible for some part of their asthmatic episodes. In the majority of patients nonimmunological mechanisms appear to predominate. Bronchial challenge with fungal, avian, and bacterial antigens implicated in the pathogenesis of hypersensitivity pneumonitis is associated with late responses believed to be mediated in large part by a precipitating antibody of the IgG class, although complement activation, cell-mediated immunity, and leukocyte histamine releasing factor(s) may be implicated.

2.2. Pathology

Both allergic and idiopathic asthma appear to produce similar anatomical changes in patients dying of status asthmaticus. Thus far the pathological observations have not helped to clarify the pathogenetic mechanisms involved. At autopsy (Hayes, 1976) the distended lungs fill the pleural cavity and obscure the lateral aspect of the mediastinum and cover the pericardial bare area. The visceral pleura usually shows distinct outlines of rib indentations. Small zones of atelectasis are present involving one or more secondary lobules. Although asthma predominantly affects the second to sixth-order divisions distal to the carina, patency is normally maintained by cartilage plates. Smaller bronchi of 2.0–10 mm are easily obstructed by combined mucosal congestion, mucous plugs, and muscle spasm.

2.2.1. Light Microscopy

The most striking microscopic changes are found in the 2.0–10 mm diameter bronchi. The plugs consist of irregular, whorled strands of *mucus* containing embedded eosinophils, ciliated epithelial cells, macrophages, and variable numbers of Charcot-Leyden crystals. The mucus may assume whorled patterns in Curschmann spirals due to coiling up of mucous plugs which are incompletely expectorated. The bronchial mucosa reveals loss of the tall ciliated mucus-secreting columnar cells, which are shed into the bronchial lumen as clumps of cells called "Creola bodies." The basal or reserve cells remain firmly attached to the basement membrane and goblet cells are increased, especially in the small airways. Hayes (1976) has speculated that mucous cell hyperplasia may be a nonspecific reparative cell response subsequent to the primary lesion of ciliated cell death. The mechanism involved in goblet cell hyperplasia is unknown.

The *basement membrane* has a characteristic eosinophilic hyaline thickening

TABLE 1. Classification of Asthma

	Allergic		
	Immediate type	Nonimmediate type	Idiopathic
Age at onset	Under 35	Adult	Under 5, over 35
Genetic influence	Familial	No	More variable
Antigens	Animal dander Pollens Fungal	Fungal Avian Bacterial	None
Antibodies	IgE reagin IgG_4 reagin	1. IgG precipitating antibody plus IgE and/or IgG_4 reagin 2. C3 activation 3. Cell-mediated immunity 4. Histamine-releasing factor? PMN, Lym?, Mono?	None
Aspirin sensitivity	No	No	Yes
Exercise induction	Yes	Yes	Yes
Bronchial provocation			
Antigen	Yes	Yes	No
Prevented by corticosteroids	No	Yes	No
Prevented by cromolyn sodium	Yes	Yes	No
Histamine	Yes	Yes	Yes
Methacholine	Yes	Yes	Yes

which is related to current activity and chronicity. The entire submucosa is congested and infiltrated with large numbers of *eosinophils* and lymphocytes, histiocytes, and plasma cells. Salvato (1968) and Connell (1971) have reported that mast cell depletion is present. Neutrophils are not characteristically present (Dunhill, 1960). Submucosal glands present in the lamina propria appear to be normal or mildly hypertrophied while the *smooth muscle* is prominent, suggesting true hyperplasia or apparent change due to contraction (Dunhill, 1960; Cardell, 1959).

2.2.2. Immunofluorescent and Electron Microscopy

Callerame *et al.* (1971a) reported that thickened basement membranes stained positively for immunoglobulins in five of 11 biopsies and six of seven autopsy specimens. IgM was the immunoglobulin most frequently seen and C3 was identified in three cases. The biopsy specimens were from the main-stem bronchi and failed to reveal an increased incidence of IgE (Callerame *et al.* 1971a). However, the peripheral location of IgE was reported by Gerber *et al.*, (1971) in six of eight patients with asthma along the epithelial aspect of the bronchial basement membrane, in the respiratory epithelium of small bronchi and bronchioles, and in the intrabronchial mucus of asthmatic lungs. The presence and distribution of IgA, IgG, IgM, complement, and fibrinogen did not differ from those in normal bronchi. This finding suggested that the bronchial mucosa might be a target tissue of IgE antibodies and site of an immunological reaction.

However, the nature of the basement membrane thickening in asthma remains uncertain. The thick basement membrane seen by light microscopy is not the same as the delicate basal lamina seen by electron microscopy. One study in an asthmatic patient suggested that the basal lamina thickening is due to deposition of collagen in the superficial submucosa (McCarter and Vazquez, 1966).

3. Normal Anatomy and Innervation

Before the interaction of immunological and nervous system mechanisms in asthma is discussed, pertinent features of pulmonary anatomy and autonomic innervation will be reviewed.

3.1. Cells of the Pulmonary Airways

3.1.1. The Epithelium

At least 13 cell types, 11 epithelial and two mesenchymal, are now recognized in the tracheobronchial epithelium (Breeze and Wheeldon, 1977). Scattered among these cells, from the trachea to the bronchioles, are intraepithelial corpuscles known as "neuroepithelial bodies." Only six cell types, the ciliated, brush, basal, K, Clara, and globule leukocyte, have been recorded in the bronchioles, where the epithelium is no longer pseudostratified. This discussion will be limited to cells which may participate in the pathogenesis of bronchial asthma.

a. Ciliated Cell. The lining of the trachea and bronchi is pseudostratified columnar ciliated epithelium which contains numerous goblet cells. Ciliated cells are present in relatively greater concentrations than goblet cells with subsequent subdivisions of the airways; goblet cells are absent by the level of the terminal bronchiole, while ciliated cells persist until the level of the respiratory bronchiole. Ciliated cells are roughly columnar, approximately 20 μm long and 7 μm wide, tapering to 2 μm at the base, where they reach the basement membrane. An irregular intercellular space surrounds the cell, except at the luminal surface, where tight cell junctions are formed. Approximately 250 cilia, each 6 μm long and 0.3 μm wide, are found on the luminal surface of each cell. Interspersed among these are one-half as many microvilli and fine cytoplasmic processes. The main function of ciliated cells is to propel the tracheobronchial secretions toward the pharynx. Another role may be in the regulation of the tracheobronchial secretions. Kilburn (1968) has pointed out that a considerable volume of these secretions must be absorbed between the periphery of the lung and the pharynx and proposed that the microvilli of ciliated cells might perform this function.

b. Goblet Cell. In normal mucosa, the mean number of goblet cells is 6800/ mm^2, and this can increase to 10,000/mm^2 in case of chronic tracheobronchitis (Ellefson and Tos, 1972). The protein moiety of mucus is synthesized in the rough-surfaced endoplasmic reticulum and passes to the Golgi apparatus, where it is combined with carbohydrates and sulfated before release. Secretion is of the apocrine type and passes through defects in the luminal cell membrane that are readily seen in scanning electron micrographs. Rhodin (1966) assumed that each goblet cell was capable of completing two secretory cycles before being sloughed or ingested by macrophages, but pointed out that the true number was unknown.

c. K Cell ("Kultschitzkylike"). K cells are found in normal lung among the exocrine bronchial mucous gland epithelium and contain "neurosecretory" granules. They are presumed to give rise to human bronchial carcinoid and oat cell carcinomas. The K cells are usually found singly in the epithelium, although they may occur in clusters of three to five cells. Fröhlich (1949) has noted intraepithelial nerve axons very closely applied to individual K cells, although confirmations have been inconsistent. Axons associated with individual or grouped K cells have been identified as sensory, cholinergic, or adrenergic (Fröhlich, 1949). In adult human beings, the cells appear to have low concentrations of 5-hydroxytryptamine (5HT) and catecholamines but can be induced to store a number of arylalkylamines after *in vitro* loading with precursor amino acids such as 5-hydroxytryptophan (5HTP) and dihydroxyphenylalanine (L-dopa) (Hage *et al.*, 1977). These procedures demonstrate a capacity for amine precursor uptake, decarboxylation, and storage in K cells. The ultrastructural and cytochemical characteristics of K cells are those of an "APUD" cell. The function of K cells is unknown. These cells might be involved in the regulation of the pulmonary circulation, smooth muscle tone in the bronchial wall, and the production of amines and kinins.

d. Nonciliated Bronchiolar Secretory Cell (Clara Cell). The epithelium of terminal bronchioles is composed mainly of low ciliated and taller nonciliated cells.

Almost all of the nonciliated cells are Clara cells, but there are also scattered brush and K cells, globule leukocytes, and sparse basal cells. Clara cells are most abundant in the bronchioles. These cells secrete a material which is not mucoid but possibly a lipoprotein. Niden (1967) proposed the controversial hypothesis that Clara cells are the source of pulmonary surfactant. It is possible that nonciliated bronchiolar secretory cells provide a form of surface-active layer in the bronchioles or a watery medium for cilia in the bronchioles similar to that on which the mucus is carried in the large airways.

e. Globule Leukocyte. Globule leukocytes have been noted in the tracheobronchial epithelium of rats, deer, cattle, and dogs but not in human airways (Breeze and Wheeldon, 1977). The globule leukocyte is an intraepithelial mononuclear cell filled with large, highly refractile, acidophilic granules that frequently indent the nucleus. It has been demonstrated that this cell is derived from the subepithelial mast cell, which it resembles ultrastructurally and histochemically. Globule leukocytes arise from subepithelial mast cells by migration through the basement membrane.

f. Neuroepithelial Body. Each neuroepithelial body is composed of a number of tall, nonciliated cells arranged more or less in parallel and forming a cone-shaped or an oval or spherical corpuscle within the epithelium (Lauweryns and Goodeeris, 1975). Neuroepithelial bodies are found throughout the entire tracheobronchial and bronchiolar epithelium and are probably most numerous in the bronchioles. The fluorescence of rabbit neuroepithelial bodies has been measured microspectrographically, and their spectra have been found to be identical with that of 5HT. Neuroepithelial bodies are well innervated by both afferent and efferent fibers. The axons originate in the lamina propria, where they are surrounded by Schwann cells. This Schwann cell sheath is lost as the axon penetrates the basement membrane and ramifies among the cells of the neuroepithelial bodies. The function of neuroepithelial bodies is not known. It has been postulated that the secretory products reach the pulmonary vein directly and may be responsible for pulmonary vasoconstriction of hypoxia and for regulation of smooth muscle tone and mucosal secretions in the bronchi (Laros, 1971).

3.1.2. The Lamina Propria

a. Subepithelial Mast Cell. There is evidence of functional differences between subepithelial and connective tissue mast cells. Immunochemical study of rat subepithelial and globule leukocytes reveals IgE both intracellularly in the granule matrix and on the cell membrane (Stimson *et al.*, 1977). The absence of IgE-synthesizing plasma cells from mucosal surfaces suggests that subepithelial mast cells and globule leukocytes may be responsible for transfer of IgE to the luminal surface secretions (Mayrhofer *et al.*, 1976). Free cells of mast cell and basophiloid type were recovered from bronchial washings of normal monkeys and dogs and of dogs allergic to ragweed antigen (Patterson *et al.*, 1974) and monkeys sensitized to *Ascaris* antigen (Ts'ao *et al.*, 1977). The cells are probably derived from globule leukocytes or subepithelial mast cells. Thus IgE-containing or -bearing cells capable of responding to specific antigen by release of biogenic amines are present *on* or *in* the respiratory epithelium.

b. Bronchus-Associated Lymphoid Tissue. Lymphoid tissue is found in the walls of conducting airways from the nasopharynx to the alveolar ducts. Multiple nodules of lymphoid tissue are scattered within the bronchial mucosa down to the level of the small bronchioles, especially at points of bifurcation. These nodules are considered to be the pulmonary anolgue of the intestinal Peyer's patch and are referred to as "bronchus-associated lymphoid tissue." Lymphoid aggregates and infiltrates are less-well-organized accumulations in the peripheral airways. The concentration of nodules around bronchial orifices suggest a role in sampling inhalant antigens deposited by airflow turbulence (Bienenstock and Johnston, 1976). Approximately 50% appear to be B cells, 20% T cells, and the remainder null cells. A direct role in antibody production is unlikely since immunization does not result in the formation of follicular immunoglobulins (Clancy and Bienenstock, 1974). This tissue may provide B cells destined to produce IgA and IgE antibodies in the lamina propria and T cells involved in cell-mediated immunity.

c. Plasma Cells. Immunoglobulin-containing plasma cells are abundant, especially around mucous gland acini and in the lamina propria. The concentration is highest in the main bronchus, moderate in the lobar bronchus and upper trachea, and sparse in the small bronchi and interalveolar septa. Approximately 70% stain for IgA and 10% for IgE (Soutar, 1976). Breeze and Wheeldon (1977) point out that a portion of the IgE-containing cells might well have been mast cells as described in the rat.

d. Lymphocytes. Lymphocytes are found in the epithelium, lamina propria, and bronchus-associated lymphoid tissue and lymphoid aggregates of the airway mucosa. Bronchoalveolar cells obtained by lavage are believed to be derived from the mucosa but differ in having B–T cell ratios similar to peripheral blood, suggesting that a large portion may have originated from blood.

e. Mucous Glands. Mucous glands of the tubuloacinar type are found in the lamina propria. It is not known why there are two components to the mucus-secreting apparatus, and separation of the two secretions has proved difficult. Estimation of the contribution to the total amount of respiratory mucus made by each of the two components, goblet cells and mucous glands, is based on an estimate by Reid (1960) that the mucous glands in man have a volume 40 times greater than that of the goblet cells. Branched secretory tubules contain mucous and serous cells and discharge their contents into large collecting and ultimately into ciliated ducts emptying through the bronchial mucosa. While the mucous cells secrete constituents of the mucous blanket, it appears that serous cells are involved in the transport of IgA across the epithelium and in the production of lysozyme.

3.1.3. Smooth Muscle Cells

Airway patency is maintained in the trachea and large bronchi by cartilage plates and in the peripheral airways by the radial traction of elastic fibers within the lung parenchyma. The muscle bundles in the large airways are mainly transverse in position, and contraction leads to circumferential narrowing. In the smaller bronchi and bronchioles the muscle bundles have a helical arrangement so that contraction results in both transverse narrowing and axial shortening. Smooth muscle does not end in the terminal bronchioles but extends to the termination of the alveolar duct and forms a terminal sphincter around the opening of the alveolar sacs.

3.2. Nerve Supply of the Lung

3.2.1. The Hypothalamus

The hypothalamus serves as an important integrating center between the brain stem–reticular system and the limbic forebrain structures (Figure 1). Ascending reticular input is conducted from the multisynaptic ascending pathways in the mesencephalic reticular nuclei via the medial forebrain bundle, dorsal longitudinal fasciculus, and mammillary peduncle. Output fibers from the lateral hypothalamic nuclei and paraventricular nuclei connect to the midbrain tegmentum and autonomic neurons in the brain stem and spinal cord. There are two reciprocally antagonistic divisions in the hypothalamus: the anterior hypothelamus, which mediates mainly cholinergic responses, and the posterior hypothalamus, the stimulation of which results largely in adrenergic responses. Hypothalamic imbalance can be produced reflexly or by direct chemical or electrical stimulation (Szentivanyi and Filipp, 1965).

3.2.2. Brain Stem

a. Control of Respiration. Lumsden (1923) concluded that three brain stem centers were associated with respiration, the pneumotaxic and apneustic centers in the pons and the medullary center. The medulla is composed of two dense bilateral aggregations of respiratory neurons, the dorsal and ventral respiratory groups. The dorsal respiratory group appears to constitute the initial intracranial processing station for many visceral reflexes affecting respiration and is the site of origin of the rhythmic respiratory drive to the central respiratory group and spinal inspiratory motoneurons (intercostal and phrenic nerves). The dorsal respiratory group is the site where vagal sensory information is first incorporated into the respiratory motor response. The ventral respiratory group contains vagal motor neurons in the nucleus ambiguous and spinal inspiratory and expiratory motoneurons in the nucleus retroambiguous. The major function of ventral respiratory group neurons is to project to distant sites and drive either spinal respiratory motoneurons (primarily intercostal and abdominal) or the auxiliary muscles of respiration innervated by the vagus nerves. Axons from the dorsal and ventral group of neurons cross the midline and descend in the ventrolateral columns of the cord to influence the rhythmic respiratory motor act. This complex subject has been concisely reviewed by Berger *et al.* (1977).

It appears that both the cough reflex and hiccup arise from structures separate from the respiratory neuron groups and traverse independent pathways until integrated at the level of the spinal respiratory motoneurons.

b. Bronchial Tone. The central nervous sites of origin of airway constrictor or dilator fibers are not known (Widdicombe, 1963). Vagal and glossopharyngeal reflexes influence airway size, supporting the presumption that constrictor fibers originate in the medulla in common with other vagal efferent nerves. It is unclear to what extent bronchomotor nervous activity is related to respiratory center discharge.

3.2.3. Efferent Pathways

a. Phrenic and Intercostal Nerves. In the somatic nervous system the efferent neuron is the ventral horn cell. Its axon leaves the central nervous system to innervate a skeletal muscle. The phrenic nerve arises from cervical roots 3–5 to

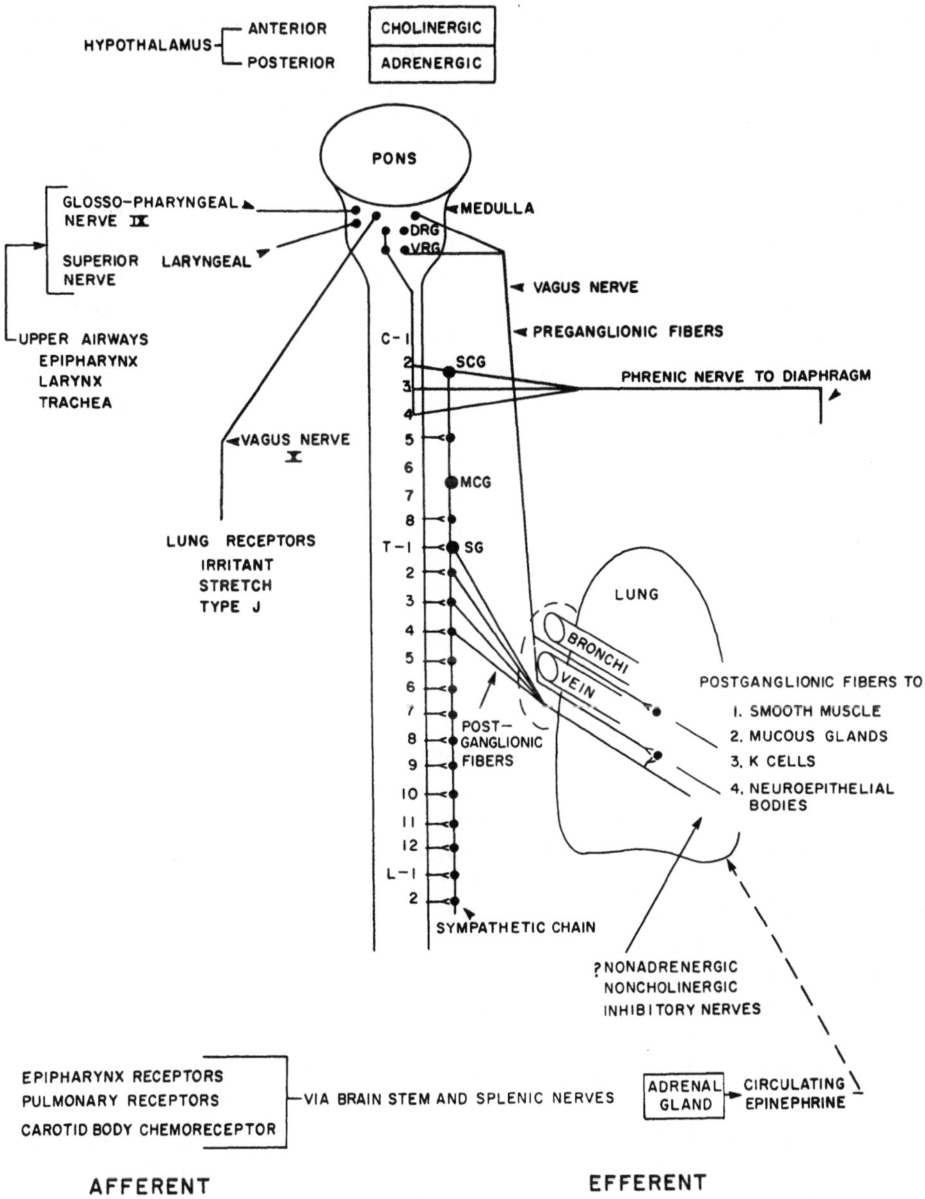

Figure 1. Afferent and efferent innervation of the lung.

innervate the diaphragm and the intercostal nerves from thoracic 1–11 to innervate the intercostal muscles. These somatic nerves effect coordinated respiration.

b. Autonomic Nervous System. The autonomic nervous system is divided into parasympathetic and sympathetic systems and includes preganglionic and postganglionic neurons. Preganglionic neurons in the pons and medulla provide fibers which travel in cranial nerves III, VII, IX, and X. The dorsal motor nucleus of the vagus nerve provides preganglionic parasympathetic innervation of post-glanglionic neurons in several organs including the pharynx, larynx, and lungs. Sympathetic preganglionic fibers originate in the intermediolateral column in the spinal cord from T_1 to L_2, exit in the white rami, and enter the paravertebral sympathetic ganglionic chain extending from the cervical to lumbar regions where nonmyelinated postganglionic fibers originate and exit via gray communicating rami to innervate visceral end organs. The ganglia of T_1–T_4 provide postganglionic fibers to the heart and lungs. Both the vagus nerve and the upper four thoracic sympathetic ganglia and possibly cervical ganglia contribute nonmyelinated fibers to the anterior and posterior pulmonary plexuses at the roots of the lungs. As the bronchi, arteries, and veins enter the lungs at the hilum, they carry with them extensions of the plexus, the largest branches accompanying the bronchi and the smallest accompanying the veins. Unmyelinated efferent fibers, predominantly parasympathetic, directly innervate bronchial smooth muscle, blood vessles, mucous glands, K cells, and neuroepithelial bodies. Goblet cells do not receive direct innervation but may be indirectly responsive via K cells and neuroepithelial body secretions (Lauweryns and Goodeeris, 1975).

By the use of histochemistry, electron microscopy, and pharmacological antagonists it has become possible to distinguish sympathetic and parasympathetic nerve endings in bronchial muscle. Three main types of synaptic vesicles or axonal varicosities have been seen (Burnstock, 1970; Burnstock *et al.*, 1972). Parasympathetic cholinergic nerves contain agranular vesicles 250–600 Å in size which store acetylcholine. The small granular vesicle accounts for over 80% of vesicles in sympathetic nerves, although 15% agranular vesicles and 5% large granular vesicles are observed as well. The dense core in the small granule vesicles is about 150 Å and the total vesicles vary in size from 250 to 600 Å. Fluorescence histochemistry and radiolabeled uptake studies indicate that these vesicles contain norepinephrine. Axons with large granular vesicles varying in size from 700 to 1600 Å are believed to contain monamines such as serotonin and 5-hydroxy-dopamine and may represent nonadrenergic, noncholinergic inhibitory nerves (Burnstock *et al.*, 1972) releasing adenosine triphosphate (ATP) as a transmitter substance. Richardson and Bouchard (1975) have demonstrated the presence of a nonadrenergic inhibitory nervous system in the trachea of the guinea pig. The studies of Silva and Ross (1974) in cat tracheobronchial muscle indicate the presence at all levels of the tracheobronchial tree of dense adrenergic and cholinergic innervation. The role of adrenergic stimulation of the tracheobronchial tree is controversial. It appears that such stimulation will inhibit the bronchoconstriction induced by vagal nerve stimulation, presumably by inhibitory innervation of vagal postganglionic neurons. In addition, some investigators report bronchodilatation following sympathetic stimulation. These effects are blocked by β-receptor antagonists, suggesting that they are responsible for any vagal antagonism or bronchodilatation. After β blockade, physiological concentrations of norepinephrine or methoxamine fail to induce bronchoconstriction, suggesting the lack of significant α-adrenergic receptor activity in the bronchial tree. Woolcock *et al.* (1969) measured the effect of β-adrenergic blocking agents on airway resistance in dogs and demonstrated increased peripheral airway resistance and bronchoconstriction after vagal stimulation. While Nadel *et al.* (1971) found that vagal stimulation produces responses in proximal airways in dogs, Woodcock *et al.* (1969) have shown that sympathetic effects are more prominent in small airways. Resting bronchial tone appears to be principally cholinergic. Following vagal stimulation, and large bronchial contraction, it is likely that β-adrenergic receptors in peripheral bronchi and bronchioles function to conteract the constrictive effect. β_2-Adrenergic receptors appear to be responsible for bronchodilatation since selective β_1-antagonists do not block this action of β-agonists. Bronchodilatation may result from the reflex release of norepinephrine as a neurotransmitter or from circulating epinephrine.

Recent studies suggest that α-receptors on smooth muscle are present and may play a physiological role in bronchial asthma. Adolphson *et al.* (1970) have demonstrated contraction of isolated tracheal and bronchial smooth muscle by epinephrine and norepinephrine after blockade by propranolol. Anthracite *et al.* (1971), using normal volunteers, showed a decrease in specific conductance by inhalation of methoxamine and antagonism by phentolamine. Additional support is provided by Simonsson *et al.* (1972), who demonstrated a decrease of specific conductance following inhalation of metaoxidrine, a specific α-adrenergic agent, in patients suffering from airway obstruction and pretreated with vagal and β-receptor antagonists.

Reflex bronchoconstriction clearly results from increased cholinergic and possible α-adrenergic receptor activation.

The bronchodilator effects of sympathetic nervous acitvity may be due principally to an inhibitory influence at the level of the parasympathetic ganglion. Evidence for such an effect includes detection of sympathetic nerve endings in parasympathetic ganglia from a variety of mammals (Mann, 1971), sympathetic inhibition of ganglionic transmission in the cat and bullfrog (Saum and De Groat 1972, Neshi 1970), and the protective effect of atropine against bronchoconstriction induced by propranolol in humans (Grieco and Pierson, 1971).

Stimulation of the vagus causes immediate discharge of the contents of the mucous glands, but the response to sympathetic stimulation is more difficult to discern. Utilizing radioactively labeled glucose and threonine in an organ culture system, Sturgess and Reed (1972) have studied the secretory mechanisms in mucous and serous cells from human bronchial glands. Acetylcholine, pilocarpine, and carbachol in concentrations from 1 to 100 μg/ml caused an increase in secretory activity blocked by atropine. Sympathomimetic and sympatholytic drugs had no effect on either mucous or serous cells. It is of further interest that bradykinin, histamine, and their antagonists did not affect bronchial secretions. Studies of nasal epithelium by Boat and Kleinerman (1975) shows no response of goblet cells to cholinergic stimulation. Although it is clear that cholinergic stimulation increases tracheobronchial gland secretion and may increase synthesis, the anatomical nervous pathways are poorly defined. Silva and Ross (1974) in their study of the innervation of cat bronchial structures have observed nerve fibers between the epithelial cells of the bronchial glands as well as between the epithelial cells of the mucosa. The nerve axons contained both agranular and large dense-cored granular vesicles both in normal animals and in those treated with 6-hydroxydopamine, a substance which produces selective degeneration of adrenergic nerve fibers. Fluorescent catecholamine-containing nerve fibers were present near and between glands but not within. Although the anatomical presence of both cholinergic and adrenergic fibers is certain, the exact function remains controversial. It is still possible that sympathetic activity may limit the mucous output caused by cholinergic stimulation.

Intraepithelial axons in airway epithelium are found in association with cells of all types but particularly adjacent to basal cells, brush cells, K cells, and neuroepithelial bodies. The proximity of fibers to K cells and neuroepithelial bodies has aroused a great deal of interest. They may function as sensory chemo- or mechanoreceptors and are candidates for a neuropharmacological role in the pathogenesis of bronchial asthma. In a quantitative study in rats (Jeffrey and Reed, 1973), approximately 33% of nonmyelinated intraepithelial axons were classified as motor adrenergic, 17% as cholinergic, and 50% as sensory. Nerve endings have also been discovered in intraalveolar septa in sites corresponding to the probable distribution of type J receptors.

3.2.4. Afferent Pathways

The upper airway and lungs possess several types of receptors that have significant effects on bronchial airways, respiration, and other visceral and somatic systems (Widdicombe, 1974; Pantal 1973) (Table 2).

a. Upper Airways. Mechanoreceptors in the epipharynx transmit via afferent nerve fibers in the pharyngeal branch of the glossopharyngeal nerve and result in inspiration, bronchodilatation, and hypertension. Irritant receptors in the larynx transmit through afferent rapidly adapting myelinated, slowly adapting myelinated, and unmyelinated fibers in the internal branch of the superior laryngeal nerve to induce cough, slow breathing, bronchoconstriction, and hypertension. The trachea also possesses irritant receptors resulting in cough and bronchoconstriction.

b. Lung Receptors. There are three major classes of lung receptors: irritant receptors, pulmonary stretch receptors, and type J receptors. It is generally accepted that all afferent nerve fibers to the central nervous system from the lungs travel in the vagus nerve. Irritant receptors are believed to lie between airway epithelial cells. They are called "rapidly adapting" because their activity markedly diminishes with sustained lung inflations or deflations. Their primary source of excitation is thought to be airway chemical irritants such as histamine and ammonia as well as mechanical irritants such as particulates. The reflex effects include bronchoconstriction, cough from central receptors, and hyperventilation from peripheral receptors. In the lung, these receptors are believed to be most abundant in 2–6 mm bronchi, especially at sites of bifurcation. This is still an area of controversy. Pantal (1973) concluded that lung irritant receptors do not have significant excitatory effects. The actual receptor sites are unknown but may be the free nonmyelinated nerve fibers in the epithelium attached to myelinated vagal nerve fibers. Slowly adapting pulmonary stretch receptors with myelinated nerves are found in the smooth muscle of bronchi, small airways, and trachea. Reflex responses include the classic Hering-Breuer inspiratory inhibition and bronchodilatation. Both the lung irritant receptors and tonically active pulmonary stretch receptors may be involved in respiration. Type J receptors activate slowly conducting nonmyelinated vagal afferent fibers. They lie close to pulmonary capillaries in the interstitium of the interalveolar septa. Pulmonary congestion may be the natural stimulus to these receptors, and it is likely that they also respond to edema, inflammation, emboli, and exercise. The main reflex effects are tachypnea, bradycardia, and laryngeal and bronchoconstriction.

Thus irritant receptors in the epithelial of the larynx, trachea, and bronchi result in reflex cough and bronchospasm and J receptor stimulation in laryngeal and bronchial constriction while stimulation of the epipharynx receptors and slowly adapting pulmonary stretch receptors is associated with reflex bronchodilatation. In addition, reflexes originating from the carotid bifurcation have opposite

TABLE 2. Upper Airway and Lung Receptors

	Receptor	Fiber type	Stimulus	Responses
Upper airways	Epipharynx	Myelinated	Mechanical	Inspiration Bronchodilatation Hypertension
	Larynx	Myelinated, both slow and rapidly adapting Nonmyelinated	Mechanical Chemical	Cough Deep breathing Bronchoconstriction Hypertension
	Trachea	Myelinated	Mechanical Chemical	Cough Bronchoconstriction Hypertension
Lung receptors	Irritant, rapidly adapting	Myelinated	Mechanical Chemical	Bronchoconstriction Cough, central Hyperventilation, peripheral; of constriction larynx on expiration
	Stretch, slowly adapting	Myelinated	Mechanical (distention)	Hering-Breuer bronchodilatation Increased heart rate Decreased peripheral vascular resistance
	Type J	Nonmyelinated	Mechanical Chemical	Rapid shallow breathing Severe constriction of larynx Hypotension Bradycardia Spinal reflex inhibition Bronchoconstriction
Carotid bifurcation	Carotid sinus baroreceptor		Rise in blood pressure	Bronchoconstriction
	Carotid body chemoreceptor		Hypoxemia	Bronchodilatation

actions; carotid sinus baroreceptors effect bronchoconstriction while carotid body receptors produce bronchodilatation. Reflex constriction results predominantly via efferent vagal activation while hyperventilation may result from phrenic and intercostal nerve transmission. Reflex bronchodilatation occurs via mechanisms which are unclear but may involve inhibitory influences at the level of the parasympathetic ganglion. In addition, it is likely that efferent impulses from the carotid body chemoreceptors and pulmonary stretch receptors are integrated in the main stem to increase splanchnic nerve discharge of epinephrine from the adrenal medulla. This catecholamine may then act directly on β_2-adrenergic receptors to bronchodilate. The adrenal gland stores catecholamines as norepinephrine, and most of this is methylated to epinephrine at the time of release.

3.3. Control Mechanisms

3.3.1. Pharmacological Control of Antigen-Induced Release of Chemical Mediators

The initial *in vitro* observation by Lichtenstein and Margolis (1968) that β-adrenergic agents and methylxanthines prevent antigen-induced release of histamine from human peripheral leukocytes was followed by confirmatory studies with human lung tissue. It is now well established in human lung that agents capable of stimulating adenylate cyclase such as β-adrenergic agonists (Orange *et al.*, 1971), histamine (H-2 receptor as determined by the agonists dimaprit and 4-methylhistamine), and prostaglandins (Tauber *et al.*, 1973) (PGE_1 and PGE_2) increase tissue concentrations of cyclic AMP and inhibit mast cell mediator generation and/or release (Figure 2). These agonists interact with specific receptor sites on the surface of a variety of cells to induce the formation of cyclic AMP from adenosine triphosphate by activation of the membrane-bound enzyme adenylate cyclase (Sutherland *et al.*, 1968). This same effect is produced by competitive inhibition of the enzyme phosphodiesterase with methylxanthines resulting in cyclic AMP increase as well as by direct action of dibutyryl cyclic AMP. The elaboration of prostaglandins as secondary chemical mediators and possible release by eosinophil phospholipase B may result in effective inhibition of primary mast cell degranulation (Hubscher, 1975).

In contrast, α-adrenergic agonists, prostaglandin $PGF_{2\alpha}$, histamine (H-1 receptor as determined by the agonists 2-methylhistamine and 2-pyridylethylamine), and cholinergic agonists result in enhancement of IgE-dependent release of chemical mediators. Both α-adrenergic agonists and low concentrations of $PGF_{2\alpha}$ result in depletion of tissue levels of cyclic AMP (Tauber *et al.*, 1973; Kaliner *et al.*, 1972). Studies with the peripheral leukocytes suggest that α-adrenergic agonists may act by increasing intracellular levels of ATPase (Coffey *et al.*, 1971). Cholinergic stimulation of sensitized lung fragments with acetylcholine or carbamylcholine chloride results in enhancement of IgE-dependent release of chemical mediators. The enhancement of the immunological release of histamine and slow-reacting substance of anaphylaxis (SRS-A) in response to the introduction of physiological amounts of acetylcholine involves specific cholinergic receptor sites of the muscarinic prototype since the action is blocked by atropine. This effect is independent of measureable changes in the tissue levels of cyclic AMP (Kaliner *et al.*, 1972). Cholinergic stimulation results in an increase in tissue concentrations of cyclic GMP, and the addition of 8-bromo-cyclic GMP to human lung fragments effects a dose-dependent enhancement of histamine release and SRS-A generation. A difference in the sensitivity of steps involved in the release of histamine and the generation of SRS-A is indicated by the fact that low concentrations of carbamylcholine chloride reverse the inhibition of histamine release from sensitized human lung fragment produced by isoproterenol but fail to inhibit SRS-A generation. In view of the sparse sympathetic innervation of the bronchial mucosa it is more likely that adrenergic modulation of mediator release is mediated by circulating catecholamines, possibly released secondary to carotid body and stretch receptor afferent impulses. In contrast, the rich cholinergic innervation of the bronchi is consistent with neural modulation of antigen-induced mediator release.

3.3.2. Bronchomotor Modulation

β_2-Adrenergic receptor stimulation as well as PGE_1 and PGE_2 results in bronchodilation in association with increased intracellular cyclic AMP (Figure 3). Resting bronchial tone is predominantly cholinergic since propranolol administration to normal subjects has only a minimal effect (Guirgis and McNeill, 1969). Bronchoconstriction in asthmatics treated with propranolol may be the result of β-adrenergic blockade on bronchial smooth muscle and/or of the apparent sympathetic inhibitory influences at the level of the sympathetic ganglion. Cholinergic

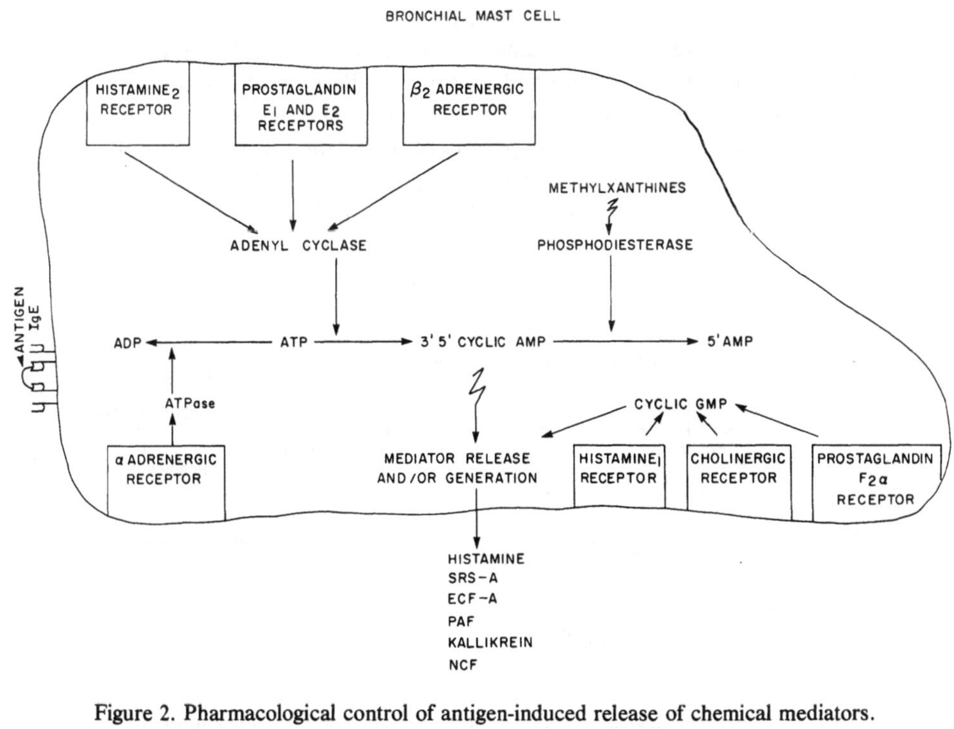

Figure 2. Pharmacological control of antigen-induced release of chemical mediators.

stimulation of isolated human bronchial smooth muscle *in vitro* does result in marked bronchoconstriction, and the inhalation of such agonists will produce bronchoconstriction in both normals and asthmatics, the latter with lower concentrations (Grieco and Pierson, 1970). In view of the rich plexus of cholinergic fibers in bronchi, the direct neural release of acetylcholine is likely, with bronchoconstriction occurring in association with elevated cyclic GMP. Stimulation of H-1 receptors by histamine in high concentrations does induce contraction. The fact that only part of the bronchoconstrictor effect of histamine injected directly into the bronchial artery of dogs is present after vagotomy suggests that histamine has both direct effects and indirect reflex action on bronchial smooth muscle (De Kock *et al.,* 1966; Brocklehurst, 1968). Both SRS-A and $PGF_{2\alpha}$ (Cuthbert, 1972) are potent bronchoconstrictors while kinins (Herxheimer and Stresemann, 1961) are not very effective in causing acute bronchoconstriction in man. The presence of α-adrenergic receptors has been controversial, but several studies suggest their presence (Adolphson *et al,* 1970; Anthracite *et al.,* 1971; Simonsson *et al.,* 1972).

While goblet cells appear to be independent of adrenergic and cholinergic modulation, the secretions of subepithelial mucous glands are increased by parasympathomimetic agents (Sturgess and Reed, 1972) while bradykinin, histamine, and their antagonists exert no significant effect.

3.4. Bronchial Airways

3.4.1. Sites of Airway Obstruction

In 1968, Hogg *et al.* utilized the retrograde catheter technique of Macklem to place a catheter into the 11th-order bronchus of 2 mm. Together with alveolar pressure and pleural pressure, the maneuver allowed the calculation of central and peripheral resistance in lungs obtained at autopsy. Peripheral resistance was 25% of the total in five normals while it was increased 4–40 times in seven emphysema patients. This demonstration that the peripheral resistance was poorly reflected by measurements of total airway resistance ignited an acute awareness of the importance of distinguishing large and small airway disease. The bronchial tree

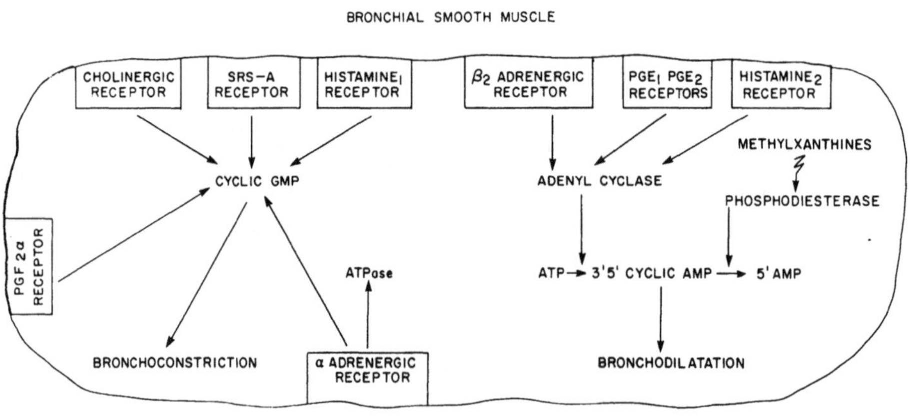

Figure 3. Pharmacological modulation of bronchial smooth muscle contraction.

consists of more than 30 orders of bronchi. Obstructive disorders may predominate in the trachea, large bronchi, small airways, and possibly the alveolar ducts. The cross-sectional diameter of the bronchial tree can be depicted as funnel shaped (Figure 4). Obstruction of bronchi of a specific cumulative diameter will have less effect on airway conduction when located in the peripheral airways. Tracheal obstruction is not detectable by measurements of airway resistance or residual volume. Hudgel *et al.* (1976) reported a patient with reversible decrease of static compliance and increase of elastic recoil suggestive of alveolar duct and sac constriction.

3.4.2. *In Vivo* Effects of Humoral Mediators

Drazen and Austen (1974b) have studied the effects of intravenous administration of SRS-A, histamine, bradykinin, and $PGF_{2\alpha}$ on the mechanics of respiration in the unanesthetized guinea pig. Using conductance as a measure of large airway function and compliance as reflecting predominantly the small airways, SRS-A resulted in a pronounced decrease of small airways while $PGF_{2\alpha}$ had an early preferential effect on large airways followed by a late equal effect on both. In contrast, both histamine and bradykinin have comparable effects on both compliance and conductance. Thus intravenously administered SRS-A alters pulmonary mechanics with a more peripheral effect than any of the other agents tested.

Using partial expiratory flow-volume maneuvers with air and HeO_2, Brown *et al.* (1977) reported that the response to histamine aerosol suggested that large airways were predominantly constricted in smokers and the small airways in nonsmokers. Although these observations could be interpreted to indicate differences in smooth muscle reactivity, they speculated that the results reflected the

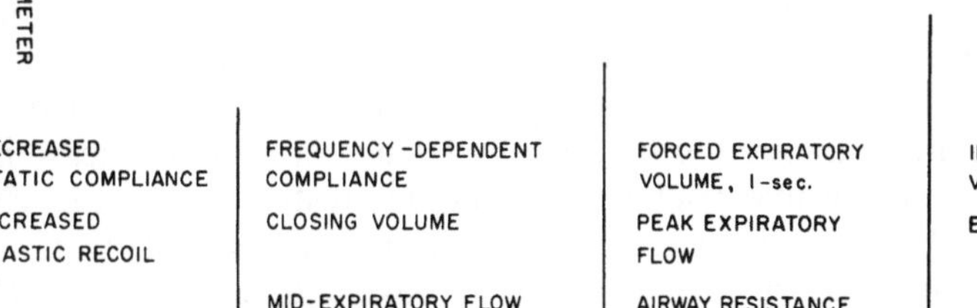

DETECTION			
DECREASED STATIC COMPLIANCE INCREASED ELASTIC RECOIL	FREQUENCY-DEPENDENT COMPLIANCE CLOSING VOLUME MID-EXPIRATORY FLOW RATE FLOW-VOLUME LOOP ROOM AIR AND HELIUM	FORCED EXPIRATORY VOLUME, 1-sec. PEAK EXPIRATORY FLOW AIRWAY RESISTANCE	INSPIRATORY FLOW-VOLUME LOOP ENDOSCOPY
RESIDUAL VOLUME NORMAL	INCREASED	INCREASED	NORMAL

Figure 4. Predominant sites of bronchial disorders.

pattern on aerosol distribution demonstrated by Dolovich *et al.* (1976) so that the aerosol penetrated less into the small airways of smokers.

3.4.3. Sites of Action of Bronchodilators

Ingram *et al.* (1977) examined the tone of normal human airways and demonstrated that although both atropine and isoproterenol produced bronchodilatation, atropine decreased density dependence while the latter was increased by isoproterenol. This suggested that atropine predominantly dilated large upstream airways and isoproterenol influenced small upstream airways. In a study of 17 patients with obstructive lung disease, Wellman *et al.* (1976) reported that density dependence, using air and HeO_2, was decreased with Sch1000, a congener of atropine, and increased with isoproterenol, again suggesting that these agents differ in the predominant site of the airways that they effect.

Thus parasympathomimetic reflexes appear to predominantly constrict the large airways while mast cell mediators act on both large and small airways. The predominant sympathomimetic effect appears to be on the small airways to induce bronchodilatation.

4. Allergic Asthma (Extrinsic)

Chapters 4, 5, and 7 have reviewed the current state of knowledge regarding the molecular definition of allergens, IgE antibodies, and mediators of immediate hypersensitivity. The discussion here will be limited to aspects of these subjects pertinent to bronchial hypersensitivity reactions.

4.1. Immunological Basis

Allergic respiratory diseases include bronchial asthma, pulmonary eosinophilia, and extrinsic alveolitis, the latter two comprising hypersensitivity pneumonitis. Bronchial provocation testing in humans allows classification of reactions into immediate, nonimmediate, and combinations of both (Pepys, 1977).

4.1.1. Immediate Asthmatic Reactions

a. IgE Antibodies. The characteristic immunological feature of atopy is the genetically determined capacity to produce specific reagininc IgE antibodies to common environmental allergens via limited immunogenic challenge. Allergic asthma is generally characterized by a family history of allergic disease including eczema and rhinitis, positive prick and intradermal tests, increased levels of IgE in the serum, and positive immediate bronchial provocation tests with suspected allergens. The family history was reported by Cooke and Vander Veer (1916) to be positive in 48.4% of 504 allergic subjects compared with only 44.5% of a control group of 76 normal persons. Total basal serum IgE levels have been shown to be clearly under the control of an IgE-regulating gene, with high IgE levels inherited as a simple Mendelian recessive trait (Bazaral *et al.*, 1974). The IgE-regulating gene can have a profound effect on specific IgE responses and mask the effects of HLA-linked Ir genes (Marsh *et al.*, 1974). Marsh *et al.* (1973, 1974) noted the association of rye grass group II antigens with HL-A8 and Ra5 of ragweed with HLA7 Creg. The Ir gene for Ra5 appeared to control production of both IgG and IgE antibodies. In contrast, Levine *et al.* (1972) reported linkage of specific HLA haplotype of the propositus and specific IgE or IgG responsiveness to antigen E of ragweed in 7 families in which there was a clear segregation of sensitivity to antigen E within the members. In addition to these genetic studies concerned with total and allergen-specific IgE, the disorder of bronchial asthma has been linked to genetic factors. Rachelefsky *et al.* (1976) reported that 88% of 30 asthma patients had B lymphocyte group 2 antigens compared with 24% of 109 controls, but they failed to identify an HLA-associated gene. Brostoff *et al.* (1976) have reported homozygosity for HLA-W6 in 21 of 26 patients with intrinsic asthma, suggesting a genetic predisposition in patients with that disorder.

As indicated in Table 1, immediate asthmatic reactions to provocation tests can be blocked by cromolyn sodium but not by corticosteroids and are effectively reversed by inhaled bronchodilators (Pepys and Hutchcroft, 1975). Such provocations lead to a bronchoconstrictive reaction which is maximal at 10–15 min and lasts for 1–2 hr. It is likely that antigenic determinants bind specific IgE antibodies which have attached to Fc receptors on the surface of basophiloid cells in the airways and subepithelial mast cells to induce mediator release. The presence of IgE on the epithelial side of basement membranes in asthmatic lungs suggests that globular leukocytes, K cells, and neuroepithelial bodies may participate in the reaction. Allergic asthmatics as a group have elevated levels of IgE, and levels of 5 times normal were found in greater than 50% (Johansson, 1967).

b. IgE_4 Antibodies. Reaginlike activity in humans has been associated with IgG class antibodies directed against horse proteins (Terr and Bentz, 1965); horse dander (Reid, 1970), milk proteins, avian antigens (Parish, 1974); and *Dermatophagoides* sp. (Bryant *et al.*, 1975). The heat-stable reaginic activity on passive transfer is short term and led to the designation by Parish (1970) as "short-term sensitizing IgG" (STS-IgG) antibody and subsequently associated with the IgG_4 subclass. Such STS-IgG appears to be less frequent and less potent in allergic mediator release. In nonatopic subjects these immunoglobulins may result in immediate skin test reactions and bronchial provocation and may act as an introductory mechanism for nonimmediate asthmatic reactions as seen in nonatopic pigeon fanciers (Pepys, 1977). Vijay and Perelmutter (1977) have demonstrated that leukocytes from 11 allergic individuals and from nine normal subjects sensitized with the serum of allergic patients were capable of releasing histamine with antihuman IgG_4, antihuman IgE, and specific allergens. This suggests a broader role for IgG_4 in immediate type I hypersensitivity reactions than has been considered previously. STS-IgG has been recorded as a familial trait and responsible for dual immediate and late (5–6 hr) skin reactions (Berry and Brighton, 1977). In addition, both IgG_2 and IgG_3 subclass antibodies cytophilic for circulating basophils have been detected in subjects with allergic bronchopulmonary aspergillosis (Assem and Turner-Warwick, 1976).

Bryant *et al.* (1975) studied 16 patients with asthma sensitive to *Dermatophagoides pteronyssimus*. In seven, cromolyn sodium was ineffective as an inhibitor of bronchial immediate allergic reactions and reaginic IgG antibodies were predominant. The presence of STS-IgG antibodies may provide one explanation for apparent failure of allergic asthmatic patients to respond to therapy with cromolyn sodium.

4.1.2. Nonimmediate (Late) Asthmatic Reactions

Nonimmediate asthmatic reactions to provocation tests are blocked by corticosteroids and cromolyn sodium and marginally reversed by aerosol bronchodilators. Inhibition of this reaction by corticosteroids contrasts with their lack of effect on immediate reactions. Pepys (1977) has distinguished three types of nonimmediate reactions: those maximal at 1 hr, those maximal at 3–4 hr, and those with recurrent nighttime exacerbations following a single aerosol provocation. The last responses have been elicited with aerosol avian antigens, gaseous formalin fumes, and chemical dusts such as ampicillin powder and interfere with the interpretation of the importance of causal exposures. The nonimmediate reactions might be considered as extrinsic nonatopic asthma. Blockade by cromolyn sodium suggests that mast cell degranulation is involved while the effectiveness of corticosteroids may implicate the participation of inflammatory cells in the pathogenesis. The ineffectiveness of aerosol bronchodilators may be due to the greater involvement of the smaller airways in these reactions. In contrast to immediate reactions, late responses are often accompanied by malaise, fever, and leukocytosis.

The pathogenesis of late nonimmediate airway responses has been controversial, as has been that involved in eosinophilic pneumonia and extrinsic allergic alveolitis. Insoluble immune complexes involving antigen and IgG precipitating antibody (type III hypersensitivity), activation of the alternative pathway of the complement system, and cell-mediated immunity have been implicated. Dual skin and inhalational test reactions with *Aspergillus fumigatus* and *Candida albicans* antigens have been attributed to IgE and $IgG_{2,3,4}$ reaginic antibodies and IgG precipitating antibodies in subjects with allergic bronchopulmonary aspergillosis and candidiosis. Late and dual bronchial responses in extrinsic allergic alveolitis have been associated with IgG^4 reaginic and precipitating antibodies in subjects sensitive to thermophylic actinomycetes and pigeon antigens. Presumable C3a and C5a act as anaphylatoxins to degranulate mast cells. Alternative pathway activaction with generation of C3a and C5a as well as macrophage activation has been suggested as a possible mechanism for disease induction by *Micropolyspora faeni* and other organic dusts (Schorlemmer *et al.*, 1977). Fink *et al.* (1975) reported that complement-fixing antibodies may play a protective role while cell-mediated immunity, as reflected by release of macrophage inhibitory factor, appears to induce alveolitis in subjects sensitive to pigeon antigens. Animal models of hypersensitivity pneumonitis suggest a primary role for delayed hypersensitivity (Moore *et al.*, 1975; Harris *et al.*, 1976) (type IV hypersensitivity). A markedly greater effect of inhaled spore particles as against antigen solutions in eliciting granulomatous pneumonitis in animals has also been shown (Salvaggio *et al.*, 1975). The late bronchial response in these instances might result from mast cell active agents released from PMSs, monocytes, or lymphocytes. This remains speculative, although it is known that lysates of human leukocytes contain heat-labile histamine-releasing factor as well as an inhibitor of release (Kelly and White, 1974). This releasing factor appears to be present in both lymphocytes and granulocytes.

Whether late reactions involve antibody or alternative pathway complement activation or reflect some aspect of cell-mediated immunity, the effect of cromolyn sodium supports the belief that mast cell degranulation is the resultant effect responsible for bronchoconstriction. In atopic patients it appears that late cutaneous allergic reactions can occur with an isolated dependence on IgE antibody, and it remains to be determined whether pure IgE reactions may result in late as well as immediate bronchial responses in such subjects. The late reaction is inhibited by prednisone (Poothullil *et al.*, 1976) and may result from the inflammatory response subsequent to mast cell mediator release.

4.2. Allergens

Protein and carbohydrates as well as low molecular weight chemicals acting as haptens may elicit allergic asthmatic responses. A partial list of major allergens and the types of bronchial reactions elicited is presented in Table 3. The size and number of antigenic determinants are important since they represent a minor component of the extrinsic agent. Ability to act as a hapten is critical for compounds such as complex salts of platinum. The 1–2 μm diameter size of *Micropolyspora faeni* allows penetration to the small airways while 10–12 μm spores of *Aspergillus fumigatus* are likely to lodge in the large bronchi.

While inhalant allergens are likely to account for most of the allergic aspects of bronchial asthma, food allergens are capable of significant contribution, especially in children. Measurement of specific IgE antibodies by RAST showed an extremely high correlation with the history of hypersensitivity in subjects allergic to peanut, bivalve mollusks, and cat (Hoffman and Haddad 1974).

Inhalants may consist of particulates, aerosols, fumes, gases, or chemical dusts. Multivalent antigens with at least two active sites are believed to react with at least two antigen-specific IgE molecules attached to the Fc receptor of basophiloid cells and epithelial mast cells and possibly on globular leukocytes, K cells, and neuroepithelial bodies and result in mast cell degranulation. Simani *et al.* (1974) have reported the penetration of intercellular spaces in the guinea pig bronchial epithelium by tracer materials after exposure to cigarette smoke. These dilated intercellular spaces and the opening of previously closed tight junctions may be the pathway for transfer of some inhaled noxious substances or allergenic macromolecules which impinge on the bronchial mucosa.

Salvaggio *et al.* (1964) found that the intranasal administration of RNase and dextran produced larger and more promptly developing wheal and erythema skin test reactivity in atopic individuals than in nonatopic subjects. They advanced the hypothesis that there is a greater absorption of antigens through the nasal mucous membranes in atopic than in nonatopic individuals. In a subsequent study (Kontou-Karakitsos *et al.*, 1975) that assessed mucosal absorption more directly, the atopic group failed to show greater or more rapid absorption of either RNase or peanut extract. The fact that tight junctions (zonula occludens) are found in the respiratory tract epithelia raises the question as to how high-molecular-weight antigens are able to get through the epithelial layer to the interstitium of the lung. In a study using the tracer protein horseradish peroxidase (40,000 daltons), sensitized guinea pigs developed significant bronchoconstriction but the antigen was superficial and did not appear to penetrate the epithelial cells, suggesting that the immunological

TABLE 3. **Partial List of Major Allergens and the Bronchial Responses Elicited by Provocation**

		Allergen		Bronchial response	
		Nature	Molecular weight	Immediate	Late
I. Inhalant aerosols					
Ragweed					
	AgE	Protein	37,800	+	
	AgK	Protein	38,200	+	
	Ra3	Protein	15,000	+	
	Ra5	Peptide	5,130	+	
	BPA-R	Protein	28,000	+	
Grasses					
	Group I	Glyco-protein	32,000	+	
	Group II	Glyco-protein	10,000	+	
	Antigen D	Peptide	5,000	+	
	Antigen B	Protein	10,500	+	
Animal dander, serum, secretions					
	Dog	Albumin	65,000	+	
	Cat	Albumin	30,000–60,000	+	
	Rat	α_2-Globulin	10,000–25,000	+	
	Mouse	Prealbumin	10,000–25,000	+	
	Guinea pig	Prealbumin	25,000	+	
	Rabbit	Albumin	18,000–38,000	+	
	Cow	Albumin	—	+	
	Horse	Albumin	22,000–60,000	+	
	Birds	—	—	+	+
	Pituitary snuff	—	—		+
	Fish meal	—	—		+
Wood dusts					
	Western red cedar			+	+
	Iroko			+	+
Molds, fungi					
	Alternaria sp.	Glycoprotein	High	+	+ occas.
	Aspergillus sp.	—	—	+	+
	Micropolyspora faeni	—	—		
	Thremoactinomyces sp.	—	—		+
	Aureobasidium sp.	—	—		+
	Cryptostroma corticale	—	—		+
	Penicillium casei	—	—		+
	Candida sp.	—	—	+	+
Insect					
	Sitophilius granarius	—	—		+
Mites					
	Dermatophagoides sp.	—	—	+	+
	Acarus siro	—	—	+	+

(continued)

TABLE 3. (*Continued*)

	Allergen		Bronchial response	
	Nature	Molecular weight	Immediate	Late
Free-living amoebae				
Acanthamoeba-polyphaga	—	—		+
Acanthamoeba castellani	—	—		+
II. Inhalant gaseous emanation, occupational				
Toluene diisocyanate[a] (TDI)	Chemical	—	+	+
Epoxy resins				
Phthalic acid anhydride	Chemical	—	+	+
Triethylene tetramine	Chemical	—	+	+
Trimellitic acid	Chemical	—	+	+
III. Inhalant chemical dusts, occupational				
Complex salts of platinum	Chemical	—	+	
Antimicrobial drugs	Chemical	—		
Ampicillin				+
Salbutamol intermediate				+

[a]No direct immunological evidence.

reaction occurred at this site (Richardson *et al.*, 1973) and that penetration to the subepithelial mast cells was not mandatory.

Ragweed pollen grains are 20 μm in diameter and too large to penetrate to the bronchi. Although they are deposited in the upper airway, reflex bronchoconstriction does not occur from this site (Hoehne and Reed, 1971). Busse *et al.* (1972) demonstrated ragweed antigen in airborne particles less than 5 μm in diameter which could penetrate to the lower airways and initiate an allergic reaction. Animal studies support the belief that it is the antigen reaching the tracheobronchial tree which is important in inducing allergic bronchoconstriction. Presumably the rapidly released Ra5 and more slowly released Ra3 and antigen E are deposited on the tracheobronchial epithelial and bind to the IgE in the epithelium and on the subepithelial mast cells.

4.2.1. Inhalant Aerosols

Table 3 lists prototype allergens which result in immediate, late, or dual bronchial responses. Late responses may occur with isolated bronchial asthma or may be associated with pulmonary eosinophilia (*Aspergillus fumigatus*, *Candida albicans*) or extrinsic allergic alveolitis (bird fancier, fish meal, rodent urine, pituitary snuff, wood dusts, spores of thermophilic actinomycetes and fungi, mite antigens, insect antigens, and free-living amoebae in contaminated water aerosols). It is of interest that α_2-globulin in the male rat and a prealbumin in the male mouse serve to induce allergic sensitization which may be reduced with the use of female animals.

4.2.2. Inhalant Gaseous Allergens

Toluene diisocyanate (TDI) use elicits both immediate and late bronchial responses, but as yet IgE antibodies have not been demonstrated. IgE antibodies have been associated with sensitivity to epoxy resins cured with phthalic acid anhydride, trimellitic acid, and triethylene tetramine.

4.2.3. Inhalant Dust Allergens

Immediate reactions occur with complex salts of platinum. Late reactions to chemical dusts are provided by workers with occupational asthma engaged in the manufacture of antimicrobial drugs including ampicillin and salbutamol due to a glycyl intermediary compound. Late reactions to chemical dusts, vapors, fumes, and ingested agents are not generally associated with systemic symptoms.

4.2.4. Occupational Asthma

Occupational asthma (Karr *et al.,* 1978) has been estimated to have a worldwide prevalence of 2% and constitutes an important group where it is possible to determine an extrinsic etiology. Allergic pathogenesis is implicated with several of the allergens listed in Table 3 as well as with the castor bean, green coffee bean, papain, pancreatic extract, enzymes from *Bacillus subtilis,* hog trypsin, phenylglycine acid chloride, and sulfone chloramides.

In other instances an irritant effect, as is the case with sulfur or nitrogen dioxide, or a pharmacological reaction, such as with byssinosis (cotton dust, direct mediator release) or TDI, may be responsible. TDI can alter the *in vitro* stimulation of lymphocyte cyclic AMP levels by isoproterenol and prostaglandin E_1 but not by histamine (Davies *et al.*, 1977). Recent dose–response studies with isoproterenol have shown that TDI may act as a partial antagonist of β-adrenergic receptors. This mechanism would not lead to asthma in a normal subject but might induce bronchospasm in a subject with a subclinical asthmatic diathesis.

4.3. Chemical Mediators

Mast cells in the lung have been localized to both the bronchial mucosal surface (globular leukocytes) and the deeper connective tissue in a perivenular distribution. These cells contain Fc receptors which bind specifically to IgE. Bridging of pairs of receptors by specific polyvalent antigen or anti-IgE initiates a series of intracellular events that results in the noncytotoxic release of the mast cell granule contents (Table 4).

4.3.1. Preformed Mediators

a. Histamine. The histamine associated with mast cells is found within the metachromatic granules as a histamine–protein–heparin complex (Unväs, 1968). Some of the established pharmacological actions of histamine relevant to its role in asthma include H-1 receptor direct and reflex (Gold *et al.*, 1972) induction of bronchoconstriction, possible mucous hypersecretion and increased vascular permeability as well as H-2 receptor dependent inhibition of IgE-mediated release of histamine (Lichtenstein and Gillespie, 1973). Histamine in low concentrations is weakly chemoattractive for eosinophils, but this effect is not clearly related to H-1 or H-2 receptors. An inhibitory effect of higher concentrations of histamine on eosinophil chemotaxis is blocked by an H-2 antagonist (Lett-Brown and Leonard, 1977).

Inhalation of histamine provokes bronchospasm in asthmatics which can be prevented in part by atropine, suggesting that reflex cholinergic efferent pathways contribute to the bronchoconstriction (Nadel, 1968). The direct effect of histamine

TABLE 4. Chemical Mediators Released from Human Lung During Allergen-IgE Hypersensitivity Reactions

Category	Mediator	Structure	Function
Preformed	Histamine	Bimidazolylethylamine	H-1 receptor
		111 daltons	a. Facilitate mediator release
			b. Stimulate vagal afferent fibers
			c. *Bronchoconstriction*
			d. $PGF_{2\alpha}$ release
			H-2 receptor
			a. Inhibit mediator release
			b. Bronchodilatation
			c. PG_{E2} release
			Effect eosinophil migration
	ECF-A	Val/Ala-Gly-Ser-Glu	a. Chemotaxis of eosinophils + PMNs
		360–390 daltons	b. Deactivation of eosinophils + PMNs
	ECF-intermediate	1300–2500 daltons	"
	NCF	Protein >160,000 daltons	"
	Heparin	Proteoglycan	a. Antithrombin
		750,000 daltons	b. Inhibit C3 amplification convertase
	Chymase	Protein 25,000 daltons	a. Proteolysis
	N-Acetyl-β-glucosamidase	50,000 daltons	
	Arylsulfatase A	15,000 daltons	
	B	60,000 daltons	
Newly generated	SRS-A	Acidic lipid 300–400 daltons	a. Direct *bronchoconstriction* and vascular permeability
	PAF	Lipid	a. Release of 5-hydroxytryptamine
		700 daltons	b. Platelet aggregation
			c. ? Platelet factor III Bronchoconstriction and fibrin deposition
	Lipid Chemo tactic factor for PMN	Lipid	a. Chemotaxis of PMNs
	Superoxide (O_2^-)	32 daltons	a. Microbial activity
			b. Tissue injury

on intrapulmonary rapidly adapting vagal afferents appears to be mediated by H-1 receptors. In addition, histamine mediates peripheral airway smooth muscle constriction via H-1 receptors while H-2 receptors, at low concentrations of histamine, may lead to bronchodilatation. In 1963 Beall reported that blood histamine levels are not elevated during an acute asthmatic attack. Bhat *et al.* (1976), Arroyave *et al.* (1977), and Stevenson *et al.* (1976) reported the transient elevation of plasma histamine and depression of complement components in venous samples taken from subjects experiencing a provoked asthmatic reaction with a skin test positive antigen or following oral challenge with aspirin in sensitive subjects. Elevated plasma histamine and fibrin split products and mildly reduced total hemolytic complement activity have been reported as well after methacholine aerosol challenge in asthmatics. Simon *et al.* (1977) demonstrated significantly elevated plasma histamine levels above 1.25 ng/ml in asthmatic patients with spontaneous severe exacerbations utilizing an enzymatic isotopic technique instead of the fluorometric assay, but this finding has not been confirmed. These studies support the role of histamine as a mediator in bronchial asthma.

b. Preformed Chemotactic Factors. Eosinophil chemotactic factor of anaphylaxis (ECF-A) (Kay and Austen, 1971), eosinophil chemotactic factor oligopeptides (ECF-oligopeptides) (Lewis and Austen, 1977), and neutrophil chemotactic factor of anaphylaxis (NCF-A) (Lewis and Austen, 1977) can be released from human lung fragments by IgE-dependent mechanisms. Each is chemotactic for eosinophils and neutrophils and acts to deactivate these cells. ECF-A extracted from human lung is composed of at least two tetrapeptides differing only in their *N*-terminal amino acid. Eosinophil chemotaxis to the tetrapeptides presumably involves binding of a hydrophobic domain of an eosinophil receptor with the *N*-terminal and activation of an ionic domain with the glutamic acid *C*-terminal.

c. Heparin. Macromolecular heparin has recently been shown to be present in rat peritoneal mast cell granules and is released with the granule by IgE-dependent mechanisms (Lewis and Austen, 1977). Although heparin has been extracted from human lung, the identity of the metachromatically staining lung mast cell granule component as heparin is unproven. Heparin may act as well to inhibit the amplification C3 convertase of the alternative complement pathway and modify C3a and C5a mast cell degranulation.

4.3.2. Newly Generated Mediators

a. Slow-Reacting Substance of Anaphylaxis (SRS-A). SRS-A, an acidic sulfur-containing lipid, acts to directly constrict bronchial smooth muscle and increase vascular permeability largely independent of cholinergic reflex mechanisms (Drazen and Austen, 1974b). Immunological *in vitro* release of SRS-A has been produced by IgE-dependent reactions in tissue fragments of human nasal polyps and lung. SRS-A is inactivated by arylsulfatases of several sources including eosinophils and mast cell rich fractions. A small amount of preformed SRS-A-like activity is extractable from some human lung preparations, and cellular SRS-A has been described in cells after IgE-dependent immunological challenge.

b. Platelet-Activating Factor (PAF). PAFs are a family of substances released by immunological activation of human lung (Bogart and Stechschulte, 1974). They release 5-hydroxytryptamine and secondarily aggregate homologous platelets and are inactivated by eosinophil phospholipase D. The elaboration of vasoactive amines and perhaps platelet factor III may result in contraction of bronchial smooth muscle and in fibrin deposition.

c. Lipid Chemotactic Factor(s) of Anaphylaxis. Lipid mediators chemotactic for neutrophils are released from human lung by IgE-dependent reactions (Lewis and Austen, 1977).

4.3.3. Secondary Mediators

a. Serotonin (5-Hydroxytryptamine). 5HT is not readily implicated in the pathogenesis of bronchial asthma because the serotonin content of human lung tissue is negligible and the isolated human bronchial ring is resistant to serotonin (Brocklehurst, 1958) (Table 5). The potential role for platelet release following PAF action must be reexamined.

b. Cellular Kallikrein. Antigen challenge of IgE-sensitized human lung fragments results in the release of mediators capable of hydrolyzing synthetic substrates such as tosyl-L-arginine methyl ester (TAMe) and cleaving bradykinin from its natural substrate, kininogen (Webster *et al.*, 1974). Cellular kallikrein may implicate the kinins as mediators of immediate hypersensitivity. Evidence that the kinins may play a role in human asthma includes induction of bronchospasm by the inhalation of kinins in asthmatics but not in nonasthmatics (Cuthbert, 1972), the elevation of kinin levels by approximately tenfold in the serum of a patient

TABLE 5. Chemical Mediators Secondarily Released from Human Lung Following Allergen-IgE Hypersensitivity Reactions

Mediator	Structure	Function
Serotonin	5-Hydroxytryptamine 176 daltons	Increased vascular permeability
Kinins	Nonapeptide	Direct bronchoconstriction and increased vascular permeability
Bradykinin		
Lysylbradykinin	Decapeptide 1000 daltons	"
Prostaglandins	20-carbon fatty acids with cyclopentane ring	
$PGF_{2\alpha}$ (from lung parenchyma)		a. Direct and reflex bronchoconstriction b. Facilitation of IgE-dependent mediator release
PG endoperoxides (PGG_2 and PGH_2)		"
TXA_2		"
PGE_1 and PGE_2 (from bronchi)		a. Direct bronchodilatation b. Inhibition of IgE-dependent mediator release
Prostacyclin (PGI)		"

during an acute asthmatic attack (Abe *et al.*, 1967), and the increased levels of components of the kinin-forming system during episodes of bronchospasm in patients with the carcinoid syndrome (Oates *et al.*, 1964).

c. Prostaglandins. Aspects of the function of prostaglandins in the lung have been reviewed recently (Hyman *et al.*, 1978; Mathe *et al.*, 1977). In *in vitro* experiments both actively and passively sensitized mammalian lung release $PGF_{2\alpha}$, PGE_1, and PGE_2, 15-keto-13,14-dihydro metabolites, and thromboxane B_2 (TxB_2 and by inference TxA_2). Small amounts of endoperoxides (PGG_2 and PGH_2) and 12-hydroxy-5,8,10-heptadecatrienoic acid (HHT) are detectable as well. TxA_2, the rabbit aorta contracting substance, has a half-life of 30 sec and is converted to the weakly active TxB_2.

$PGF_{2\alpha}$, 15β-$PGF_{2\alpha}$, PG endoperoxides, and TxA_2 are potent human bronchoconstrictive agents acting on smooth muscle via a PG receptor. This direct action is antagonized by the bronchodilator PGEs. As aerosols, PGE_1 and PGE_2 are about 10 times more potent bronchodilators than isoproterenol. *In vitro* studies indicate that β_2-adrenergic antagonists potentiate while atropine diminishes the response to $PGF_{2\alpha}$, suggesting the role of parasympathetically mediated reflexes (Mathe *et al.*, 1977).

Histamine and SRS-A both act to liberate prostaglandins. Antagonism of H-1 receptors by pyrilamine diminishes the subsequent response to histamine, predominantly decreasing the flow of $PGF_{2\alpha}$ from the lung parenchyma. In contrast, antagonism of H-2 receptors by metiamide reduces the subsequent flow of PGE_2 from sensitized airways. The observation that eicosatetraenoic acid inhibits prostaglandin formation but does not affect SRS-A release whereas cromolyn sodium inhibits the release of SRS-A and prostaglandins supports the view that prostaglandins are not formed by a pathway common to the primary mediators (Dawson and Tomlinson, 1974). However, it has recently been suggested that SRS-A may be formed from arachidonic acid via the activity of a lipoxygenase acting at a step proximal to cycloxygenase.

The secondarily released prostaglandins can influence the IgE-dependent release of mediators from human lung fragments. PGs of the E type increase cyclic AMP and inhibit release while very low concentrations of both PGE and $PGF_{2\alpha}$ have been found to decrease the level of cyclic AMP and enhance anaphylactic release (Tauber *et al.*, 1973).

In asthmatic patients an increase in the plasma level of the main metabolite of $PGF_{2\alpha}$ has been found after an attack (Green *et al.*, 1974), although the level of $PGF_{2\alpha}$ is not significantly altered (Okazaki *et al.*, 1976). There is a remarkable difference in the sensitivity of asthmatic and control subjects to aerosol $PGF_{2\alpha}$. The dose eliciting a 50% decrease in conductance ranged from 4 to 1024 ng in asthmatic patients while 128,000–1,024,000 ng was required in control subjects (Mathe and Hedquist, 1975). While in healthy and asthmatic subjects PGE_1 and PGE_2 produce bronchodilatation, in some PGE_2 may bronchoconstrict. This constrictive response might reflect a cholinergically mediated reflex, conversion of PGE_2 to $PGF_{2\alpha}$, or release of $PGF_{2\alpha}$, histamine, or acetylcholine. While the effect of PGs on the basal tone of airways and the hyperreactivity to $PGF_{2\alpha}$ in asthma imply participation in allergic asthma, their role remains uncertain. The relative amounts of prostaglandins and not the actual concentration of any single compound derived from arachidonic acid may be determinative. Mathe *et al.* (1977) speculate that $PGF_{2\alpha}$ could be bound to tissue or plasma proteins and hence protected from degradation by 15PGDH. After an acute episode of asthma there might be gradual dissociation of bound $PGF_{2\alpha}$ to account for prolonged bronchoconstriction. The fact that indomethacin does not prevent or ameliorate asthmatic attacks in man may be due to the activity of $PGF_{2\alpha}$ in nanogram amounts produced by the remaining capacity for synthesis. Szczeklik *et al.* (1975) has proposed that aspirinlike drugs may induce an asthmatic attack by inhibiting PG synthesis in patients dependent on PGE bronchodilatation. Recently (Moncada *et al.*, 1976) a new product of PG endoperoxides called "prostacyclin" (PGI) has been detected. It is a potent inhibitor of platelet aggregation and a bronchodilator. Only small quantities appear in the lung, but its role in IgE-dependent mediator release has not been determined.

4.3.4. Recruitment of Cells and Plasma Effector Systems

Eosinophils, platelets, and neutrophils are recruited by the preformed and generated chemical mediators. Eosinophils are rich in histaminase, which destroys histamine, arysulfatase B, which is capable of inactivating SRS-A, phospholipase D, which inactivates PAF, and phospholipase B, which leads to the production of PGE_1, the eosinophil-derived inhibitor of mast cell degranulation (Hubscher, 1975). This antimediator role of eosinophils is presumed to account for their recruitment at sites of IgE-dependent reactions and presence in bronchial asthma and eosinophilic pneumonias. Platelets may contribute to pathogenesis by elaborating vasoactive amines and platelet factor III, which may result in bronchoconstriction and fibrin deposition (Austen and Orange, 1975). The plasma protein effector systems including clotting (platelet factor III), fibrinolysis, and kinin generation (cellular kallikrein) may participate in the persisting inflammatory reaction to alter bronchial reactivity to nonimmunological stimuli long after subsidence of an acute IgE-dependent allergic reaction.

It was noted above that late cutaneous allergic reactions can occur with an isolated dependence on IgE antibody. The initial cutaneous wheal-and-flare response reflects altered vascular permeability, whereas the later erythematous, warm, and painful reaction is accompanied by an intense cellular infiltration. Immunochemical studies have not revealed deposition of immune complexes or complement components during this late inflammatory phase (Lewis and Austen, 1977). Elicitation of both inflammatory phases by injection not only of specific antigen but also of anti-IgE indicates that mast cell activation can contribute to both acute and chronic processes. The dual response of airways to inhaled antigen has a time course compatible with that of the biphasic cutaneous response to IgE-dependent mast cell degranulation. While late bronchial response may be IgE induced, other mechanisms enumerated above may be responsible as well.

4.3.5. Pulmonary Endothelial Cells

Pulmonary endothelial cells have numerous metabolic functions beyond the scope of this chapter. It may be relevant to the pathogenesis of bronchial asthma that epinephrine and histamine are allowed free passage and prostaglandins are synthesized while some mediators such as norepinephrine, bradykinin, serotonin, and prostaglandins of the PGE and PGF series are inactivated (Ryan and Ryan, 1977). In addition, both ATP and cyclic AMP are metabolized during passage through the lungs. Alteration of pulmonary endothelial metabolic function might be significant in contributing to a basic defect in chronic bronchial asthma.

4.3.6. Non-IgE-Mediated Mast Cell Degranulation

Studies with peripheral leukocytes indicated that IgG reagin (Petersson, 1975), activation of either the alternative or classical pathway of complement (Grant *et al.*, 1977; Petersson *et al.*, 1975; Siraganian and Hook, 1976) and leukocyte lysates can release histamine and presumably the other chemical mediators. C5a is far more potent than C3a and accounts for the majority of classical anaphylatoxin. Activated complement releases histamine from both nonallergic and allergic individuals and is not restricted to atopics. A second pathway for initiating inflammation, not dependent on the presence of antibody, is via the 5000-dalton human leukocyte factor of Kelly and White (1974). Either or both mechanisms for mast cell degranulation may explain some late bronchial responses and may participate in the pathogenesis of nonallergic bronchial asthma.

4.4. Cholinergic Reflex Pathways

Aerosol or parenteral atropine is an antagonist of muscarinic parasympathetic receptors and partially (Itkin and Anand, 1970) or totally (Yu *et al.*, 1972) prevents airway obstruction after antigen inhalation in susceptible asthmatics, suggesting that the antigen-induced mediators may be acting to stimulate afferent epithelial irritant receptors. Gold *et al.* (1972) used dogs allergic to known antigens, exposing them to these by inhalation. A sharp rise in airway resistance was thus induced; this was eliminated by vagal blockade, both afferent and efferent. Furthermore, unilateral challenge of one lung with antigen resulted in bronchoconstriction which was bilateral; this was inhibited by vagal blockade on the challenged side. The difficulty of clinical studies based on atropine antagonism is that pretreatment often results in bronchodilatation and an altered baseline. Fish *et al.* (1977), in a study of six asthmatic subjects sensitive to ragweed, reported that atropine pretreatment improved pulmonary function parameters but did not prevent the response to antigen; it maintained a better level of function only compared to when antigen was given alone. There was a suggestion that there might be a cholinergic effect of antigen at low doses. Ruffin *et al.* (1978) demonstrated that a β_2-adrenergic agonist, such as fenoterol, was more effective than cholinergic antagonists, such as Sch1000, in preventing the early asthmatic response induced by inhaled antigen in ten subjects. These two studies cast doubt on a major role for the parasympathetic system on the allergen-induced early asthmatic response. The fact that recent studies of the canine model of allergic asthma with *Ascaris suum* antigen indicate that unilateral blockade of the vagus nerve is effective in preventing respiratory distress (Zimmerman *et al.*, 1976) while atropine is not (Krell *et al.*, 1976) suggests that vagal afferent irritant receptors may still be stimulated but that the efferent response is not susceptible to pharmacological antagonism.

There is evidence to support the participation of reflex cholinergic pathways in the bronchoconstriction resulting from histamine (Breeze and Wheeldon, 1977) and serotonin in dogs and histamine (Nadel, 1968) and $PGF_{2\alpha}$ (Patel, 1975) in humans. As with antigen-induced bronchoconstriction, β_2-adrenergic agonists are more effective than atropine in protecting against histamine-induced asthma (Cockcroft *et al.*, 1977; Casterline *et al.*, 1976), but atropine does appear to exert a moderate protective effect which is more detectable in ragweed-sensitive asthmatics than in hay fever subjects.

With both antigen- and histamine-induced bronchospasm, the direct effect appears to outweigh the indirect influence on the efferent cholinergic reflexes. The potential role of the vagus may be important in the early stages of an attack or when the asthma is not severe but is probably less so as the lung is burdened with secretions and edema, and contains high levels of directly acting mediators.

An alternate hypothesis is that of interaction of constricting agents such as histamine with smooth muscle receptor sites for cholinergic and adrenergic influences. Bouhuys (1976) suggests that under physiological conditions low-level β-adrenergic and cholinergic stimuli, insufficient to affect airway caliber by themselves, impinge on airway smooth muscle and influence its response to other contractile agents. The observation that histamine exerted a direct effect in an experimental model after 5–10 sec while firing of vagal efferents occurred only after a latency of at least 30 sec suggested that the vagal afferent firing might be the result rather than the cause of the response to histamine and account for the diminished histamine response with atropine and hexamethonium. Nonetheless, cholinergic reflex mechanisms do appear to be operative, as cause or result of the histamine response. The existence of such a reflex was clearly demonstrated by De Kock *et al.* (1966) in animals since atropine prevented the effects of histamine not only in the airways where histamine was delivered but also in a bypassed tracheal segment whose nerve supply was intact but which received no histamine.

5. Idiopathic Asthma (Intrinsic)

In the majority of patients with chronic bronchial asthma the symptom complex does not appear to be the result of immune mechanisms. Several defects have been proposed as basic in pharmacogenesis but the evidence supporting each remains inconclusive. These defects have been presented to explain the adverse responses in both allergic and idiopathic asthmatic patients to airway irritants, histamine, methacholine, $PGF_{2\alpha}$, exercise, infection, and emotional factors.

5.1. Hyperresponsive Cholinergic Receptors

The possibility that hyperresponsive vagal afferent receptors or smooth muscle muscarinic cholinergic receptors might play a significant role in pathogenesis is suggested by the dense cholinergic innervation of airway smooth muscle, the canine asthma model, and the effects of aerosolized methacholine and atropine in human asthmatics.

5.1.1. Canine Asthma Model

In the anesthetized, natively allergic dog, aerosols of specific antigen (buffered aqueous extracts of mixed grass pollen, *Toxocara canis*, or *Ascaris suum* cause increased airflow resistance and moderately decreased static lung compliance. Studies in the intact animal suggest that indirect, neural reflex mechanisms, in addition to direct mediator effects, are involved in the initiation and modulation of IgE-mediated airway reactions. It is unlikely that vagal reflexes are responsible for the entire sequence of reactions induced by antigen, because under appropriate conditions bronchoconstriction is evident in these dogs despite complete blockade of cholinergic mechanisms (Cotton *et al.*, 1977; Kessler *et al.*, 1973). Interaction between antigen and IgE antibody is essential to initiate the reaction sequence since neither methacholine or electrical stimulation of the vagus nerves alone causes degranulation of mast cells or release of histamine. In studies of anaphylaxis, Mills *et al.* (1969; Mills and Widdicombe, 1970) showed that antigen-induced bronchoconstriction in sensitized guinea pigs and rabbits depended on stimulation of rapidly adapting vagal sensory endings and resulted in reflex airway constriction. In allergic dogs, the airway reaction induced by antigen is abolished by vagotomy and by atropine administered either intravenously or by aerosol, indicating that vagal *efferent* pathways are involved. Under these experimental conditions, when isoproterenol was administered after atropine, only a small additional airway dilation occurred. When the vagus nerves were cooled to 7–10°C, conduction of action potentials from the rapidly adapting vagal sensory receptors in the airways was blocked, but efferent pathways remained intact, as indicated by the presence of a bronchoconstrictor response to asphyxia. This cold block inhibited the reflex bronchoconstriction induced by histamine aerosols and antigen-induced bronchoconstriction, indicating that *afferent* pathways in the vagus nerve were involved in the airway reaction to antigen (Gold *et al.*, 1972). Bilateral bronchoconstriction induced by unilateral antigen administration was blocked as well by cooling the ipsilateral nerve to 0°C. Subsequently Vidruk *et al.* (1976) showed that antigen as well as histamine aerosols stimulate rapidly adapting vagal sensory receptors even in the presence of large doses of isoproterenol, suggesting that mediators released by antigen can stimulate *afferent* nerve endings directly rather than indirectly by airway smooth muscle deformation. Pulmonary arterial infusion of histamine, acetylcholine, and antigen into vagotomized dogs during propranolol infusion resulted in alveolar duct constriction and increased tissue levels of cyclic AMP and cyclic GMP. The changes in smooth muscle tone appeared to precede the cyclic nucleotide changes, suggesting that the latter were triggered by the muscle contraction rather than causing it (Gold, 1977).

These studies appear to establish the role of vagal reflexes in antigen- and mediator-induced bronchoconstriction but do not provide any information regarding a basic defect applicable to bronchial asthma in humans. Studies in humans indicate that the reflex-induced bronchoconstriction secondary to an allergen is less important than the direct end-organ effect.

5.1.2. Hyperresponsiveness to Aerosol Methacholine

Humans with bronchial asthma are hyperreactive to a variety of pharmacological agents, including methacholine. Studies published by Dautrebande and Philpott in 1941 and Tiffeneau in 1945 demonstrated bronchoconstriction with aerosol cholinergic agonists. The failure to produce significant sensitivity to methacholine with intravenous (Zaid and Beall, 1966) or aerosol (Townley *et al.*, 1976) propranolol suggests that β_2-adrenergic blockade is an unlikely explanation for the methacholine response. In contrast, asthmatic patients show a marked increased sensitivity to methacholine after propranolol but not after practolol (Ryo and Toronley, 1976). Only 1 mg of propranolol in asymptomatic asthmatic subjects produced a marked increase of bronchial sensitivity to methacholine. Fifteen-minute aerosol of methacholine results in significant bronchoconstriction in normal subjects (Grieco and Pierson, 1970), but the effect of concomitant propranolol has not been investigated.

While both hay fever and asthmatic subjects demonstrate reduction of specific conductance following aerosol methacholine, Fish *et al.* (1976) reported that only asthmatics were likely to experience FEV_1 reduction. They concluded that there is hypersensitivity of both central and peripheral airways in asthmatics and in the larger central airways of nonasthmatic allergic subjects.

Allen *et al.* (1977) reported that histamine was elevated in plasma of six of seven asthmatic patients between 1 and 10 min after aerosol challenge while plasma complement hemolytic activity (CH50) was reduced, suggesting activation of mediator systems.

Aerosol methacholine sensitivity appears to be increased after influenza vaccine (Ouellette and Reed, 1965; Anand *et al.*, 1968), endotoxin (Ouellette *et al.*, 1967), corticosteroid therapy (Arkins *et al.*, 1968), and respiratory tract infections (Parker and Bilbo, 1965).

5.1.3. Atropine Blockade

Hyperirritability of the airways is a descriptive characteristic of asthma whose mechanism is unknown. It could be due to prior bronchoconstriction, increased airway smooth muscle, biochemical abnormalities in airway smooth muscle, or reflex stimulation via rapidly adapting sensory receptors in the airways. Nadel (1977) has proposed that a decreased threshold of sensory receptors in the airway epithelium exists in these patients. This could explain not only bronchoconstriction but also cough and hyperventilation responses. The principal evidence in favor of this hypothesis is the blocking effect of atropine on the bronchoconstrictive effects of aerosols of histamine (Simonsson *et al.*, 1967), methacholine (Grieco and Pierson, 1970), citric acid, cold air, prostaglandin $PGF_{2\alpha}$, particulate dusts, hypoxemia (Astin and Penman, 1967), placebo allergens (Luparello *et al.*, 1970), propranolol (Grieco and Pierson, 1971), some cases of exercise-induced asthma (Ingram *et al.*, 1977), viral infection (Empey *et al.*, 1976), and influenza vaccine (Laitinen *et al.*, 1976) effect on histamine challenge in healthy subjects. Damage to epithelium might explain why bronchial hyperreactivity occurs during recovery from acute viral respiratory infection.

A similar blocking effect of efferent responses occurs with hexamethonium while lidocaine may interrupt neural afferent receptors (Weiss and Patwardhan, 1977).

The fact that vagal interruptions and glomectomy (Segal and Dulfano, 1965) have not proved to be efficacious in the management of bronchial asthma is probably due to reinnervation of vagal efferent pathways. Since cholinergic ganglia are located in the bronchial airways, this procedure interrupts preganglionic nerves. Regenerating fibers probably need to grow only a few centimers to contact cholinergic ganglia. Using NaCN response as a measure of carotid body sensitivity and pressure as a measure of carotid sinus sensitivity, Takino and Takino (1968) claimed to be able to select patients with reversible "pulmonary vagotonia" likely to benefit from glomectomy.

5.1.4. Eccrine Sweat Responses

Human eccrine sweat glands are innervated by cholinergic fibers traveling in the sympathetic thoracolumbar chain. Kaliner (1976) reported that 90 patients with allergic rhinitis and/or asthma demonstrated statistically significant increases in sweat responses to essentially all concentrations of methacholine examined. There was no difference in the sweat responses of patients with allergic rhinitis alone as compared to those with both rhinitis and asthma.

5.2. Partial β-Adrenergic Blockade

In 1963 Szentivanyi proposed that the increased irritability of the airways in asthma might be due to diminished response to β-adrenergic stimulation. The injection of *Bordetella pertussis* organisms increases the normal sensitivity of certain strains of mice and rats but not rabbits and guinea pigs to histamine in the order of 30- to 300-fold and to serotonin about 20- to 50-fold. This histamine sensitivity is associated with diminished response to β-stimulation and enhanced response to α-stimulation. Partially purified histamine-sensitizing factor (HSF) appears to be a lipoprotein of about 90,000 daltons which also contains leukocytosis-promoting activity and adjuvant activity for hemagglutinating and reaginic antibodies (Lehrer *et al.*, 1974). Increased histamine sensitivity and decreased β-adrenergic responsiveness appear to accompany pertussis vaccination in humans (Sen *et al.*, 1974). Despite the fact that propranolol does not significantly affect the response of normal persons to histamine or cholinergic aerosols, suggesting that β-blockade is not the primary defect in asthmatics, numerous studies *in vivo* and *in vitro* do appear to demonstrate reduced beta adrenergic responsiveness.

5.2.1. Cardiovascular and Metabolic Responses

In 1963 Cookson and Reed reported diminished hyperglycemia and peripheral vasodilatation but normal cardiac responses to β-adrenergic stimulation. Asthmatic persons have a diminished rise in blood sugar and lactate (Middleton *et al.*, 1968) as well as a decreased eosinopenic response. The cardiac responses are normal (Grieco *et al.*, 1968), and most observers reported normal rise in free fatty acids. Nelson *et al.* (1975) noted reduced responses to epinephrine infusions in seven normal individuals induced by 1 week of oral ephedrine and interpreted this as an adaptive response to prolonged excessive stimulation. While Morris *et al.* (1972) recorded normal increase of urinary epinephrine and norepinephrine with stress in chronic asthma, Mathe and Knapp (1969) demonstrated decreased plasma free fatty acids and urinary epinephrine excretion. Urinary excretion of vanillyl mandelic acid has been reported as low in asthmatic children. Selective β_2-adrenergic blockade was suggested but not established by these *in vivo* studies.

5.2.2. Plasma and Urinary Cyclic AMP

Apold and Aknes (1977) reported a correlation between increased bronchial responsiveness to histamine and diminished plasma cyclic AMP response after epinephrine in asthmatic children. The defect appears to be permanent since it persists during asymptomatic periods. Urinary cyclic AMP levels are decreased in asthmatic children and normalized by glucocorticoids, suggestive of restoration of β-adrenergic responsiveness (Coffey *et al.*, 1974). Both extrinsic and intrinsic asthmatic patients studied by Jenne *et al.* (1977a) had a significant reduction of urinary cyclic AMP/creatinine ratio and responses of eosinophils, plasma lactate, blood sugar, and plasma cyclic AMP to oral terbutaline, a relatively selective β_2-adrenergic agonist. The β_2-dysfunction was noted even in patients with minimal inhaler use, suggesting a primary defect rather than one induced by therapy.

5.2.3. Leukocyte Cyclic AMP Response

Parker and Smith (1973) showed that leukocytes from asthmatics, when incubated with isoproterenol in the presence of theophylline, generated deficient amounts of cyclic AMP. This phenomenon was not shared by appropriate stimulation of prostaglandin PGE_1 receptors. This leukocyte subresponsiveness has been confirmed by Alston *et al.* (1974), Gillespie *et al.* (1974), and Logsdon *et al.* (1972). The response of leukocytes of asthmatics is impaired, and the degree of impairment appears to vary with the severity of asthma. Recent studies suggest that previous or concurrent sympathomimetic therapy may produce tolerance of the β-receptor, as has been demonstrated *in vitro* by Lefkowitz (1976). Terbutaline has been shown to affect *in vitro* leukocyte cyclic AMP responses tested 24 hr following its discontinuation (Spaulding *et al.*, 1975). Morris *et al.* (1974) have shown that the *in vitro* cyclic AMP responses of peripheral leukocytes are markedly impaired within 120 min of subcutaneous injection. They have recently extended this observation to chronic ephedrine administration, and even more strikingly following terbutaline or carbuterol treatment (Morris *et al.*, 1977). Jenne *et al.* (1977b) reported moderate tolerance induced by oral terbutaline maintenance in the response of plasma lactate, blood sugar, eosinophils, and plasma and urine cyclic AMP with return to normal within a week of discontinuing the drug. Even excessive inhaler use must be considered since large doses of inhaled isoproterenol may confer some tolerance on myocardial rate receptors (Paterson *et al.*, 1968), and data by Comolly and Greenacre (1976) suggest that large doses of inhaled adrenergic agents will suppress *in vitro* lymphocyte cyclic AMP responses. When these inhaled agents were replaced by inhaled beclomethasone and cromolyn sodium, lymphocyte responses were said to return to normal. However, the asthmatics had lower baseline cyclic AMP values and subnormal absolute increases, suggestive of a persistent defect. It is clear that leukocyte cyclic AMP responses to β_2-adrenergic agonists are blunted in asthma. Whether this is a primary defect or solely due to tolerance induction remains to be settled.

5.2.4. Human Asthmatic Bronchial Muscle

The *in vitro* data on human asthmatic bronchial muscle are sparse. Svedmyr *et al.* (1976) found no alteration of the dose–response curve for isoproterenol relaxation in three intrinsic asthmatics. Normal smooth muscle β-responses would not preclude an impairment of homeostatic control mediated through sympathetic receptors.

5.2.5. Leukocyte Catecholamine Receptors

Leukocyte epinephrine receptors were compared by Sokol and Beall (1975) in ten asthmatics and nine normal individuals and found not to be substantially different in number (1.0×10^6) or binding affinity. However, decreased [^{3}H]dihydroalprenolol binding to lymphocytes in asthmatics has been reported by Kariman and Lefkowitz (1977). This decrease was apparent in patients not receiving adrenergic bronchodilators.

5.2.6. T-Lymphocyte E-Rosette Formation

A study with peripheral lymphocyte active E-rosette formation in 19 asthmatics demonstrated diminished isoproterenol inhibition and carbamylcholine augmentation, suggesting hyporesponsiveness of the function of both receptors. Eight of the patients had been off all medications for at least 3 weeks, and yet the β-response was significantly abnormal (Lang *et al.*, 1978).

5.2.7. Platelet Aggregation

Epinephrine-induced aggregation of platelets was reportedly reduced in asthmatic subjects (Solinger *et al.*, 1973), but results have been conflicting. A study (Maccia *et al.*, 1977) of second-wave platelet aggregation revealed abnormal responses to epinephrine, ADP, collagen, and thrombin in patients with allergic asthma and high serum IgE levels as compared to those in nonimmunological asthmatics and controls, suggesting that the allergic state may affect platelet membrane responsiveness to multiple aggregating agents.

5.2.8. Lysosomal Enzyme Release

Isoproterenol inhibits zymoson-stimulated release of lysosomal enzymes from granulocytes. Busse (1977) noted significantly decreased response to isoproterenol in patients with mild asthma who had not taken bronchodilators for 2 weeks before study and also in patients with severe asthma requiring bronchodilators and corticosteroids. During viral respiratory infections the granulocyte response to isoproterenol was further decreased, suggesting alteration of β-receptor function. Decreased isoproterenol responsiveness has been noted as well in volunteers following symptomatic rhinovirus 16 infection, further supporting this as a possible mechanism for virus-induced asthma.

5.3. Hyperresponsive α-Adrenergic Receptors

Increased α-adrenergic responsiveness, possibly in concert with reduced β-adrenergic function, is a plausible possibility as well. Ahlquist (1948) had proposed the concept of α- and β-adrenergic receptors to account for the opposing actions of sympathetic agents in various organs. However, the existence and potency of the α-adrenergic receptors in the bronchi have been questioned.

5.3.1. Effects of α-Adrenergic Agonists and Antagonists on Bronchoconstriction

Stimulation of the thoracic sympathetic nerves after β-adrenergic blockade did not narrow airways, suggesting that insignificant α-adrenergic receptors are present (Cabezas *et al.*, 1971). *In vivo*, Anthracite *et al.* (1971) did report a decrease in specific conductance with phentolamine. In asthmatics Simonson *et al.* (1972) demonstrated a decrease in conductance on inhalation of metaoxidrine, an α-adrenergic agonist, following pretreatment with cholinergic and β-adrenergic antagonists. The use of α-adrenergic antagonists may be confused by the fact that this group of drugs acts not only to block α-adrenergic receptors but also to prevent the reuptake of catecholamines which could potentiate bronchodilator effects. Patel and Kerr (1975) showed that allergen-induced bronchospasm in ten patients was significantly inhibited by the α-receptor blocking drug thymoxamine given intravenously in all and as an aerosol in two.

5.3.2. Isolated Bronchial Smooth Muscle

Several studies with normal isolated smooth muscle have provided evidence for the existence of α-adrenergic receptors, but human asthmatic bronchial muscle has not been examined. Contraction of isolated tracheal and bronchial smooth muscle has been elevated by epinephrine and epinephrine after blockade of β-receptors by propranolol (Mathe *et al.*, 1971).

5.3.3. Effect of Agonists and Antagonists on Leukocytes

a. Adenylate Cyclase. In acute asthma it has been shown that diminished leukocyte adenylate cyclase responses to isoproterenol can be restored toward normal by α-receptor blocking drugs, phentolamine and thymoxamine, suggesting an enhanced adrenergic response. Lodgsdon *et al.* (1973) and Alston *et al.* (1974) reported that *in vitro* phentolamine or thymoxamine permitted an enhanced stimulation of adenylate cyclase by isoproterenol in leukocytes of asthmatics so that the latter effect reached the range seen with nonasthmatics. In these studies it was not clear whether these drugs acted to unblock β-receptors or to block hypersensitive α-receptors.

b. ATPase. Divalent cation-dependent ATPase activity appears to be stimulated by α-adrenergic activity and blocked by an α-antagonist and may represent the enzyme for α-adrenergic modulation (Coffey *et al.*, 1971). Studies in non-steroid-treated asthmatic children reveal significantly elevated magnesium- and calcium-dependent ATPase activity in the particulate and soluble fractions of leukocytes and platelets (Coffey *et al.*, 1974; Coffey and Middleton, 1975). Glucocorticosteroid treatment is associated with partial restoration of normal β-adrenergic responsiveness and a reduction of ATPase activities in these cells. These data have supported the hypothesis that an adrenergic imbalance in asthma may result in part from imbalance in the activities and sensitivities of two adrenergically responsive membrane enzymes—adenylate cyclase and ATPase.

c. Guanylate Cyclase. Lymphocyte guanylate cyclase is reported to rise in normals in response to *in vitro* norepinephrine plus propranolol in normal subjects but not in active asthmatics (Haddock *et al.*, 1975), suggesting a diminished α-adrenergic response. Our own studies with lymphocyte E-rosette formation fail to reveal a significant increase of phenylephrine responsiveness (Lang *et al.*, 1978).

These *in vitro* studies and the reports of clinical efficacy of phentolamine (Marcelle *et al.*, 1968; Gross *et al.*, 1974), thymoxamine (Griffin *et al.*, 1972), and dibenzamine (Klotz and Berstein, 1950) support continued examination of this hypothesis.

5.4. Alternative Hypotheses

5.4.1. Cyclic Nucleotide Interaction

In several mammalian tissues the increase in cyclic AMP following isoproterenol is associated with an attenuated response of cyclic GMP to acetylcholine while the increase in cyclic GMP following a cholinergic agonist is associated with an attenuated response of cyclic AMP to a β-adrenergic agonist (Lee *et al.*, 1972; Gallin *et al.*, 1978). The interaction between cyclic nucleotides is complex as evidenced by the observations that low concentrations of cyclic GMP stimulate phosphodiesterase hydrolysis of cyclic AMP whereas with higher concentrations of the former there is inhibition of cyclic AMP hydrolysis (Beavo *et al.*, 1971).

5.4.2. Defective Nonadrenergic Inhibitory Nervous System

The nonadrenergic inhibitory nervous system, which has been demonstrated in the guinea pig trachea (Richardson and Bouchard, 1975), may play a role in the pathogenesis of the hyperreactive airways in asthma, although the existence of this system in human bronchi remains to be documented.

5.4.3. The Prostaglandin Hypothesis

The effects of several prostaglandins on human lungs have been reviewed in a previous section. A number of mechanisms, alone or in combination, could account for the hyperreactivity of airways to $PGF_{2\alpha}$. The failure of pretreatment with indomethacin to ameliorate asthmatic attacks in man might be due to residual $PGF_{2\alpha}$/PGE synthesis. At present the exact role of the prostaglandins is uncertain.

5.4.4. Hyporesponsive Histamine-2 Receptors

Increased bronchial sensitivity to inhaled histamine in asthma is well known and involves, in part, H-1 receptors on bronchial smooth muscle and bronchial mast cells. Busse and Sosman (1977) studied cyclic AMP and lysosomal enzyme release from peripheral leukocytes of asthmatic subjects and showed diminished H-2 receptor response to histamine. They suggested that decrease of H-2 receptor responsiveness in the lung could enhance the H-1 bronchoconstrictor effect of histamine as well as hinder the H-2 receptor inhibition of both mast cell degranulation and PMN lysosomal enzyme release.

5.5. Aspirin Sensitivity

Adverse reactions to aspirin are frequently associated with nasal polyps and sinusitis, occurring in 20% of severely ill adult asthmatics (Farr, 1970) and from 3% to 8% of unselected asthmatic populations (Stevenson *et al.*, 1976). There are a predominance of female and middle-aged patients, usually an absence of reaginic antibody, and normal serum IgE levels, but eosinophilia is frequent. The problem is further complicated by the fact that nonsteroidal antiinflammatory drugs such as indomethacin as well as aminopyrine and tartrazine induce asthma in aspirin-intolerant patients. Thus far, only analgesics which inhibit prostaglandin synthesis, such as diclofac and naproxen, produce bronchospasm in aspirin-sensitive patients (Szczeklik *et al.*, 1977). In aspirin-sensitive patients it may be that PGE is preferentially inhibited, leaving the effects of endogenous bronchoconstrictors unopposed. The action of SRS-A, which may be generated from arachidonic acid, would also be unopposed. The lack of PGEs would promote the release of histamine and might explain the observations of Stevenson *et al.* (1976) that aspirin challenge leads to a significant rise in plasma histamine. Cromolyn sodium may protect against or reduce the response to aspirin (Szczeklik *et al.*, 1977). Okazaki *et al.* (1977) report a positive correlation between *in vitro* leukocyte PGE basal level inhibition and antigen-induced histamine release enhancement following incubation with aspirin, supporting the regulatory role of PGE. Histamine may well be one of the mediators of bronchospasm precipitated by inhibitors of PGE biosynthesis in aspirin-sensitive patients with bronchial asthma.

5.6. Exercise-Induced Asthma

Using density dependence of maximal expiratory flow rates during bronchospasm in 12 subjects, McFadden *et al.* (1977) distinguished patients in whom there was predominantly large airway obstruction and others in whom the response was principally in the small airways. In the five subjects in the large airways group, pharmacological vagal efferent blockade totally abolished the bronchospastic response to exercise. In the seven in the small airways group, anticholinergic drugs produced marked bronchodilatation but did not alter the response to exercise; yet this response was blunted after mediator release was inhibited by cromolyn sodium. Cromolyn sodium has clearly been shown to be effective in ameliorating the effects of exercise-induced bronchospasm in some children and adults (Wallace and Grieco, 1976), suggesting the role of mast cell degranulation. The protective effect of atropine and Sch1000 has been demonstrated in selected patients (Kiviloog, 1975; Chan-Yeung, 1977) as well, supporting the role of vagal reflexes. This variation in responsiveness appears to reflect differences in mechanism and predominant site of bronchoconstriction. Improvement of the understanding of pathogenesis is likely to lead to more effective specific therapy. Lactic acidemia does not appear to be the cause of exercise-induced asthma (Strauss *et al.*, 1977). In addition, no significant changes in peripheral blood PGE and $PGF_{2\alpha}$ levels have been detected (Field *et al.*, 1976).

5.7. Viral Infections Inducing Asthma

Respiratory infections are potent provocative agents of asthmatic attacks and may be predominant in more than 25% of patients (Stevenson *et al.*, 1975). There appears to be no association between recovery of bacteria, pathogenic or otherwise, from the respiratory tract of asthmatic patients and exacerbation of asthmatic symptoms (McIntosh *et al.*, 1973). Several studies have detected viral respiratory infections in children and in some adults (Berman *et al.*, 1975; Berkovitz *et al.*, 1970; Mitchell *et al.*, 1976). In a study from Denver (McIntosh *et al.*, 1973) 42% of all wheezing episodes in 32 hospitalized children were associated with viruses, with an increase to 85% during periods of community prevalence of viral infections. Minor *et al.* (1974) studied a group of 16 outpatient asthmatic children and noted exacerbations of asthma associated with 50% of viral infections. Implicated viral agents in several studies include myxoviruses [respiratory syncytial virus (RSV), influenza A_2, influenza B, parainfluenza], enteroviruses (rhinovirus, coronavirus), and the adenovirus group. RSV appears to be a prominent cause of infectious asthma in children of preschool age, particularly in those under the age of 3 years, whereas rhinoviruses apparently account for the majority of attacks in children between the ages of 3 and 12 years. In adults, rhinoviruses and influenza A appear to be the most common viral pathogens identified (Minor *et al.*, 1976).

The mechanism(s) by which viral infections cause exacerbation of asthma is unclear. There is no published evidence that an IgE response to viral antigens is involved, although this possibility has not been excluded. Several lines of evidence support the hypothesis that nonimmunological mechanisms are operative.

5.7.1. Induction of Bronchial Hyperreactivity and Small Airways Disease

The detrimental effects of viral respiratory tract disease on small airway function are well established in normal individuals with rhinovirus, influenza, and common cold infections (Johanson *et al.*, 1969; Cate *et al.*, 1973; Picken *et al.*, 1972; Hall *et al.*, 1976; Blair *et al.*, 1976). The adverse effects of viral infection in asthmatic subjects are most likely due to an exaggeration of this response seen in normals. Because viral respiratory tract infections cause transient damage to the airway epithelium, Empey *et al.* (1976) studied the effect of inhalation of histamine aerosol on airway resistance in otherwise healthy subjects with colds. Inhalation of histamine aerosol produced a greater increase in airway resistance in subjects with colds while atropine sulfate aerosol reversed or prevented these exaggerated bronchomotor responses, implicating postganglionic cholinergic pathways. Airway epithelial damage induced by infection presumably sensitizes the rapidly adapting airway receptors to inhaled irritants, causing increased bronchoconstriction via a vagal reflex. Aerosol live attenuated influenza A and B virus administered to nonimmune healthy subjects resulted in aerosol histamine hypersensitivity. The bronchial reactivity was maximal on the second day, disappeared by the ninth day, and was prevented and reversed by atropine sulfate aerosol (Laitinen *et al.*, 1976).

Bronchial hypersensitivity to methacholine has been shown to be increased in asthmatic subjects after administration of killed influenza vaccine and live measles vaccine (Anand *et al.*, 1968; Kumar and Newcomb, 1970).

5.7.2. Enhancement of IgE-Mediated Histamine Release

Ida *et al.* (1977) have reported enhancement of IgE-mediated histamine release from virus-treated human basophils. Herpes simplex type 1, influenza A and adenovirus-1 were incubated with peripheral leukocytes from patients allergic to ragweed and enhanced both ragweed antigen E and anti-IgE histamine release. Examination of the culture fluids revealed that the enhancement of histamine release was associated with a soluble factor that had the properties of interferon, a substance shown to directly enhance histamine release.

5.7.3. Leukocyte β-Adrenergic and Histamine-2 Receptor Hypofunction

During viral respiratory infections, granulocyte responsiveness to isoproterenol has been reported to be diminished (Busse, 1977) and suggests alteration of

β_2-receptor function. Induction of symptomatic rhinovirus 16 infection appears to reduce granulocyte β_2-adrenergic and histamine-2 receptor function while influenza and rhinovirus *in vitro* may have the same effects (Busse *et al.*, 1978).

5.8. Emotions and Bronchial Asthma

The putative roles of the parasympathetic nervous system and of the sympathetic nerves and adrenergic receptor responses to circulating catecholamines in the pathogenesis of bronchial asthma may well underlie the physiological expression of emotions in this disorder. It has been shown that suggestion accompanying administration of a diluent can precipitate either bronchoconstriction or bronchodilatation (Luparello *et al.*, 1970). Subsequently, suggestion has been shown to have a greater effect on large airways, implying a role for the vagus (Spector *et al.*, 1976). A great deal remains to be learned about this important provocative factor of asthma exacerbation.

6. References

Abe, K., Watanabe, N., Kumagai, M., Mouri, T., Seki, T., and Yoshinaga, K., 1967, Circulating plasma kinin in patients with bronchial asthma, *Experientia* **23**:626–631.

Adolphson, R. L., Abern, S. B., and Townley, R. G.N 1970, Demonstration of alpha adrenergic receptors in human respiratory smooth muscle, *Clin. Res.* **18**:629–633.

Ahlquist, R. P., 1948, A study of the adrenergic receptors, *Am. J. Physiol.* **153**:586–606.

Allen, D. H., Mathison, D. A., Wagner, P. D., Arroyave, C. M., Ploy, E., and Tan, E. M., 1977, Mediator release during methacholine-induced bronchoconstriction in asthmatic patients, 34 Annual Meeting, American Academy of Allergyn Feb. 27–Mar. 1, Abstr. 40.

Alston, W. C., Patel, K. R., and Kerr, J. W., 1974, Response of leukocyte adenyl cyclase to isoprenaline and effect of alpha-blocking drugs in extrinsic asthma, *Br. Med. J.* **1**:90–93.

American Thoracic Society Committee on Diagnostic Standards for Nontuberculous Diseases, 1962, Definitions and classification of chronic bronchitis, asthma, and pulmonary emphysema, *Am. Rev. Respir. Dis.* **85**:762–766.

Anand, S. C., Itkin, I. H., and Kind, L. S., 1968, Effect of influenza vaccine on methacholine (mecholyl) sensitivity in patients with asthma of known and unknown origin, *J. Allergy* **42**:187–92.

Anthracite, R. F., Vachon, L., and Knapp, P. H., 1971, Alpha-adrenergic receptors in the human lung, **33**:481–488.

Apold, J., and Asknes, L., 1977, Correlation between increased bronchial responsiveness to histamine and diminished plasma cyclic adenosine monophosphate response after epinephrine in asthmatic children, *J. Allergy Clin. Immunol.* **59**:343–347.

Arkins, J. A., Schleuter, D. P., and Fink, J. N., 1968, The effect of corticosteroids on methacholine inhalation in symptomatic bronchial asthma, *J. Allergy* **41**:209–216.

Arroyave, C. M., Stevenson, D. D., and Vaughan, J. H., 1977, Plasma complement changes during bronchospasm provoked in asthmatic patients, *Clin. Allergy* **7**:173–180.

Assem, E. S. K., and Turner-Warwick, M., 1976, Cytophilic antibodies in bronchopulmonary aspergilloma and cryptogenic pulmonary eosinophilia, *Clin. Exp. Immunol.* **26**:67–77.

Astin, T. W., and Penman, R. W. B., 1967, Airway obstruction due to hypoxemia in patients with chronic lung disease, *Am. Rev. Respir. Dis.* **95**:567–577.

Austen, K. F., and Orange, R. P., 1975, Bronchial asthma: The possible role of the chemical mediators of immediate hypersersivivity in the pathogenesis of subacute chronic disease, *Am. Rev. Respir. Dis.* *112*:423–436.

Bazaral, M., Orgel, H. A., and Hamburger, R. N., 1974, Genetics of IgE and allergy: Serum IgE levels in twins, *J. Allergy Clin. Immunol.* **54**:288–304.

Beall, G. N., 1963, Plasma histamine concentrations in allergic diseases, *J. Allergy* **34**:8–16.

Beavo, J. A., Hardman, J. G., and Sutherland, E. W., 1971, Stimulation of adenosine 3′,5′-monophosphate hydrolysis by guanosine 3′-5′ monophosphate, *J. Biol. Chem.* **246**:3841–3847.

Berger, A. J., Mitchell, R. A., and Severinghaus, J. W., 1977, Regulation of respiration, *N. Engl. J. Med.* **297**:92–97, 138–143, 194–201.

Berkovitz, S., Millian, S. J., and Snyder, R. D., 1970, The association of viral and mycylosma infections with recurrence of wheezing in the asthmatic child, *Ann. Allergy* **28**:43–49.

Berman, S. Z., Mathison, D. A., Stevenson, D. D., Tan, E. M., and Vaughan, J. H., 1975, Transtracheal aspiration studies in asthmatic patients in relapse with "infective" asthma and in subjects without respiratory disease, *J. Allergy Clin. Immunol.* **56**:206–214.

Berry, J. B., and Brighton, W. D., 1977, Familial human short-term sensitizing (IgG S-TS) antibody, *Clin. Allergy* **7**:401–406.

Bhat, K. N., Arroyave, C. M., Marney, S. R., Jr., Stevenson, D. D., and Tan, E. M., 1976, Plasma histamine changes during provoked bronchospasm in asthmatic patients, *J. Allergy Clin. Immunol.* **58**:647–656.

Bienenstock, J., and Johnston, N., 1976, A morphologic study of rabbit bronchial lymphoid aggregate and lymphoepithelium, *Lab. Invest.* **35**:343–349.

Blair, T. H., Grensberg, S. B., and Stevens, P. M., 1976, Effects of rhinovirus infection on pulmonary function of healthy human volunteers, *Am. Rev. Resp. Dis.* **114**:95–102.

Boat, T., and Kleinerman, J., 1975, Human respiratory tract secretions. 2. Effect of cholinergic and adrenergic agents on *in vitro* release of protein and mucous glycoprotein, *Chest* **67**:325–329.

Bogart, D. B., and Stechschulte, D. J., 1974, Release of platelet activating factor from human lung, *Clin. Res.* **22**:652 (abstr.).

Bouhuys, A., 1976, Experimental asthma in man and in animals, in: *Bronchial Asthma: Mechanisms and Therapeutics* (E. B. Weiss and M. S. Segal, eds.), pp. 457–470, Little, Brown, Boston.

Breeze, R. G., and Wheeldon, E. B., 1977, The cells of the pulmonary airways, *Am. Rev. Respir. Dis.* **116**:705–777.

Brocklehurst, W. E., 1958, The action of 5-hydroxytryptamine on smooth muscle, in: *5-Hydroxytryptamine* (G. P. Lewis, ed.), Pergamon, New York.

Brocklehurst, W. E., 1968, Pharmacological mediators of hypersensitivity reaction, in: *Clinical Aspects of Immunology* (P. G. H. Gell and R. R. A. Coombs, eds.), Blackwell, Oxford.

Brostoff, J., Mowbray, J. F., Kapoor, H., Hollowell, S. J., Rudolf, M., and Saunders, K. B., 1976, 80% of patients with intrinsic asthma are homozygous for HLA W6, *Lancet* **2**:872–873.

Bryant, D. H., Burns, M. W., and Lazarus, L., 1975, Identification of IgG antibody as a carrier of reaginic activity in asthmatic subjects, *J. Allergy Clin. Immunol.* **56**:417–428.

Brown, N. E., McFadden, E. R., Jr., and Ingram, R. H., Jr., 1977, Relative contribution of large and small airways to flow limitation in normal subjects before and after atropine and isoproterenol, *J. Clin. Invest.* **59**:696–701.

Burnstock, G., 1970, *Smooth Muscle* (E. Bullbring, A. F. Brading, A. W. Jones, and T. Tometa, eds.), pp. 1–16, Williams and Wilkins, Baltimore.

Burnstock, G., Satchell, D. L., and Smythe, A., 1972, A comparison of the excitatory and inhibitory effects of nonadrenergic, noncholinergic nerve stimulation and exogenously applied ATP on a variety of smooth muscle preparations from different vertebrate species, *Br. J. Pharmacol.* **46**:234–241.

Busse, W. W., 1977, Decreased granulocyte response to isoproterenol in asthma during upper respiratory infections, *Am. Rev. Respir. Dis.* **115**:783–791.

Busse, W. W., and Sosman, J., 1977, Decreased H2 histamine response of granulocytes of asthmatic patients, *J. Clin. Invest.* **59**:1080–1087.

Busse, W. W., Reed, C. E., and Hoehne, J. H., 1972, II. Demonstration of ragweed antigen in airborne particules smaller than pollen, *J. Allergy Clin. Immunol.* **50**:289–293.

Busse, W. W., Cooper, W., Warshauer, D., Dick, E., and Albrecht, R., 1978, Altered granulocyte isoproterenol and H-2 histamine response by *in vitro* influenza virus, 34th Annual Meeting, American Academy of Allergy, Abstr. 68.

Cabezas, G. A., Graf, P. D., and Nadel, J. A., 1971, Sympathetic versus parasympathetic nervous regulation of airways in dogs, *J. Appl. Physiol.* **51**:651–655.

Callerame, M. L., Condemi, J. J., Ishizaka, K., Johansson, S. G. O., and Vaughan, J. H., 1971a, Immunoglobulins in bronchial tissues from patients with asthma with special reference to immunoglobulin E, *J. Allergy* **47**:187–194.

Callerame, M. L., Condemi, J. J., Bohrod, M. G., and Vaughan, J. H., 1971b, Immunologic reactions of bronchial tissues in asthma, *N. Engl. J. Med.* **284**:459–464.

Cardell, B. S., and Pearson, R. S. B., 1959, Death in asthmatics, *Thorax* **14**:341–346.

Casterline, C. L., Evans, R., III, and Ward, G. W., Jr., 1976, The effect of atropine and albuterol aerosols on the human bronchial response to histamine, *J. Allergy Clin. Immunol.* **58**:67–613.

Cate, T. R., Roberts, J. S., Russ, M. A., and Pierce, J. A., 1973, Effects of common colds on pulmonary function, *Am. Rev. Respir. Dis.* **108**:858–865.

Chan-Yeung, M., 1977, The effect of Sch 1000 and disodium cromoglycate on exercise-induced asthma, *Chest* **71**:320–323.

Clancy, R., and Bienenstock, J., 1974, The proliferative response of bronchus-associated lymphoid tissue after local and systemic immunization, *J. Immunol.* **112**:1997–2001.

Cockcroft, D. W., Killian, D. N., Mellon, J. J. A., and Hargreave, F. E., 1977, Protective effect of drugs on histamine-induced asthma, *Thorax* **32**:429–437.

Coffey, R. G., and Middleton, E., Jr., 1973, Relrease of histamine from mast cells by lysosomal cationic proteins: Possible involvement of adenylate cyclase and adenosine triphosphatase in pharmacologic regulation, *Int. Arch. Allergy* **45**:593–599.

Coffey, R. G., and Middleton, E., Jr., 1974, Effects of glucocorticosteroids on the urinary excretion of cyclic AMP and electrolytes by asthmatic children, *J. Allergy Clin. Immunol.* **54**:41–53.

Coffey, R. G., and Middleton, E., Jr., 1975, Increased adenosine triphosphatase activity in platelets of asthmatic children, *Int. Arch. Allergy Immunol.* **48**:171–181.

Coffey, R. G., Hadden, J. W., Hadden, E. M., and Middleton, E., Jr., 1971, Stimulation of ATPase by norepinephrine: An alpha-adrenergic receptor mechanisms, *Fed. Proc.* **30**:497 (abstr.).

Coffey, R. G., Hadden, J. W., and Middleton, E., Jr., 1974, Increased adenosine triphosphatase in leukocytes of asthmatic children, *J. Clin. Invest.* **54**:138–146.

Connell, J. T., 1971, Asthmatic deaths: Role of the mast cell, *J. Am. Med. Assoc.* **215**:769–776.

Conolly, M. E., and Greenacre, J. K., 1976, The lymphocyte beta adrenergic receptor in normal subjects and patients with bronchial asthma, *J. Clin. Invest.* **58**:1307–1316.

Cooke, R. A., and Vander Veer, A., 1916, Human sensitization, *J. Immunol.* **1**:216–226.

Cookson, D. U., and Reed, C. E., 1963, A comparison of the effects of isoproterenol in the normal and asthmatic subject, *Am. Rev. Respir. Dis.* **88**:636–641.

Cotton, D. J., Bleecker, E. R., Fischer, S. P., Graf, P. D., Gold, W. M., and Nadel, J. A., 1977, Rapid shallow breathing after *Ascaris suum* antigen inhalation: Role of vagus nerves, *J. Appl. Physiol.* **42**:107–111.

Cuthbert, M. F., 1972, Prostaglandins and bronchial smooth muscle, *Thorax* **27**:263–274.

Davies, R. J., Butcher, B. T., O'Neil, C. E., and Salvaggio, J. E., 1977, The *in vitro* effect of toluene diisocyanate on lymphocyte cyclic adenosine monophosphate production by isoproterenol, prostaglandin and histamine, *J. Allergy Clin. Immunol.* **60**:223–228.

Dawson, W., and Tomlinson, R., 1974, Effect of cromoglycate and eicosatrienoic acid on the release of prostaglandins and SRS-A from immunologically challenged guinea pig lungs, *Br. J. Pharmacol.* **52**:107–112.

De Kock, M. A., Nadel, J. A., Zui, S., Colebatch, H. J. H., and Olsen, C. R., 1966, New method for perfusing bronchial arteries: Histamine bronchoconstriction and apnea, *J. Appl. Physiol.* **21**:185–192.

Dolovich, M. B., Sanchis, J., and Rossman, C., 1976, Aerosol penetrance: A sensitive index of peripheral airways obstruction, *J. Appl. Physiol.* **40**:468–472.

Drazen, J. M., and Austen, K. F., 1974a, Atropine modification of the pulmonary effects of chemical mediators in the guinea pig, *J. Appl. Physiol.* **38**:834–837.

Drazen, J. M., and Austen, K. F., 1974b, Effects of intravenous administration of slow-reacting substance of anaphylaxis, histamine, bradykinin, and prostaglandin $F_{2\alpha}$ on pulmonary mechanics in the guinea pig, *J. Clin. Invest.* **53**:1679–1685.

Dunhill, M. S., 1960, The pathology of asthma, with special reference to changes in the bronchial mucosa, *J. Clin. Pathol.* **13**:27–39.

Ellefsen, P., and Tos, M., 1972, Goblet cells in human trachea: Quantitative studies of a pathological biopsy material, *Arch. Otolaryngol.* **95**:547–555.

Empey, D. M., Laitinen, L. A., Jacobs, L., Gold, W. M., and Nadel, J. A., 1976, Mechanisms of bronchial hyperactivity in normal subjects after upper respiratory tract infection, *Am. Rev. Respir. Dis.* **113**:131–139.

Eppinger, H., and Hess, L., 1915, *Vagotonia: A Clinical Study in Vegetative Neurology,* Nervous and Mental Disease Publishing Co., New York.

Farr, R. S., 1970, The need to re-evaluate acetylsalicylic acid (aspirin), *J. Allergy* **45:**321–328.

Field, J., Allegra, J., Trautlein, J., Demers, L., Gillin, M., and Zelis, R., 1976, Measurement of plasma prostaglandins during exercise-induced bronchospasm, *J. Allergy Clin. Immunol.* **58:**581–585.

Fink, J. N., Moore, V. L., and Barboriak, J. J., 1975, Cell-mediated hypersensitivity in pigeon breeders, *Int. Arch. Allergy Immunol.* **49:**831–837.

Fish, J. E., Rosenthal, R. R., Batra, G., Menkes, H., Summer, W., Permutt, S., and Norman, P., 1976, Airway responses to methacholine in allergic and nonallergic subjects, *Am. Rev. Respir. Dis.* **113:**579–586.

Fish, J. E., Rosenthal, R. R., Summer, W. R., Menkes, H., Norman, P. S., and Permutt, S., 1977, The effect of atropine on acute antigen-mediated airway constriction in subjects with allergic asthma, *Am. Rev. Respir. Dis.* **115:**371–379.

Frohlich, F., 1949, Die "Helle Zelle" der Bronchialschleimhaut und ihre Beziehungen zum Problem des Chemoreceptoren, *Frankfurt Z. Pathol.* **60:**517–543.

Gallin, J. I., Sandler, J. A., Clyman, R. I., Manganiello, V. C., and Vaughan, M., 1978, Agents that increase cyclic AMP inhibit accumulation of cGMP and depress human monocyte locomotion, *J. Immunol.* **120:**492–496.

Gerber, M. A., Paronetto, F., and Kochwa, S., 1971, Immunohistochemical localization of IgE in asthmatic lungs, *Am. J. Pathol.* **62:**339–349.

Gillsepie, E., Valentine, M. D., and Lichtenstein, L. M., 1974, Cyclic AMP metabolism in asthma: Studies with leukocytes and lymphocytes, *J. Allergy Clin. Immunol.* **53:**27–33.

Goetzl, E. J., and Austen, K. F., 1976, Structural determinants of the eosinophil chemotactic activity of the acidic tetrapeptides of eosinophil chemotactic factor of anaphylaxis, *J. Exp. Med.* **144:**1424.

Gold, W. M., 1977, Neurohumoral interactions in airways, *Am. Rev. Respir. Dis. Suppl.* **115:**127–137.

Gold, W. M., Kessler, G. R., and Yu, D. Y. C., 1972, Role of vagus nerve in experimental asthma in allergic dogs, *J. Appl. Physiol.* **33:**719–725.

Grant, J. A., Dupree, E., and Thueson, D. O., 1977, Complement-mediated release of histamine from human leukocytes. III. Possible regulatory role of microtubules and microfilaments, *J. Allergy Clin. Immunol.* **60:**306–311.

Green, K., Hedqvist, P., and Svanborg, N., 1974, Increased plasma levels of 15-keto-13,14 dehydro-prostaglandin $F_{2\alpha}$ after allergen-provoked asthma in man, *Lancet* **2:**1419–1422.

Grieco, M. H., and Pierson, R. N., Jr., 1970, Cardiopulmonary effects of methacholine in asthmatic and normal subjects, *J. Allergy* **45:**195–207.

Grieco, M. H., and Pierson, R. N., 1971, Mechanism of bronchoconstriction due to beta adrenergic blockade, *J. Allergy Clin. Immunol.* **48:**143–152.

Grieco, M. H., Pierson, R. N., Jr., and Pi-Sunyer, F. X., 1968, Comparison of the circulatory and metabolic effects of isoproterenol, epinephrine and methoxamine in normal and asthmatic subjects, *Am. J. Med.* **44:**863–872.

Griffin, J. P., Kamburoff, P. L., and Prime, P. J., 1972, Thymoxamine and airway obstruction, *Lancet* **1:**1288–1294.

Gross, G. N., Souhrada, J. F., and Farr, R. S., 1974, The long-term treatment of an asthmatic patient using phentolamine, *Chest* **66:**397–401.

Guirgis, H. M., and McNeill, R. S., 1969, The nature of the adrenergic receptors in isolated human bronchi, *Thorax* **24:**613–615.

Haddock, A. M., Patel, K. R., Alston, W. C., and Kerr, J. W., 1975, Response of lymphocyte guanyl cyclase to propranolol, noradrenaline, thymoxamine, and acetylcholine in extrinsic bronchial asthma, *Br. Med. J.* **1:**357–359.

Hage, E., Hage, J., and Juel, G., 1977, Endocrine-like cells of the pulmonary epithelium of the human adult lung, *Cell. Tissue Res.* **1978:**39–45.

Hall, W. J., Douglas, R. G., Jr., and Hyde, R. W., Roth, F. K., Cross, A. S., and Speers, D. M., 1976, Pulmonary mechanics after uncomplicated influenza, *Am. Rev. Respir. Dis.* **113:**141–147.

Harris, J. O., Bice, D., and Salvaggio, J. E., 1976, Cellular and humoral bronchopulmonary immune response of rabbits immunized with thermophilic actinomyces antigen, **114:**29–43.

Hayes, J. A., 1976, The pathology of bronchial asthma, in: *Bronchial Asthma Mechanisms and Therapeutics* (E. B. Weiss and M. S. Segal, eds.), pp. 347–381, Little, Brown, Boston.

Herxheimer, H., and Stresemann, E., 1961, The effect of bradykinin aerosol in guinea-pigs and in man, *J. Physiol. (London)* **158:**38.

Hoehne, J. H., and Reed, C. E., 1971, Where is the allergic reaction in ragweed asthma? *J. Allergy Clin. Immunol.* **48:**36–39.

Hoffman, D. R., and Haddad, Z. H., 1974, Diagnosis of IgE-mediated reactions to food antigens by radioimmunoassay, *J. Allergy Clin. Immunol.* **54:**165–173.

Hogg, J. C., Macklem, P. T., and Thurlbeck, W. M., 1968, Site and nature of airway obstruction in chronic obstructive lung disease, *N. Engl. J. Med.* **278:**1355–1360.

Hubscher, T., 1975, Role of the eosinophil in the allergic reactions. I. EDI- an eosinophil-derived inhibitor of histamine release, J. Immunol. **114:**1379–1384.

Hudgel, D. W., Cooper, D., and Souhrada, J., 1976, Reversible restrictive lung disease simulating asthma, *Ann. Intern. Med.* **85:**328–332.

Hyman, A. L., Spannhake, E. W., and Kadowitz, P. J., 1978, Prostaglandins and the lung, *Am. Rev. Respir. Dis.* **117:**111–136.

Ida, S., Hooks, J. J., Siraganian, R. P., and Notkins, A. L., 1977, Enhancement of IgE-mediated histamine release from human basophils by viruses—Role of interferon, *J. Exp. Med.* **145:**892–898.

Ingram, R. H., Jr., Wellman, J. J., McFadden, E. R., Jr., and Mead, J., 1977, Relative contribution of large and small airways to flow limitation in normal subjects before and after atropine and isoproterenol, *J. Clin. Invest.* **59:**696–703.

Itkin, I. H., and Anand, S. C., 1970, The role of atropine as a mediator blocker of induced bronchial obstruction, *J. Allergy* **45:**178–186.

Jeffrey, P., and Reid, L., 1973, Intraepithelial nerves in normal rat airways: A quantitative electron microscopic study, *J. Anat.* **114:**35–42.

Jenne, J. W., Chick, T. W., Strickland, R. D., and Wall, F. J., 1977a, A comparison of beta adrenergic function in asthma and chronic bronchitis, *J. Allergy Clin. Immunol.* **60:**341–356.

Jenne, J. W., Chick, T. W., Strickland, R. D., and Wall, F. J., 1977b, Subsensitivity of beta responses during treatment with a long-acting beta-2 preparation, *J. Allergy Clin. Immunol.* **59:**383–390.

Johanson, W. G., Jr., Pierce, A. K., and Sanford, J. P., 1969, Pulmonary function in uncomplicated influenza, *Am. Rev. Respir. Dis.* **100:**141–146.

Johansson, S. G. O., 1967, Raised levels of a new immunoglobulin class (IgND) in asthma, *Lancet* **2:**951–955.

Kaliner, M., 1976, The cholinergic nervous system and immediate hypersensitivity. I. Eccrine sweat responses in allergic patients, *J. Allergy Clin. Immunol.* **58:**308–315.

Kaliner, M. A., Orange, R. P., and Austen, K. F., 1972, Immunological release of histamine and slow reacting substance of anaphylaxis from human lung. IV. Enhancement of cholinergic and alpha adrenergic enhancement of mediator release, *J. Exp. Med.* **1936:**556–567.

Kariman, K., and Lefkowitz, R. J., 1977, Decreased beta-adrenergic receptor bindings in lymphocytes from patients with bronchial asthma, *Clin. Res.*,503A (abstr.).

Karr, R. M., Davies, R. J., Butcher, B. T., Lehrer, S. B., Wilson, M. R., Dharmarajan, V., and Salvaggio, J. E., 1978, Occupational asthma, *J. Allergy Clin. Immunol.* **61:**54–65.

Kay, A. B., and Austen, K. F., 1971, The IgE-mediated release of eosinophil chemotactic factor from human lung, *J. Immunol.* **107:**899–902.

Kelly, M. T., and White, A., 1974, An inhibitor of histamine release from human leukocytes, *J. Clin. Invest.* **53:**1343–1348.

Kessler, G. F., Austin, J. H. M., Graf, P. D., Gamsu, G., and Gold, W. M., 1973, Airway constriction in experimental asthma in dogs: Tantalum bronchographic studies, *J. Appl. Physiol.* **35:**703–709.

Kilburn, K. H., 1968, A hypothesis for pulmonary clearance and its applications, *Am. Rev. Respir. Dis.* **98:**449–453.

Kiviloog, J., 1975, The effect of pretreatment with atropine in exercise-induced bronchoconstriction, *Pediatrics. Suppl.* **56:**940–941.

Klotz, S. D., and Berstein, C., 1950, The use of dibenamine in the severe asthmatic state and related chronic pulmonary conditions, *Ann. Allergy* **8:**767–771.

Kontou-Karakitsos, K., Salvaggio, J. E., and Mathews, K. P., 1975, Comparative nasal absorption of allergens in atopic and nonatopic subjects, *J. Allergy Clin. Immunol.* **55:**241–248.

Krell, R. D., Chakrin, L. W., and Wardell, J. R., Jr., 1976, The effect of cholinergic agents on a canine model of allergic asthma, *J. Allergy Clin. Immunol.* **58:**19–30.

Kumar, L., and Newcomb, R. W., 1970, Effect of living measles vaccine on bronchial sensitivity of asthmatic children to methacholine, *J. Allergy* **45:**104 (abstr.).

Laitinen, L. A., Elkin, R. B., Empey, D. W., Jacobs, L., Mills, J., Gold, W. M., and Nadel, J. A., 1976, Changes in bronchial reactivity after administration of live attenuated influenza virus, *Am. Rev. Respir. Dis.* **113:**194 (abstr.).

Lang, P., Goel, Z., and Grieco, M. H., 1978, Subsensitivity of T lymphocytes to sympathomimetic and cholinergic stimulation in bronchial asthma, *J. Allergy Clin. Immunol.* **61:**248–254.

Laros, C. D., 1971, Local chemical regulation of the flow resistance in the bronchial tree and pulmonary circulation, *Respiration* **28:**120–128.

Lauweryns, J. M., and Goodeeris, P., 1975, Neuroepithelial bodies in the human child and adult lung, *Am. Rev. Respir. Dis.* **111:**469–476.

Lee, T.-P., Kue, J. F., and Greengard, P., 1972, Role of muscarinic cholinergic receptors in regulation of guanosine 3′5′-cyclic monophosphate content in mammalian brain, heart muscle and intestinal smooth muscle, *Proc. Natl. Acad. Sci.* **69:**3287–3291.

Lefkowitz, R. J., 1976, *β*-Adrenergic receptors, recognition and regulation, *New Engl. J. Med.* **295:**323–328.

Lehrer, S. B., Tan, E. M., and Vaughan, J. H., 1974, Extraction and partial purification of the histamine-sensitizing factor of *Bordetella pertussis*, *J. Immunol.* **113:**18–26.

Lett-Brown, M. A., and Leonard, E. J., 1977, Histamine-induced inhibition of normal basophil chemotaxis to C5a, *J. Immunol.* **118:**815–821.

Levine, B. B., Stember, R. H., and Fotino, M., 1972, Ragweed hay fever: Genetic control and linkage to Hl-A haplotypes, *J. Allergy Clin. Immunol.* **51:**81 (abstr.).

Lewis, R. A., and Austen, K. F., 1977, Nonrespiratory functions of pulmonary cells: The mast cell, *Fed. Proc.* **36:**2676–2682.

Lichtenstein, L. M., and Gillespie, E., 1973, Inhibition of histamine release by histamine controlled by H-2 receptor, *Nature (London)* **244:**287–292.

Lichtenstein, L. M., and Margolis, S., 1968, Histamine release *in vitro:* Inhibition by catecholamines and methylxanthines, *Science* **161:**902–906.

Logsdon, P. J., Middleton, E., Jr., and Coffey, R. G., 1972, Stimulation of leukocyte adenyl cyclase by hydrocortisone and isoproterenol in asthmatic and non-asthmatic subjects, *J. Allergy Clin. Immunol.* **50:**45–56.

Logsdon, P. J., Carnright, D. V., Middleton, E., Jr., and Coffey, R. G., 1973, The effect of phentolamine on adenylate cyclase and on isoproterenol stimulation in leukocytes from asthmatic and nonasthmatic subjects, *J. Allergy Clin. Immunol.* **52:**148–157.

Lumsden, T., 1923, Observations on the respiratory centres in the cat, *J. Physiol. (London)* **57:**153–162.

Luparello, T. J., Leist, N., Laurie, E. J., and Sweet, P., 1970, The interaction of psychologic stimuli and pharmacologic agents on airway reactivity in asthmatic subjects, *Psychosom. Med.* **32:**509–515.

Maccia, C. A., Gallagher, J. S., Ataman, G., Glueck, H. I., Brooks, S. M., and Bernstein, I. L., 1977, Platelet thrombopathy in asthmatic subjects with elevated immunoglobulin E, *J. Allergy Clin. Immunol.* **59:**101–108.

Mann, S. P., 1971, The innervation of mammalian bronchial smooth muscle: The localization of catecholamines and cholinesterases, *Histochem. J.* **3:**319–325.

Marcelle, R., Bottin, R., and Jiechmes, J., 1968, Réactions bronchomatrices de l'homme sans après blocage des récepteurs *β* adrénergiques, *Acta Allergol.* **23:**11–17.

Marsh, D. G., and Bias, W. B., 1974, Control of specific allergic response in man: HL-A associated and IgE-regulatory genes, *Fed. Proc.* **33:**774 (abstr.).

Marsh, D. G., Bias, W. B., Hse, S. H., and Goodfriend, L., 1973, Association of the HL-A 7 cross-reacting group with a specific reaginic antibody response in allergic man, *Science* **179:**691–696.

Marsh, D. G., Bias, W. B., and Ishizaka, K., 1974, Genetic control of basal serum immunoglobulin E level and its effect on specific reaginic sensitivity, *Proc. Natl. Acad. Sci.* **71:**3588–3593.

Mathe, A. A., 1977, Prostaglandins and the lung in: *The Prostaglandins,* Vol. 3 (P. W. Ramwell, ed.), pp. 169–180, Plenum, New York.

Mathe, A. A., and Hedqvist, P., 1975, Effect of prostaglandins $F_{2\alpha}$ and E_2 on airway conductance in healthy subjects and asthmatic patients, *Am. Rev. Respir. Dis.* **111**:313–320.

Mathe, A. A., and Knapp, P. H., 1969, Decreased plasma free fatty acids and urinary epinephrine in bronchial asthma, *N. Engl. J. Med.* **281**:234–238.

Mathe, A. A., Aström, A., and Persson, N. A., 1971, Some bronchodilating responses of human isolated bronchi: Evidence for the existence of alpha adrenoreceptors, *J. Pharm. Pharmacol.* **23**:905–911.

Mathe, A. A., Hedqvist, P., Strandberg, K., and Leslie, C. A., 1977, Aspects of prostaglandin function in the lung, *N. Engl. J. Med.* **296**:850–855, 910–914.

Mayrhofer, G., Bazin, H., and Gowans, J. L., 1976, Nature of cells binding anti-IgE in rats immunized with *Nippostrongylus brasiliensis:* IgE synthesis in regional nodes and concentration in mucosal mast cells, *Eur. J. Immunol.* **6**:537–544.

McCarter, J. H., and Vazquez, J. J., 1966, The bronchial basement membrane in asthma, *Arch. Pathol.* **82**:328–336.

McFadden, E. R., Jr., Ingram, R. H., Jr., and Haynes, R. L., 1977, Predominant site of flow limitation and mechanisms of post-exertional asthma, *J. Appl. Physiol.* **42**:746–752.

McIntosh, K., Ellis, E. R., and Hoffman, L. S., 1973, The association of viral and bacterial respiratory infections with exacerbations of wheezing in young asthmatic children, *J. Pediatr.* **82**:578–582.

Middleton, E., Jr., and Finke, S. R., 1968, Metabolic response to epinephrine in asthma, *J. Allergy* **42**:288–299.

Mills, J. E., and Widdicombe, J. G., 1970, Role of the vagus nerve in anaphylaxis and histamine-induced bronchoconstriction in guinea pigs, *Br. J. Pharmacol.* **39**:724–728.

Mills, J. E., Sellick, H., and Widdicombe, J. G., 1969, Activity of lung irritant receptors in pulmonary microembolism anaphylaxis and drug-induced bronchoconstriction, *J. Physiol. (London)* **205**:337–341.

Minor, T. E., Dick, E. C., De Meo, A. N., Ouellette, J. J., Cohen, M. P., and Reed, C. E., 1974, Viruses as precipitants of asthmatic attacks in children, *J. Am. Med. Assoc.* **227**:292–298.

Minor, T. E., Dick, E. C., Baker, J. W., Ouellette, J. J., Cohen, M., and Reed, C. E., 1976, Rhinovirus and Influenza type A infections as precipitants of asthma, *Am. Rev. Respir. Dis.* **113**:149–153.

Mitchell, I., Inglis, H., and Simpson, H., 1976, Viral infection in wheezing bronchitis and asthma in children, *Arch. Dis. Child.* **15**:707–711.

Moncada, S., Gryglewski, R. J., Bunting, S., *et al.*, 1976, A lipid peroxide inhibits the enzyme in blood vessel microsomes that generates from prostaglandin endoperoxides the substance (prostaglandin X) which prevents platelet aggregation, *Prostaglandins* **12**:715–718.

Moore, V. L., Hensley, G. T., and Fink, J. N., 1975, An animal mode of hypersensitivity pneumonitis in the rabbit, *J. Clin. Invest.* **56**:937–944.

Morris, H. G., DeRoche, G., and Earle, M. R., 1972, Urinary excretion of epinephrine and norepinephrine in asthmatic children, *J. Allergy Clin. Immunol.* **50**:138–145.

Morris, H. G., DeRoche, G. C., and Caro, C. N., 1974, Response of leukocyte cyclic AMP to epinephrine stimulation *in vivo* and *in vitro, J. Allergy Clin. Immunol.* **53**:98 (abstr.).

Morris, H. G., Rusnak, S. A., and Barzens, K., 1977, Leukocyte cyclic adenosine monophosphate in asthmatic children: Effects of adrenergic therapy, *Clin. Pharmacol. Ther.* **22**:352–356.

Nadel, J. A., 1968, Mechanisms of airway response to inhaled substances, *Arch. Environ. Health* **16**:171–178.

Nadel, J. A., 1977, Autonomic control of airway smooth muscle and airway secretions, *Am. Rev. Respir. Dis. Suppl.* **115**:117–126.

Nadel, J. A., Cabezas, G. A., and Austin, J. H. M., 1971, *In vivo* roentgenographic examination of parasympathetic innervation of small airways: Use of powdered tantalum and a fine focal spot X-ray tube, *Chest Radiol.* **6**:9–16.

Nelson, H. S., Black, J. W., Branch, L. B., Pfuetze, B., Spaulding, H., Summers, R., and Wood, D., 1975, Subsensitivity to epinephrine following the administration of epinephrine and ephedrine to normal individuals, *J. Allergy Clin. Immunol.* **55**:299–309.

Neshi, S., 1970, Cholinergic and adrenergic receptors at sympathetic preganglion nerve terminals, *Fed. Proc.* **29**:1957 (abstr.).

Niden, A. H., 1967, Bronchiolar and large alveolar cell in pulmonary phospholipid metabolism, *Science* **158:**1323–1327.

Oates, J. A., Melmon, K., Sjoerdsma, A., Gillespie, L., and Mason, D. T., 1964, Release of a kinin peptide in the carcinoid syndrome, *Lancet* **1:**514–518.

Okazaki, T., Vervloet, D., Attallah, A., Lee, J. B., and Arbesman, C. A., 1976, Prostaglandins and asthma: The use of blood components for metabolic studies, *J. Allergy Clin. Immunol.* **57:**124–133.

Okazaki, T., Ilea, V. S., Rosario, N. A., Reisman, R. R., Arbesman, C. E., Lee, J. B., and Middleton, E., Jr., 1977, Regulatory role of prostaglandin E in allergic histamine release with observations on the responsiveness of basophil leukocytes and the effect of acetylsalicylic acid, *J. Allergy Clin. Immunol.* **60:**360–366.

Orange, R. P., Austen, W. G., and Austen, K. R., 1971, Immunological release of histamine and slow reacting substance of anaphylaxis from human lung. I. Modulation by agents influencing cellular levels of cyclic 3′,5′-adenosine monophosphate, *J. Exp. Med.* **134:**136–145.

Ouellette, J. J., and Reed, C. E., 1965, Increased response of asthmatic subjects to methacholine after influenza vaccine, *J. Allergy* **36:**558–563.

Ouellette, J. J., Chosy, J. J., and Reed, C. E., 1967, Catecholamine execretion and bronchial response to methacholine after *Salmonella enteriditis* endotoxin in a normal and an asthmatic subject, *J. Allergy* **39:**234–237.

Pantal, A. S., 1973, Vagal sensory receptors and their reflex effects, *Physiol.Rev.* **53:**159–164.

Parish, W. E., 1970, Short term anaphylactic antibodies in human sera, *Lancet* **2:**591–592.

Parish, W. E., 1974, Skin sensitizing non-IgE antibodies: Association between human IgG S-TS and IgG4, *Progr. Immunol.* **4:**19–25.

Parker, C. D., and Bilbo, R. E., 1965, Methacholine aerosol as a test for bronchial asthma, *Arch. Intern. Med.* **115:** 452–455.

Parker, C. W., and Smith, J. W., 1973, Alterations in cyclic adenosine monophosphate metabolism in human bronchial asthma, *J. Clin. Invest.* **52:**48–59.

Patel, K. R., 1975, Atropine, sodium cromoglycate, and thymoxamine in $PGF_{2\alpha}$-induced bronchoconstriction in extrinsic asthma, *Br. Med. J.* **2:**360–362.

Patel, K. R., and Kerr, J. W., 1975, Effect of alpha receptor blocking drug, thymoxamine, on allergen induced bronchoconstriction in extrinsic asthma, *Clin. Allergy* **5:**311–316.

Paterson, J. W., Conolly, M. E., and Davies, D. S., 1968, Isoprenaline resistance and the use of pressurized aerosols in asthma, *Lancet* **2:**426–431.

Patterson, R., Tomita, Y., Oh, S. H., Susyko, I. M., and Pruzansky, J. J., 1974, Respiratory mast cells and basophiloid cells. I. Evidence that they are secreted into the bronchial lumen, morphology degeneration and histamine release, *Clin. Exp. Immunol.* **16:**223–229.

Pepys, J., 1977, Clinical and therapeutic significance of patterns of allergic reactions of the lungs to extrinsic agents, *Am. Rev. Respir. Dis.* **116:**573–588.

Pepys, J.,and Hutchcroft, B. J., 1975, Bronchial provocation tests in etiologic diagnosis and analysis of asthma, *Am. Rev. Respir. Dis.* **112:**829–859.

Petersson, B. A., 1975, Induction of histamine release and desensitization in human leukocytes: IgG-mediated histamine release, *Scand. J. Immunol.* **4:**777–784.

Petersson, B. A., Nilsson, A., and Stalenheim, G., 1975, Induction of histamine release and desensitization in human leukocytes, *J. Immunol.* **114:**1581–1584.

Picken, J. J., Niewoehner, D. E., and Chester, E. H., 1972, Prolonged effects of viral infections of the upper respiratory tract upon small airways, *Am. J. Med.* **52:**738–746.

Poothullil, J., Umemoto, L., Dolovich, J., Hargreave, F. E., and Day, R. P., 1976, Inhibition by prednisone of late cutaneous allergic responses induced by antiserum to human IgE, *J. Allergy Clin. Immunol.* **57:**164–167.

Rachelefsky, G., Park, M. S., Siegel, S., Terasaki, P. I., Katz, R., and Saito, S., 1976, Strong association between B-lymphocyte group-2 specificity and asthma, *Lancet* **2:**1042–1044.

Reid, L. M., 1960, Measurement of the bronchial mucus gland layer: A diagnostic yardstick in chronic bronchitis, *Thorax* **15:**132–141.

Reid, R. T., 1970, Reaginic activity associated with immunoglobulins other than IgE, *J. Immunol.* **104:**935.

Rhodin, J. A. G., 1966, The ciliated cell: Ultrastructure and function of the human tracheal mucosa, *Am. Rev. Respir. Dis.* **93:**1–11.

Richardson, J. B., and Bouchard, T., 1975, Demonstration of a nonadrenergic inhibitory nervous system in the trachea of the guinea pig, *J. Allergy Clin. Immunol.* **56:**473–480.

Richardson, J. B., Hogg, J. C., Bouchard, T., and Hall, D. L., 1973, Localization of antigen in experimental bronchoconstriction in guinea pigs, *J. Allergy Clin. Immunol.* **52:**172–181.

Ruffin, R. E., Cockcroft, D. W., and Hargreave, F. E., 1978, A comparison of the protective effects of fenoterol and Sch 1000 on allergen-induced asthma, *J. Allergy Clin. Immunol.* **61:**42–47.

Ryan, J. W., and Ryan, U. S., 1977, Pulmonary endothelial cells, *Fed. Proc.* **36:**2686–2690.

Ryo, U. Y., and Townley, R. G., 1976, Comparison of respiratory and cardiovascular effects of isoproterenol propranolol and practolol in asthmatic and normal subjects, *J. Allergy Clin. Immunol.* **57:**12–24.

Salvaggio, J. E., Cavenaugh, J. J. A., Lowell, F. C., and Leskowitz, S., 1964, A comparison of the immunologic responses of normal and atopic individuals to intranasally administered antigen, *J. Allergy* **35:**62–67.

Salvaggio, J., Phanuphak, P., Stanford, R., Bice, D., and Claman, H., 1975, Experimental production of granulomatous pneumonitis, *J. Allergy Clin. Immunol.* **56:**364–380.

Salvato, G., 1968, Some histological changes in chronic bronchitis and asthma, *Thorax* **23:**168–173.

Saum, W. R., and De Groat, W. C., 1972, Parasympathetic ganglion: Activation of an adrenergic inhibitory mechanism by cholinomimetic agents, *Science* **1975:**659–664.

Schorlemmer, H. Y., Edwards, J. H., Davies, P., and Allison, A. C., 1977, Macrophage responses to mouldy hay dust, *Micropolyspora faeni* and zymosan, activators of complement by the alternate pathway, *Clin. Exp. Immunol.* **27:**198–204.

Segal, M. S., and Dulfano, M. J., 1965, Glomectomy in the treatment of chronic bronchial asthma, *N. Engl. J. Med.* **272:**57–63.

Sen, D. K., Arora, S., Gupta, S., and Sanyal, R. K., 1974, Studies of adrenergic mechanisms in relation to histamine sensitivity in children immunized with *Bordetella pertussis* vaccine, *J. Allergy Clin. Immunol.* **54:**25–31.

Silva, D. G., and Ross, G., 1974, Ultrastructure and fluorescence histochemical studies on the innervation of the tracheobronchial muscle of normal cats and cats treated with 6-hydroxydopamine, *J. Ultrastruct. Res.* **47:**310–318.

Simani, A. S., Inouel, S., and Hogg, J. C., 1974, Penetration of the respiratory epithelium of guinea pigs following exposure to cigarette smoke, *Lab. Invest.* **31:**75–81.

Simon, R. A., Stevenson, D. D., Arroyave, C. M., and Tan, E. M., 1977, The relationship of plasma histamine to the activity of bronchial asthma, *J. Allergy Clin. Immunol.* **60:**312–316.

Simonsson, B. G., Jacobs, F. M., and Nadel, J. A., 1967, Role of autonomic nervous system and the cough reflex in the increased responsiveness of airways in patients with obstructive airway disease, *J. Clin. Invest.* **46:**1812–1818.

Simonsson, B. G., Svedmyer, N., Anderson, R., and Bergh, N. P., 1972, *In vivo* and *in vitro* studies on alpha-receptors in human airways; potentiation with bacterial endotoxins, *Scand. J. Respir. Dis.* **58:**227–236.

Siraganian, R. P., and Hook, W. A., 1976, Complement-induced histamine release from human basophils. II. Mechanism of the histamine release reaction, *J. Immunol.* **116:**639–646.

Sokol, W. N., and Beall, G. N., 1975, Leukocyte epinephrine receptors of normal and asthmatic individuals, *J. Allergy Clin. Immunol.* **55:**310–324.

Solinger, A., Bernstein, D. L., and Glueck, H. I., 1973, The effect of epinephrine on platelet-aggregation in normal and atopic subjects, *J. Allergy Clin. Immunol.* **51:**29–34.

Soutar, C. A., 1976, Distribution of plasma cells and other cells containing immunoglobulin in the respiratory tract of normal man and class of immunoglobulin contained therein, *Thorax* **31:**158–164.

Spaulding, H. S., Jr., Nelson, A. S., and Branch, B., 1975, Altered cardiovascular and metabolic responses to epinephrine following the administration of ephedrine and terbutaline to normal men, *J. Allergy Clin. Immunol.* **55:**97 (abstr.).

Spector, S., Luparello, T. J., Kopetzky, M. T., Souhrada, J., and Kinsman, R. A., 1976, Response of asthmatics to methacholine and suggestion, *Am. Rev. Respir. Dis.* **113:**43–50.

Stevenson, D. D., Mathison, D. A., Tan, E. M., and Vaughan, J. H., 1975, Provoking factors in bronchial asthma, *Arch. Intern. Med.* **135:**777–783.

Stevenson, D. D., Arroyave, C. M., Bhat, K. N., and Tan, E. M., 1976, Oral aspirin challenges in asthmatic patients: A study of plasma histamine, *Clin. Allergy* **6:**493–499.

Stimson, J. A. V., Hintz, D. S., Minster, A. M., and Spicer, S. S., 1977, Immunocytochemical evidence for antibody binding to mast cell granules, *Exp. Mol. Pathol.* **26:**85–94.

Strauss, R. H., Ingram, R. H., Jr., and McFadden, E. R., Jr., 1977, A critical assessment of the roles of circulating hydrogen ion and lactate in the production of exercise-induced asthma, *J. Clin. Invest.* **60:**658–664.

Sturgess, J., and Reed, L., 1972, An organ culture study of the effect of drugs on the secretory activity of the human bronchial submucosal gland, *Clin. Sci.*, **43:**533–541.

Sutherland, E. W., Robison, G. A., and Butcher, R. W., 1968, Some aspects of the biological role of adenosine 3′,5′-monophosphate (cyclic AMP), *Circulation* **37:**299–306.

Svedmyr, N. L. V., Larsson, S. A., and Thiringer, G. K., 1976, Development of "resistance" in beta-adrenergic receptors of asthmatic patients, *Chest* **69:**479–484.

Szczeklik, A., Gryglewski, R. J., and Czerneawska-Mysik, G., 1975, Relationship of inhibiton of prostaglandin in biosyntheses by analgesics to asthma attacks in aspirin-sensitive patients, *Br. Med. J.* **1:**67–73.

Szczeklik, A., Gryglewski, R. J., and Czerniawska-Mysik, G., 1977, Asthmatic attacks induced in aspirin-sensitive patients by dicloferae and naproxen, *Br. Med. J.* **2:**321.

Szentivanyi, A., and Filipp, G., 1965, Anaphylaxis and the nervous system. Part II, *Ann. Allergy* **16:**143–151.

Szentivanyi, A., Fishel, C. W., and Talmage, D. W., 1963, Adrenalin mediation of histamine and serotinin hyperglycemia in pertussis sensitized mice, *J. Infect. Dis.* **113:**86–98.

Takino, M., 1946, Findings in bronchial asthma, *Sogiogaku (Japan)* **3:**456–468.

Takino, M., and Takino, Y., 1968, Indication for glomectomy and postoperative treatment of asthma, *Tokuku J. Exp. Med.* **94:**257–273.

Tauber, A. E., Kaliner, M., Stechschulte, D. J., and Austen, K. F., 1973, Immunological release of histamine and slow reacting substance of anaphylaxis from human lung. V. Effects of prostaglandins on release of histamine, *J. Immunol.* **111:**27–32.

Terr, A. I., and Bentz, J. D., 1965, Skin sensitizing antibodies in serum sickness, *J. Allergy* **36:**433–445.

Townley, R. G., McGeady, S., and Bewtra, A., 1976, The effect of beta adrenergic blockade on bronchial sensitivity to acetyl-beta-methacholine in normal and allergic rhinitis subjects, *J. Allergy Clin. Immunol.* **57:**358–366.

Ts'ao, C. H., Patterson, R., McKenna, J. M., and Suszko, I. M., 1977, Ultrastructural identification of mast cells obtained from human bronchial lumens, *J. Allergy Clin. Immunol.* **59:**320–326.

Unväs, B., 1968, Histamine release in allergic conditions, in: *Allergology* (B. Rose, M. Richater, A. Sehon, and A. W. Frankland, eds.), pp. 127–141, Excerpta Medica Foundation, Amsterdam.

Vidruk, E. H., Hahn, H. L., Nadel, J. A., and Sampson, S. R., 1976, Mechanism of stimulation of rapidly adapting receptors of histamine in dog lung, *Fed. Proc.* **35:**841 (abstr.).

Vijay, H. M., and Perelmutter, L., 1977, Inhibition of reagin-mediated PCA reactions in monkeys and histamine release from human leukocytes by human IgG_4 subclass, *Int. Arch. Allergy Appl. Immunol.* **53:**78–87.

Walker, I. C., 1918, A clinical study of 400 patients with bronchial asthma, *Boston Med. Surg. J.* **1979:**288–294.

Wallace, D., and Grieco, M. H., 1976, Double-blind cross-over study of cromolyn sodium inhibition of exercise-induced bronchospasm in adults, *Ann. Allergy* **37:**153–163.

Webster, M. E., Horakova, Z., Beaver, M. A., Takahashi, H., and Newball, H. H., 1974, Release of arginine esterase and histamine from human lung passively sensitized with ragweed antibody, *Fed. Proc.* **33:**761 (abstr.).

Weiss, E. B., and Patwardhan, A. W., 1977, The responses to lidocaine in bronchial asthma, *Chest* **72:**429–438.

Wellmann, J. J., McFadden, E. R., Jr., and Ingram, R. H., Jr., 1976, Density-dependence of maximal expiratory flow rates before and after bronchodilators in patients with obstructive airways disease, *Clin. Sci. Mol. Med.* **51:**133–138.

Widdicombe, J. C., 1963, Regulation of tracheobronchial smooth muscle, *Physiol. Rev.* **43:**1–37.

Widdicombe, J. C., 1974, Reflex control of breathing, in: *Respiratory Physiology: MTP International Review of Science,* Ser. 1, Vol. 2 (J. G. Widdicombe, ed.), pp. 273–301, Butterworth, London.

Woolcock, A. J., Macklem, P. T., and Hogg, J. C., 1969, Influence of autonomic nervous system on airway resistance and elastic recoil, *J. Appl. Physiol.* **26:**814–821.

Yu, D. Y. C., Galant, S. P., and Gold, W. M., 1972, The role of the parasympathetic nervous system in human asthma: Inhibition of antigen-induced bronchoconstriction by atropine sulfate, *J. Appl. Physiol.* **32**:823–828.

Zaid, G., and Beall, G. N., 1966, Bronchial response to beta-adrenergic blockade, *New Engl. J. Med.* **275**:580–584.

Zimmerman, I., Islam, M. S., and Ulmer, W. T., 1976, Effect of unilateral vagus blockade on antigen-induced airway obstruction, *Respiration* **33**:359–365.

14

Immunological Features of Infiltrative Pulmonary Disease

REYNOLD M. KARR and JOHN E. SALVAGGIO

1. Introduction

Until recently, purely clinical criteria have been used to define infiltrative pulmonary disease. The criteria include the identification of an inhaled etiological antigen, a prior sensitizing exposure to this antigen, the subsidence of symptoms following antigen avoidance, and the development of disease in only a small number of exposed individuals. Gell and Coombs (1969) have defined four major immunological mechanisms of tissue injury, all of which may play a role in a variety of hypersensitivity pulmonary disorders, that do not strictly conform to these classical clinical criteria. Consequently, it is now known that certain forms of allergic pneumonitis may persist for some time after cessation of an etiological exposure and may involve auto antigens (intrinsic) rather than extrinsic antigens, as in the case of the autoimmune diseases.

Allergic infiltrative diseases of lung are composed of three main pathologic entities: hypersensitivity pneumonitis, the eosinophilic pneumonias, and diffuse pulmonary fibrosis. Common to all three entities is an inflammatory or fibrotic infiltration of lung parenchyma producing impairment of gas exchange. Although overlap may occur—e.g., eosinophilic granuloma often progresses to diffuse interstitial pulmonary fibrosis—this classification has proved to be clinically useful. Certain distinct immunopathological features of hypersensitivity are found in many types of these three major forms of allergic pneumonitis and will be discussed in detail in this chapter.

REYNOLD M. KARR and JOHN E. SALVAGGIO • Clinical Immunology Section, Department of Medicine, Tulane University School of Medicine, New Orleans, Louisiana 70112.

2. Hypersensitivity Pneumonitis (Extrinsic Allergic Alveolitis)

An inflammatory reaction in the distal segments of lung may occur when sensitized human subjects inhale a variety of organic dusts and finely disbursed animal proteins of appropriate particle size. The condition, now known in America as ''hypersensitivity pneumonitis'' and in Great Britain as ''extrinsic allergic alveolitis,'' was first recognized by Ramazzini (1713). More than two centuries later, it received renewed attention when Campbell (1932) described farmer's lung, characterized by features of acute pneumonitis following repeated exposure to moldy hay. Pigeon breeders exposed to avian proteins may experience a similar disorder (Fink *et al.*, 1968), and currently the number of etiological agents known to produce disease is increasing with greater awareness and recognition. The various types of hypersensitivity pneumonitis are identified by euphemistic terms or eponyms describing the exposure condition or the suspected etiological agent. For additional information, the reader is referred to recent reviews of the subject by Salvaggio (1976), Schatz *et al.* (1977), and Roberts and Moore (1978).

2.1. Etiology

The list of occupational, avocational, and iatrogenic conditions of antigen exposure is continually expanding (Table 1). Sources of antigen are numerous and may include microorganisms (bacteria, fungi, amoebae), animals, and plants. Drugs, as well as certain low-molecular-weight industrial chemicals, have been found to produce disease. Antigens of actinomycete and avian origin have been most intensively studied and merit detailed consideration.

2.1.1. Actinomycete Antigens

Certain thermophilic and mesophilic actinomycete organisms have been shown to produce disease in such diverse situations as home central heating, farming, mushroom picking, and processing of sugar cane fiber. Although they are often wrongly identified as fungi because of their similar morphology, they are actually true bacteria or Eubacteriales. Their growth is supported best in decaying organic matter such as hay or bagasse at elevated temperatures in the range between 37°C and 60°C. With the use of Anderson samplers and qualitative culture plating techniques, Gregory and Lacey (1963a,b) and Seabury *et al.* (1969) have studied the flora of hay and bagasse. Actinomycete organisms grow particularly well in compost with a neutral pH of 7.0. The higher moisture content of old hay and bagasse (about 40%) more consistently maintains a temperature between 40°C and 60°C and therefore supports the growth of thermophilic organisms much better than in fresh hay or bagasse. Gregory and Lacey (1963a,b) have detected up to 1.6×10^9 actinomycete spores in the ambient atmosphere following the handling of moldy hay. Hargreave (1973) has determined particle sizes to be smaller than $6 \mu m$, and it has been estimated that a farmer working in this environment might inhale and retain 750,000 spores per minute in the alveolar spaces of his lungs (Lacey and Lacey, 1964). Salvaggio (1970) has reported similar figures for moldy bagasse. Thermophilic actinomycetes grow well in compost, but they may also occur ubiquitously in soil, foods, fresh water, the atmosphere, and other natural sources.

TABLE 1. Etiology of Hypersensitivity Pneumonitis

Offending agent	Source	Disorder
Thermophilic actinomycetes		
Micropolyspora faeni	Moldy hay	Farmer's lung
Thermoactinomyces vulgaris	Moldy sugarcane (bagasse)	Bagassosis
Thermoactinomyces candidus	Contaminated home humidifier and air-conditioning ducts	Humidifier lung
Thermoactinomyces viridis	Cattle	Fog fever
	Moldy cork	Suberosis
	Vineyards	Vineyard sprayer's lung
	Ventilation system	
Thermoactinomyces sacchari	Moldy compost	Mushroom worker's disease
True fungi		
Alternaria sp.	Moldy wood pulp	Wood pulp worker's disease
Cryptostroma corticale	Maple bark	Maple bark stripper's lung
Pencillium casei	Cheese mold	Cheese worker's lung
Cryptostroma corticale	Moldy maple logs	Maple bark disease
Aspergillus clavatus	Moldy cheese	Cheese washer's lung
	Moldy barley	Malt worker's lung
Mucor stolonifer	Moldy paprika pods	Paprika slicer's lung
Pullularia sp.	Moldy wood dust	Sequoiosis
Graphium sp.	Moldy wood dust	Sequoiosis
Animal proteins		
Parrot serum proteins	Parrot droppings	Budgerigar fancier's disease
Pigeon serum proteins	Pigeon droppings	Pigeon breeder's disease
Turkey proteins	Turkey products	Turkey handler's disease
Duck proteins	Feathers	Duck fever
Bovine and porcine proteins	Pituitary snuff	Pituitary snuff taker's lung
Chicken proteins	Chicken products	Feather plucker's disease
Bat serum protein	Bat droppings	Bat lung
Rat serum protein	Rat urine	—
Insect products		
Ascaris siro (mite)	Dust	—
Sitophilus granarius (wheat weevil)	Contaminated grain	Miller's lung
Amoebae		
Naegleria gruberi	Contaminated water	—
Acanthamoeba castellani		
Acanthamoeba polyphaga		
Vegetable derivatives		
Unknown	Tea plants	Tea grower's disease
	Cloth wrappings of mummies	Coptic disease
	Tobacco plants	Tobacco grower's disease
	Cereal grain	Grain measurer's lung
	Dried grass and leaves	Thatched roof disease
	Sawdust (redwood, maple, red cedar)	Sequoiosis
Chemical agents		
Nitrofurantoin	Iatrogenic	—
Hydrochlorthiazide	Iatrogenic	—
Toluene diisocyanate	Urethane foaming	—
Sodium cromolyn	Iatrogenic	—

The most important source of actinomycete antigen in moldy hay is *Micropolyspora faeni*. Edwards (1972b) studied its antigenic components using immunoelectrophoresis. He identified eight major antigens and labeled them according to their electrophoretic mobility. Further purification and analysis then led to partial characterization. The major precipitin line in the "C" region has been called "antigen 1," which is a heat-stable (100°C) glycopeptide with an average molecular weight of 85,000 associated with the mycelial cell wall. The major precipitin line in the "A" region has been called "antigen 2," which is a heat-labile protein with a molecular weight of 44,000 demonstrating chymotrypsin-like activity. The major precipitin line in the "B" region has been called "antigen 3," which is a heat-labile protein with a molecular weight of 77,000 also demonstrating enzymatic activity. A fast anodally migrating line, "antigen 4," is a heat-labile protein with a high sugar content and a molecular weight of 101,000. Using a discontinuous gel gradient polyacrylamide electrophoresis technique, Roberts (1978) has identified 20–30 different protein bands, with each actinomycete species demonstrating a unique electrophoretic pattern. Some of these proteins can lyse casein. Diisopropylfluorophosphate (DPF) inhibits the reaction, identifying these enzymes as serine proteases. Further characterization of the molecular structure and biological activity of actinomycete antigen is a major area of intensive research.

2.1.2. Avian (Pigeon) Antigens

Hypersensitivity pneumonitis has been related to antigens derived from feathers, serum, and excrement of several avian species (Table 1). Sensitized subjects may develop disease following exposure to antigens in pigeon serum and droppings (Fink *et al.*, 1968). Fredricks (1978) performed analyses on a soluble, nondialyzable pigeon dropping extract (PDE). Immunoelectrophoresis of this material produced four dominant precipitin arcs which he labeled serially "PDE_1" through "PDE_4," with increasing mobility. All of these components were acidic. Another antigen was detected by simple gel diffusion and labeled "PDE_B" because it was found to be basic. PDE_1 was determined to be a glycoprotein with a molecular weight of 200,000 containing 88% protein and 12% carbohydrate. Ouchterlony gel diffusion studies with PDE_1 demonstrated lines of identity with chicken α-chains, which suggested that PDE_1 may be a pigeon IgA molecule or derivative. PDE_3 was found to be a heat-stable molecule composed of 30% protein and 70% carbohydrate with an average molecular weight of 16,000. Stabilizing disulfide and hydrogen bonds are probably present in PDE_3, because it is susceptible to treatment with β-mercaptoethanol and urea. The antigen, therefore, is probably a mucopolysaccharide-protein conjugate, or mucin. PDE_B was shown to be a glycoprotein with a molecular weight of 42,000. It cross-reacted with PDE_1, suggesting that it may be an Fab or Fc breakdown product of pigeon IgA. PDE_1 and PDE_B are contained in pigeon serum as well as pigeon droppings. PDE_3 is likely present in droppings but not in serum since rabbit antipigeon serum precipitated only with PDE_1 and PDE_B, not with PDE_3. When PDE was passed through a DEAE-cellulose column, eluates demonstrated esterase activity in two adjacent peaks; the first peak eluted with PDE_B and indicated an enzymatic function for this antigen. Intensive study is currently in progress to elucidate molecular structure and biological properties of these potent avian antigens.

2.2. Clinical Features: Disease Presentation

The clinical categories of acute, subacute, and chronic disease are thought to be determined by the intensity and frequency of exposure to etiological antigens. Pigeon breeder's disease, which often presents as acute hypersensitivity pneumonitis, generally results from a brief, intensive antigen exposure and may present similarly to acute bacterial or viral pneumonia. Patients typically describe the rapid onset of cough, fever, chills, aches, and dyspnea. There may also be cyanosis and hemoptysis in severe cases. Symptoms generally start several hours after an exposure and may resolve within several hours to weeks unless reexposure occurs. A misdiagnosis of bacterial or viral pneumonia is often made. The patient may be hospitalized, and treatment with antibiotics is generally followed by improvement, which would otherwise have resulted spontaneously with antigen avoidance. The patient is then discharged unknowingly back to his occupation or site of exposure only to again experience an exacerbation followed by a repetition of the same course of events. When the diagnosis remains unrecognized, repeated exposures may produce irreversible damage to the lung. A careful history often reveals onset of symptoms several hours after beginning work or sometimes not until the patient returns home in the evening. With this type of occupational exposure, symptoms may abate on weekends only to recur again on Monday following a return to work. However, if the exposure is in the home, as is the case with actinomycete contamination of central heating ducts or home humidifiers, a reverse temporal pattern of symptoms can result. Inquiry into a patient's hobbies may reveal the presence of a pigeon coop or a home woodshop and suggest an avocational source of antigen. A careful drug history is also important since certain medications may produce a picture of acute pneumonitis in susceptible subjects. Such medications include nitrofurantoin, procarbazine, and rifampin, among others. Subacute or chronic disease may result from less intensive exposure to an offending antigen over a longer period of time. Typical symptoms include insidious onset of cough, exertional dyspnea, anorexia, weight loss, and easy fatiguability. Often medical attention is sought only after diffuse interstitial fibrosis with pulmonary insufficiency has occurred. Advanced pulmonary fibrosis with right-sided congestive heart failure has been reported in certain rare forms of hypersensitivity pneumonitis such as thatched roof disease in natives of New Guinea (Blackburn and Greer, 1966).

2.3. Diagnosis

Basic to the diagnosis of hypersensitivity pneumonitis is the establishment of an association between a specific inhalant exposure, usually an organic dust or animal protein, and the development of symptoms with pneumonitis. Further diagnostic support is provided when removal of the subject from the particular suspect exposure results in remission of signs and symptoms. It may also be useful, after prolonged antigen avoidance and remission of disease, to intentionally reintroduce the subject for a brief period of time to the offending environment in order to further document a relationship with the development of disease. Physical findings are not specific since they may be identical in bacterial or viral pneumonia; however, they do serve to clinically confirm the existence of lung inflammation. Several laboratory procedures may further aid in establishing a diagnosis and in identifying a specific etiology.

2.3.1. Immunological Studies

Antibodies that specifically precipitate with an offending organic dust or animal protein antigen are commonly found in the serum of subjects with hypersensitivity pneumonitis. Serum precipitating antibodies to thermophilic actinomycetes were found by Pepys and Jenkins (1965) to be present in about 90% of patients with farmer's lung. Greater than 95% of these precipitating antibodies exhibited specificity for *Micropolyspora faeni*. Conventional Ouchterlony double diffusion techniques are easily used to identify these antibodies. Commercially available extracts of actinomycete species, certain true fungi, organic dusts, and avian proteins are available for patient screening and may be useful, although it should be understood that they are poorly standardized. The diagnostic accuracy of this procedure is somewhat limited by the finding of serum precipitating antibody in significant numbers of exposed, asymptomatic subjects. Fink *et al.* (1972) studied 200 pigeon breeders and found that 40% demonstrated serum precipitins without evidence of disease. Pepys and Jenkins (1965) reported that as many as 18% of normal farmers with a history of moldy hay exposure without symptoms demonstrated serum precipitins to a hay antigen. Less commonly, false-negative reactions may occur, possibly because of the relative insensitivity of the assay. An alternative explanation is that different subjects may produce antibodies with specificity for different antigenic components of the same organism. Consequently, a diagnostic antigen extract containing some but not all antigenic components might produce false-negative reactions in some individuals with disease. Of equal importance is the finding that precipitin titers tend to decrease with prolonged antigen avoidance and disease remission, so that subjects without recent exposure may have lost detectable levels of precipitating antibody. Because of the recognition of an increasing number of offending agents and the limited number of commercially available antigens, it is reasonable to screen suspected organic dusts for antigen activity by double gel diffusion analysis using the patient's serum, a positive reference control serum, and a negative control serum from an unexposed subject. Demonstration of precipitating antibody in the patient's serum, along with proper controls, may indicate the existence of an offending antigen in the crude dust extract. Further purification of antigenic components may then be facilitated by double gel radioimmunodiffusion analysis using the patient's serum. When microorganisms are suspected as sources of antigen, special cultures may aid in precise identification and provide a source of diagnostic antigen.

Many antigen preparations when injected intradermally in appropriate concentrations produce a variety of types of skin reactions only in sensitized subjects. Other antigenic preparations, including crude extracts of actinomycete organisms, tend to be nonspecifically irritating and, as such, do not differentiate sensitized from nonsensitized subjects. Salvaggio *et al.* (1975) have successfully used extensively dialyzed nonirritating crude thermophilic actinomycete extracts for skin testing in experimental animals. Further characterization and purification of these extracts may lead to the development of diagnostically useful skin test reagents for man. However, other diagnostic antigens of animal origin such as pigeon serum and pigeon dropping extract are not irritating in appropriate concentrations and may be used for skin testing in man. Positive skin reactions typically occur 4–8 hr after application of antigen and consist of an Arthus-type reaction, although immediate 20-min wheal-and-flare reactions have been reported by Fink (1973) to occur in 80% of patients with pigeon breeder's disease when skin tested with pigeon protein. Moore *et al.* (1974), Caldwell *et al.* (1973), and Fink *et al.* (1975) all demonstrated migration inhibition factor (MIF) production by peripheral blood leukocytes of symptomatic pigeon breeders. Demonstration of MIF appeared to correlate with disease activity, despite the usual absence of delayed 48-hr skin reactions to these antigens.

2.3.2. Chest X-ray

The X-ray changes seen in the chest in hypersensitivity pneumonitis have been reviewed (Hargreave *et al.*, 1972; Staines and Forman, 1961; Unger *et al.*, 1968). Interstitial and alveolar micronodular infiltrates appearing in a patchy or diffuse distribution are common in acute disease. Nodule size may range from one to several millimeters in diameter. Nodules may be discrete or coalesce. Acinar shadows may also be seen. The intensity of the chest X-ray abnormality frequently reflects severity of symptoms. Hilar adenopathy may occur infrequently and suggest a mistaken diagnosis of sarcoidosis. Linear interstitial densities and an acinar pattern often coexist in subacute disease. A "hilar haze" with a symmetrical "ground glass" appearance resembling pulmonary edema may often be apparent, since infiltrates occur less commonly in the apices and bases. On rare occasions, the chest X-ray in acute disease, especially if taken very soon after exposure, may be entirely normal.

2.3.3. Histopathology

The intensity of antigenic exposure and the stage of disease at the time biopsy is taken are thought to be the main factors determining the histopathological changes seen in most varieties of hypersensitivity pneumonitis. The characteristic finding is an intense alveolar and interstitial inflammation with frequent involvement and narrowing of bronchioles, as may be seen in bronchiolitis obliterans. Infiltrating cells consist of lymphocytes, plasma cells, and alveolar macrophages. The cytoplasm of these macrophages may appear finely vacuolated, lending it a foamy appearance. Eosinophils are rarely seen in significant number. As disease persists and a subacute phase develops, noncaseating granulomas appear which closely resemble those found in sarcoidosis. Ultimately, the granulomas may persist or disappear as interstitial fibrosis develops. Short exposures to antigen, however, generally resolve without residual pulmonary damage.

Immunofluorescent studies on lung tissue from patients with farmer's lung have been performed by Wenzel *et al.* (1971). The presence of actinomycete antigen in the walls of bronchioles was suggested by the finding of positive staining in this location using globulin isolated from patient sera and labeled with fluorescein. Infiltrating plasma cells and lymphocytes were found to contain IgG, IgA, and IgM, and C3 was demonstrated in histiocytes. There was no evidence of pulmonary blood vessel inflammation, and there was no specific immunofluorescent staining of vessel walls. However, there are isolated reports of biopsy-proven pulmonary vasculitis within several days following an acute episode (Barrowcliff and Arblaster, 1968).

2.3.4. Pulmonary Function Tests

Several nonspecific physiological changes are seen during the course of hypersensitivity pneumonitis. The acute disease is usually characterized by a significant decrease in lung volumes with little change in spirometric function, although a mild fall in FEV_1 coincident with a decrease in FVC may be observed. Interstitial inflammation produces increased stiffness of lung, resulting in a decrease in lung compliance. These are also marked ventilation/perfusion abnormalities which are reflected in a decreased diffusion capacity and arterial oxygen tension. As with clinical and X-ray changes, these functional abnormalities of acute disease are reversible. In chronic disease with extensive pulmonary fibrosis, both obstructive and restrictive ventilatory defects become irreversible.

2.3.5. Provocative Inhalation Challenge

Diagnosis of an offending exposure may be facilitated by bringing the patient back to the suspected environment during an asymptomatic period. Signs and symptoms of disease may develop over the ensuing 24-hr period and provide important clues to the etiological agent. A controlled provocative inhalation challenge, performed in the laboratory, may also be used to diagnose hypersensitivity pneumonitis. The technique has also been used to identify etiological antigens by proving a direct "cause-and-effect" relationship, and to investigate pathogenetic mechanisms (Karr *et al.*, 1978a,b). Only water-soluble antigens should be used. They may be administered by any suitable pressurized nebulizer producing small droplet sizes less than 10 μ in diameter. One challenge is performed every 24 hr with progressive tenfold increases of antigen concentration until either the maximum concentration of 10 mg/ml is reached or a reaction occurs. The most important parameters to monitor include pulmonary functions, body temperature, white blood cell count, vital signs, lung ascultation, and chest X-ray films when appropriate. Frequent assessment during the 24-hr period following a challenge is essential for the detection and documentation of late pulmonary reactions.

Certain undiagnosed cases, where repeated clinical episodes occur without demonstrable serum precipitins, are especially suitable for this type of testing. It should be emphasized, however, that positive challenge results must be critically interpreted since endotoxins and other irritant materials found in crude dust extracts may produce febrile reactions in some normal subjects. Although unlikely, there is always the possibility of producing a severe pneumonitis which might ultimately lead to permanent lung damage. In most cases, the benefit of early recognition and consequent avoidance of the offending agent generally outweighs any potential risks. For these reasons, the provocative inhalation challenge technique has become a frequently used tool for both clinical diagnosis and research.

2.4. Therapy

Recognition of the etiological antigen and particular condition of exposure is necessary for the adequate management of the patient with hypersensitivity pneumonitis. With this information, an attempt can be made to eliminate antigen inhalation. The approach will not only control disease in sensitized subjects but will also prevent sensitization in susceptible previously unexposed individuals. Disease prevention is always the best long-term approach. For example, in occupations where composts are used, such as farming and sugar cane processing, dispersion of thermophilic actinomycete spores can be markedly diminished by wetting of composts before handling and grinding. Another approach is to suppress growth of these organisms with a nontoxic 1% solution of propionic acid. A pasteurization process has been described (Buechner, 1971) which renders certain organic dust fibers sterile. Frequent cleaning and water change of indoor air humidifier units may also prevent growth of microorganisms. Respirable dusts may be greatly diminished with effective indoor ventilation systems in industries such as lumber where large quantities of dust are produced. A decreased incidence of bagassosis and maple bark stripper's disease has resulted from the use of some of these procedures.

In certain situations there may be very strong socioeconomic pressures preventing the elimination of etiological respirable antigens from the work environment. The task may be further complicated since etiological antigens may not always be readily identifiable, as is often the case with chronic interstitial lung diseases. The best approach under these circumstances is to remove the subject from the offending work environment and retrain him for a job in a different location. When a change in jobs is not feasible, and the patient has no reasonable alternative than to continue working despite exposure, a protective face mask may serve to diminish the amount of respirable antigen. However, the very small particle size (1–6 μm) of these offending dusts makes this measure at best only partially effective. Corticosteroid therapy may be effective in the control of hypersensitivity pneumonitis, although the evidence for this is largely anecdotal. It does appear that long-term maintenance on corticosteroids, of an individual subject to chronic exposure, may diminish progression of disease. In order to minimize long-term steroid side effects, an alternate-day corticosteroid regimen has been useful in the treatment of chronic disease and is usually indicated if systemic symptoms are present with pulmonary consolidation and arterial blood hypoxemia. Mild episodes rapidly resolve spontaneously without treatment if antigen exposure is eliminated.

There is little information about the natural history of hypersensitivity pneumonitis in the face of chronic exposure. However, a 5-year morbidity rate of 30%, with respiratory disability due mainly to pulmonary fibrosis, has been reported (NHLI Task Force Report, 1972). The enormous impact of this disease on industry and individual workers in terms of loss of time from work and personal hardship makes it essential for physicians to be thoroughly familiar with the diagnosis and management of the many forms of hypersensitivity pneumonitis.

2.5. Pathogenesis

2.5.1. Human Studies

Some of the etiological antigens of hypersensitivity pneumonitis have been found to exhibit certain biological properties such as activation of complement or macrophages, enhancement of immune response through an adjuvant effect, elicitation of a specific immune response as a potent antigen, and enzymatic destruction of certain tissue components. Host susceptibility factors are likely important since only a minority of regularly exposed subjects contract disease (Christensen *et al.*, 1975; Chemlik *et al.*, 1974). Total peripheral blood eosinophil counts and IgE levels in subjects with hypersensitivity pneumonitis are typically normal (Pepys, 1973). Additionally, there does not appear to be any increase in the prevalence of atopic disease and immediate-type wheal-and-flare skin reactions to common aeroallergens, making atopy an unlikely predisposing factor. However, HLA typing has provided evidence for genetically determined susceptibility. An increased frequency of HLA-B8 has been found in subjects with farmer's lung and pigeon breeder's disease (Flaherty *et al.*, 1975; Rittner *et al.*, 1975). Also, HLA-BW40 has been found with increased frequency in pigeon breeder's disease (Allen *et al.*, 1977). Since the HLA-B locus is thought to be located geographically close to immune response genes in the major histocompatibility complex on chromosome 6, the association of these alleles with disease is thought to indicate the presence of a closely linked immune response gene governing abnormal immune response to these unique antigens producing hypersensitivity pneumonitis.

The nonspecific irritative property of some antigens involved in hypersensitivity pneumonitis may be an important part of their pathogenic potential. Several studies in animals have shown that nonspecific lung irritation augments pulmonary sensitization (Moore *et al.*, 1975; Bice *et al.*, 1977; Salvaggio, 1976). Moore *et al.* (1975) have shown that, in the rabbit, long-term immunization with pigeon dropping extract (PDE) produces only an antibody response without inflammatory lesions; however, if BCG is used to prior inflame the lung, then inhalation challenge with PDE produces granulomatous lesions resembling those of hypersensitivity pneumonitis. This occurs in association with demonstrable cell-mediated hypersensitivity to the inhaled antigen.

Studies in humans and the development of animal models have contributed greatly to our current understanding of the specific immune response to etiological antigens in this disease. Immune mechanisms have been considered largely in terms of the Gell and Coombs (1969) type I–IV classification. As previously stated, the type I reagin-mediated hypersensitivity reaction appears to be of little importance in classical hypersensitivity pneumonitis; however, it has been noted that as many as 80% of patients with pigeon breeder's disease may demonstrate wheal-and-flare skin reactions to pigeon antigens (Fink, 1973) which may also be associated with immediate-type bronchospastic reactions following bronchoprovocation (Hargreave and Pepys, 1972). The same kind of association has been reported in a variant of farmer's lung (Karr *et al.*, 1978b). Despite these several exceptions, most patients studied do not demonstrate an increased prevalence of asthma or atopy. Wenzel *et al.* (1971) have demonstrated *Micropolyspora faeni* antigen, immune globulin, and complement in bronchiolar walls and mononuclear cells of lung biopsy specimens from patients with farmer's lung and have interpreted the data to indicate a type II cytotoxic mechanism. They proposed that antigen combines directly with cell surface antigens and in the presence of complement reacts with specific antibody, resulting directly in tissue damage. Their view, however, has not found substantial support to date. Evidence for a type III immune complex mechanism is greater. Serum precipitating antibodies specific for the etiological antigen are found in most varieties of hypersensitivity pneumonitis, and the level of antibody appears to correlate with intensity of exposure and severity of disease (Fink *et al.*, 1967). Also, the late (4–8 hr) Arthus-type skin reactions which are produced by many of these antigens such as the avian antigen histologically consist of small vessel necrotizing vasculitis with deposition of complement and immunoglobulin in vessel walls (Pepys, 1969; Fink *et al.*, 1968). Other supporting evidence includes the late 4–8 hr pulmonary reaction following bronchoprovocation with antigen, which follows the time course observed with the Arthus reaction and the immunofluorescent studies of lung biopsy material which usually demonstrate tissue deposition of antigen, immunoglobulin, and complement, all necessary constituents of an immune complex reaction. However, there is great controversy concerning the interpretation of these data. The fact that precipitins may be present in a sizable percentage of exposed asymptomatic subjects suggests that an antibody response may be necessary but not sufficient to produce disease. Alternatively, it may be that the antibody response is a normal consequence of antigen exposure having little relationship to disease. Also, there may be qualitative differences in the precipitins, as shown by Hollingdale (1974). He reported that subjects with farmer's lung demonstrate precipitins against only the glycoprotein moiety of *Micropolyspora faeni,* while asymptomatic exposed subjects demonstrate precipitins against both the glycoprotein and protein fractions. Another argument against an immune complex mechanism is the striking lack of vasculitic lesions which are so typical of type III hypersensitivity. However, it may be necessary to biopsy the lung early in the progression of the lesion in order to demonstrate necrotizing vasculitis (Ghose *et al.*, 1974; Barrowcliff and Arblaster, 1968). Moreover, the frequent finding of granulomas, which are thought to be most typical of type IV hypersensitivity, has been shown by Spector and Heesom (1969) and Germuth (1961) to result also from insoluble antigen–antibody complexes not readily digested by lysosomal enzymes. Complement studies too have added to the controversy. Serum complement levels typically drop during acute immune complex disease such as serum sickness; however, in acute pigeon breeder's disease serum complement levels either remain within the normal range or increase following natural exposure or bronchoprovocation (Stiehm *et al.*, 1967; Moore *et al.*, 1974, 1975). An unexpected finding has been a decrease of serum complement levels in asymtomatic subjects following antigen exposure. Recent studies (Marx and Flaherty, 1975) indicate that organic dusts can directly activate the alternative complement pathway. Pigeon dropping extract has been shown by Huis *et al.* (1976) to consume total hemolytic complement. Activation of both classical and alternative complement pathways is thought to be contributory. From these major arguments for and against the existence of an immune complex mechanism in hypersensitivity pneumonitis, it is apparent that its precise role still remains poorly defined.

The characteristic granulomas and other histopathological features resembling a tuberculin-like reaction have directed the focus of attention toward defining a possible role for cell-mediated hypersensitivity in the pathogenesis of this disease. Studies in humans have shown that peripheral blood lymphocytes from symptomatic subjects with bird antigen induced hypersensitivity pneumonitis will produce *in vitro* MIF following avian antigen stimulation, while lymphocytes from asymptomatic exposed subjects do not respond (Caldwell *et al.*, 1973; Moore *et al.*,

1974). Antigen-induced [^{3}H]thymidine uptake by peripheral blood lymphocytes from symptomatic subjects, but not from asymptomatic exposed subjects, further supports a role for a type IV hypersensitivity reaction (Hansen and Penny, 1974). The degree of lymphocyte stimulation appears to correlate with disease activity (Schatz *et al.*, 1976). Delayed 24- to 72-hr skin reactivity is generally an unusual finding; however, Warren and Woolf (1972) have reported this type of skin reaction to a feather extract when administered together with an antihistamine. Since the antihistamine blocks the immediate and possibly also the late immune response, antigen may persist at the skin test site, allowing for the development of the classical delayed response.

2.5.2. Animal Models

In order to study further the biological response to antigens known to produce hypersensitivity pneumonitis, a number of animal models have been developed by various investigators. The animal models most often discussed in the literature are listed in Table 2. Many of these models have contributed greatly to our understanding of the pathogenesis of this disease. For example, Bice *et al.* (1976a) were able to transfer sensitivity using lymphoid cells, but not serum, from sensitized rabbits to previously unexposed rabbits. This adoptive transfer resulted in the production of disease following antigen challenge by inhalation. In support of these observations are the findings of other workers that serum from sensitized animals is not capable of transferring the challenge-induced pulmonary lesions (Tuft *et al.*, 1972; Joubert *et al.*, 1976). Other animal models have been described using a parenteral sensitizing dose of either avian or dust antigen alone or with complete Freund's adjuvant (CFA). Following antigen challenge by inhalation, lesions characteristic of hypersensitivity pneumonitis have developed (Bice *et al.*, 1976b; Miyamato and Kabe, 1971; Fink *et al.*, 1973).

More recent studies have shown that local, organ-restricted immune mechanisms may involve the lung with or without systemic evidence of sensitization. In the past, such local organ-specific reactivity may have been overlooked because human studies of type IV hypersensitivity have been generally restricted to peripheral blood leukocytes. A recent study indicates that bronchoalveolar cells from a patient with pigeon breeder's disease transformed and produced MIF *in vitro* in response to pigeon antigen stimulation, while peripheral blood lymphoid cells taken from the same individual at the same time demonstrated no reactivity to the same antigen (Schuyler *et al.*, 1978). Reynolds *et al.* (1977) found a higher proportion of lymphocytes, higher IgG and IgM levels, and higher T/B cell ratios in bronchoalveolar washings from hypersensitivity pneumonitis patients than in those from subjects without this disease. In support of this finding, the work of Salvaggio *et al.* (1975) indicates that production of peripheral, humoral, and cell-mediated immune responses to offending antigens is not sufficient to induce pulmonary lesions following inhalation challenge, unless local cell-mediated immunity is also present. The suggestion is that specific immunological reactivity of the skin or peripheral circulation may not accurately reflect the immunological reactivity of the lung. Thus, although the Gell and Coombs classification of immune injury has generally been clinically useful, its artificial separation of related immune functions may not be directly applicable to certain disorders such as hypersensi-

TABLE 2. Animal Models of Hypersensitivity Pneumonitis

Investigators	Animal	Antigen	Sensitization	Immunological aspects
Richerson *et al.* (1971)	Rabbit	Ovalbumin	Active parenteral	Production of alveolitis, vasculitis, and peribronchitis following aerosol challenge
Kawai *et al.* (1972)	Rabbit	*M. faeni*	Active intratracheal	Production of precipitating antibody, delayed skin reactivity, antigen-induced lymphocyte transformation, and alveolar macrophage migration inhibition associated with mononuclear cell infiltrates of lung
Brentjens *et al.* (1974)	Rabbit	BSA[a]	Active parenteral	Maintenance of antigen–antibody equivalence, producing pulmonary lesions with deposition of antigen, immune globulin, complement, and fibrinogen
Moore *et al.* (1975)	Rabbit	PDE[b]	Active insufflation	Enhancement of antigen-specific cell-mediated hypersensitivity by prior inflammation of the lung with BCG
Salvaggio *et al.* (1975)	Rabbit	BSA *M. faeni*	Active intratracheal	Comparison of sequential changes in disease induced by intratracheal soluble and particulate antigens
Bice *et al.* (1976a)	Rabbit	Ovalbumin	Passive parenteral	Passive transfer of hypersensitivity pneumonitis with sensitized lymph node cells following intrabronchial antigen challenge
Harris *et al.* (1976b)	Rabbit	*M. faeni*	Active intratracheal	Induction of specific cellular and humoral hypersensitivity in association with pulmonary lesions
Peterson *et al.* (1977)	Rabbit	PDE	Active insufflation	Enhancement of antigen-specific cell-mediated hypersensitivity by prior inflammation of the lung with carrageenan
Miyamoto and Kabe (1971)	Guinea pig	Tuberculin	Active parenteral Passive parenteral	Production of mononuclear cell infiltrates following aerosol challenge and passive transfer with sensitized lymphoid cells

[a] Bovine serum albumin.
[b] Pigeon dropping extract.
[c] Azobenzene arsonate.

(continued)

TABLE 2. *(Continued)*

Investigators	Animal	Antigen	Sensitization	Immunological aspects
Richerson (1972)	Guinea pig	Ovalbumin Tuberculin ABA[c]	Active parenteral	Influence of different antigens in various combinations with adjuvants on the basic cellular or humoral characteristics of the resultant immune response
Wilkie *et al.* (1973)	Guinea pig	*M. faeni*	Active parenteral	Passive transfer of disease with both sensitized cells and serum
Santives *et al.* (1976) Roska *et al.* (1977)	Guinea pig	PDE Ovalbumin Pigeon serum	Active parenteral Passive parenteral	Production of immune complex disease following aerosol antigen challenge in both actively sensitized animals and animals passively sensitized with serum
Wilkie (1976,1977)	Guinea pig	*M. faeni*	Active parenteral Passive parenteral	Passive transfer with sensitized cells or plasma of tachypneic response to antigen challenge and abolishment of response by specific antigen desensitization
Fink *et al.* (1970)	Rat	PDE	Active insufflation	Production of interstitial granulomatous lesions and precipitating antibody
Johnson and Ward (1974)	Rat	BSA	Passive intrabronchial	Interstitial deposits of antigen and antibody and requirement of C3 and neutrophils for tissue damage
Fink *et al.* (1973)	Monkey	PDE	Passive parenteral	Unique aspects of disease influenced by passive transfer of either sensitized lymphoid cells or serum

tivity pneumonitis. The continuing difficulty in fully characterizing the pathogenesis of hypersensitivity pneumonitis in terms of a discrete mechanism of injury would support this thesis. Kaltreider (1976) has reviewed "local" immune mechanisms of the lung.

This emerging concept of local immunological reactivity of the lung and the accessibility of cells and fluid from both humans and animals by bronchial lavage are providing new approaches to the study of this disease. For example, repeated respiratory tract exposure of rabbits to *Micropolyspora faeni* leads to the development of pulmonary lesions histologically comparable to those of human hypersensitivity pneumonitis (Harris *et al.*, 1976b; Stankus *et al.*, 1978). In these studies, infiltration of mononuclear cells into the interstitial, peribronchial, and intraalveolar spaces is characteristic of recent lesions while the development of granulomas and giant cells is seen more commonly with mature lesions. Lavage of the lungs produces bronchoalveolar cells demonstrating small numbers of phagolysosomes and suggests that these cells are immature phagocytes that have been recruited in response to immunization. These lesions typically contain over 10 times as many "activated" alveolar macrophages as are found in unimmunized animals. The presence of this unique macrophage morphology correlates well with metabolic parameters of activation such as increased glucose oxidation and *in vitro* cellular killing of *Listeria monocytogenes*. Intratracheal challenge of these animals with *Micropolyspora faeni* antigen can specifically recall both the intense granulomatous pulmonary lesions and the marked increase in numbers of activated alveolar macrophages. Macrophage activation, in this respect, may occur as an immunologically specific event.

One of the many biological properties of most of these organic antigens is their ability to activate the alternative complement pathway, and it is known that complement products such as C3b may induce lysosomal enzyme release from alveolar macrophages (Figure 1). These enzymes may further cleave C3, generating more chemotactic complement products and C3b, which then further recruit and activate macrophages, forming an "amplification loop" of inflammation. Such a mechanism could explain the development of pulmonary granulomas where large numbers of macrophages with ingested *M. faeni* or other antigens accumulate. Schorlemmer *et al.* (1977) have proposed a hypothesis for the development of hypersensitivity pneumonitis implicating complement activation by inhaled antigen and consequent generation of chemotactic factors and C3b. Phagocytosis of antigen by alveolar macrophages might result in release of lysosomal enzymes which could further cleave C3, thus forming more chemotactic factors and C3b. Factor B interacts with C3b to further cleave C3. Concurrently, sensitized B lymphocytes mature into plasma cells and secrete antibody. Inhaled antigen might then lead to the formation of immune complexes which may also be ingested by macrophages that become activated. There is evidence to indicate that sensitized T cells contribute by secreting lymphokines such as macrophage-activating factor, resulting in further macrophage activation. Repeated introduction of antigen producing continued inflammation eventually results in fibrosis through a macrophage-mediated regulation of fibroblasts. The activated alveolar macrophage is the pathogenetic focal point in this hypothesis and serves as a functional link between an inhaled offending antigen and the resulting elicitation of pulmonary lesions. Several immunological and nonimmunological processes developing simultaneously at the bronchoalveolar level are involved and result in inflammation whenever antigen is introduced. Hypersensitivity pneumonitis therefore likely involves a complex interaction between local and systemic immune and nonimmune mechanisms, unique antigen characteristics, and host response.

3. The Eosinophilic Pneumonias

One of the first analyses of pulmonary infiltration on chest X-ray accompanied by blood eosinophilia was provided by Crofton *et al.* (1952) in Great Britain, who identified five categories of disease. These included Loeffler's syndrome, prolonged pulmonary eosinophilia without asthma, pulmonary eosinophilia with asthma, tropical pulmonary eosinophilia, and polyarteritis nodosa. They emphasized the necessity of excluding such disorders as classical infectious pneumonia, hydatid disease of the lung, Hodgkin's disease, and sarcoidosis. Reeder and Goodrich (1952), in the United States, coined the term "PIE syndrome" (pulmonary infiltrates with eosinophilia) but excluded Loeffler's syndrome and tropical eosinophilia from being included in this term. Evolution of the British and American classifications has extended the term "PIE syndrome" to include the original five categories of disease. With increased availability of diagnostic lung biopsy material, recent studies have recognized the diagnostic importance of the histopathological findings, which frequently include marked infiltration of lung tissue with eosinophils (Liebow and Carrington, 1969; Weinberg, 1972; Kazemi, 1977).

We have tried to reconcile these varying points of view and accumulated data by adopting the term "eosinophilic pneumonias" used by Liebow and Carrington

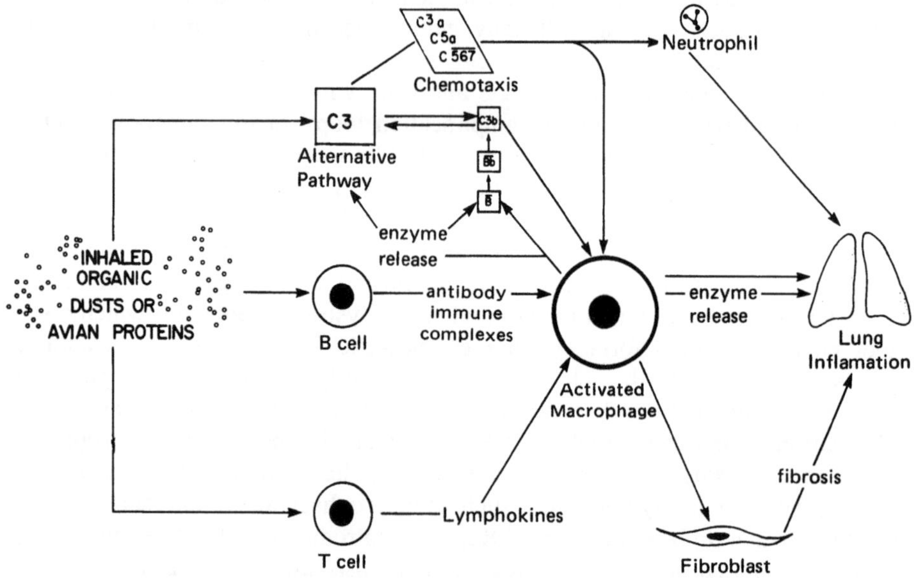

Figure 1. Pathogenesis of hypersensitivity pneumonitis. When susceptible individuals inhale certain organic dusts, alveolar macrophages become functionally activated through both immune and nonimmune mechanisms. Release of lysosomal enzymes from these cells produces direct tissue damage and further potentiates the inflammatory response. (See text for details.)

(1969) to describe all lung disease characterized by X-ray evidence of pulmonary infiltration accompanied by either peripheral blood eosinophilia or histopathological evidence of lung tissue infiltration by large numbers of eosinophils. It seems to us that production of disease is dependent not only on characteristics of a specific etiological agent but also on host susceptibility factors such as airway lability. Consequently, we have constructed a classification of the eosinophilic pneumonias based on these considerations (Table 3). The importance of airway lability as a host susceptibility factor forms the basis of our division of the eosinophilic pneumonias into asthmatic and nonasthmatic categories. Certainly there are occasional exceptions to this classification. For example, pulmonary involvement in polyarteritis nodosa may occur in the absence of asthma. Also, asthma has been reported in two patients with eosinophilic granuloma (Fifer, 1963). Despite some exceptions, the separation of eosinophilic pneumonias into asthmatic and nonasthmatic categories has proved useful clinically and in the understanding of disease mechanisms. The most rapid advances in our understanding of the eosinophilic pneumonias have been in those diseases associated with asthma, such as allergic bronchopulmonary aspergillosis (ABA). This section will present an overview of each of the recognized clinical entities composing the eosinophilic pneumonias, with emphasis on those diseases that are best understood.

3.1. Eosinophilic Pneumonias with Asthma

3.1.1. Allergic Bronchopulmonary Aspergillosis (ABA)

There are five basic types of pulmonary disease known to be caused by the ubiquitous *Aspergillus* species. First, the aspergillus organism may produce an infectious pneumonitis in subjects who are immunologically compromised from lymphatic neoplasia or treatment with cytotoxic agents. In this situation, aspergillus organisms invade lung tissue and are directly responsible for consolidation and parenchymal damage. Second, subjects with a prior history of pulmonary tuberculosis, with a residual lung cavity, may develop a "fungus ball" in the cavity composed predominantly of aspergillus organisms. Third, several cases of classical hypersensitivity pneumonitis without asthma or eosinophilia have been found to result from occupational exposure to antigens derived from *Aspergillus clavatus*

TABLE 3. Eosinophilic Pneumonias

	Asthmatic
1.	Allergic bronchopulmonary aspergillosis
2.	Tropical eosinophilia
3.	Pulmonary vasculitis (polyarteritis nodosa and allergic granulomatous angiitis)
	Nonasthmatic
1.	Infection and infestation (Loeffler's syndrome and chronic eosinophilic pneumonia)
2.	Drugs and chemicals
3.	Eosinophilic granuloma of lung
4.	Leukocytic neoplasms

growing in malt and barley (Riddle and Grant, 1967; Pepys, 1969) and *Aspergillus flavus* growing in moldy corn (Patterson *et al.*, 1974). Fourth, conventional allergic asthma without interstitial lung disease may occur in certain sensitive subjects when exposed to aspergillus and other deuteromycete spores. Fifth, a local allergic reaction to noninvading aspergillus organisms resident in the airway may produce a form of asthmatic eosinophilic pneumonia known as "allergic bronchopulmonary aspergillosis" (ABA).

The first report of ABA by Hinson *et al.* (1952) described diagnostic tests for detecting the disease. Many years later, McCarthy and Pepys (1971a) found that in the United Kingdom about 80% of cases of eosinophilic pneumonia were in fact ABA. Although ABA seems to be relatively more common in Great Britain, greater numbers of cases are being recognized in the United States with improved diagnostic tests and criteria (Rosenberg *et al.*, 1977; Patterson, 1978). Unfortunately, many cases likely remain undiagnosed because of the general lack of familiarity with this syndrome and with the simple *in vitro* diagnostic procedures.

a. Clinical Presentation. The most common presentation is that of episodic pulmonary infiltrates developing in an established asthmatic subject with associated marked peripheral blood and sputum eosinophilia. It is important not to confuse ABA with a complicating viral or bacterial pneumonitis occurring in an asthmatic subject, where significant peripheral blood and sputum eosinophilia may merely reflect the activity of asthma already aggravated by the viral infection. However, an asthmatic subject exhibiting chronic intermittent or persistent pulmonary infiltrates should lead suspicion to ABA. Most patients with ABA are highly atopic, exhibiting broad patterns of positive wheal-and-flare skin reactivity to common inhalant allergens. This is especially true of young patients. However, when ABA develops later in life, this broad pattern of wheal-and-flare skin reactivity may be absent, and the patient may react only to a skin test with the aspergillus antigen (McCarthy and Pepys, 1971b). In Great Britain, disease activity may become worse during the winter months, when the atmospheric counts of aspergillus spores are particularly high (McCarthy and Pepys, 1971a). A high prevalence of antecedent asthma in these patients has been reported by Pepys (1969, 1977); however, Patterson (1978) in America has found that some patients experience only minimal asthmatic symptoms. Central bronchiectasis is the hallmark of this disease (Scadding, 1967) and develops in most active and untreated cases. Therefore, the importance of diagnosing this condition, even when only mild symptoms are present, lies in preventing this serious sequela by appropriate treatment.

b. Chest X-ray. Evidence of pulmonary consolidation, often in a patchy distribution, may be found initially on chest X-ray in about one-third of patients (McCarthy *et al.*, 1970). Less common findings include "parallel lines" or "tubular shadows" which represent dilated bronchi (Simon, 1975). Tubular shadows may be replaced by "bandlike" or "toothpaste" shadows. These represent secretions in a dilated bronchus. A V-shaped shadow may represent mucous plugs in two bronchi joining toward the hilum. A similar shadow, the "gloved-finger" opacity, is either expanded at its distal end or expanded and then tapered. The intensity of intrabronchial densities or gross parenchymal consolidation may often correlate with disease activity. Repeated collapse of varying sites of lung may be caused by mucous plugs obstructing proximal bronchi. Consequently, atelectasis is a common finding on chest X-ray. Bronchography may readily demonstrate the characteristic central bronchietasis which is usually present in longstanding or severe disease.

c. Histopathology. Interstitial granulomatous infiltration with large numbers of eosinophils is commonly found in biopsies of consolidated lung tissue. Eosinophils may fill alveolar spaces. At autopsy, the presence of mucous plugs in the bronchi may correlate with tubular shadows seen on previous chest X-rays. Mucous gland hypertrophy, infiltration with neutrophils and eosinophils, atrophy of cilia, and squamous metaplasia of bronchial walls are other common histopathological findings (McCarthy and Pepys, 1971a).

d. Physiology. Pulmonary function tests in acute disease demonstrate findings typical of asthma such as decreased FEV_1 and PFR with increased RV. Total lung capacity, as determined by body plethysmography, has been variable. Although reduced steady-state DL_{CO} is unusual in asthma, it has been found frequently in ABA (McCarthy and Pepys, 1971a). Airways obstruction is commonly reversible early in the disease process. As the disease persists, reversibility is lost; however, cor pulmonale and pulmonary hypertension are infrequently observed.

e. Skin Tests and Precipitins. Although there is no adequate standard of antigen potency, crude extracts of the mat and spores from aspergillus cultures can be obtained from commercial sources for skin tests and precipitin studies. There are no adequate studies comparing culture filtrates with mycelial extracts. Despite these admitted limitations, certain purified extracts of aspergillus organisms have proved to be quite useful diagnostically. In ABA, the characteristic positive skin reaction to aspergillus antigen consists of an immediate wheal-and-flare followed by a late Arthus-type reaction. In a study of 20 subjects with ABA, Rosenberg *et al.* (1977) in the United States have found that all demonstrated the immediate-type skin reaction, whereas only about one-third demonstrated the late Arthus-type reaction. Reed (1978), in comparing skin reactivity to aspergillus antigen in conventional asthmatic subjects with that in normal subjects, found 12% and 4% positive immediate-type skin reactions, respectively. A significant problem with the diagnostic skin test therefore is its lack of specificity for ABA. The problem of specificity ultimately may be solved by standardization of antigens. This might allow for more precise determination of quantitative differences in sensitivity.

Another important diagnostic test for ABA is the demonstration of precipitating serum antibody against *Aspergillus fumigatus* antigen by Ouchterlony double gel diffusion. However, antifungal antibody may merely reflect environmental exposure to this ubiquitous antigen, since Bardana *et al.* (1972) have detected precipitins in the serum of a few non-ABA subjects and have found antiaspergillus antibodies in the sera of many other subjects by using more sensitive primary binding assay procedures. Analogous data come from the finding of serum precipitins specific for certain other microorganisms such as *Hemophilus influenza, Pneunoccus pneumoniae,* and *Staphylococcus aureus* in patients infected with these agents (McCarthy and Pepys, 1971b). Species differences may be important in the development of disease. *Aspergillus fumigatus* has been most commonly associated with ABA; however, other *Aspergillus* species have also been implicated. Although there may be certain antigenic differences between species, Reed *et al.* (1978), using several different strains of *A. fumigatus, A. clavatus, A. flavus, A. terreus,* and *A. niger,* have noted that a serum reacting to one species may react to many of the other species as well. Therefore, the presence of precipitins in the serum of a normal subject does not by itself indicate a diagnosis of ABA, but neither does the absence of a precipitin reaction in the serum of a symptomatic subject exclude the diagnosis. Nevertheless, in the majority of cases, this simple diagnostic test is quite useful.

f. Diagnosis. Diagnostic criteria for ABA have appeared in the British and American literature. In a review of 143 cases of ABA, McCarthy and Pepys (1971b) described the following diagnostic features: (1) marked peripheral blood and sputum eosinophilia, (2) wheezing and transitory pulmonary infiltrates, (3) immediate and late skin reactions to *Aspergillus fumigatus* antigen; (4) positive sputum cultures for *Aspergillus fumigatus* in over 50% of cases, (5) expectoration of brown sputum plugs containing fungal mycelia; (6) serum precipitating antibody to *Aspergillus fumigatus* by double gel diffusion; (7) dual (immediate and late) asthmatic reactions to bronchoprovocation testing with *Aspergillus fumigatus* antigen; and (8) markedly elevated levels of total serum IgE antibody reflecting activity of disease. Rosenberg *et al.* (1977), based on a study of 20 patients, have proposed a precise set of criteria including episodic bronchial obstruction, peripheral blood eosinophilia, immediate skin reactivity to aspergillus antigen, precipitating antibodies against aspergillus antigen, elevated total serum IgE antibody concentrations, and a history of transient or fixed pulmonary infiltrates. The presence of all six criteria makes the diagnosis of ABA very probable. If central bronchiectasis is also present, the diagnosis becomes certain. These investigators also acknowledged the importance of demonstrating aspergillus in the sputum, a history of brown plugs in the sputum, and a late skin reaction to aspergillus antigen; however, they felt that these criteria were less helpful since they were infrequently present in the patients studied. They also found that the high levels of total serum IgE antibody do not exhibit specificity for the aspergillus antigen when analyzed by RAST. The finding may represent a possible nonspecific IgE adjuvant effect of aspergillus antigen, or it may reflect an artifact of the assay procedure.

Subjects with ABA have been challenged by bronchoprovocation with aspergillus antigen (McCarthy and Pepys, 1971b). Immediate asthmatic reactions occurring within 10–20 min following challenge, late asthmatic reactions occurring 7–8 hr following challenge, or dual asthmatic reactions including both the immediate and late responses have frequently been demonstrated in these subjects. The temporal pattern of airway response may reflect the pattern of skin response. Bronchoprovocation with aspergillus antigen has been used investigatively for the most part; however, in certain cases where other criteria are incompletely fulfilled, the elicitation of a dual asthmatic response following antigen challenge may add diagnostic support for ABA.

g. Therapy. Favorable responses to the treatment of ABA with prednisone, 20–40 mg/day, have been reported by McCarthy and Pepys (1971a). This treatment apparently resulted in clearing of chest X-ray evidence of atelectasis and bronchial shadows, reduction of sputum production, elimination of demonstrable aspergilli from sputum, and a reduction of sputum plug expectoration in the majority of patients. Specific antifungal agents such as nystatin (Stark, 1967) and amphotericin B (Slavin *et al.*, 1970) have been reported effective; however, most authorities still favor primary treatment with corticosteroids (Rosenberg *et al.*, 1977). Although fungal invasion of lung parenchyma might constitute a theoretical objection to the use of corticosteroids in these patients, this appears to be a rare occurrence. Rosenberg *et al.* (1977) have shown that prednisone in a dosage of 0.5 mg/kg body weight taken on an alternate-day schedule is usually effective. The alternate-day schedule has been clearly shown to minimize adrenal suppression and potential corticosteroid side effects with long-term therapy. Nonabsorbable inhalant steroid preparations such as beclomethasone may also hold some promise, but anecdotal evidence suggests that they are not as effective as oral corticosteroid in reducing pulmonary infiltrates. There are still few data on criteria for periodic follow-up of patients, and indeed the optimal duration of corticosteroid therapy is unknown. The long-term complications of this disease, including central bronchiectasis and pulmonary fibrosis, and the fact that a high proportion of subjects with ABA are below the age of 20 years make effective but safe treatment most important.

h. Pathogenesis. The dual asthmatic reaction following bronchoprovocation with aspergillus antigen has been thought to be due to two separate disease mechanisms (Pepys, 1969). The immediate reaction is thought to be mediated by homocytotropic IgE antibody specific for aspergillus and the late response by immune complexes composed of aspergillus antigen and host immunoglobulin. The latter reaction is frequently accompanied by leukocytosis and fever. A relationship between the two mechanisms of immune injury has been suggested by the work of Cochrane *et al.* (1968). Working with rabbits, they demonstrated that antigen-induced IgE-mediated release of histamine allowed for egress of serum immune complexes into vascular walls and tissues with resultant production of inflammation through activation of the classical complement pathway. There is some clinical support for this mechanism in ABA since disodium cromoglycate (DSCG), a known inhibitor of the IgE-mediated release of histamine and other effector substances, blocks both immediate and late asthmatic reactions resulting from bronchoprovocation, while prior administration of cortisone acetate typically inhibits only the late response. Furthermore, Golbert and Patterson (1970) infused serum from a patient with ABA, who demonstrated both serum reagin and precipitins, into a primate. Both skin tests and bronchoprovocation with aspergillus antigen elicited dual reactions. When the same experiment was repeated using another patient's serum containing reagins but no precipitins, there was no transfer of lesions following challenge. Although these data suggested a humoral mechanism of disease, recent evidence indicates a possible role for cell-mediated hypersensitivity. Lymphocyte transformation studies using the whole blood method with aspergillus antigen have been performed in six patients by Rosenberg *et al.* (1977). Lymphocyte transformation was found in five of these ABA subjects; however, no transformation occurred in three non-ABA asthmatics with only immediate skin reactivity to aspergillus antigen. In a study of patients with aspergilloma, Goldstein (1978) noted a low prevalence of wheal-and-flare skin reactivity, a low degree of lymphocyte transformation, but high levels of precipitating antibody to the aspergillus antigen. Contrasting findings in patients with ABA included immediate wheal-and-flare skin reactions, a high degree of antigen-induced lymphocyte transformation, and low levels of precipitating antibody. These data suggest that the pathogenesis of ABA involves interrelationships of several of the mechanisms of hypersensitivity described by Gell and Coombs (1969). Host susceptibility factors such as labile airways and perhaps an abnormal immune response to the aspergillus organism may lead to persistence of saprophytic aspergilli in the airways. The resultant continuing antigen stimulation may lead to the development of specific reagins, precipitating antibodies, and lymphokine production, all interacting as either contributing or resulting manifestations of the immune damage.

3.1.2. Tropical Eosinophilia

The syndrome of peripheral blood eosinophilia, chronic cough, and miliary pulmonary infiltrates has been often noted to occur in the tropics but was first clearly recognized as a distinct entity by Frimodt-Moller and Barton (1940). The condition was also recognized by Weingarten (1943), who coined the term "tropical eosinophilia" and reported the therapeutic use of arsenic. The fortuitous discovery that diethycarbamazine was effective in the treatment of pulmonary manifestations led to the identification of an etiological helminth infestation, later identified by Danaraj (1958) as predominantly filaria. He stressed the diagnostic importance of antifilarial antibody studies since it was often difficult to demonstrate microfilariae in the blood of many cases. Wong (1964) and Neva *et al.* (1975) feel that tropical eosinophilia may result from an immunological host response to infestation that traps microfilariae in tissues, making them less accessible to the circulation. Unique host susceptibility factors are likely important since certain ethnic groups are predisposed to the pulmonary manifestations of this disease. As with certain other types of infestation, tropical eosinophilia is characterized by markedly elevated serum IgE levels (Ezeoke *et al.*, 1973). Ultimately, an appreciation of the etiological role for IgE antifilarial antibody and its occurrence in great quantities in only a minority of subjects infected may eventually identify a useful purpose for IgE antibodies in general. The most frequent cause of tropical eosinophilia appears to be infestation with filaria; however, other organisms such as *Necator, Toxacara, Ascaris, Strongyloides, Ancylostoma braziliensis, Trichuris trichiuria,* and *Fasciola hepatica* may also produce this syndrome. The treatment of choice appears to be diethylcarbamazine since Neva *et al.* (1975) have shown that this agent is effective in alleviating symptoms, decreasing eosinophil counts, and diminishing CF titers of antifilarial antibody. Tropical (filarial) eosinophilia has been recently reviewed by Neva and Ottesen (1978).

3.1.3. Pulmonary Vasculitis

There are two major forms of pulmonary vasculitis that may be associated with asthma and eosinophilic pulmonary infiltrates. These are polyarteritis (Wilson and Alexander, 1945) and allergic granulomatous angiitis (Churg and Strauss, 1951). Although granulomas with giant cells, often containing Charcot-Leyden crystals, are characteristic of allergic granulomatous angiitis, both polyarteritis and allergic granulomatous pneumonitis are characterized histopathologically by leukocytoclasis with fibrinoid necrosis of small vessel walls.

Polyarteritis is a rapidly progressive generalized necrotizing vasculitis producing inflammation of the media and adventitia of medium- and small-sized blood vessels. Localized aneurysmal dilatations result from weakening of vessel walls and are readily demonstrable with renal arteriography. An infectious etiology and an immune complex pathogenesis in some cases have been suggested by the demonstration of the hepatitis B surface antigen (HB_s) along with immune globulins in involved vessel walls (Sergent *et al.*, 1976). The original description of the disease by Kussmaul and Maier (1866) failed to mention lung involvement; however, Wilson and Alexander (1945) reported an 18% frequency of bronchial asthma in a survey of 300 cases with the disease. The asthma generally preceded development of vasculitis, and most of these subjects appeared to be nonatopic. Peripheral blood eosinophilia was found in 95% of patients with asthma but was generally absent in those patients with only vasculitis. Other investigators have reported lung involvement in 29% of cases (Rose and Spencer, 1957) and 10% of cases (Divertie and Olsen, 1960).

Allergic granulomatous angiitis was originally described by Churg and Strauss (1951) as a varient of classical polyarteritis. The major differences are that most subjects with allergic granulomatous angiitis are atopic and asthma is present in nearly all cases (Rosenberg *et al.*, 1975). Widespread involvement of many organs such as kidney, liver, integument, and nervous system is frequently found in both diseases.

3.2. Eosinophilic Pneumonias without Asthma

3.2.1. Infection and Infestation

A syndrome of pulmonary infiltration with peripheral blood eosinophilia without asthma and not necessarily related to residence in the tropics may be associated with various infectious agents including viruses, bacteria, fungi, and helminths. Normally, the infected host responds immunologically to control or eliminate the invading organism. Appropriate pharmacotherapy may aid in this process. The infestation generally clears, and the prognosis is good. Therefore, it is not surprising that Loeffler (1932) originally described a syndrome of transient migratory or successive pulmonary infiltrates associated with blood eosinophilia and lasting for only 20 days or less. Subsequently, the disease was shown to be commonly associated with infestations with such agents as *Ascaris lumbricoides, Strongyloides spp.*, *Necator americanus*, *Fasciola hepatica*, and *Entamoeba histolytica*. The syndrome may result also from drug reactions, fungal infections, and allergic vasculitis. Consequently, "Loeffler's syndrome" has become an anachronism and has been replaced by more precise terminology based on etiological agents and specific host response. Pulmonary infiltration with eosinophilia may be found in association with other infectious diseases including tuberculosis, brucellosis, histoplasmosis, and coccidiomycosis. Pulmonary infiltration in these diseases may be transient or chronic depending on the host response to infection.

A form of chronic eosinophilic pneumonia, not usually associated with asthma, has been described by Weinberg (1972). Pulmonary infiltrates and peripheral blood eosinophilia persist for months to years and are commonly associated with episodic fever, cough, and dyspnea. Cavitation and parenchymal destruction are uncommon findings. Women are affected more often than men, and the disease responds well to corticosteroid therapy (Pepys and McCarthy, 1973).

3.2.2. Drugs

Under appropriate conditions, most subjects taking a particular drug may experience side effects, toxicity from overdosage, or adverse drug interactions. In contrast, hypersensitivity reactions to drugs or their metabolites occur in only a small proportion of subjects taking the medication. With first exposure, there is usally a significant latent period before the reaction develops. However, with reexposure, the reaction develops more rapidly. Since there are often no demonstrable changes in circulating antibodies or cellular reactivity, the hypersentitivity nature of the reaction has been often inferred by these unique clinical characteristics. The frequent finding of peripheral blood eosinophilia may additionally suggest a hypersensitivity mechanism, although the true significance of this observation is not yet appreciated. Several examples of interstitial pulmonary reaction caused by drugs will be presented. For more detailed reviews, the reader is referred to Rosenow (1972) and Whitcomb (1973).

a. Nitrofurantoin. Two pulmonary syndromes caused by nitrofurantoin have been identified. An acute syndrome develops 3–10 days following initiation of the drug and is characterized by fever, chills, and dyspnea, commonly associated with elevated peripheral blood eosinophil counts (Hailey *et al.*, 1969). Interstitial, predominantly basilar pulmonary infiltrates on chest X-ray, along with auscultory evidence of crepitant rales, are usually present but rapidly subside when the drug is discontinued. They appear again if the drug is reintroduced. There is no evidence that corticosteroid therapy accelerates recovery. In contrast, the chronic syndrome presents with cough and dyspnea beginning 6 months to 6 years following chronic continuous or intermittent use of nitrofurantoin. Lung histopathology reveals interstitial fibrosis with variable mild mononuclear cell infiltration. Withdrawal of the drug and administration of corticosteroids often result in marked improvement. Skin rashes, pleural effusion, and eosinophilia seen in the acute syndrome are generally absent. An immune mechanism has not been demonstrated in either the acute or the chronic form of this disease.

b. Busulfan. An alkylating agent used mainly in the treatment of chronic myelogenous leukemia, bulsulfan may cause diffuse interstitial and alveolar infiltrates with characteristic expectoration of damaged type II alveolar cells (Heard and Cooke, 1968). Lung biopsy is often necessary to exclude infectious or leukemic processes. Diffuse interstitial fibrosis often occurs despite cessation of the drug and corticosteroid therapy. There are other cytotoxic drugs which have been shown to cause interstitial lung disease and associated peripheral blood eosinophilia. These include methotrexate, bleomycin, and cyclophosphamide. Interstitial fibrosis may result if the inflammatory process continues unabated.

c. Sulfonamides. Nearly all sulfonamide compounds are capable of producing interstitial pulmonary infiltrates with peripheral blood eosinophilia (Fiegenberg *et al.*, 1967). Common manifestations include fever, cough, and dyspnea which resolve after the drug is discontinued. The same pattern of disease may also be produced by penicillin, phenylbutazone, tolbutamide, chlorpropamide, diphenylhydantoin, paraaminosalicylic acid, imipramine, and mephenesin.

d. Heroin. Drug addicts often present in the hospital emergency room with acute pneumonitis following the intravenous use of newly acquired heroin (Steinberg and Karliner, 1968). Whether heroin or some contaminant is the responsible agent has not been resolved; however, a similar syndrome has been seen with propoxyphene and methadone.

e. Gold. Rheumatoid arthritis patients receiving gold may develop interstitial infiltration with peripheral blood eosinophilia (Winterbauer *et al.*, 1976). When the drug is discontinued, it may be 3–5 months before disease remits. Gold-induced lymphocyte transformation has been reported in patients with gold-induced pulmonary disease (Geddes and Brostoff, 1976). Other drugs known to be capable of causing interstitial lung disease include D-penicillamine, hexamethonium, hydrochlorthiazide, and methylsergide.

3.2.3. Pulmonary Eosinophilic Granuloma

There is a group of diseases with the common histopathology of infiltrating histiocytes and eosinophils, often interspersed with multinucleated giant cells. The term "histiocytosis-X" has been used to describe three main categories of these diseases, which include Letterer–Siwe disease, a virulent multisystem involvement of infants; Hand–Schuller–Christian disease, a benign multisystem disease of adults; and eosinophilic granuloma, a unifocal disease involving only one organ, usually either bone or lung. Eosinophilic granuloma involving lung may affect both infants and adults and typically begins with insidious onset of cough and exertional dyspnea (Smith *et al.*, 1974; Strieder, 1978). Peripheral blood eosinophilia and asthma are unusual. Pulmonary infiltration seen by chest X-ray, often creating a nodular honeycomb pattern, is associated with diabetes insipidus in about 20% of cases. Skeletal surveys of bone using X-ray or scanning procedures detect typical bone lesions in 20% of cases. Pulmonary infiltrates usually resolve spontaneously but may also progress to produce a diffuse interstitial fibrosis, cor pulmonale, and respiratory failure. Although good objective data are lacking, treatment with corticosteroids in severe cases has been reported to be effective. The great variability in prognosis is similar to that seen in sarcoidosis.

3.2.4. Neoplasia

Eosinophils may diffusely infiltrate several organs at once without any obvious underlying cause. This has led to a general category of disease termed "hypereosinophilic syndrome" (Chused *et al.*, 1975). The characteristic widespread distribution of lesions, often involving heart, bone marrow, liver, skin, kidney, and nervous system, has led to consideration of an underlying leukemic process of eosinophils. Since there has been a lack of correlation between abnormal myelopoiesis and clinical course, criteria for diganosis have been imprecise (Resnik and Myerson, 1970). Part of the difficulty may lie in distinguishing eosinophilic leukemia from neutrophilic chronic granulocytic leukemia with accompanying peripheral blood eosinophilia (Flannery *et al.*, 1972). Localization of eosinophilic infiltration and fibrosis to heart (Loeffler's endocarditis), lungs (chronic PIE syndrome), or gastrointestinal tract (eosinophilic gastroenteritis) may be useful differentiating features. Response to corticosteroid therapy is variable and prognosis is generally poor. A few patients may survive with minimal disability for many years, while rapid debilitating disease develops in others. Parrillo *et al.* (1977) have found that patients not responding to corticosteroids often respond to the DNA inhibitor hydroxyurea.

4. Pulmonary Fibrosis

A syndrome of rapidly progressive diffuse pulmonary fibrosis commonly resulting in respiratory failure and death was first described by Hamman and Rich (1934, 1944). Despite the occurrence of occasional cases presenting a more indolent clinical course of 15–20 years (Scadding, 1960), the average life span of most patients is about 47 months from the onset of dyspnea (Stack *et al.*, 1972). It is now known that diffuse pulmonary fibrosis may occur in association with connective tissue disease and/or autoimmune phenomena, develop from exposure to certain industrial agents, appear as a residuum of certain pulmonary infections, or occur as a manifestation of certain well-described lung disorders of unknown etiology (Table 4).

Based on a variety of histopathological lung findings, Liebow and Carrington (1967) subdivided interstitial lung disease and attempted to relate lung histopathology to clinical characteristics. The largest group of subjects demonstrate desquamative interstitial pneumonia (DIP) or usual interstitial pneumonia (UIP). Diffuse cellular infiltration with little fibrosis or necrosis characterizes DIP, whereas significant fibrosis with little cellular infiltration characterizes UIP. Corticosteroid therapy is thought to be effective in reversing the inflammatory cellular process of DIP but ineffective in altering the predominantly fibrotic change found in UIP. Bronchiolitis obliterans with alveolar damage (BIP), lymphoid interstitial pneumonia (LIP), and giant cell interstitial pneumonia (GIP) are examples of other less common types of interstitial pneumonitis which may potentially evolve into interstitial fibrosis. Carrington *et al.* (1978) have concluded that this histological

TABLE 4. Etiology of Pulmonary Fibrosis

Connective tissue diseases	Infectious diseases
Systemic lupus erythematosus	Tuberculosis
Progressive systemic sclerosis	Coccidiomycosis
Rheumatoid arthritis	Histoplasmosis
Polymyositis	Cryptococcosis
Goodpasture's syndrome	Helminths
Idiopathic fibrosing alveolitis	Viruses?
Occupational diseases	Idiopathic diseases
Silicosis	Eosinophilic granuloma
Berylliosis	Sarcoidosis
Asbestosis	Alveolar proteinosis
Hypersensitivity pneumonitis	Alveolar microlithiasis
Pharmaceutical reactions	Pulmonary hemosiderosis
	Neoplasm

classification predicts response to treatment and prognosis. However, other investigators have shown that histological changes characteristic of DIP and UIP may be found in different areas of the same lung biopsy section and that DIP may evolve into UIP. The most common approach now is to categorize these diseases according to etiology and immunological characteristics and to determine the stage of progression and possible degree of reversibility by assessing the relative presence of cellular infiltration *vis-à-vis* fibrotic change (Crystal *et al.*, 1976; Fishman, 1978). Diffuse pulmonary fibrosis therefore appears to be composed of a diverse group of diseases with different etiologies and probably different pathogeneses, but all resulting in diffuse scarring of lung parenchyma.

4.1. Connective Tissue Diseases

4.1.1. Systemic Lupus Erythematosus (SLE)

Young women are most often affected by systemic lupus erythematosus, which may involve the connective tissue in virtually every organ of the body, most commonly the synovial membrane of joints, serous membranes lining the lungs and heart, the skin, and the blood vessels. The course is generally quite variable. Disease may be acute and fulminant, episodic and variable, or chronic and indolent. When death occurs, it usually results from renal failure, damage to the central nervous system, or overwhelming infection. The most unique laboratory feature of this disease is the frequent occurrence of several types of antinuclear antibodies. The serum level of one of these, anti-double-stranded DNA (anti-dsDNA), has been found to reflect activity of this disease, especially the renal involvement. Pathogenesis is unknown. C-type viruses have been implicated. Also, it has been suggested that defective or low numbers of suppressor T cells may be responsible for an inadequate control of immunological response to self antigens.

Pulmonary involvement, including effusion, focal atelectasis, and acinar or interstitial infiltrates located predominantly at the lung bases, probably occurs in 50–70% of SLE patients (Huang *et al.*, 1965; Fraser and Pare, 1970). In a study of lung section specimens taken at autopsy, Gross *et al.* (1972) found a 98% frequency of interstitial pneumonitis, 70% interstitial fibrosis, 19% vasculitis, and 93% chronic pleuritis. Eisenberg *et al.* (1973) studied the clinical manifestations of this disease in 18 subjects with SLE and chronic diffuse interstitial pneumonitis and noted symptoms of dry cough, pleuritic chest pain, and dyspnea. Physical examination revealed diminished diaphragmatic excursion and basilar rales. A restrictive ventilatory defect, hypoxemia, and a reduced diffusing capacity were detected by pulmonary function tests. These physiological abnormalities are known to occur also in the absence of clinical symptoms or chest X-ray changes (Huang *et al.*, 1965). Whether the antinuclear antibodies or immune complexes commonly present in this disease play an important role in development of interstitial fibrosis requires further investigation. However, when rabbits are immunized with BSA and maintained in a state of relative antigen–antibody equivalence, membranous and proliferative pulmonary lesions develop with deposition of antigen, host immunoglobulin, complement, and fibrinogen (Brentjens *et al.*, 1974). More recently, Dreisin *et al.* (1978) have demostrated that subjects in the cellular phase of idiopathic pulmonary fibrosis exhibit circulating immune complexes. These observations add further support for the general pathogenetic importance of immune complexes in the production of interstitial inflammation culminating in fibrosis.

4.1.2. Progressive Systemic Sclerosis (PSS)

Production of abnormal collagen fibers is an important aspect of progressive systemic sclerosis, which is associated with atrophy and sclerosis of skin, gastrointestinal tract, muscles, kidneys, heart, and lungs. As in SLE, the presence of serum autoantibodies is a common finding. About 25–30% of patients demonstrate positive agglutination tests for rheumatoid factor and about 90% of patients demonstrate positive fluorescent tests for antinuclear antibodies (Rodnan, 1972). Females are affected 3 times more commonly than males with a peak incidence in the fourth to sixth decades of life. Pulmonary symptoms are found in about one-half of patients (Fraser and Pare, 1970; Barnett, 1974); however, 95% of patients have been found to exhibit abnormal pulmonary function tests (Barnett, 1974). Clinically, patients exhibit dyspnea, cough and fine basilar rales. Pulmonary hypertension and cor pulmonale may develop in association with severe vascular and intersititial damage. A diffuse interstitial reticular pattern, most prominent at the lung bases, is the most frequent abnormality seen on chest X-ray. Micronodulation is often present, and honeycombing with subpleural cyst formation is seen in advanced cases. Cysts are generally small, less than 5 mm in diameter. They are found bilaterally, predominantly in the basal and paravertebral areas, but occasionally become large and rupture, producing a pneumothorax (Fraser and Paré, 1970; Barnett, 1974). In addition, abnormal esophageal motility may lead to regurgitation of gastric contents, resulting in recurrent aspiration pneumonia. Pulmonary function tests commonly demonstrate a restrictive defect with reduced lung volumes as well as a reduced compliance; however, in mild disease there may be no demonstrable physiological abnormalities. An isolated reduced diffusing capacity of carbon monoxide is often the first sign of lung disease.

In a study of PSS cases at autopsy, Sackner (1966) found a 77% prevalence of pulmonary fibrosis. In a study of 28 cases, Weaver *et al.* (1968) found bilateral interstitial fibrosis with bronchiolectasis and cyst formation. Norton and Nardo (1970) have described frequent involvement of pulmonary arterioles and capillaries, but it is still unclear whether a relationship exists in PSS between pulmonary vasculitis and interstitial fibrosis.

4.1.3. Rheumatoid Arthritis

Rheumatoid arthritis is predominantly a disease of synovial joints; however, it may often affect other tissues and organs, including the lungs. Lung involvement is characterized by pleuritis, vasculitis with pulmonary hypertension, diffuse interstitial pneumonitis, fibrosis, and nodulation. Serum complement levels in these patients are generally normal; however, an important diagnostic feature is the common finding of a significantly depressed complement level in the pleural fluid. Although diffuse interstitial lung disease in rheumatoid arthritis is generally uncommon, when it does occur it typically affects the lung bases. In a review of 516 chest X-rays of patients with rheumatoid arthritis, Walker and Wright (1968) found only eight with diffused interstial lung disease. Lung function testing may be more sensitive in detecting disease since Frank *et al.* (1973) found the much higher prevalence of 41% of lung involvement with this approach. The most common change observed was a restrictive defect with reduced diffusing capacity, occurring more often in men than in women. Intrapulmonary nodules are commonly seen on chest X-ray and are histologically identical to the subcutaneous rheumatoid nodules so characteristic of this disease. The pulmonary nodules may cavitate and precede clinical arthritis by many years, as has been described by Caplan (1953) in the case of rheumatoid pneumoconiosis.

4.1.4. Polymyositis

Although polymyositis and dermatomyositis are inflammatory diseases of striated muscle, they usually present with painless weakness and atrophy of proximal muscle groups. The diseases affect women about twice as commonly as they affect men and show two peak incidences, one during the first decade and the second during the fifth and sixth decades of life. The prevalence of interstitial lung involvement has been estimated to be about 5% (Frazier and Miller, 1974). Forty percent of patients develop pulmonary disease 1–24 months before there are any manifestations of skin and muscle involvement (Schwarz *et al.*, 1976). When symptomatic the disease presents as an acute pneumonitis reflecting the activity of the skin and muscle disease, or when asymptomatic it may be found incidently on routine chest X-ray. Commonly, symptoms consist of insidious onset of cough and dyspnea, coincident with diffuse interstitial infiltration, predominantly at the lung bases. Without treatment, these cases commonly progress to severe restrictive lung disease with cor pulmonale. However, administration of corticosteroids may lead to significant improvement in clinical, X-ray, and pulmonary function parameters in about 50% of patients (Schwarz *et al.*, 1976). An overlap syndrome has been described exhibiting features of SLE, PSS, and polymyositis. Approximately 95% of patients with this mixed connective tissue disease (MCTD) exhibit high titer anti-ribonuclear protein antibody in their sera (Sharp *et al.*, 1972). Proliferative glomerulonephritis is unusual and prognosis following corticosteroid treatment is generally good. About 50% of cases have been associated with the development of diffuse pulmonary fibrosis.

4.1.5. Goodpasture's Syndrome

Goodpasture (1919) described a case of hemorrhagic pneumonia and nephritis occurring in a young man recovering from influenza during the great pandemic of 1918–1919. Subsequently, many cases have been described. About 80% of patients are young males with a median age of 21 years. The disease often begins with hemoptysis, generally associated with cough and exertional dyspnea. Rapidly progressive nephritis develops within several weeks to months. Chest X-ray generally reveals perihilar pulmonary infiltrates extending to the middle or lower lobes. These findings are associated with hemoptysis and often resolve when bleeding has ceased. Death occurs from renal failure, hypertension, or massive hemoptysis. Histopathological examination of the lung generally reveals intraalveolar hemorrhage, siderophages, and nodular thickening of alveolar septae. The absence of interstitial deposition of iron distinguishes this disease from idiopathic pulmonary hemosiderosis (Rusby and Wilson, 1960).

Proliferative glomerulitis with epithelial crescents is evident on renal biopsy specimens. Characteristic linear deposition of IgG and complement components along the glomerular basement membrane is often demonstrated by fluorescent staining. This IgG has been found to exhibit antiglomerular basement membrane (GBM) specificity, and passive transfer experiments have demonstrated its pathogenetic potential (Dixon, 1971). Some investigators using immunofluorescent techniques have claimed to demonstrate anti-GBM antibody in the lung (Beirne *et al.*, 1968; Sturgill and Westervelt, 1965), but other workers dispute this finding (Duncan *et al.*, 1965; Scheer and Grossman, 1964). Although anti-GBM antibody may exert direct complement-mediated cytotoxic damage to both kidney and lung, the exact relationship between the hemorrhagic pneumonitis and the nephritis remains unclear. Corticosteroid and antibiotic treatment has generally produced poor results. Bilateral nephrectomy has been advocated following a report by Maddock *et al.* (1967) of improved control of pulmonary hemorrhage following this procedure. No consistently effective treatment is currently available.

4.1.6. Idiopathic Fibrosing Alveolitis (IFA)

A large group of patients with diffuse interstitial pulmonary fibrosis has been recognized in whom there does not appear to be any underlying connective tissue disease, occupational exposure, or other etiological factor. Accumulating evidence suggests a possible underlying immunological aberration in this group, characterized by the presence of autoantibodies such as rheumatoid factors and antinuclear antibodies in sera from over 50% of cases. *In vitro* MIF production in response to type 1 collagen (Crystal *et al.*, 1976) and DNA (Haslam *et al.*, 1975) has been demonstrated in over 95% of cases. Immunoglobulin and complement have been demonstrated in the lungs of patients with IFA (Schwarz *et al.*, 1977; Eisenberg *et al.*, 1977). Finally, circulating immune complexes have been found in a majority of patients with the cellular phase of disease (Dreisin *et al.*, 1978). Many of the connective tissue diseases such as rheumatoid arthritis, systemic lupus erythematosus, and Raynaud's disease may ultimately develop in some of these patients. Caplan (1953) recognized an association between nodular lung fibrosis on chest X-ray and rheumatoid arthritis in pneumoconiotic coal miners. Miall *et al.* (1953) have subsequently shown that over 50% of miners with this X-ray pattern have rheumatoid arthritis. Additionally, Caplan *et al.* (1962) reported that 70% of coal miners with nodular pneumoconiosis, but without clinical arthritis, had positive serological tests for rheumatoid factor. Although a relationship may exist between the inhalation of silica and the formation of rheumatoid factors and immune complexes, it still does not explain the high incidence of autoantibodies in the sera of IFA patients, the majority of whom have never been massively exposed to silica or inorganic dusts. Histopathological examination of lung tissue reveals interstitial fibrosis; however, total collagen is not increased. Rather, there is an alteration of ratios of collagen types, with fibrillar type I collagen being increased relative to type III collagen. Type I collagen is more rigid and more easily seen by light microscopy, possibly accounting for the observed decrease in lung compliance. Important procedures in the diagnostic evaluation for IFA include pulmonary function tests, autoantibody screen including rheumatoid factor and antinuclear antibody, lung biopsy, and serial assessment by gallium-67 scanning and bronchial lavage analysis (Crystal *et al.*, 1976). Static recoil pressure measured at maximal inspiration and an increased alveolar capillary O_2 gradient accentuated with exercise are the physiological studies which best correlate with extent of fibrosis. Treatment with corticosteroids may reduce inflammation and prevent subsequent irreversible fibrotic lung damage if a significant cellular phase is present. There are few data on the efficacy of cytotoxic agents such as azothioprine and cyclophosphamide.

4.2. Occupational Diseases

4.2.1. Silicosis and Anthracosis

Recurrent or persistent inhalation of free crystalline silicon dioxide may result in silicosis. This most common form of pneumoconiosis occurs in such occupations as mining, sand blasing, quarrying, and many other industries where respirable crystalline silica dust is generated. There are several major molecular forms of free crystalline silica which, in decreasing order of fibrogenic potential, include tridymite, cristolbilite, coesite, quartz, and stishovite (King *et al.,* 1953). A tetrahedral atomic configuration is thought to be important for fibrogenicity. The only form of free crystalline silica not tetrahedral is stishovite, which is octahedral and entirely nonfibrogenic (Zaidi *et al.,* 1956).

Two types of disease have been recognized, the most common of which presents insidiously after prolonged silica dust exposure and cigarette smoking. Symptoms include recurrent cough and sputum with progressive dyspnea on exertion, often indicating an associated chronic bronchitis or emphysema. Nodulation and interstitial fibrosis are evident on chest X-ray. The other type of presentation follows massive exposure and generally results in acute onset of dyspnea, fever, malaise, and signs of systemic toxicity. Chest X-ray reveals a less striking nodular interstitial and acinar infiltrative pattern.

The outstanding histopathological feature is the presence of nodules which are laminated and hyalinized. Advanced cases demonstrate coalescence of nodules to form conglomerate hyalinized masses, often obliterating large portions of lung. Over 50% of patients with this conglomerate process have been found to have tuberculous infection as well. Because of the frequency of this complication and the fact that mediastinal lymph nodes in conventional silicosis may demonstrate noncaseating granulomas, it is always important to consider complicating tuberculosis. Experimentally, the production of conglomerate disease requires the combined presence of silica and tubercle bacilli. Tubercle bacilli appear to greatly enhance the fibrotic process, probably by exerting a potent immunological adjuvant effect, as has been demonstrated for tubercle derivatives such as complete Freund's adjuvant. The existence of an immunological aberration in the mechanism of disease is suggested by the high prevalence of autoantibodies, specifically antinuclear antibody, in the general population of silicotic patients (Jones *et al.,* 1977) and the autoimmune features of Caplan's syndrome as described above. In an assessment of *in vitro* parameters of cellular immunity in 16 patients with silicosis,

Schuyler *et al.* (1977) found that skin tests for delayed hypersensitivity, peripheral blood T- and B-cell quantitation, and lymphocyte transformation with pokeweed mitogen and phytohemagglutinin were all comparable to control group values; however, there was a distinct depression in lymphocyte transformation with low-dose concanavalin A. There may also be impaired production of MIF following lymphocyte stimulation with specific antigens such as SKSD. Additionally, the finding of large numbers of type II alveolar cells in bronchial lavage specimens may suggest a selective effect of silica on this cell population. The complex interrelationship of silica, autoantibodies, immune complexes, and interstitial pulmonary fibrosis may ultimately be shown to relate to a defect in T-cell regulatory function.

Coal worker's pneumoconiosis, also known as "anthracosis," is a disease of lung, distinct from silicosis, which may develop from prolonged inhalation of coal dust. Two forms have been recognized, including a simple lesion or coal macule with focal emphysema and a diffuse progressive pulmonary fibrosis. It is frequent to find features of both anthracosis and silicosis occurring in the same subject, since many coal beds contain silica as well. The coal macule form of disease is characteristic of anthracosis; however, it has been suggested that concurrent exposure to silica dust is necessary for the development of the typical lesion. True nodular lesions are not seen unless other histopathological features of both silicosis and anthracosis are also observed. The diffuse pulmonary fibrotic disease usually results from prolonged exposure to coal dust, and large confluent areas of fibrosis commonly are found predominantly in the apical lobes but also extending to the middle lobes of the lung. Hyalinized, pigmented masses of collagen may be present, although the nodular lesions of silicosis are not always seen. James (1954) has reported a 40% incidence of superinfection with tubercle bacilli in cases involving massive interstitial fibrosis. Since Caplan first described the connection between pneumoconiosis and rheumatoid disease in four coal miners, immune mechanisms have been thought to be operative in this disease. The nodular lesions seen in Caplan's syndrome may indicate prior exposure to silica so that these immunological phenomena are probably not directly related to pure coal dust but rather to the inhalation of silicone dioxide.

4.2.2. Berylliosis

There are two independent forms of lung disease which have been associated with beryllium inhalation. One is an acute chemical pneumonitis due to large exposure to metallic beryllium or any of the several beryllium salts, and the other is a chronic disease characterized by cough and progressive dyspnea. The finding that as few as 10% of patients with the chronic form of berylliosis have a history of one or more prior episodes of acute berylliosis suggests a separate mechanism for each of these two types of disease. Acute berylliosis either completely resolves or results in death within 1–4 months. The mean length of survival in chronic disease is generally 8–11 years. Workers manufacturing fluorescent lightbulbs were exposed to beryllium phosphor and were among the first cases reported. Currently, chronic berylliosis is most often seen in the beryllium extraction and smelting industry and also found, although somewhat less commonly, in metal alloy production, metal machining and fabrication, ceramic manufacturing, and atomic research. Disease may also develop in local residents living near a factory using beryllium.

Noncaseating granulomas characterize the lung histopathology in chronic berylliosis. Asteroid and Schaumann bodies along with hyalinized nodules may also be seen. Granulomatous inflammation has been found in other organs such as kidneys and liver. Advanced cases of chronic berylliosis may involve pulmonary hypertension and cor pulmonale, a common cause of death. Although complicating bronchogenic carcinoma is rearely seen, pulmonary embolism with infarction occurs in as many as 15% of advanced cases. Unique to berylliosis is the finding that total exposure dose does not appear to correlate with severity of disease, suggesting a probable hypersensitivity pathogenesis. The low incidence of disease in exposed workers and the frequent improvement following treatment with corticosteroids add further support to this hypothesis. Delayed skin responses and *in vitro* MIF production using beryllium salts have been demonstrated in both sensitized man and guinea pig (Marx and Burrell, 1973). Hypersensitivity to beryllium has also been transferred with sensitized lymphoid cells (Curtis, 1951). However, studies demonstrating lymphocyte transformation with beryllium salts in man and guinea pig (Marx and Burrell, 1973; Hanifin *et al.*, 1970; Henderson *et al.*, 1972) have been challenged by other reports of suppression of lymphocyte transformation by beryllium salts in the guinea pig (Jones and Amos, 1975) and in the rabbit (Kang *et al.*, 1977). Additionally, it is apparent that beryllium salts are both immunogenic and toxic, a characteristic common to certain other antigens capable of inducing a cell-mediated hypersensitivity response.

4.2.3. Asbestosis

In recent years, considerable attention has been given to the disease resulting from exposure to asbestos fibers. Iron and magnesium silicate with variable amounts of calcium and free iron are the main constituents of asbestos. There are two basic forms of this mineral, serpentine and amphibole, which are further divided into six types. Chrysotile, a member of the serpentine group, is composed of long fibers and is easily woven. These characteristics have made it the most commonly used in industry. Crocidolite, amosite, anthrophyllite, tremolite, and actinolite belong to the amphibole group and are chemically stable and resistant to acid. Asbestos has important antithermal properties and therefore has been used in countless products predominantly as an insulator. Large amounts of dust are generated from the production and use of asbestos. Chronic exposure commonly results in interstitial fibrotic lung disease. Frequent complications include tuberculosis, bronchiectasis, emphysema, or lung cancer, especially pleural mesothelioma (Wagner *et al.*, 1960; Selikoff *et al.*, 1965). A minimum of 7–10 years following onset of exposure usually elapses before typical symptoms of dry cough and exertional dyspnea appear. A nonnodular, diffuse interstitial infiltrate, most prominent at the lung bases, is evident on chest X-ray. Histopathologically, interstititial and alveolar fibrosis with small, 20–50 μm, iron-containing ferruginous bodies appear. These ferruginous bodies, formerly called "asbestos bodies," are thought to represent asbestos fibers coated with ferritin-containing proteins which may protect against further tissue reaction. Hyaline and calcified pleural plaques involving the visceral pleura, but not the parietal pleura, are frequently seen (Becklake, 1976).

Investigation of the biological properties of asbestos has revealed that it can induce the *in vitro* release of lysosomal enzymes from macrophages (Allison, 1971). Asbestos may also be cytolytic, but, in contrast to the rapid lytic action of silica on biologic membranes, asbestos may be tolerated as an intracellular inclusion for hours without noticeable effect on the phagocytosing cell. Additionally, unlike silica, asbestos activates the alternative complement pathway (Wilson *et al.,* 1977) and induces biochemiluminescence in peripheral blood neutrophils (H. R. Gaumer, personal communication). These unique biological properties of asbestos may be important in the pathogenesis of asbestosis.

A fourfold increased prevalence of antinuclear antibodies and rheumatoid factors as well as an increased prevalence of HLA-B27 antigen in asbestos patients has been reported by Turner-Warwick and Parkes (1970), who have proposed that antinuclear antibodies act as disease accelerators, once the fibrosis has been initiated by some separate event. The high prevalence of HLA-B27 has also been found in certain axial arthropathies where exessive fibrosis of ligamentous structures is characteristic. The HLA-B27 antigen, therefore, may represent a host susceptibility factor for an exaggerated fibrotic response. The rare occurrence of antinuclear antibodies and rheumatoid factors in the HLA-B27-positive arthropathies casts some doubt on the validity of this finding. Although the pathogenesis of asbestosis is still incompletely understood, the roles of host genetic factors and the immune system appear to be important.

Diffuse pulmonary fibrosis may result from other diseases caused by occupational exposure, including the various chronic forms of hypersensitivity pneumonitis discussed earlier in this chapter, acute and chronic reactions to various pharmaceutical agents following exposure in the manufacturing process or therapeutic administration, and excessive exposure to radiation. It is known that excessive irradiation of lung parenchyma produces tissue damage with consequent inflammation and scarring; however, immunological mechanisms have not been demonstrated to play a role in this process.

4.3. Infectious and Idiopathic Diseases

Granulomatous inflammation of lung leading to interstitial fibrosis, nodulation, and calcification may result from primary tuberculosis, histoplasmosis, coccidiomycosis, blastomycosis, and cryptococcosis. In the United States, histoplasmosis is endemic to the Mississippi River Valley. Coccidiomycosis is endemic to the San Joaquin Valley in California, while blastomycosis is found predominantly in the central and southeastern portions of the country. In the active phase of these diseases, smears of sputum and sections of tissue, along with cultures, may reveal the diagnosis. Delayed-type intradermal skin reactions to tuberculin, coccidioidin, and histoplasmin indicate prior exposure but not necessarily active disease. The advisability of applying diagnostic fungal skin tests must always be considered since histoplasmin may alter subsequent serological reactivity. The blastomycin skin test is an unreliable indicator of sensitization or disease. In the case of the mycoses, serological analysis for precipitating and complement-fixing antibodies also provides important diagnostic inflammation. With regard to histoplasmosis, there are currently three useful serological tests. The complement fixation (CF) test, employing either mycelial (histoplasmin) or yeast antigens, is usually positive in active infection. A titer of 1:8 or greater is considered presumptive evidence of histoplasmosis, and titers of 1:32 or greater are highly suggestive of infection. A fourfold or greater rise in titer suggests disease progression, while a fourfold fall in titer generally indicates disease regression. However, the height of the antibody titer does not correlate with the degree of dissemination of disease. The histoplasmin skin test, when applied to a positive reactor, may cause a rise in histoplasmin CF titer in up to 20% of cases. Cross-reactions may occur with blastomycosis. Gel diffusion, using a concentrated histoplasmin antigen, is less sensitive than the CF test but more specific for acute disease. There are two precipitin bands, an H band which is specific for active disease and an M band which may develop following a histoplasmin skin test and persist even after the patient has recovered. The histoplasmin latex agglutination test detects acute pulmonary disease but is positive in only 50% of chronic cases. While the histoplasmin skin test has been useful in epidemiological surveys and for the general evaluation of a patient's cell-mediated immune status, its lack of specificity for active disease and its affect on serology limit its applicability for evaluating suspected cases of histoplasmosis.

Serological tests available for detecting coccidiomycosis include agglutination, CF, and gel diffusion. Most patients with active disease demonstrate a rapid rise in CF titer, which remains high when dissemination occurs. The agglutination test becomes positive 2–3 weeks following exposure in patients developing active disease. The demonstration of precipitating antibody by gel diffusion generally indicates acute disease. The coccidioidin skin test does not appear to alter serological reactivity and may be positive in active disease or merely reflect prior infection in a normal, asymptomatic subject.

The CF test has been used in the evaluation of blastomycosis due to infection with *B. dermatitidis,* but sensitivity is low and cross-reactivity high, so that the test is of no practical value in the diagnosis of this infection. A gel immunodiffusion test using a yeast phase antigen is very specific, with a sensitivity of 80%. The immunological diagnosis of these diseases has been reviewed by Heinlen and Salvaggio (1976).

Some of these individual diseases have unique clinical and radiographic characteristics. Diffuse pulmonary fibrosis accompanied by widespread punctate parenchymal calcifications is typically found in healed or chronic histoplasmosis. Coccidiomycosis is more often characterized by thin-walled cavities or cysts; and the common Ghon complex, occasionally with apical pleural thickening, is found in healed pulmonary tuberculosis. All these diseases represent infectious disorders capable of producing diffuse pulmonary fibrosis. Certainly, if these infectious processes are adequately controlled by either host immune mechanisms or chemotherapy, then inflammation seldom progresses to the diffuse fibrotic stage. The inflammatory response, occurring as a consequence of a cell-mediated immune reaction to the infecting organism, represents an important immunological host response facilitating the containment and killing of organisms. However, this same inflammatory response may also lead to diffuse scarring of lung, often observed with extensive infection.

Other lung disorders of unknown etiology have been associated with diffuse interstitial pulmonary fibrosis. Eosinophilic granuloma of lung, characterized by histiocytic proliferation, may present few symptoms or chest X-ray changes, or may result in diffuse fibrosis with honeycombing, predominantly of the upper lobes. Another idiopathic granulomatous disease of lung is sarcoidosis, which frequently produces enlargement of hilar lymph nodes. Although commonly a benign condition, it may produce linear and nodular interstititial pulmonary infiltrates which can evolve into extensive diffuse fibrosis with honeycombing. Secondary emphysema may develop from fibrous traction and hilar bronchial compression. Alveolar proteinosis is characterized by the accumulation of periodic acid-Schiff positive proteinacious material in the alveoli, producing ventilation-perfusion defects. This disease may often resolve with only minimal residual interstitial fibrosis. Alveolar microlithiasis gets its name from the deposition of multiple minute calcifications in alveoli and occasionally in bronchioles. These may persist for a long time producing no functional change, but ultimately inflammatory and fibrous damage to alveolar walls results in ventilation-perfusion imbalance. Pulmonary hemosiderosis may present with recurrent episodes of hemoptysis, respiratory distress, and anemia. It usually affects children. The histopathology of siderotic nodules reveals siderophages, giant cells, and fibroblasts infiltrating alveolar walls, ducts, and respiratory bronchioles. Metastatic lymphangiitic carcinomatoses, lymphomas, and leukemias may also infiltrate lung parenchyma and produce respiratory insufficiency. Alveolar cell carcinoma, bronchiolar adenomatosis, bronchiolar carcinoma, and diffuse epithelial hyperplasia may all extend outward from their origin to diffusely line alveolar walls. When this occurs, pulmonary insufficiency results from a true alveolar–capillary block. Most of these diseases are relatively rare. Since there are few data on their etiologies or pathogeneses, very little information is available on possible immunological mechanisms.

ACKNOWLEDGMENT

We wish to thank Miss Velda Force for the great amount of work and care she contributed in the preparation of the manuscript.

5. References

Allen, D. H., Basten, A., Williams, G. V., and Woolcock, A. J., 1975, Familial hypersensitivity pneumonitis, *Am. J. Med.* **59:**505.

Allen, D. H., Basten, A., Woolcock, A. J., and Guinan, J., 1977, HLA and bird breeder's hypersensitivity pneumonitis, *Monogr. Allergy* **11:**7.

Allison, A. C., 1971, Effects of silica and asbestos on cells in culture, in: *Inhaled Particles III* (W. H. Walton, ed.), p. 437, Unwin Bros. Ltd. Gresham Press, England.

Bardana, E. J., McClatchy, J. K., Farr, R. S., and Minden, P., 1972, The primary interaction of antibody components of Aspergillus. II. Antibodies in sera from normal persons and from patients with aspergillosis, *J. Allergy Clin. Immunol.* **50:**208.

Barnett, A. J., 1974, *Scleroderma,* Thomas, Springfield, Ill.

Barrowcliff, D. F., and Arblaster, P. G., 1968, Farmer's lung: A study of an early fatal case, *Thorax* **23:**490.

Becklake, M. R., 1976, Asbestos-related diseases of the lung and other organs: Their epidemiology and implications for clinical practice, *Am. Rev. Resp. Dis.* **114:**187.

Beirne, G. J., Octaviano, G. N., Kopp, W. L., and Burns, R. O., 1968, Immunohistology of the lung in Goodpasture's syndrome, *Ann. Intern. Med.* **69:**1207.

Berrens, L., and Maesen, F. P. V., 1972, An immunochemical study of pigeon breeder's disease. II. The specific antigens, *Int. Arch. Allergy Appl. Immunol.* **43**:327.
Berrill, W. T., and vanRood, J.J., 1977, DW6 and avian hypersensitivity pneumonitis, *Lancet* **2**:248.
Bice, D. E., Salvaggio, J. E., and Hoffman, E., 1976a, Passive transfer of experimental hypersensitivity pneumonitis with lymphoid cells in the rabbit, *J. Allergy Clin. Immunol.* **58**:250.
Bice, D. E., Salvaggio, J., Hoffman, E., and McCarron, K., 1976b, Adjuvant properties of *Micropolyspora faeni*, *J. Allergy Clin. Immunol.* **57**:207 (abstr.).
Bice, D. E., McCarron, K., Hoffman, E. O., and Salvaggio, J. E., 1977, Adjuvant properties of *Micropolyspora faeni*, *Int. Arch. Allergy Appl. Immunol.* **55**:267.
Blackburn, C., and Greer, W., 1966, Precipitins against extracts of thatched roofs in the sera of New Guinea natives with chronic lung disease, *Lancet* **2**:1396.
Brentjens, J. R., O'Connell, D. W., Pawlowski, I. B., Hsu, K. C., and Andres, G. A., 1974, Experimental immune complex disease of the lung, *J. Exp. Med.* **140**:105.
Buechner, H. A., 1971, *The Management of Fungus Disease of the Lungs,* Thomas, Springfield, Ill.
Caldwell, J. R., Pearce, C. E., Spencer, C., Leder, T., and Waldman, R. H., 1973, Immunologic mechanisms in hypersensitivity pneumonitis, *J. Allergy Clin. Immunol.* **52**:225.
Campbell, J. M., 1932, Acute symptoms following work with hay, *Br. Med. J.* **2**:1143.
Caplan, A., 1953, Certain unusual radiological appearances in chests of coal miners suffering from rheumatoid arthritis, *Thorax* **8**:29.
Caplan, A., Payne, R. B., and Withey, G. L., 1962, A broader concept of Caplan's syndrome related to rheumatoid factors, *Thorax* **17**:205.
Carrington, C. B., Gaensler, E. A., Coutu, R. E., Fitzgerald, M. S., and Gupta, R. G., 1978, Natural history and treated course of usual and desquantitative interstitial pneumonia, *N. Engl. J. Med.* **298**:801.
Chemlik, F., doPico, G., Reed, C. E., and Dickie, H., 1974, Farmer's lung, *J. Allergy Clin. Immunol.* **54**:180.
Christensen, L. T., Schmidt, C. D., and Robbins, L., 1975, Pigeon breeder's disease—A prevalence study and review, *Clin. Allergy* **5**:417.
Churg, J., and Strauss, L., 1951, Allergic granulomatosis, allergic angiitis, and periarteritis nodosa, *Am. J. Pathol.* **27**:277.
Chusid, M. J., Dale, D. C., West, B. C., and Wolff, S. M., 1975, The hypereosinophilic syndrome, *Medicine* **54**:1.
Claman, H. N., Karr, R. M., Kohler, P. F., Mass, M. F., McIntosh, R. M., Sams, W. M., Small, P., Stanford, R. E., and Thorne, E. G., 1974, Systemic (allergic?) vasculitis, *J. Allergy Clin. Immunol.* **54**:54.
Cochrane, C. G., Hawkins, D., and Kniker, W. T., 1968, Mechanisms involved in the localization of circulating immune complexes in blood vessels, in: *Immunopathology* (P. A. Miescher and P. Graber, eds.), p. 32, Sixth International Symposium on Mechanisms of Inflammation Induced by Immune Reactions, Schwabe.
Crofton, J. W., Livingstone, J. L., Oswald, N. C., and Roberts, A. T. M., 1952, Pulmonary eosinophilia, *Thorax* **7**:1.
Crystal, R. G., Fulmer, J. D., Roberts, W. C., Moss, M. L., Line, B. R., and Reynolds, H. Y., 1976, Idiopathic pulmonary fibrosis, *Ann. Intern. Med.* **85**:769.
Curtis, G. H., 1951, Cutaneous hypersensitivity due to beryllium: A study of 13 cases, *Arch. Dermatol. Syph.* **64**:470.
Danaraj, T. J., 1958, Treatment of eosinophilic lung (tropical eosinophilia) with diethyl carbamazine, *Q. J. Med.* **27**:243.
Divertie, M., and Olsen, A., 1960, Pulmonary infiltration associated with blood eosinophilia (PIE): A clinical study of Loeffler's syndrome and of periarteritis nodosa with PIE syndrome, *Proc. Mayo Clin.* **37**:340.
Dixon, F. J., 1971, Glomerulonephritis and immunopathology, in: *Immunobiology* (R. A. Good and D. W. Fisher, eds.), p. 167, Sinauer Associates, Stamford, Conn.
Dreisin, R., Schwarz, M., Theofilopoulos, A., and Stanford, R., 1978, Circulating immune complexes in the idiopathic interstitial pneumonias, *N. Engl. J. Med.* **298**:353.
Duncan, D. A., Drummond, K. N., Michael, A. F., and Vernier, R. L., 1965, Pulmonary hemorrhage and glomerulonephritis, *Ann. Intern. Med.* **62**:920.
Edwards, J. H., 1972a, The double dialysis method of producing farmer's lung antigens, *J. Lab. Clin. Med.* **79**:683.

Edwards, J. H., 1972b, The isolation of antigens associated with farmer's lung, *Clin. Exp. Immunol.* **11**:341.

Edwards, C., and Luntz, G., 1974, Budgerigar-fancier's lung: A report of a fatal case, *Br. J. Dis. Chest* **68**:57.

Edwards, J. H., Baker, J. T., and Davies, B. H., 1974, Precipitin test negative farmer's lung—Activation of the alternative pathway of complement by mouldy hay dust, *Clin. Allergy* **4**:379.

Eisenberg, H., Dubois, E. L., Sherwin, R. P., and Balchum, O. J., 1973, Diffuse interstitial lung disease in systemic lupus erythematosus, *Ann. Intern. Med.* **79**:37.

Eisenberg, H., Barnett, E., and Simmons, H., 1977, Diffuse pulmonary interstitial disease, an immune complex disease, *Clin. Res.* **25**:132A.

Ezeoke, A., Perera, A. B. V., and Hobbs, J. R., 1973, Serum IgE elevation with tropical eosinophilia, *Clin. Allergy* **3**:33.

Fiegenberg, D., Weiss, H., and Kirshman, H., 1967, Migratory pneumonia with eosinophilia associated with sulfonamide administration, *Arch. Intern. Med.* **120**:85.

Fifer, W. R., 1963, A typical primary pulmonary histiocytosis-X, *Am. Rev. Resp. Dis.* **87**:568.

Fink, J. N., 1973, Hypersensitivity pneumonitis, *J. Allergy Clin. Immunol.* **52**:309.

Fink, J. N., Barboriak, J. J., and Dosman, A. J., 1967, Immunologic studies of pigeon breeder's disease, *J. Allergy* **39**:214.

Fink, J. N., Sosman, A. J., Barboriak, J. J., Schlueter, D. P., and Holmes, R. A., 1968, Pigeon breeder's disease—A clinical study of a hypersensitivity pneumonitis, *Ann. Intern. Med.* **68**:1205.

Fink, J. N., Hensley, G. T., and Barboriak, J. J., 1970, An animal model of a hypersensitivity pneumonitis, *J. Allergy* **46**:156.

Fink, J. N., Schlueter, D. P., Sosman, A. J., Unger, G. F., Barboriak, J. J., Rimm, A. A., Arkins, J. A., and Dhaliwal, K. S., 1972, Clinical survey of pigeon breeder's, *Chest* **62**:277.

Fink, J., Hensley, G., and Barboriak, J., 1973, A primate model of hypersensitivity pneumonitis, *J. Allergy Clin. Immunol.* **51**:125.

Fink, J. N., Moore, V. L., and Barboriak, J. J., 1975, Cell-mediated hypersensitivity in pigeon breeder's, *Int. Arch. Allergy Appl. Immunol.* **49**:831.

Fishman, A. P., 1978, UIP, DIP, and all that (editorial), *N. Engl. J. Med.* **298**:843.

Flaherty, D. K., Iha, T., Chemlik, F., Dickie, H., and Reed, C. E., 1975, HLA-8 and farmer's lung disease, *Lancet* **2**:507.

Flannery, E., Dillon, D., Freeman, M., Levy, J., D'Ambrosio, V., and Bedynek, J., 1972, Eosinophilic leukemia with fibrosing endocarditis and short Y chromosome, *Ann. Intern. Med.* **77**:223.

Frank, S. T., Weg, J. G., Harkleroad, L. E., and Fitch, R. F., 1973, Pulmonary dysfunction in rheumatoid disease, *Chest* **63**:27.

Fraser, R. G., and Paré, J. A., 1970, Disease of altered immunologic activity, in: *Diagnosis of Disease of the Chest,* p. 866, Saunders, Philadelphia.

Fraser, R. G., and Paré, J. A. P., 1975, Extrinsic allergic alveolitis, *Sem. Roentgenol.* **10**:31.

Frazier, A. R., and Mitler, R. D., 1974, Interstitial pneumonitis in association with polymyositis and dermatomyositis, *Chest* **65**:403.

Fredricks, W., 1978, Antigens in pigeon dropping extracts, NIAID Workshop on Antigens in Hypersensitivity Pneumonitis (J. Fink and J. Salvaggio, eds.), *J. Allergy Clin. Immunol.* **61**:221.

Frimodt-Moller, C., and Barton, R. M., 1940, Pseudo-tuberculous condition associated with eosinophilia, *Indian Med. Gaz.* **75**:607.

Geddes, D., and Brostoff, J., 1976, Pulmonary reaction to chryotherapy, *N. Engl. J. Med.* **295**:507.

Gell, P. G. H., and Coombs, R. R. A., 1969, *Clinical Aspects of Immunology,* F. A. Davis, Philadelphia.

Germuth, F. G., 1961, The biologic significance of experimentally induced allergic granulomas, *Am. Rev. Resp. Dis.* **84**:84.

Ghose, T., Landrigan, P., Killeen, R., and Dill, Jr., 1974, Immunopathological studies in patients with farmer's lung, *Clin. Allergy* **4**:119.

Golbert, T. M., and Patterson, R., 1970, Pulmonary allergic aspergillosis, *Ann. Intern. Med.* **72**:395.

Goldstein, R. A., 1978, Cellular immune responses in aspergillosis, in: Proceedings of NIAID Workshop on Antigens in Hypersensitivity Pneumonitis (J. Salvaggio and J. Fink, eds.), *J. Allergy Clin. Immunol.* **61**:229.

Goodpasture, E. W., 1919, The significance of certain pulmonary lesions in relation to the etiology of influenza, *Am. J. Med. Sci.* **158:**863.

Gregory, P. H., and Lacey, M. E., 1963a, Liberation of spores from mouldy hay, *Tr. Bort. Mycol. Soc.* **46:**73.

Gregory, R. P., and Lacey, M. E., 1963b, Mycological examination of the dust from mouldy hay associated with farmer's lung disease, *J. Gen. Microbiol.* **30:**75.

Gross, M., Esterly, J. R., and Earle, R. H., 1972, Pulmonary alterations in systemic lupus erythematosus, *Am. Rev. Resp. Dis.* **105:**572.

Hailey, F., Glassock, H., and Hewitt, W., 1969, Pleuropneumonic reactions to nitrofurantoin, *N. Engl. J. Med.* **281:**1087.

Hamman, L., and Rich, A. R., 1935, Fulminating diffuse interstitial fibrosis of the lungs, *Tr. Am. Clin. Climatol. Assoc.* **51:**154.

Hamman, L., and Rich, A. R., 1944, Acute diffuse interstitial fibrosis of the lungs, *Bull. Johns Hopkins Hosp.* **74:**177.

Hanifin, J. M., Epstein, W. L., and Cline, M. J., 1970, *In vitro* studies of granulomatous hypersensitivity to beryllium, *J. Invest. Dermatol.* **55:**284.

Hansen, P. J., and Penny, R., 1974, Pigeon breeder's disease: Study of the cell-mediated immune response to pigeon antigens by the lymphocyte culture technique, *Int. Arch. Allergy Appl. Immunol.* **47:**498.

Hargreave, F. E., 1973, Review article: Extrinsic allergic alveolitis, *Can. Med. Assoc. J.* **108:** 1150.

Hargreave, F. E., and Pepys, J., 1972, Allergic respiratory reactions in bird fancier's provoked by allergen inhalation provocation tests, *J. Allergy Clin. Immunol.* **50:**157.

Hargreave, F., Hinson, K. F., and Reid, L., 1972, The radiological appearances of allergic alveolitis due to bird sensitivity (bird fancier's lung), *Clin. Radiol.* **23:**1.

Harris, J. O., Bice, D., and Salvaggio, J. E., 1976a, Cellular and humoral bronchopulmonary immune response of rabbits immunized with thermophilic actinomycetes antigen, *Am. Rev. Resp. Dis.* **114:**29.

Harris, J., Bice, D., and Salvaggio, J., 1976b, Experimental granulomatous pneumonitis: Bronchopulmonary response to *M. faeni* in the rabbit, *Chest* **69:**287.

Haslam, P., Turner-Warwick, M., and Lukoszek, A., 1975, Antinuclear antibody and lymphocyte responses to nuclear antigens in patients with lung disease, *Clin. Exp. Immunol.* **20:**379.

Heard, B., and Cook, R., 1968, Busulfan lung, *Thorax* **23:**187.

Heinlen, B., and Salvaggio, J., 1976, Molds, spores, and fungal allergens: Diagnostic skin tests and serologic procedures, in: *Clinical Laboratory Science* (D. Seligson, ed.), CRC Press, Cleveland.

Henderson, W. R., Fukuyama, K., Epstein, W. C., and Spitler, L. E., 1972, *In vitro* demonstration of delayed hypersensitivity in patients with berylliosis, *J. Invest. Dermatol.* **58:**5.

Hinson, K. F. W., Moon, A. J., and Plumber, N. S., 1952, Bronchopulmonary aspergillosis, *Thorax* **7:**317.

Hollingdale, M. R., 1974, Antibody response in patients with farmer's lung disease to antigens from *Micropolyspora faeni*, *J. Hyg.* **72:**79.

Horn, B., Robin, E., Theodore, J., and VanKessel, A., 1975, Total eosinophil counts in the management of bronchial asthma, *N. Engl. J. Med.* **292:**1152.

Huang, C. T., Hennigar, G. R., and Lyons, H. A., 1965, Pulmonary dysfunction in systemic lupus erythematosus, *N. Engl. J. Med.* **272:**288.

Huis, J., Veld, T., and Berrens, L., 1976, Inactivation of hemolytic complement in human serum by an acylated polysaccharide from a gram-positive rod: Possible significance in pigeon breeder's disease, *Infect. Immun.* **13:**1619.

James, W. R. L., 1954, The relationship of tuberculosis to the development of massive pneumoconiosis in coal workers, *Br. J. Tuberc.* **48:**89.

Johnson, K. J., and Ward, P. A., 1974, Acute immunologic pulmonary alveolitis, *J. Clin. Invest.* **54:**349.

Jones, J. M., and Amos, H. E., 1975, Contact sensitivity *in vitro*. II. The effect of beryllium preparations on the proliferative responses of specifically allergized lymphocytes and normal lymphocytes stimulated with PHA, *Int. Arch. Allergy Appl. Immunol.* **48:**22.

Jones, R. N., Turner-Warwick, M., Ziskind, M., and Weill, H., 1977, High prevalence of antinuclear antibodies in sandblaster's silicosis, *Am. Rev. Resp. Dis.* **113:**393.

Joubert, J. R., Ascah, K., Moroz, L. A., and Hogg, J. C., 1976, Acute hypersensitivity pneumonitis in the rabbit, *Am. Rev. Resp. Dis.* **113:**503.

Kaltreider, H. B., 1976, Expression of immune mechanisms in the lung, *Am. Rev. Resp. Dis.* **113:**347.

Kang, K., Bice, D., Hoffman, E., D'Amato, R., and Salvaggio, J., 1977, Experimental studies of sensitization to beryllium, zirconium, and aluminum compounds in the rabbit, *J. Allergy Clin. Immunol.* **59:**425.

Karr, R. M., Davies, R. J., Butcher, B. T., Lehrer, S. B., Wilson, M. R., Dharmarajan, V., and Salvaggio, J. E., 1978a, Occupational asthma, *J. Allergy Clin. Immunol.* **61:**54.

Karr, R. M., Kohler, P. F., and Salvaggio, J. E., 1978b, Hypersensitivity pneumonitis and extrinsic asthma, *Chest* **74:**98.

Kawai, T., Salvaggio, J., Lake, W., and Harris, J., 1972, Experimental production of hypersensitivity pneumonitis with bagasse and thermophilic actinomycetic antigen, *J. Allergy Clin. Immunol.* **50:**276.

Kazemi, H., 1977, Case records of the Massachusetts General Hospital, *N. Engl. J. Med.* **297:**155.

King, E. J., Mohanty, G. P., Harrison, C. V., and Nagelschmidt, G., 1953, The action of different forms of pure silica on the lungs of rats, *Br. J. Ind. Med.* **10:**9.

Kleinerman, J., 1974a, Industrial pulmonary diseases: Silicosis, asbestosis, and talc pneumoconiosis, in: *Textbook of Pulmonary Diseases* (G. L. Baum, ed.), p. 489, Little, Brown, Boston.

Kleinerman, J., 1974b, Industrial pulmonary diseases: Coal-worker's pneumoconiosis, berylliosis and miscellaneous causes, in: *Textbook of Pulmonary Diseases* (G. L. Baum, ed.), p. 509, Little, Brown, Boston.

Kussmaul, A., and Maier, R., 1866, Ueber eine Bisher nicht beschriebene eigenthumliche Arterienerkrankung, die mit, Morbis Brightii und rapid Fortschreten dass allgemeiner Muskellahmung einherght, *Deutsch. Arch. Klin. Med.* **1:**484.

Lacey, J., and Lacey, M. E., 1964, Spore concentrations in the air of farm buildings, *Tr. Br. Mycol. Soc.* **47:**547.

Liebow, A., and Carrington, C., 1969, The eosinophilic pneumonias, *Medicine* **48:**251.

Liebow, A. A., and Carrington, C. B., 1967, Alveolar diseases: The interstitial pneumonias, in: *Frontiers of Pulmonary Radiology* (M. Simon, ed.), p. 102, Grune and Stratton, New York.

Liebow, A. A., and Carrington, C. B., 1969, The eosinophilic pneumonias, *Medicine* **48:**251.

Loeffler, W., 1932, Zur Differential-diagnose der Lungeninfiltrierung. III. Ueber fluechtigue Succedan-infiltrate (mit Eosinophilie), *Beitr. Klin. Tuberk.* **79:**368.

Maddock, R. K., Jr., Stevens, L. E., Reemstma, K., and Bloomer, H. A., 1967, Goodpasture's syndrome: Cessation of pulmonary hemorrhage after bilateral nephrectomy, *Ann. Intern. Med.* **67:**1258.

Marx, J. J., and Burrell, R., 1973, Delayed hypersensitivity to beryllium compounds, *J. Immunol.* **111:**590.

Marx, J. J., and Flaherty, D. J., 1975, Alternate pathway activation of complement by antigens associated with hypersensitivity pneumonitis, *J. Allergy Clin. Immunol.* **55:**70.

McCarthy, D. S., and Pepys, J., 1971a, Allergic bronchopulmonary aspergillosis, clinical immunology (I), clinical features, *Clin. Allergy* **1:**261.

McCarthy, D. S., and Pepys, J., 1971b, Allergic bronchopulmonary aspergillosis, clinical immunology. 2. Skin, nasal, and bronchial tests, *Clin. Allergy* **1:**415.

McCarthy, D. S., Simon, G., and Hargreave, F. E., 1970, The radiological appearance in allergic bronchopulmonary aspergillosis, *Clin. Radiol.* **21:**366.

McIntosh, K., Ellis, E. F., Hoffman, L. S., Lybass, T. G., Eller, J. J., and Fulginiti, V. A., 1973, The association of viral and bacterial respiratory infections with exacerbations of wheezing in young asthmatic children, *J. Pediatr.* **82:**578.

Miall, W. E., Caplan,. A., Cochrane, A. L., Kilpatrick, G. S., and Oldham, P. D., 1953, An epidemiologic study of rheumatoid arthritis associated with characteristic chest X-ray appearances in coal-workers, *Br. Med. J.* **2:**1231.

Miyamoto, T., and Kabe, J., 1971, The lungs as the site of delayed-type hypersensitivity reactions in guinea pigs, *J. Allergy Clin. Immunol.* **47:**181.

Miyamoto, T., Kabe, J., Node, M., Kobayashi, N., and Miura, K., 1971, Physiologic and pathologic respiratory changes in delayed-type hypersensitivity reactions in guinea pigs, *Am. Rev. Resp. Dis.* **103:**509.

Moore, V. L., Fink, J. N., Barboriak, J. J., Ruff, L. L., and Schlueter, D. P., 1974, Immunologic events in pigeon breeder's disease, *J. Allergy Clin. Immunol.* **55:**319.

Moore, V. L., Hensley, G. T., and Fink, J. N., 1975, An animal model of hypersensitivity pneumonitis in the rabbit, *J. Clin. Invest.* **56:**937.

Neva, F. A., and Ottesen, E. A., 1978, Current concepts in parasitology: Tropical (filarial) eosinophilia, *N. Engl. J. Med.* **298:**1129.

Neva, F. A., Kaplan, A. P., Pacheco, G., Gray, L., and Danaraj, T. J., 1975, Tropical eosinophilia, *J. Allergy Clin. Immunol.* **55:**422.

NHLI Task Force Report, 1972, National Institutes of Health, Department of Health, Education and Welfare, Washington, D. C.

Norton, W. L., and Nardo, J. M., 1970, Vascular disease in progressive systemic sclerosis (scleroderma), *Ann. Intern. Med.* **73:**317.

Parrillo, J. E., Fauci, A. S., and Wolff, S. M., 1977, The hypereosinophilic syndrome: Dramatic response to therapeutic intervention, *Tr. Assoc. Am. Phys.* **90:**135.

Patterson, R., 1978, Studies of hypersensitivity lung disease with emphasis on a solid phase radioimmunoassay as a potential diagnostic aid in: Proceedings of NIAID Workshop on Antigens in Hypersensitivity Pneumonitis (J. Salvaggio and J. Fink, eds.), *J. Allergy Clin. Immunol.* **61:**216.

Patterson, R., and Roberts, M., 1974, IgE and IgG antibodies against *Aspergillus fumigatus* in sera of patients with bronchopulmonary allergic aspergillosis, *Int. Arch. Allergy* **46:**150.

Patterson, R., Sommers, H., and Fink, J. N., 1974, Farmer's lung following inhalation of *Aspergillus flavus* growing in mouldy corn, *Clin. Allergy* **4:**79.

Patterson, R., Schatz, M., Fink, J. N., deSwarte, R. S., Roberts, M., and Cugell, D., 1976, Pigeon breeder's disease. I. Serum immunoglobulin concentrations: IgG, IgM, IgA, and IgE antibodies against pigeon serum, *Am. J. Med.* **60:**144.

Pepys, J., 1966, Pulmonary hypersensitivity disease due to inhaled organic antigens (editorial), *Ann. Intern. Med.* **64:**943.

Pepys, J., 1969, Hypersensitivity diseases of lungs due to fungi and organic dusts, in: *Monographs in Allergy,* Vol. 4, Karger, Basel.

Pepys, J., 1973, Immunopathology of allergic lung disease, *Clin. Allergy* **3:**1.

Pepys, J., 1977, Clinical and therapeutic significance in patterns of allergic reactions of the lungs to extrinsic agents, *Am. Rev. Resp. Dis.* **116:**573.

Pepys, J., and Jenkins, P. A., 1965, Precipitin (FLH) test in farmer's lung, *Thorax* **20:**21.

Pepys, J., and McCarthy, D. S., 1973, Crytogenic pulmonary eosinophilias, *Clin. Allergy* **3:**339.

Peterson, L. B., Thrall, R. S., Moore, V. L., Stevens, J. O., and Abramoff, P., 1977, An animal model of hypersensitivity pneumonitis in the rabbit: Induction of cellular hypersensitivity to inhaled antigens using carrageenan and BCG, *Am. Rev. Resp. Dis.* **116:**1007.

Ramazzini, B., 1713 (1940), *DeMorbus artificum diatriba,* University of Chicago Press, Chicago.

Reed, C., 1978, Variability of antigenicity of *Aspergillus fumigatus,* in: Proceedings of NIAID Workshop on Antigens in Hypersensitivity Pneumonitis (J. Salvaggio and J. Fink, eds.), *J. Allergy Clin. Immunol.* **61:**227.

Reeder, W. H., and Goodrich, B. E., 1952, Pulmonary infiltration with eosinophilia (PIE syndrome), *Ann. Intern. Med.* **36:**1217.

Resnick, M., and Myerson, R., 1970, Hypereosinophilic syndrome, *Am. J. Med.* **51:**560.

Reynolds, H. Y., Fulmer, J. D., Kazierowski, J. A., Roberts, W. C., Frank, M. M., and Crystal, R. G., 1977, Analysis of cellular and protein content of bronchoalveolar lavage fluid from patients with idiopathic pulmonary fibrosis and chronic hypersensitivity pneumonitis, *J. Clin. Invest.* **59:**165.

Richerson, H. B., 1972, Acute experimental hypersensitivity pneumonitis in the guinea pig, *J. Lab. Clin. Med.* **79:**745.

Richerson, H. B., Cheng, F. H. F., and Bauserman, S. C., 1971, Acute experimental hypersensitivity pneumonitis in rabbits, *Am. Rev. Resp. Dis.* **104:**568.

Riddle, H. F. V., and Grant, I. W. B., 1967, Allergic alveolitis in a malt worker, *Thorax* **22:**478.

Rittner, C., Sennekamp, J., and Vogel, F., 1975, HLA-B8 in pigeon fancier's lung, *Lancet* **2:**1303.

Roberts, R., 1978, Fractionation and characterization of thermophilic actinomycetes, in: Proceedings of NIAID Workshop on Antigens in Hypersensitivity Pneumonitis (J. Salvaggio and J. Fink, eds.), *J. Allergy Clin. Immunol.* **61:**234.

Roberts, R. C., and Moore, V. L., 1978, Immunopathogenesis of hypersensitivity pneumonitis, *Am. Rev. Resp. Dis.* **116:**1075.

Rodnan, G.P., 1972, Progressive systemic sclerosis, in: *Arthritis* (J.L. Hollander and D.J. McCarty, eds.), Lea and Febiger, Philadelphia.

Rose, G., and Spencer, H., 1957, Polyarteritis nodosa, *Q. J. Med.* **26:**1.

Rosenberg, M., Patterson, R., Mintzer, R., Cooper, B. J., Roberts, M., and Harris, K. E., 1977, Clinical and immunologic criteria for the diagnosis of allergic bronchopulmonary aspergillosis, *Ann. Intern. Med.* **86:**405.

Rosenberg, T., Medsger, T., DeCicco, F., and Fireman, P., 1975, Allergic granulomatous angiitis, *J. Allergy Clin. Immunol.* **55:**56.

Rosenow, E. C., 1972, The spectrum of drug induced pulmonary disease, *Ann. Intern. Med.* **77:** 977.

Rosenow, E., DeRemee, R., and Dines, D., 1968, Chronic nitrofurantoin pulmonary reactions, *N. Engl. J. Med.* **219:**1258.

Roska, A. K., Garancis, J. C., Moore, V. L., and Abramoff, P., 1977, Immune-complex disease in guinea pigs. I. Elicitation by aerosol challenge, suppression with cobra venom factor, and passive transfer with serum, *Clin. Immunol. Immunopathol.* **8:**213.

Rusby, N. L., and Wilson, C., 1960, Lung purpura with nephritis, *Q. J. Med.* **29:**501.

Sackner, M. A., 1966, *Scleroderma,* Grune and Stratton, New York.

Saltzman, P. W., West, M., and Chomet, B., 1962, Pulmonary hemosiderosis and glomerulonephritis, *Ann. Intern. Med.* **56:**409.

Salvaggio, J. E., 1970, Hypersensitivity pneumonitis: Pandora's box, *N. Engl. J. Med.* **283:**314.

Salvaggio, J. E., 1976, *Proceedings of the IX International Congress of Allergology, Allergy and Clinical Immunology,* Buenos Aires, Excerpta Medica International Congress, Series No. 414.

Salvaggio, J., Phanuphak, P., Stanford, R., Bice, D., and Claman, H., 1975, Experimental production of granulomatous pneumonitis, *J. Allergy Clin. Immunol.* **56:**364.

Santives, T., Roska, A. K., Hensley, G. T., Moore, V. L., Fink, J. N., and Abramoff, P., 1976, Immunologically induced lung disease in guinea pigs: A comparison of ovalbumin and pigeon serum as antigens, *J. Allergy Clin. Immunol.* **57:**582.

Scadding, J. G., 1960, Chronic diffuse interstitial fibrosis of the lungs, *Br. Med. J.* **1:**443.

Scadding, J. G., 1967, The bronchi in allergic aspergillosis, *Scand. J. Resp. Dis.* **48:**372.

Schatz, M., Patterson, R., Fink, J., and Moore, V., 1976, Pigeon breeder's disease. II. Pigeon antigen induced proliferation of lymphocytes from symptomatic and asymptomatic subjects, *Clin. Allergy* **6:**7.

Schatz, M., Patterson, R., and Fink, J., 1977, Immunopathogenesis of hypersensitivity pneumonitis, *J. Allergy Clin. Immunol.* **60:**27.

Scheer, R. L., and Grossman, M. A., 1964, Immune aspects of the glomerulonephritis associated with pulmonary hemorrhage, *Ann. Intern. Med.* **60:**1009.

Schorlemmer, H. V., Edwards, J. H., Davies, P., and Allison, A. C., 1977, Macrophage responses to mouldy hay dust, *Micropolyspora faeni* and zymosan, activators of complement by the alternative pathway, *Clin. Exp. Immunol.* **27:**198.

Schuyler, M., Ziskind, M., and Salvaggio, J., 1977, Cell-mediated immunity in silicosis, *Am. Rev. Resp. Dis.* **116:**147.

Schuyler, M. R., Thigpen, T. P., and Salvaggio, J. E., 1978, Local pulmonary immunity in pigeon breeder's disease, *Ann. Intern. Med.* **88:**355.

Schwarz, M. I., Matthay, R. A., Sahn, S. A., Stanford, R. E., Marmorstein, B. L., and Scheinhorn, D. J., 1976, Interstitial lung disease in polymyositis and dermatomyositis, *Medicine* **55:**89.

Schwarz, M. I., Dreisen, R. B., and Stanford, R. E., 1977, The role of immune complexes in idiopathic interstitial pneumonia, *Clin. Res.* **25:**422A.

Seabury, J., Salvaggio, J., Buechner, H., and Kundur, V. G., 1969, Bagassosis. III. Isolation of thermophilic and mesophilic actinomycetes and fungi from moldy bagasse, *Proc. Soc. Exp. Biol. Med.* **129:**351.

Selikoff, I. J., Churg, J., and Hammond, E. C., 1965, Relation between exposure to asbestos and mesothelioma, *N. Engl. J. Med.* **272:**560.

Sergent, J., Lockshin, M., Christian, C., and Gocke, D., 1976, Vasculitis with hepatitis B antigenemia, *Medicine* **55:**1.

Sharp, G. C., Irvin, W. S., Tan, E. M., Gould, R. G., and Holman, H. P., 1972, Mixed connective tissue disease—An apparently distinct rheumatic disease syndrome associated with a specific antibody to an extractable nuclear antigen (ENA), *Am. J. Med.* **148:**159.

Simon, G., 1975, Type I immunologic reactions in the lung, *Sem. Roentgenol.* **10:**21.

Simonian, S., Krockey, E., and Boyd, D., 1977, Chronic interstitial pneumonitis with fibrosis after long-term therapy with nitrofurantoin, *Ann. Thor. Surg.* **24:**284.

Slavin, R. G., Million, L., and Cherry, J., 1970, Allergic bronchopulmonary aspergillosis: Characterization of antibodies and results of treatment, *J. Allergy* **46:**150.

Smith, M., McCormack, L. J., and Van Ordstrand, H. S., 1974, "Primary" pulmonary histiocytosis-X, *Chest* **65:**176.

Spector, W. G., and Heeson, W., 1969, The production of granulomata by antigen-antibody complexes, *J. Pathol.* **98:**31.

Stack, H. R., Choo-Kang, Y. F. J., and Heard, B. E., 1972, The prognosis of cryptogenic fibrosing alveolitis, *Thorax* **27:**535.

Staines, F. H., and Forman, J. A., 1961, A survey of "Farmer's lung," *J. Coll. Gen. Practit.* **4:**351.

Stankus, R. P., Cashner, F. M., and Salvaggio, J. E., 1978, Bronchopulmonary macrophage activation in the pathogenesis of hypersensitivity pneumonitis, *J. Immunol.* **120:**685.

Stark, J. E., 1967, Allergic pulmonary aspergillosis successfully treated with inhalation of nystatin: Report of a case, *Dis. Chest* **51:**96.

Steinberg, A., and Karliner, J., 1968, The clinical spectrum of heroin pulmonary edema, *Arch. Intern. Med.* **122:**122.

Stiehm, E. R., Reed, C. E., and Tooley, W. H., 1967, Pigeon breeder's lung in children, *Pediatrics* **39:**904.

Strieder, D. J., 1978, Case records of the Massachusetts General Hospital, *N. Engl. J. Med.* **298:**327.

Sturgill, B. C., and Westervelt, F. B., 1965, Immunofluorescent studies in a case of Goodpasture's syndrome, *J. Am. Med. Assoc.* **194:**914.

Thigpen, T., Salvaggio, J., and Schuyler, M., 1978, Evidence of bronchoalveolar lymphocyte sensitization in pigeon breeder's disease, *Ann. Intern. Med.* **88:**355.

Tuft, D. S., Giddens, W. E., Fairchild, G. A., and VanArsdel, P. P., 1972, The mechanism of hypersensitivity pneumonitis in the rabbit, *J. Allergy Clin. Immunol.* **49:**103 (abstr.).

Turner-Warwick, M., and Parkes, R., 1970, Circulating rheumatoid and antinuclear factors in asbestos workers, *Br. Med. J.* **3:**492.

Unger, J. D., Fink, J. M., and Unger, G. F., 1968, Pigeon breeder's disease: A review of the roentgenographic pulmonary findings, *Radiology* **90:**683.

Wagner, J. C., Sleggs, C. A., and Marchand, P., 1960, Diffuse pleural mesothelioma and asbestos exposure in the North West Cape Province, *Br. J. Ind. Med.* **17:**260.

Walker, W. C., and Wright, V., 1968, Pulmonary lesions and rheumatoid arthritis, *Medicine* **47:**501.

Warren, W. P., and Woolf, C. R., 1972, Avian-induced hypersensitivity pneumonitis, *J. Can. Med. Assoc.* **107:**1196.

Weaver, A. L., Divertie, M. B., and Titus, J. L., 1968, Pulmonary scleroderma, *Dis. Chest* **54:**490.

Weinberg, A. N., 1972, Case records of the Massachusetts General Hospital, *N. Engl. J. Med.* **286:**1205.

Weingarten, R. J., 1943, Tropical eosinophilia, *Lancet* **1:**103.

Wenzel, F. J., Emanuel, D. A., and Gray, R. L., 1971, Immunofluorescent studies in patients with farmer's lung, *J. Allergy* **48:**224.

Whitcomb, M., 1973, Drug-induced lung disease, *Chest* **63:**418.

Wilkie, B. N., 1976, Experimental hypersensitivity pneumonitis: Humoral and cell-mediated immune response of cattle to *Micropolyspora faeni* and clinical response to aerosol challenge, *Int. Arch. Allergy Appl. Immunol.* **50:**359.

Wilkie, B. N., 1977, Experimental hypersensitivity pneumonitis: Reduced severity of clinical response following repeated injections of *Micropolyspora faeni* antigens, *Int. Arch. Allergy Appl. Immunol.* **53:**389.

Wilkie, B., Pauli, B., and Gygax, M., 1973, Hypersensitivity pneumonitis: Experimental production in guinea pigs with antigens of *Micropolyspora faeni*, *Pathol. Microbiol.* **39:**393.

Wilson, K., and Alexander, H., 1945, The relationship of periarteritis nodosa to bronchial asthma and other forms of hypersensitivities, *J. Lab. Clin. Med.* **30:**195.

Wilson, M. R., Gaumer, H. R., and Salvaggio, J. E., 1977, Activation of the alternative complement pathway and generation of chemotactic factors by asbestos, *J. Allergy Clin. Immunol.* **60:**218.

Winterbauer, R., Wilske, K., and Wheelis, R., 1976, Diffuse pulmonary injury associated with gold treatment, *N. Engl. J. Med.* **294:**919.

Wong, M. M., 1964, Studies on microfilaremia in dogs. II. Levels of microfilaremia in relation to immunologic responses of the host, *Am. J. Trop. Med. Hyg.* **13:**66.

Zaidi, S. H., King, E. J., Harrison, C. V., and Nagelschmidt, G., 1956, Fibrogenic activity of different forms of free silica, *Arch. Ind. Health* **13:**122.

15

Augmented Immunoglobulin E Synthesis in Primary Immunodeficiency

REBECCA H. BUCKLEY

1. Introduction

In addition to evidence presented in the preceding chapters that IgE biosynthesis is increased in the atopic allergic diseases, there is increasing documentation that augmented IgE production often occurs in certain of the primary immunodeficiency disorders. The association of allergy with immunodeficiency has been suspected on clinical grounds for some time, although it seems more likely that many symptoms in immunodeficient patients thought to be allergic in nature merely mimic them, such as the "wheezing" of patients with pneumonia or the "hay fever" in others with infectious nasopharyngitis. In this regard, earlier claims of the frequent occurrence of "hay fever," "asthma" (Goldfarb and Fudenberg, 1961), and "eczema" (Peterson *et al.*, 1962) in agammaglobulinemic patients have not been supported by observations in larger groups of such patients, by results of skin tests for reaginic antibody, or by serum IgE concentrations, which have usually been extremely low (Figure 1 and Table 1) (Polmar *et al.*, 1972b; Buckley and Fiscus, 1975). Similarly, the "eczema" reported in patients with ataxia-telangiectasia did not have the typical clinical features of atopic dermatitis (Reed *et al.*, 1966), and serum IgE concentrations are uniformly very low in these patients (Polmar *et al.*, 1972a; Buckley and Fiscus, 1975).

REBECCA H. BUCKLEY • Departments of Pediatrics and Microbiology and Immunology, Duke University School of Medicine, Durham, North Carolina 27710. This work was supported in part by Asthma and Allergic Diseases Centers Grant No.P50 AI12026-04. The author is the recipient of Allergic Diseases Academic Award No.K07 AI70830-05.

Nevertheless, certain immunodeficiency states are characterized by overproduction of IgE antibodies (Table 1) (Buckley *et al.*, 1972; Polmar *et al.*, 1972b; Waldmann *et al.*, 1972, Buckley and Fiscus, 1975). The regular occurrence of increased IgE biosynthesis with a particular immunodeficiency disorder was first noted in patients with the Wiskott–Aldrich syndrome (Berglund *et al.*, 1968; Waldmann *et al.*, 1972). Later, the author and her associates (Buckley *et al.*, 1972) described two adolescent boys with a lifelong history of severe recurrent staphylococcal abscesses involving the skin, lungs, and joints who had exceptionally high serum IgE concentrations but normal concentrations of the other immunoglobulins. Polmar *et al.* (1972b) reported that an infant with DiGeorge's syndrome consistently had an elevated serum IgE concentration, and Kikkawa *et al.* (1973) first described a high serum IgE concentration in an infant with a variant of thymic alymphoplasia (the so-called Nezelof syndrome). A high frequency of elevated serum IgE was also noted by the author among 75 patients with selective IgA deficiency (Buckley, 1975).

Since the discovery of IgE and delineation of the biological properties of antibodies in this class (Ishizaka and Ishizaka, 1970), many investigators have searched for a useful function for these antibodies. From the evidence mentioned above that increased IgE synthesis is found not only in the allergic diseases but also in certain primary immunodeficiency disorders, it would appear that IgE

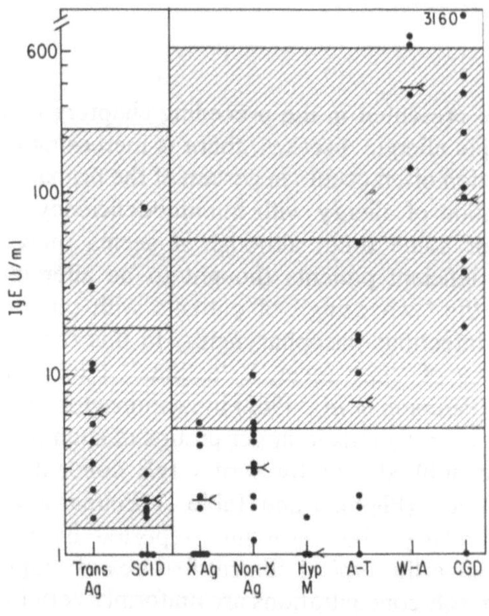

Figure 1. Serum IgE concentrations in X Ag, non-X Ag, trans Ag, HypM, SCID, A-T, W-A, and CGD. The cross-hatched area on the left represents the 95% confidence interval for 12 normal infants; the normal geometric mean of 18 U/ml is indicated by the middle horizontal line. The cross-hatched area on the right represents the 95% confidence interval for 106 normal children and adults; the normal geometric mean of 55 U/ml is indicated by the middle horizontal line. Individual immunodeficient patient IgE values are depicted by the dots and the geometric means of the patient groups by the horizontal arrows. From Buckley and Fiscus (1975).

TABLE 1. Serum IgE Concentrations in Immunodeficiency Patients[a]

Group	Number	Age	Range (U/ml)	Geometric mean	p value (t test)	Median	p value (Mann–Whitney)
1. Transient hypogammaglobulinema	8	3–20 mo	2–31	6	0.05	5	0.0269
2. Severe combined immunodeficiency	9	3–17 mo	<1–82	2	<0.0001	2	0.0018
3. X-linked agammaglobulinemia	10	3–16 yr	<1–5	2	<0.0001	1	<0.0001
4. Non-X-linked agammaglobulinemia	15	6–35 yr	1–10	3	<0.0001	3	<0.0001
5. X-linked immunodeficiency with hyper-IgM	3	7 mo–21 yr	<1–2	1	<0.0001	1	0.0016
6. Selective IgA deficiency	74	5 mo–50 yr	3–3800	124	<0.0001	174	0.0001
7. Ataxia-telangiectasia syndrome	7	5–14 yr	<1–54	7	<0.0001	10	0.0005
8. Nezelof syndrome	3	8 mo–3 yr	5–7000	55	NS	5	NS
9. Wiskott–Aldrich syndrome	4	8 mo–12 yr	135–720	381	<0.0001	487	0.0020
10. Extreme hyperimmunoglobulinemia E	11	3–31 yr	2150–40,000	11,305	<0.0001	12,362	<0.0001
11. Other variable immunodeficiency	6	1–14 yr	11–2880	142	NS	70	NS
12. Chronic granulomatous disease	10	6 mo–17 yr	<13160	88	NS	100	NS
13. Normal infants	12	2–19 mo	3–81	18 (1–222)[b]	—	25	—
14. Normal children and adults	106	2–55 yr	2–549	55 (5–621)[b]	—	55	—

[a]From Buckley and Fiscus (1975).
[b]95% confidence interval.

contributes little or no beneficial function. Nevertheless, from a teleological standpoint it does not seem likely that IgE would have survived in evolution on the basis of its harmful properties. One of the first roles evaluated was whether IgE may have a protective function in host defense against infectious agents. Interest in this role was stimulated by the report of Ammann *et al.* (1969) that susceptibility to infection in patients with ataxia-telangiectasia was correlated with a combined deficiency of IgA and IgE but not with IgA deficiency alone. This correlation was not confirmed in a larger group of patients with ataxia-telangiectasia studied by Polmar *et al.* (1972a). Indeed, the converse was found, e.g., there was a very high frequency of respiratory tract disease in those who were IgA deficient but not IgE deficient. The latter authors as well as others (Buckley and Fiscus, 1975; Van der Giessen *et al.,* 1976) did, however, find lower than normal mean serum IgE concentrations in patients with ataxia-telangiectasia as well as those with a variety of other categories of immunodeficiency. In the author's studies, concentrations of IgE were measured in sera from 165 patients with a variety of well-defined primary immunodeficiency disorders in an effort to find information possibly relevant to the role of antibodies of this class in host defense (Buckley and Fiscus, 1975). IgE concentrations were significantly lower than normal in patients who had marked deficiencies in all three major immunoglobulin classes, such as those with transient hypogammaglobulinemia of infancy, severe combined immunodeficiency disease, and X-linked agammaglobulinemia (Figure 1 and Table 1). In addition, IgE concentrations were depressed in patients with X-linked immunodeficiency with hyper IgM and in those with ataxia-telangiectasia.

Since there are multiple host deficiencies in all of the above categories of immunodeficiency, it is impossible to assign a role for IgE deficiency in the infection susceptibility of any of these patients. Possibly relevant to this question is the report by Levy and Chen (1970) of a healthy IgE-deficient person and a number of similar healthy IgE-deficient individuals who have been identified by the present author (unpublished).

The predominant production of both IgA and IgE immunoglobulins by plasma cells in lymphoid tissues adjacent to mucosal surfaces suggests that, if IgE antibodies do have a protective role, it would be as a mediator of local immunity (Tada and Ishizaka, 1970). It has been postulated that vasoactive substances released following the interaction of antigen with mast cell or basophil-fixed IgE antibodies may alter vascular permeability so as to facilitate the passage of other components of the immune system into sites where they are needed. Studies in rats experimentally infested with *Nippostrongylus brasiliensis* or *Schistosoma mansoni* have implicated other important roles for IgE antibodies in host defense against those parasites (Dineen *et al.,* 1973; Capron *et al.,* 1977; Butterworth *et al.,* 1977). It is well known that IgE antibody–antigen reactions result in the influx of eosinophils into the local site. Butterworth *et al.* (1977) have demonstrated antibody-dependent eosinophil cytotoxicity against ^{51}Cr-labeled schistosomula that appears to be mediated by IgG antibody and is inhibited by antigen–antibody complexes. In addition, there is some evidence that IgE antibodies can interact with membrane receptors on macrophages to increase the binding of these cells to *Schistosoma mansoni* schistosomules and enhance the lethal effect of IgG antibody-dependent macrophage-mediated cytotoxicity (Capron *et al.*, 1975). Similar evidence for a beneficial or protective role for IgE in man remains to be discovered.

2. Potential Mechanisms for Augmented IgE Synthesis in Immunodeficiency

Two obvious mechanism that possibly could account for increased IgE synthesis in primary immunodeficiency are (1) that it occurs as a result of infection or infestation with organisms or parasites that preferentially stimulate IgE antibody synthesis or (2) that it occurs as a result of faulty immunoregulation due to unique characteristics of the primary disease. It has been known for some time that parasitic infestation or administration of parasitic antigens or adjuvants, such as killed *Bordetella pertussis* or *Corynebacterium parvum* organisms or aluminum hydroxide gel, to animals will facilitate the production of reaginic or homocytotropic antibodies. In addition, serum IgE concentrations have been elevated in patients with parasitic infestation (Johansson *et al.*, 1968) and in those with certain bacterial (Green *et al.*, 1976) and fungal (Jones *et al.*, 1974) infections. This indicates that environmental influences as well as genetic factors are important in determining tendencies for excessive production of IgE. One clinical characteristic shared by many patients with primary immunodeficiency who have elevated IgE levels is their tendency to have infections with staphylococcal organisms, raising the question of whether staphylococcal infections stimulate excessive IgE production. Against this possibility is the fact that most patients with chronic granulomatous disease of childhood or with cystic fibrosis, frequently infected with staphylococci, were found to have normal IgE concentrations (Figure 1 and Table 1) (Buckley and Fiscus, 1975).

Until recently, little was known about host factors that influence IgE antibody formation. Important observations bearing on this point were made by Tada and his associates in 1971 when they demonstrated enhancement of ongoing IgE antibody production in the rat by treatment of the animals with small doses of antithymocyte serum, 400 R whole-body irradiation (Tada *et al.*, 1971), adult thymectomy and splenectomy (Okumura and Tada, 1971a) or by administration of various immunosuppressive drugs before or shortly after immunization (Taniguchi and Tada, 1971). The common facilitating factor in these treatments was revealed by further studies in which these investigators found that administration of carrier-specific T lymphocytes could inhibit ongoing hapten-specific homocytotropic antibody formation (Okumura and Tada, 1971b). The augmentation of ongoing homocytotropic antibody production by immunosuppressive manipulations was surprising and paradoxical, since these workers had shown earlier that priming of carrier-specific T-helper cells was necessary for production of homocytotropic antibody by hapten-specific antibody-forming B cells (Tada and Okumura, 1971). These studies provide strong evidence that IgE synthesis, while requiring T-helper cells for initiation, is also under active T-suppressor cell control. Thus it can be seen that patients with partial deficiencies in their thymic-dependent systems could have sufficient numbers of T-helper cells for initiation of IgE antibody formation but an inadequate number of T-suppressor cells, resulting in augmented IgE biosynthesis. On the other hand, states where thymus-dependent function is either completely lacking or relatively unaffected might be expected to be accompanied by little or no or normal IgE antibody production.

3. Excessive IgE Synthesis in Primary Immunodeficiency Disorders

In the studies cited above (Buckley and Fiscus, 1975) of serum IgE concentrations in patients with well-defined primary immunodeficiency diseases, IgE values were significantly elevated in patients with Wiskott–Aldrich syndrome, with the Nezelof syndrome, with selective IgA deficiency, and with the hyper-IgE syndrome (Table 1). Subsequent to that study, the author found one patient with non-X-linked agammaglobulinemia whose IgE concentration was above the 95% confidence interval for normal subjects; all other agammaglobulinemics studied have had very low concentrations of IgE. In a study of the metabolism of IgE in patients with primary immunodeficiency states, Iio *et al.* (1977) found that, in general, IgE levels correlated with the IgE synthetic rate and that abnormalities in the catabolic rate did not exert an important effect. Except for the patients with selective IgA deficiency and the one with non-X-linked agammaglobulinemia, all immunodeficiency patients with excessive IgE production in this and other reports have had impaired but not absent cell-mediated immunity (Waldmann *et al.*, 1972; Polmar *et al.*, 1972b; Kikkawa *et al.*, 1973).

3.1. The Wiskott–Aldrich Syndrome

The Wiskott–Aldrich syndrome is characterized by megakaryocytic thrombocytopenic purpura, dermatitis, undue susceptibility to infection, low to absent isohemagglutinins, and a progressive acquisition of cellular immunodeficiency (Huntley and Dees, 1957; Cooper *et al.* 1968). Abnormal immunoglobulin concentrations have been reported in these patients, the predominant dysgammaglobulinemia being characterized by an elevated IgE (Figure 1 and Table 1) (Waldmann *et al.*, 1972; Buckley and Fiscus, 1975), a low IgM, an elevated IgA, and a normal or slightly low IgG concentration (Blaese *et al.*, 1971).

In keeping with the elevated serum IgE concentrations, the dermatitis seen in these patients resembles very closely that of atopic eczema (Figure 2) and tends to have a similar distribution. Moreover, skin tests with inhalant and food allergens yield frequent positive immediate wheal-and-flare reactions (Huntley and Dees, 1957), and RAST studies on sera from such patients have demonstrated the presence of IgE antibodies to a variety of food and inhalant allergens (Caplin *et al.*, 1977). The thymus and lymphoid tissues are morphologically normal early in life, but a progressive depletion occurs with age of cells in thymus-dependent areas of peripheral lymphoid tissues, and susceptibility to viral and fungal agents develops (Cooper *et al.*, 1968). Whether the progressive impairment of thymic function is always related to augmented IgE production in these children is not known, but concentrations of IgE have been noted to increase with age, and most of the elevated levels have been found in older patients (Waldmann *et al.*, 1972). The pattern of dysgammaglobulinemia is not constant even within the same patient, however; thus it is not a reliable diagnostic criterion. The immunoglobulin deficiencies when they occur may be due in part to the hypercatabolism of IgG and IgM that has been documented in these patients, along with hypercatabolism of albumin and IgA (Blaese *et al.*, 1971).

Patients with the Wiskott–Aldrich syndrome usually manifest their disorder early in life with bloody diarrhea and recurrent respiratory infections. This sex-linked recessive trait usually leads to death in childhood, primarily from infection. Like patients with ataxia-telangiectasia, children with this syndrome have a high incidence of lymphoreticular malignancy and this is frequently the cause of death.

A failure of immune recognition of polysaccharide antigens has been demonstrated in this condition, and undue susceptibility to bacterial infections has been attributed to an inability to respond to bacterial polysaccharide antigens (Cooper *et al.*, 1968). The *in vitro* responses of cultured peripheral blood lymphocytes to phytohemagglutinin and antigens have been variable but often normal (Schiff *et al.*, 1974).

3.2. DiGeorge's Syndrome

The thymic hypoplasia or third and fourth pharyngeal pouch syndrome has also been associated with augmented IgE production (Polmar *et al.*, 1972b). Embryologically the thymus and parathyroids arise from the third and fourth pharyngeal pouches and are fused for a time during development. DiGeorge's syndrome occurs as a result of failure of normal development of these pouches (DiGeorge, 1968) and is usually manifested in the newborn period by hypocalcemic tetany due to congenital hypoparathyroidism. There is often an early appearance of mucocutaneous moniliasis, which persists despite conventional therapy. Despite

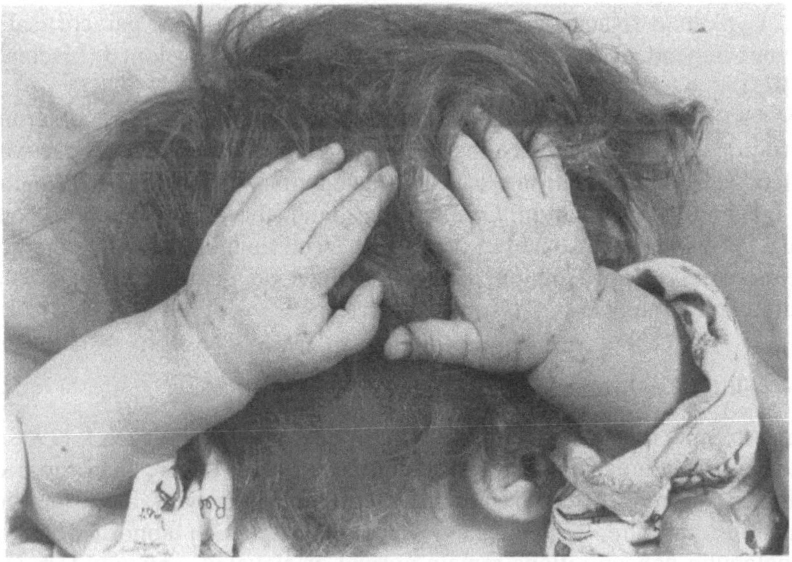

Figure 2. Pruritic eczematoid dermatitis over dorsum of hands of a patient with the Wiskott–Aldrich syndrome. Scattered petachiae are seen at sites of excoriation. From Buckley (1974).

the above-noted tendency for some of these patients to have elevated serum IgE concentrations, no allergic signs or symptoms have been described thus far. Antibody formation may be normal early in infancy but usually diminishes with time, despite persistence of normal immunoglobulin concentrations—probably due to the deficiency of T-helper cells (Lischner and Huff, 1975). Afflicted infants have characteristic facies as well as associated anomalies of the trachea, esophagus, heart, or great vessels. Patients with "complete" DiGeorge syndrome are usually unable to survive beyond infancy because of their extreme susceptibility to opportunistic agents which afflict those with a severe deficiency of "T"-cell function (i.e., fungi, viruses, *Pneumocystis carinii,* and gram-negative bacteria) or because of their cardiac abnormalities. Affected infants have depressed or absent cell-mediated immune reactions *in vivo,* and allograft rejection is markedly impaired. Circulating lymphocyte counts may be normal early in infancy, but the lymphocytes of many such patients respond poorly to the T-cell mitogens phytohemagglutinin (PHA) and concanavalin A (Con A) (Lischner and Huff, 1975). This is undoubtedly related to the fact that a majority of the circulating lymphocytes in these patients have been found to carry B-cell differentiation markers. Contrary to what is written in most texts about these infants, however, rarely is there complete absence of T-cell function (Lischner and Huff, 1975). Most DiGeorge infants who have been studied by the newer methods available for detecting and enumerating peripheral blood lymphocyte subpopulations have been found to have some T cells. Moreover, *in vitro* lymphocyte stimulation studies have been normal or near normal in a number of these infants. In reviewing serial mediastinal sections from autopsy material of 16 infants with DiGeorge's syndrome, Lischner and Huff (1975) found very small amounts of thymic tissue in 12 of these infants (referred to as having the "partial" form), and, except for varying degrees of involution, the tissue was histologically normal, containing both thymocytes and Hassall's corpuscles. Lymphoid follicles appeared normal, but lymph node paracortical areas and thymus-dependent regions of the spleen were poorly developed (Lischner and Huff, 1975).

The fact that some but not all of these infants have had elevated serum IgE concentrations may be related to the degree of thymic hypoplasia. Those with the "complete" DiGeorge syndrome may not have sufficient T-helper cell function to initiate IgE antibody formation. On the other hand, those with the more common "partial" form who have some but depressed T-cell function would be more likely to have increased IgE production, as they may have adequate numbers of T-helper cells but deficient numbers of T-suppressor cells.

3.3. Nezelof's Syndrome

This thymic dysplasia syndrome, first described by Nezelof (1968), has immunological features similar to but quantitatively less severe than those of the DiGeorge syndrome. Affected individuals do not, however, have parathyroid abnormalities and the thymus gland is present although abnormal. Although immunoglobulin concentrations remain normal or elevated, antibody formation is depressed or even lacking for certain antigens. Greatly elevated concentrations of serum IgE have been described in some but not all of these patients (Kikkawa *et al.,* 1973; Buckley and Fiscus, 1975), but allergy has not been a consistent finding.

Again, the tendency to augmented IgE production may be related to the degree of thymic dysfunction, with the most severely affected being incapable of manifesting this feature.

The condition has a familial occurrence, affects members of both sexes, and is thought to be an autosomal trait. Some such patients have been found to be deficient in the purine salvage pathway enzyme nucleoside phosphorylase (Giblett *et al.*, 1975). The clinical courses of these children have been quite variable, with some dying in infancy from viral or fungal infections and others remaining relatively well as late as 8 years of age. These individuals experience unduly severe infections with vaccinia and varicella viruses, remain lymphopenic, and have markedly depressed cell-mediated immune responses; half of the reported patients have also had an associated neutropenia. There is often continuous diarrhea which sometimes responds to treatment with disaccharide-free diets. At postmortem examinations the thymus glands are found to be extremely small and lack corticomedullary distinction or Hassall's corpuscles. Thymus-dependent areas of peripheral lymphoid tissues are also depleted.

3.4. Selective IgA Deficiency

Selective IgA deficiency is the fourth type of well-defined primary immunodeficiency disorder in which elevated serum IgE concentrations have been noted (Schwartz and Buckley, 1971; Buckley and Fiscus, 1975). In keeping with this, a high frequency of atopy (55%) was noted among a group of 75 such patients (Buckley, 1975). This condition is thought to be not only the most common type of dysgammaglobulinemia (i.e., deficiency of one or more but not all of the classes of immunoglobulins) but also the most frequent type of immunodeficiency (Buckley, 1975). It has an observed incidence of 0.2% in normal populations and of over 1% among patients referred because of recurrent infections or allergic respiratory problems (Buckley and Dees, 1969). There is a strong familial occurrence of this defect, and although an autosomal mode of inheritance appears certain it is unclear whether the trait is recessive or dominant with variable expressivity. Synthesis of other immunoglobulins is usually normal, accounting for the fact that this diagnosis is missed when γ-globulin levels are determined by serum electrophoresis.

While IgA deficiency has been reported in apparently healthy individuals, there is abundant evidence to indicate that it is more commonly associated with ill health (Buckley, 1975). Among the various clinical entities with which it has been associated are atopic hypersensitivity, recurrent sinopulmonary and ear infections, recurrent urinary tract infections, sprue, rheumatoid arthritis, lupus erythematosus, and other collagen diseases; idiopathic pulmonary hemosiderosis; and ataxia-telangiectasia (Buckley, 1975). In addition, a high frequency of autoantibody formation has been reported, as well as a peculiar propensity of these patients to produce antiruminant antibodies (Buckley and Dees, 1969). The latter often interfere with accurate performance of immunological studies employing ruminant heteroantisera (Buckley and Fiscus, 1975).

Possibly related to their propensity to have augmented IgE and allergic disorders is the well-known tendency of these patients to have severe or fatal anaphylactic reactions when they have been given blood or plasma transfusions from normal donors (Vyas *et al.*, 1968). These reactions are generally considered to be due to preformed class-specific antibodies to IgA present in these patients. Although the rapidity of the reactions suggests that they may be mediated by IgE antibodies, such antibodies to IgA have never been demonstrated in these patients. This could be because tests for IgE anti-IgA antibodies are inadequate, as antibodies to IgA have been found in high titer in other immunoglobulin classes in these patients (Vyas and Fundenberg, 1974). Caution should be exercised in concluding that either allergy or augmented IgE production is a feature of all patients with selective absence of serum and secretory IgA, however, since no data are available on the incidence of these features in non-hospital-referred IgA deficients. The increased incidence of allergy and elevated IgE noted among the author's patients would have to be considered a possible function of selection created by the fact that most of the patients were discovered in the allergy clinic. Nevertheless, it is of interest that the predominant distribution of both IgA- and IgE-containing plasma cells is in paragut and pararespiratory lymphoid tissues (Tada and Ishizaka, 1970). This raises the question of whether IgA antibodies may have a role in limiting mucosal permeability to antigens and whether the absence of such antibodies might permit greater stimulation of IgE antibody formation. Alternately, as with the other immunodeficiency states discussed previously, augmented IgE production seen in IgA-deficient patients could be due to a deficiency of a subpopulation of T cells important in regulating IgE-forming B cells. The only evidence in support of a T-cell deficiency in patients with selective IgA deficiency has been the finding of a slightly decreased percentage of sheep erythrocyte rosetting lymphocytes in some of these patients (Schiff *et al.*, 1974) and impaired interferon production by PHA-stimulated lymphocytes from others (Epstein and Ammann, 1974).

3.5. The Hyper-IgE Syndrome

In 1972 the author and her associates described two adolescent boys with lifelong histories of recurrent skin, lung, and joint abscesses (Buckley *et al.*, 1972). Although extensive studies of their immunological functions failed to demonstrate abnormalities consistent with any of the then-defined immunodeficiency disorders, certain unique features were revealed. These patients were found to have exceptionally high serum concentrations of IgE, pronounced blood and sputum eosinophilia, delayed cutaneous anergy to ubiquitous antigens, abnormally low anamnestic antibody responses following booster immunizations, and poor antibody and cell-mediated responses to neoantigens. Despite their markedly elevated IgE concentrations and positive immediate skin tests to a number of food, inhalant, and pollen allergens, neither boy had symptoms of respiratory allergy. One had a history of a generalized pruritic dermatitis for the first 4 years of his life and the other had a similar dermatitis chronically.

Since these first two patients were reported, the author has evaluated 18 additional patients with strikingly similar clinical and immunological features. Before describing them, it should be noted that a number of patients have been reported subsequently by others (Clark *et al.*, 1973; Hill and Quie, 1974; Van Scoy *et al.*, 1975; Church *et al.*, 1976; Blum *et al.*, 1977; Weston *et al.*, 1977) as having this syndrome, many but not all of whom had clinical features closely resembling those of our first two patients. Each of the later-reported patients, except one of the two reported by Blum *et al.* (1977) and the one by Weston *et al.* (1977), was described as having defective polymorphonuclear chemotactic responsiveness. Because of these reports, the suggestion was made that defective polymorphonuclear chemotaxis was the basis for the patients' infection susceptibility. As will be described below, however, chemotactic abnormalities have been highly variable, inconstant features in the 20 patients evaluated by the author. Moreover, many of the case descriptions reported were more in keeping with merely infected atopic dermatitis rather than this entity, as the infections were described as superficial (Hill and Quie, 1974; Hill *et al.,* 1976a; Dahl *et al.,* 1976; Fontan *et al.,* 1976; Jacobs and Norman, 1977). Relevant to this point are recent reports of chemotactic abnormalities in patients with urticaria (Hill *et al.,* 1976a), asthma, eczema (Jacobs and Norman, 1977; Snyderman *et al.,* 1977), and allergic rhinitis (Hill *et al.,* 1976b). In addition, however, such abnormalities have been described in nonallergic dermatitis (Pincus *et al.,* 1975), chronic mucocutaneous candidiasis (Snyderman *et al.,* 1973), and otitis media and chronic diarrhea (Hill *et al.,* 1977). In the last three conditions there was no associated dermatitis, and serum IgE concentrations were not elevated. To add to the confusion, polymorphonuclear chemotactic defects have also been described in two red-haired siblings, both of whom had histories of recurrent infection but neither of whom had eczema or elevated serum IgE (Witemeyer and Van Epps, 1976). Thus the inconstancy of polymorphonuclear chemotactic defects in this syndrome and the association of them with so many other conditons lead one to believe that they are not basic to this disease. As will become evident, however, the patients who have this syndrome represent a distinct clinical entity and one that is not defined by the presence or absence of either a polymorphonuclear or mononuclear chemotactic defect.

3.5.1. Clinical Manifestations

Some general features of the 20 patients with the hyper-IgE syndrome evaluated by the author are listed in Table 2. The patients ranged in age from 2 to 31 years, 13 were male and 7 female, and 8 were black and 12 white. They came from a very wide geographic area. It is important to emphasize that this is a rare disorder and that these are not merely individuals with atopic eczema who have repeated superficial infections of their skin lesions. These patients invariably have had recurrent severe bouts of furunculosis and pneumonia secondary to *Staphylococcus aureus* from early infancy, some from day 1 of life, and all had pneumatocoeles develop as a result of their recurrent pneumonias. Often the pneumatocoeles persisted or, in those in whom they resolved, remained evident roentgenographically for an unusually long time (Figure 3). Seven of these patients required thoracic surgery because of chronic infection—two underwent complete pneumonectomies, four had lobes removed because of lung abscesses, one had an empyema drained, and one had a candida granuloma removed from his anterior mediastinum. All patients have been plagued by infections with *Staphylococcus aureus,* but some have had problems with recurrent *Hemophilus influenzae,* pneumococcal, group A streptococcal, gram-negative, and fungal infections as well. The sites of infections in the 20 patients studied by the author are listed in Table 3. Infections of the skin and lungs have predominated, but the ears, eyes, oral mucosa, sinuses, joints, blood, and even viscera have been involved in some.

TABLE 2. General Features of 20 Patients with the Hyper-IgE Syndrome

Patient	Age (yr)	Sex	Race	Age at first infection	Dermatitis	Asthma	IgE (IU/ml)
BS	14	M	W	6 wk	+	−	22,300
RB	14	M	W	Newborn	+	−	6,600
AY	16	M	B	Newborn	+	−	40,000
CC	13	M	W	18 mo	+	−	6,400
TF	11	M	W	Newborn	+	−	9.000
AT	6	M	W	Infancy	+	−	5,000
LH	12	M	B	10 mo	+	−	22,000
JB	2	M	W	1 day	+	−	11,600
DS	17	M	W	Infancy	+	−	46,000
SE	12	M	W	Infancy	+	+	26,500
EN	31	F	B	Infancy	+	+	15,600
VD	11	F	W	1 mo	+	−	38,400
PD	7	F	B	Newborn	+	−	25,600
GD	13	F	B	Infancy	+	−	2,150
FD	3	M	B	4 mo	+	−	2,788
FK	22	M	W	Infancy	+	−	12,362
JM	2	F	W	Infancy	+	−	5,000
AC	10	F	B	Infancy	+	−	51,200
RT	7	M	W	1 day	+	−	33,000
CH	5	F	B	3 wk	+	−	24,000

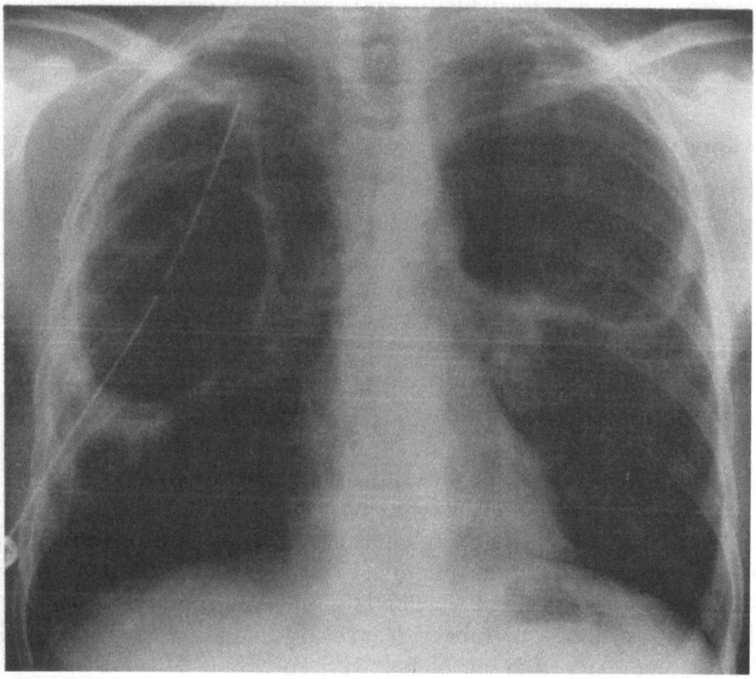

Figure 3. Chest roentgenogram of 12-year-old boy with the hyper-IgE syndrome. Giant pneumatocoeles were present for more than 1 year. A putrid abscess due to *Enterobacter cloacae* led to chest tube insertion on the right. The left cyst required emergency excision due to massive hemoptysis and was found to contain an aspergilloma. From Buckley (1979).

TABLE 3. Sites of Infections in 20 Patients with the Hyper-IgE Syndrome

Skin	20/20
Abscesses	20/20
Deep cellulitis	2/20
Lung	20/20
Pneumatocoeles	20/20
Resection of lobes	4/20
Total pneumonectomy	2/20
Ears	13/20
Mastoidectomy	2/20
Oral mucosa	7/20
Sinuses	8/20
Eyes	9/20
Joints	4/20
Viscera	3/20
Blood	3/20

A peculiar tendency for the abscesses to localize about the scalp, face, and neck has been observed in infants and younger children with the disorder (Figure 4). Sites that have not been foci of infections include the urinary and gastrointestinal tracts, the meninges, and the bones (except the mastoids).

All 20 patients had either dermatitis at the time of their evaluation or, more often, a history of pruritic dermatitis earlier in life. Although the lesions resembled those of an eczematoid dermatitis and the skin was often lichenified, the distribution and characteristics of the lesions were not those of typical atopic eczema. None of the patients had histories of allergic rhinitis, and only two were ever noted to wheeze. Even in the latter two patients, asthma was not a prominent symptom.

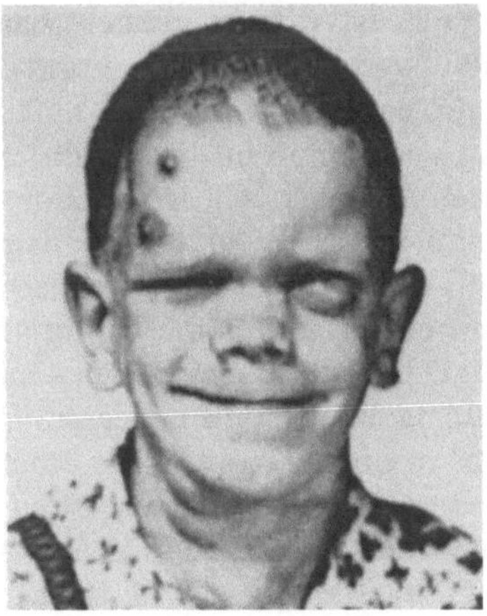

Figure 4. Photograph of patient with hyper-IgE syndrome showing multiple abscesses of the face and neck and coarse facial features. From Buckley *et al.* (1972), reproduced by permission from Bristol Laboratories.

Two of the patients without a history of wheezing were given methacholine inhalation challenges without a significant drop in their FEV_1. Thus there was little or no evidence of respiratory allergy in these patients. None had a history or clinical evidence of parasitic infestation at the time he or she was evaluated.

Several of these patients have retarded growth, predominantly those with chronic lower respiratory tract disease, and all but one evaluated by the author have had coarse facial features (Figure 4). There have been no red-haired, fair-skinned females among these 20 patients; these were physical features mentioned by Davis *et al.* (1966) in describing two patients with what they called "Job's" syndrome. These patients were also described as having "cold" nontender abscesses. Most abscesses observed by the author in patients with the hyper-IgE syndrome have been tender and warm, although often the patients have had large deep-seated abscesses without manifesting much evidence of systemic toxicity. Although serum IgE concentrations were later found by Hill *et al.* (1974) to be elevated in the two original patients with Job's syndrome and in two more, from the limited clinical and immunological data given in those four, the only reported cases (Davis *et al.*, 1966; Hill *et al.*, 1974), it is unclear whether that syndrome and the hyper-IgE syndrome are closely related or possibly even the same entity.

Seven instances of the familial occurrence of the hyper-IgE syndrome were noted among the above 20 patients, and there are additional reports of this in the literature (Van Scoy *et al.*, 1975; Blum *et al.*, 1977). The fact that both males and females have been affected, as have members of succeeding generations, suggests an autosomal dominant form of inheritance with incomplete penetrance. A summary of the most important clinical features of these patients is presented in Table 4.

3.5.2. Laboratory Findings

Eosinophilia of blood and sputum has been a consistent finding in all 20 patients evaluated by the author. Blood eosinophilia as high as 55–60% has occured in some infants with the disorder, and in most patients both the percentage and the absolute number of eosinophils have been greater than in the average atopic patient. Total white counts have ranged from normal to markedly elevated (50,000–60,000/mm^3), but no patients were ever noted to be neutropenic or lymphopenic. Anemia is not uncommon in those with chronic lower respiratory infections but is not a feature of patients whose infections are controlled.

Investigations of humoral immunity in the 20 patients noted above have consistently shown serum IgE concentrations to be exceedingly high, ranging from 3 to 82 times the upper limit of normal for the author's laboratory (Table 2). In addition, concentrations of IgD have been elevated in a majority, with 14 of the 20 having values greater than 10 mg/dl and some concentrations being in the range of 50–159 mg/dl. Concentrations of one or more of the other three immunoglobulins have also been elevated in some patients, but more often they have been normal. Serum IgE concentrations have been measured in all available first-degree relatives of eight of these patients, and the values were all found to be within the normal range for this laboratory (Table 5). Consistent with the finding of poor anamnestic antibody responses to diphtheria and tetanus and a lack of a response to the neoantigen KLH in the first two patients, diphtheria and tetanus antibody titers

TABLE 4. Clinical Features of 20 Patients with the Hyper-IgE Syndrome

Severe infections of the skin and lower respiratory tract from infancy. All have had furunculosis, staphylococcal pneumonia, and pneumatoceoles. Most have also had infections of ears, sinuses, eyes, and oral mucosa. Fewer have had infections of joints, viscera, and blood.

Staphylococcus aureus, coagulase positive, has caused infections in all. *Candida albicans, Hemophilus influenzae,* pneumococci, and streptococci, group A, isolated in from one-half to one-fourth; miscellaneous gram-negative rods and other fungi in some.

Pruritic dermatitis chronically or (more often) in past; little or no respiratory allergy. Rash is not typical atopic eczema.

Both sexes affected (males 13, females 7); 12 were white, 8 black.

Familial occurrence in 7/20 families studied; IgE normal in nonaffected relatives. Pattern in families suggests autosomal dominant trait with incomplete penetrance. No increased frequency of any HLA-A or -B locus antigens.

were found to be low initially in all 20 patients, and only one of 11 given booster immunizations with DPT or DT showed a normal anamnestic antibody response to either antigen. Isohemagglutinin titers were normal in most but low in some and elevated in others. Serum antibodies to staphylococcal and candida organisms were detected in the serum of one of the first two patients evaluated (Buckley *et al.*, 1972), but sera from the other 18 have not been tested for antibodies to these organisms. In keeping with their markedly elevated total serum IgE concentrations, the patients when tested have been found to have strongly positive immediate

TABLE 5. Serum IgE Concentrations in Hyper-IgE Patients and Their Relatives[a]

Patient and relatives	IgE (IU/ml)	Patient and relatives	IgE (IU/ml)
1. AY	40,000	5. AT	5,000
Fa	96	Fa	13
Bro	116	Mo	10
		Sis_1	15
2. TF	9,000	Sis_2	6
Fa	52		
Mo	46	6. JB	11,600
Bro_1	49	Fa	8
Bro_2	49	Mo	84
		Bro_1	8
3. RB	6,600	Bro_2	4
Fa	42		
Mo	315	7. LH	22,000
Bro	110	Mo	170
		Sis_1	83
4. CC	6,400	Sis_2	190
Fa	110		
Mo	46	8. SE	26,500
Bro	560	Mo	52
Sis	210	Fa	107
		Bro	425
		Sis	48

[a]106 normal children and adults: 55 (5–621) IU/ml.

wheal-and-flare reactions to a number of inhalant, food, and pollen allergens, as well as to candida, staphylococcal, and other bacterial and fungal antigens. IgE was isolated from the serum of one of the first two patients and found to contain both κ- and λ-chains on gel diffusion analysis, thus ruling against the likelihood that the IgE in the sera of these patients is paraprotein in nature.

Rosette formation and membrane immunofluorescence studies were done by the author to identify and enumerate lymphocyte subpopulations in the peripheral blood of patients with the hyper-IgE syndrome. The results failed to demonstrate a subpopulation deficiency or excess. In particular, the percentages of cells forming spontaneous erythrocytes with untreated and neuraminidase-treated sheep erythrocytes were normal in all tested, and there was no evidence to suggest an increased percentage of IgE-bearing B lymphocytes.

Although delayed cutaneous anergy to ubiquitous antigens, such as candida and streptokinase-streptodornase, was found in the first two patients described with this condition (Buckley *et al.*, 1972), this has been a feature in only approximately one-half of the subsequent patients in the author's series evaluated for *in vivo* evidence of cellular immunocompetence (Table 6). *In vitro* studies of cell-mediated immunity in the patients in whom these have been conducted have revealed normal lymphocyte proliferative responses to the mitogens phytohemagglutinin (PHA), concanavalin A (Con A), and pokeweed (PWM) by mononuclear cells from all but two. In contrast, lymphocyte proliferative responses to the antigens *Candida albicans* and tetanus toxoid have been absent or very low in all tested, when compared to simultaneous dose–response and time–course study results in normal control subjects (Table 6). Since antigen-induced proliferation of lymphocytes is considered to be primarily by thymus-dependent (T) cells, mixed lymphocyte culture studies were conducted in eight of the author's patients to further evaluate their capacity to mount a specific T-cell response. In support of an abnormality in specific immune responsiveness in this syndrome, an inability of patients' lymphocytes to proliferate when stimulated by mitomycin-C-treated mononuclear cells from one or more genetically different members of their own

TABLE 6. Studies of Cellular Immunity in Nine Patients with the Hyper-IgE Syndrome

	In vivo		*In vitro*: Percent of normal[a] proliferation to				
Patient	Candida	SK-SD	PHA	ConA	PWM	Candida	Tetanus
RB	–	–	67.84	89.24	81.48	0	0
AY	+	–	38.68	46.15	47.40	1.16	0
CC	–	–	76.45	85.75	77.50	0.46	0
TF	–	+	104.82	70.43	116.66	—	17.18
AT	–	–	102.28	103.29	105.57	0	13.69
LH	+	+	275.9	162.60	396.85	0	–
JB	+	+	105.85	93.94	158.69	0	0
DS	+	+	130.59	168.66	215.82	38.57	0
SE	–	–	94.51	49.33	51.85	0	0

[a]Normalized values were computed using the following formula:

$$\text{response} = \frac{\text{cpm (stimulated)} - \text{cpm (unstimulated) patient} \times 100}{\text{cpm (stimulated)} - \text{cpm (unstimulated) normal control}}$$

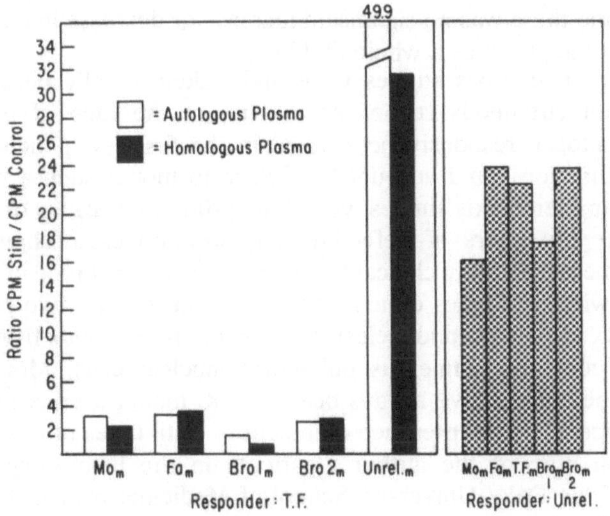

Figure 5. Results of mixed leukocyte culture studies with mononuclear blood cells from a patient (TF) with the hyper-IgE syndrome. Sources of responding cells are indicated on the abscissa, as are the sources of the mitomycin-C-treated stimulating cells. The patient's cells failed to respond to cells from the genetically different members of his family but responded briskly to those from an unrelated normal control. The effectiveness of the various stimulator cells in stimulating the unrelated control's cells is shown in the right panel. From Buckley and Becker (1978).

families has been found in six of eight evaluated (Figure 5). In contrast, lymphocytes from five of the six exhibiting unresponsiveness in intrafamilial mixed leukocyte cultures proliferated vigorously when stimulated by unrelated mitomycin-C-treated mononuclear cells. This disparate response could be explained on the basis of striking antigenic differences between the related and unrelated stimulator cells or by differences in the functional capacities of the monocytes in the two mixed cell populations. HLA-A and -B locus typing has been done on eight of the author's patients and their first-degree relatives. No unusual antigens

TABLE 7. HLA-A and -B Locus Antigens in Eight Patients with the Hyper-IgE Syndrome

Patient	Antigens
RB	3,5/10,5
AY	1,40/w28,?
CC	3,17/w24,w35
TF	2,12/2,15
AT	11,5/1,12
LH	w30,7/w31,40
JB	2,40/?,13
SE	26,w21/w31,40

were found, and there was no significant increase or decrease in any of the antigen frequencies in the group as a whole (Table 7).

Monocyte chemotaxis studies were undertaken initially because of the impaired delayed cutaneous responses *in vivo* in the face of normal *in vitro* lymphocyte mitogen responsiveness noted in the first few patients. A defect in effector cell function could account for failure to mount such a response. Polymorphonuclear chemotaxis studies were done primarily because of the abovementioned reports by others of defective polymorphonuclear chemotaxis in this disorder, not because of any clinical features to suggest that type of defect. Indeed, Rebuck skin window studies done by the author in the first two patients showed a normal influx of polymorphonuclear cells, and purulent fluids from infected sites have always contained numerous polymorphonuclear cells. Moreover, patients followed by the author have always been able to mount a brisk peripheral blood neutrophil response in the presence of infection. Both types of chemotaxis studies were done on nine of the author's patients in the laboratory of Dr. Ralph Snyderman of the Duke University School of Medicine; over half of the patients have had studies done on more than one occasion. The results can be summarized by saying that only three of the nine patients have had consistent depressions of either polymorphonuclear or mononuclear chemotaxis (one of each type and one with both). In some patients demonstrating defective chemotaxis, repeat studies were normal and there appeared to be no correlation of the abnormality with drug intake or the presence or absence of infection. Plasma from some but not all of these patients has been noted to inhibit chemotaxis of normal control monocytes. As noted above, the significance of these and other abnormal chemotactic features is far from clear, but the fact that they are not present in every patient makes it almost certain that chemotactic abnormalities do not represent the basic problem in these patients.

Studies of total hemolytic complement activity have been carried out in virtually all patients described with this disorder and have all been normal. In addition, the first two patients had quantitative measurements of each of the nine complement components and these were also all normal (Buckley *et al.*, 1972). Serum from each of the patients studied has been capable of generating C5a chemotactic factor normally.

Studies of phagocytic cell ingestion, metabolism, and killing have been normal in all of the patients evaluated by the author and in those reported in the literature. Because of clinical histories so strongly resembling those of patients with chronic granulomatous disease of childhood (CGD), these were among the first tests to be done. They have included studies of nitroblue tetrazolium dye reduction, hexose monophosphate shunt activity, phagocytic capacity, bacterial killing capacity, and chemiluminescence.

Histological sections of lymph nodes, spleen, and lung cysts obtained from surgery on several of these patients have all been unique in their striking degree of tissue eosinophilia. This was particularly true in the spleen of one boy who underwent splenectomy because of traumatic rupture and in the wall of a giant lung cyst excised from another patient. Hassall's corpuscles and normal thymic architecture were observed at postmortem examination of one patient.

A summary of the major immunological features of these patients is presented in Table 8.

TABLE 8. Major Immunological Features of 20 Patients with the Hyper-IgE Syndrome

Markedly elevated IgE; IgD also elevated in a majority; other immunoglobulins may be elevated but are usually normal.
Positive immediate wheal-and-flare reactions to a variety of food, inhalant, bacterial, and fungal antigens.
Eosinophilia in blood and sputum.
Impaired anamnestic (IgG) antibody responses.
Depressed cell-mediated immunity to ubiquitous antigens *in vivo* in one-half and to specific antigens *in vitro* in all studied. Responses to mitogens are normal, as are lymphocyte subpopulations.
Abnormal intrafamilial mixed leukocyte responses in 6/8 studied.
Highly variable chemotactic abnormalities (only 3/9 studied have had consistent depressions of polymorphonuclear or monocyte chemotaxis); plasma inhibitors of monocyte chemotaxis in some.

3.5.3. Treatment

Since the primary defect in these patients is unknown, no definitive therapy is available. The most successful therapy consists of lifelong chronic dicloxacillin therapy to prevent staphylococcal infections, by far the most frequent clinical problems. If pneumatocoeles form and persist for more than 6 months, surgical excision should be strongly considered, since the cysts tend to enlarge with time and compress adjacent normal lung as well as become infected with other organisms, leading to lung abscesses and fungus balls (Figure 3). Cutaneous abscesses rarely occur when patients receive dicloxacillin regularly, but if furuncles do form, incision and drainage are usually necessary. Immunostimulants such as transfer factor and levamisole have been used in some of these patients prior to their being referred to the author. No patients experienced any measurable benefit from such agents, and, in some, deterioration occurred during these treatments as a result of failure to administer dicloxacillin or to intervene surgically when needed.

3.5.4. Prognosis

If this disorder is recognized early in life and the patient is kept on chronic dicloxacillin therapy, the prognosis is quite good. Several such patients have reached maturity, indicating that the defect is compatible with life into adulthood. If the diagnosis is not made early in life, however, chronic lung disease may develop and problems with infectious agents other than staphylococci, such as *Hemophilus influenzae,* candida, and aspergillus, become more frequent. Putrid lung abscesses may develop within the persistent cystic lung cavities, and aspergilloma formation with accompanying massive hemoptysis may occur. The latter can lead to sudden death. One patient in the author's series developed Hodgkin's disease at age 19; this is the only known case of malignancy to have developed in this disorder thus far.

3.5.5. Potential Immunosuppressive Action of Excess IgE Antibody

The possibility has been suggested by Hill and Quie (1974) that patients with augmented IgE production might have depression of other types of immune function secondary to the chronic release of histamine by IgE antigen–antibody reactions. They proposed that the histamine so released could interact with H-2 receptors on leukocytes to effect an increase in intracellular cyclic 3′,5′-adenosine monophosphate, resulting in an overall antiinflammatory effect. In support of their postulate, they reported that histamine in concentrations of 10^{-3} and 10^{-5} M caused significant inhibition of polymorphonuclear chemotactic responsiveness. However, this finding could not be confirmed by Snyderman *et al.* (1977), who also failed to find inhibition of monocyte chemotaxis in the presence of histamine in concentrations ranging from 10^{-3} to 10^{-8} M. A more attractive hypothesis to the author is that the other immunological abnormalities found are related to whatever the as yet undefined primary defect is in such patients, which in turn may also be responsible for their tendency to have augmented IgE synthesis.

4. References

Ammann, A. J., Cain, W. A., Ishizaka, K,, Hong, R., and Good, R. A., 1969, Immunoglobulin E deficiency in ataxia-telangiectasia, *N. Engl. J. Med.* **281**:469–472.

Berglund, G., Finnstrom, O., Johansson, S. G. O., and Moller, K. L., 1968, Wiskott-Aldrich syndrome: A study of 6 cases with determination of the immunoglobulins A, D, G, M, and ND, *Acta Paediatr. Scand.* **57**:89–97.

Blaese, R. M., Strober, W., Levy, A. L., and Waldmann, T. A., 1971, Hypercatabolism of IgG, IgA, IgM and albumin in the Wiskott-Aldrich syndrome: A unique disorder of serum protein metabolism, *J. Clin. Invest.* **50**:2331–2338.

Blum, R., Geller, G., and Fish, L. A., 1977, Recurrent severe staphylococcal infections, eczematoid rash, extreme elevation of IgE, eosinophilia and divergent chemotactic responses in two generations, *J. Pediatr.* **90**:607–609.

Buckley, R. H., 1974, Allergic eczema, in: *Brenneman's Practice of Pediatrics,* Vol. II, Harper and Row, Hagerstown, Md.

Buckley, R. H., 1975, Clinical and immunologic features of selective IgA deficiency, in: *Immunodeficiency in Man and Animals* (D. Bergsma, R. A. Good, J. Finstad, and N. W. Paul, eds.), pp. 134–142, Sinauer Associates, Sunderland, Mass.

Buckley, R. H., 1979, Hyperimmunoglobulinemia E, undue susceptibility of infection, and depressed immunologic function, in: *Pediatric Immunology* (B. N. Kagan and H. Hodes, eds.), Science and Medicine Publishing, New York.

Buckley, R. H., and Becker, W. G., 1978, Abnormalities in the regulation of human IgE synthesis, *Immunol. Reviews* **41**:288–314.

Buckley, R. H., and Dees, S. C., 1969, Correlation of milk precipitins with IgA deficiency, *N. Engl. J. Med.* **281**:465–469.

Buckley, R. H., and Fiscus, S. A., 1975, Serum IgD and IgE concentrations in immunodeficiency diseases, *J. Clin. Invest.* **55**:157–165.

Buckley, R. H., Wray, B. B., and Belmaker, E. Z., 1972, Extreme hyperimmunoglobulinemia E and undue susceptibility to infection, *Pediatrics* **49**:59–70.

Butterworth, A. E., Remold, H. G., Houba, U., David, J. R., Franks, D., David, P. H., and Sturrock, R. F., 1977, Antibody-dependent eosinophil-mediated damage to ^{51}Cr-labelled schistosomula of *Schistosoma mansoni:* Mediation by IgG and inhibition by antigen-antibody complexes, *J. Immunol.* **118**:2230–2236.

Caplin, J. A., Capriles, A., Straub, D. L., Neiburger, J. B., Wilkinson, J. H., and Dockhorn, R. J., 1977, Allergy in the Wiskott-Aldrich syndrome: A case report, *Ann. Allergol.* **39**:43–44.

Capron, A., Dessaint, J.-P., Capron, M., and Bazin, H., 1975, Specific IgE antibodies in immune adherence of normal macrophages to *Schistosoma mansoni* schistosomules, *Nature (London)* **253**:474–475.

Capron, A., Dessaint, J.-P., Joseph, M., Torpier, G., Capron, M., Rousslaux, R., Santoro, F., and Bazin, H., 1977, IgE and cells in schistosomiasis, *Am. J. Trop. Med. Hyg.* **26**:39–47.

Church, J. A., Frenkel, L. D., Wright, D. G., and Bellanti, J. A., 1976, T lymphocyte dysfunction, hyperimmunoglobulinemia E, recurrent bacterial infections, and defective neutrophil chemotaxis in a Negro child, *J. Pediatr.* **88:**982–985.

Clark, R. A., Root, R. K., Kimball, H. R., and Kirkpatrick, C. H., 1973, Defective neutrophil chemotaxis and cellular immunity in a child with recurrent infections, *Ann. Intern. Med.* **78:**515–519.

Cooper, M. D., Chase, H. P., Lowman, J. T., Krivit, W., and Good, R. A., 1968, Wiskott-Aldrich syndrome: An immunologic deficiency disease involving the afferent limb of immunity, *Am. J. Med.* **44:**499–513.

Dahl, M. V., Greene, W. G., and Quie, P. G., 1976, Infection, dermatitis, increased IgE and impaired neutrophil chemotaxis, *Arch. Dermatol.* **112:**1387–1390.

Davis, S. D., Schaller, J., and Wedgwood, R. J., 1966, Job's syndrome: Recurrent "cold," staphylococcal abscesses, *Lancet* **1:**1013–1015.

DiGeorge, A. M., 1968, Congenital absence of the thymus and its immunologic consequences: Concurrence with congenital hypoparathyroidism, in: *Immunologic Deficiency Diseases in Man* (D. Bergsma, ed.), pp. 116–123, National Foundation Press, White Plains, N.Y.

Dineen, J. K., Ogilvie, B. M., and Kelly, J. D., 1973, Expulsion of *Nippostrongylus brasilienses* from the intestine of rats: Collaboration between humoral and cellular components of the immune response, *Immunology* **24:**467–475.

Epstein, L. B., and Ammann, A. J., 1974, Evaluation of T lymphocyte effector function in immunodeficiency diseases: Abnormality in mitogen-stimulated interferon production in patients with selective IgA deficiency, *J. Immunol.* **112:**617–626.

Fontan, G., Lorente, F., Garcia Rodriguez, M. C., and Ojeda, J. A., 1976, Defective neutrophil chemotaxis and hyperimmunoglobulinemia E—a reversible defect? *Acta Pediatr. Scand.* **65:**509–511.

Giblett, E. R., Ammann, A. J., Wara, D. W., Sandman, R., and Diamond, L. K., 1975, Nucleoside phosphorylase deficiency in a child with severely defective T cell immunity and normal B cell immunity, *Lancet* **1:**1010–1013.

Goldfarb, A. A., and Fundenberg, H., 1961, Hypogammaglobulinemia and its relationship to the allergic diathesis, *N. Y. J. Med.* **61:**2721–2731.

Green, R. L., Scales, R. W., and Kraus, S. J., 1976, Increased serum immunoglobulin E concentrations in venereal diseases, *Br. J. Vener. Dis.* **52:**257–260.

Hill, H. R., and Quie, P. G., 1974, Raised serum IgE levels and defective neutrophil chemotaxis in three children with eczema and recurrent bacterial infections, *Lancet* **1:**183–187.

Hill, H. R., Ochs, H. D., Quie, P. G., Clark, R. A., Pabst, H. F., Klebanoff, S. J., and Wedgwood, R. J., Defect in neutrophil granulocyte chemotaxis in Job's syndrome of recurrent "cold" staphylococcal abscesses, *Lancet* **2:**617–619.

Hill, H. R., Estensen, R. D., Hogan, N. A., and Quie, P. G., 1976a, Severe staphylococcal disease associated with allergic manifestations, hyperimmunoglobulinemia E and defective neutrophil chemotaxis, *J. Lab. Clin. Invest.* **88:**796–806.

Hill, H. R., Williams, P. B., Krueger, G. G., and Janis, B., 1976b, Recurrent staphylococcal abscesses associated with defective neutrophil chemotaxis and allergic rhinitis, *Ann. Intern. Med.* **85:**39–43.

Hill, H. R., Book, L. S., Hemming, V. G., and Herbst, J. J., 1977, Defective neutrophil chemotactic responses in patients with recurrent episodes of otitis media and chronic diarrhea, *Am. J. Dis. Child.* **131:**433–436.

Huntley, C. C., and Dees, S. C., 1957, Eczema associated with thrombocytopenic purpura and purulent otitis media: Report of five fatal cases, *Pediatrics* **19:**351–361.

Iio, A. Strober, W., Broder, S., Polmar, S. H., and Waldmann, T. A., 1977, The metabolism of IgE in patients with immunodeficiency states and neoplastic conditions, *J. Clin. Invest.* **59:**743–755.

Ishizaka, K., and Ishizaka, T., 1970, Biological function of γE antibodies and mechanisms of reaginic hypersensitivity, *Clin. Exp. Immunol.* **6:**25–42.

Jacobs, J. C., and Norman, M. C., 1977, A familial defect of neutrophil chemotaxis with asthma, eczema, and recurrent skin infections, *Pediatr. Res.* **11:**732–736.

Johansson, S. G. O., Mellbin, T., and Vahlquist, B., 1968, Immunoglobulin levels in Ethiopian preschool children with special reference to high concentrations of immunoglobulin E (IgND), *Lancet* **1:**1118–1121.

Jones, H. E., Reinhardt, J. H., and Rinaldi, M. G., 1974, Immunologic susceptibility to chronic dermatophytosis, *Arch. Dermatol.* **110**:213–220.

Kikkawa, Y., Kamimura, K., Hamajjima, T., Sekiguichi, T., Kawai, T., Takenada, M., and Tada, T., 1973, Thymic alymphoplasia with hyper-IgE-globulinemia, *Pediatrics* **51**:690–696.

Levy, D. A., and Chen, J., 1970, Healthy IgE-deficient person, *N. Engl. J. Med.* **283**:541–542.

Lischner, H. W., and Huff, D. S., 1975, T cell deficiency in DiGeorge syndrome, in: *Immunodeficiency in Man and Animals* (D. Bergsma, R. A. Good, J. Finstad, and N. W. Paul, eds.), pp.16–21, Sinauer Associates, Sunderland, Mass.

Nezelof, C., 1968, Thymic dysplasia with normal immunoglobulins and immunologic deficiency: Pure alymphocytosis, in: *Immunologic Deficiency Diseases in Man* (D. Bergsma, ed.), pp. 104–115, National Foundation Press, White Plains, N.Y.

Okumura, K., and Tada, T., 1971a, Regulation of homocytotropic antibody formation in the rat. III. Effect of thymectomy and splenectomy, *J. Immunol.* **106**:1019–1026.

Okumura, K., and Tada, T., 1971b, Regulation of homocytotropic antibody formation in the rat. VI. Inhibitory effect of thymocytes on the homocytotropic antibody response, *J. Immunol.* **107**:1682–1689.

Peterson, R. D. A., Page, A. R., and Good, R. A., 1962, Wheal and erythema allergy in patients with agammaglobulinemia, *J. Allergy* **33**:406–411.

Pincus, S. H., Thomas, I. T., Clark, R. A., and Ochs, H. D., 1975, Defective neutrophil chemotaxis with variant ichthyosis, hyperimmunoglobulinemia E, and recurrent infections, *J. Pediatr.* **87**:908–911.

Polmar, S. H., Waldmann, T. A., Balestra, S. T., Jost, M. C., and Terry, W. D., 1972a, Immunoglobulin E in immunologic deficiency diseases. I. Relation of IgE and IgA to respiratory tract disease in isolated IgE deficiency, IgA deficiency, and ataxia telangiectasia, *J. Clin. Invest.* **51**:326–330.

Polmar, S. H., Waldmann, T. A., and Terry, W. D., 1972b, IgE in immunodeficiency, *Am. J. Pathol.* **69**:499–512.

Reed, W. B., Epstein, W. L., Boder, E., and Sedgewick, R., 1966, Cutaneous manifestations of ataxia-telangiectasia, *Am. Med. Assoc.* **195**:746–753.

Schiff, R. I., Buckley, R. H., Gilbertsen, R. B., and Metzgar, R. S., 1974, Membrane receptors and *in vitro* responsiveness of lymphocytes in human immunodeficiency, *J. Immunol.* **112**:376–386.

Schwartz, D. P., and Buckley, R. H., 1971, Serum IgE concentrations and skin reactivity to anti-IgE antibody in IgA-deficient patients, *N. Engl. J. Med.* **284**:513–517.

Snyderman, R., Altman, L. C., Frankel, A., and Blaese, R. M., 1973, Defective mononuclear leukocyte chemotaxis: A previously unrecognized immune dysfunction. Studies in a patient with chronic mucocutaneous candidiasis, *Ann. Intern. Med.* **78**:509–513.

Snyderman, R., Rogers, E., and Buckley, R. H., 1977, Abnormalities of leukotaxis in atopic dermatitis, *J. Allerg. Clin. Immunol.* **60**:121–126.

Tada, T., and Ishizaka, K., 1970, Distribution of γE-forming cells in lymphoid tissues of the human and monkey, *J. Immunol.* **104**:377–387.

Tada, T., and Okumura, K., 1971, Regulation of homocytotropic antibody formation in the rat. V. Cell cooperation in the anti-hapten homocytotropic antibody response, *J. Immunol.* **107**:1137–1145.

Tada, T., Taniguichi, M., and Okumura, K., 1971, Regulation of homocytotropic antibody formation in the rat. II. Effect of X-irradiation, *J. Immunol.* **106**:1012–1018.

Taniguchi, M., and Tada, T., 1971, Regulation of homocytotropic antibody formation in the rat. IV. Effects of various immunosuppressive drugs, *J. Immunol.* **107**:579–585.

Van der Giessen, M., Reerink-Brongers, E. E., and Veen, T. A., 1976, Quantitation of Ig classes and IgG subclasses in sera of patients with a variety of immunoglobulin deficiencies and their relatives, *Clin. Immunol. Immunopathol.* **5**:388–398.

Van Scoy, R. E., Hill, H. R., Ritts, R. E., and Quie, P. G., 1975, Familial neutrophil chemotaxis defect, recurrent bacterial infections, mucocutaneous candidiasis, and hyperimmunoglobulinemia E, *Ann. Intern. Med.* **82**:766–771.

Vyas, G. N., and Fudenberg, H. H., 1974, Immunobiology of human IgA: A serologic and immunogenetic study of immunization to IgA in transfusion and pregnancy, *Clin. Genet.* **1**:45–64.

Vyas, G. N., Perkins, H. A., and Fudenberg, H. H., 1968, Anaphylactoid transfusion reactions associated with anti-IgA, *Lancet* **2**:312–315.

Waldmann, T. A., Polmar, S. H., Balestra, S. T., Jost, M. C., Bruce, R. M., and Terry, W. D., 1972, Immunoglobulin E in immunologic deficiency diseases. II. Serum IgE concentration of patients with acquired hypogammaglobulinemia, thymoma and hypogammaglobulinemia, myotonic dystrophy, intestinal lymphangiectasia, and Wiskott-Aldrich syndrome, *J. Immunol.* **109**:304–310.

Weston, W. L., Humbert, J. R., August, C. S., Harnett, J., Mass, M. F., Dean, P. B., and Hagan, I. M., 1977, A hyperimmunoglobulin E syndrome with normal chemotaxis *in vitro* and defective leukotaxis *in vivo*, *J. Allerg. Clin. Immunol.* **59**:112–119.

Witemeyer, S., and Van Epps, D., 1976, A familial defect in cellular chemotaxis associated with redheadedness and recurrent infection, *J. Pediatr.* **89**:33–37.

16

Hypersensitivity Vasculitis: The Acute Phase of Leukocytoclastic (Necrotizing) Lesions

W. E. PARISH

1. Properties of Complexes and Immune-Complex-Mediated Responses

1.1. Introduction: Arthus-Like Responses and Vasculitis

There is no inflammatory event in which blood vessels do not participate. There are few allergic responses in which changes in blood vessels are not the main histological feature, as in anaphylaxis, Arthus responses, delayed hypersensitivity, and some cytotoxic reactions. A consideration of "hypersensitivity vasculitis" in the widest interpretation of the term is a review of allergic responses, but the designation tends to be restricted to vasculitis resulting from Arthus or the Arthus-like immune-complex-mediated disorders.

The classical Arthus response results from the local injection of antigen that binds with precipitating antibody to form complexes that activate the complement system. Among the several properties of complement is the release of fragments that are chemoattractant for neutrophils. The neutrophils while ingesting the complexes release the lysosomal enzymes that mediate much of the tissue damage, resulting in the characteristic histological features—the characteristic lesion being a severe infiltration by neutrophils which degenerate leaving remnants and fine particles of DNA, leukocyte-platelet thrombi, fibrinoid necrosis, and disruption of the basement membrane and elastic lamina of larger vessels.

W. E. PARISH • Environmental Safety Division, Unilever Research, Sharnbrook, Bedfordshire, England.

The essential requirements for the reaction are precipitating antibody, complement, and neutrophils. Tissue changes occur in animals depleted of complement or neutrophils, but there is no acute vasculitis. The severity of the reaction depends much on the amounts of antigen and antibody, their relative proportions, and the nature of the antigen.

Responses due to deposition of immune complexes from the blood may be considered to be a modified form of generalized Arthus phenomenon, but the potential of the complexes to induce tissue damage is more restricted. The antigen needs to be in slight to moderate excess of equivalence to antibody, and the complexes have to be above a critical size and present in sufficient amount. The affinity of the antibody for antigen influences the biological activity; complexes containing firm-binding antibody tend to be quickly and harmlessly removed, whereas complexes containing weakly binding antibody appear to be associated with tissue disorders. Circulating complexes are frequently found in most persons if sufficiently sensitive methods are used to detect them, but they are quickly and harmlessly removed. Complexes will induce vasculitis only if they are deposited in sufficient amount beneath the endothelium, and this results from increased vascular permeability which could be stimulated by anaphylactic sensitivity to the antigen of the complex, by anaphylatoxin fragments of activated complement, or by processes unrelated to the particular complex.

Reactions induced by complexes are not confined to deposition of preformed complexes in the blood. They may also occur when circulating antibody binds with antigen previously deposited in or autologous antigen exposed in the susceptible tissue, and also may be formed when antibody is locally synthesized to persist as cell-bound antibody to react with circulating or locally released antigen.

Small amounts of immune complexes are frequently formed in normal persons, contributing to the rapid removal of exogenous substances ingested, inhaled, or absorbed through the skin or to clearance of commensal or weakly infective bacteria and viruses. In persons with damaged tissues the amounts of the complexes in the blood are much increased and more readily detectable. The antigens may be exogenous from infecting organisms or endogenous (organ specific or nonspecific) from the damaged tissue (see Table 3). Drugs used in treatment increase the potential for circulating complexes as haptens or antigens or make vessels more susceptible to deposition by affecting platelets, mast cells, or the endothelium. They may also suppress some of the natural inhibitors of inflammation and thereby enhance the tissue damage. Changes in immunoglobulin and formation of complexes induce synthesis of rheumatoid-type antiglobulins which modify existing antigen–antibody complexes or form new complexes of immunoglobulins (e.g., IgG–anti-IgG) and complement only. These may fortuitously bind other substances, e.g., DNA, either by mechanical trapping or because part of the complexed immunoglobulin is anti-DNA antibody.

It appears that most circulating complexes in patients with chronic diseases are removed harmlessly, and although they may have a potential to cause tissue damage there is no evidence that they do so. In some patients, however, the complexes contribute to further tissue damage, particularly in the skin, kidney, joints, and, experimentally in rabbits, the heart. The blood vessels are most susceptible to the activity of immune complexes in the skin, but in some disorders, as in systemic lupus erythematosus or dermatitis herpetiformis, the damage associated with the complexes is more widespread. Rheumatoid arthritis is an excellent example of a disorder affecting several organs and tissues, and in which there are many immunological abnormalities, some of which contribute to the tissue damage. Immune complexes are formed and may contain rheumatoid factors and anti-DNA antibodies, which are synthesized in many patients, especially those with extraarticular lesions. Although much research has been done on the properties of the complexes, there is no definite evidence that they initiate the cutaneous lesions.

There are a large number of clinical designations for cutaneous vasculitis, but several of the disorders, although differing in clinical manifestations, probably have a similar etiology. When parts of the same lesion, or lesions of different duration in the same patient, are examined, a considerable variation in histological features is observed, and evidence of complexes is not confined to any particular stage of lesion development. Until the differences in clinical signs can be related to differences in causation, in the laboratory there is much to recommend the grouping together of acute mainly neutrophil-infiltrated lesions as leukocytoclastic or necrotizing vasculitis and the grouping of mainly mononuclear cell-infiltrated lesions separately.

This chapter presents a brief description of immune complex mediated reactions and the presence of immunoglobulins and complement in human cutaneous vasculitis, and considers the possible identity of the antigens forming the complexes.

1.2. Properties of Immune Complexes in Relation to Tissue Damage

There are several reviews (e.g., Weigle, 1961; Ishizaka, 1963) from which may be obtained references to much of the detail concerning the relation of immune complexes and tissue damage.

Immune complexes are formed of one or more molecules of antigen combining with one or more molecules of antibody. When formed *in vitro* a mixture of complexes containing free antigen determinants may interact with Fab portion of antibody to form visible aggregates, floccules, or precipitates. Complexes formed of the appropriate antibodies fix and activate complement components, so the complexes acquire greater mass due to the complement components, C1q and C3b determinants which modify the activity of the complex. Rheumatoid factors and other anti-IgG antibodies may enlarge the complexes, make soluble complexes insoluble, convert non-complement-fixing to complement-fixing complexes, and when forming larger aggregates combine with complexes containing antibody of other antigenic specificities. Furthermore, other substances may be trapped in the lattice of the complexes, e.g., DNA, lipoprotein, or viral particles.

The class or subclass of immunoglobulin modifies the activity of the complexes, particularly those that bind and activate complement, as in human IgM, IgG_1, IgG_3, and weakly by IgG_2. The affinity of the antibody is also important. Complexes with firm-binding antibody are readily removed if there is sufficient antibody in the complex. Weak-binding antibodies, particularly those that tend to dissociate and reassociate with antigen, may form tissue-damaging complexes if deposited within tissues, but are not bound well by macrophage receptors preliminary to ingestion. Size is also an important influence on biological activity of complexes inducing tissue damage, which have to be 19 S or greater as determined by the ultracentrifuge.

Several other properties influence the biological activity of complexes. These include the nature of the antigen, particularly differences between low molecular weight proteins forming sharply defined equivalence points and polysaccharides and viruses forming broad zones of equivalence. Also, the number of antigenic determinants and their availability to the antibodies to form a lattice determine their susceptibility to form complexes or larger aggregates.

Complexes vary in ratios of antigen to antibody, and the composition of the complex has much influence on their biological activities (Figure 1). Complexes formed in extreme antigen excess with the composition 1Ag:1Ab or 2Ag:1Ab are soluble with little biological activity unless subsequently modified by rheumatoid factors. They do not fix complement, for which two or more antibody molecules have to be bound in the complex. In moderate antigen excess of antibody, e.g., in complexes of 3Ag:2Ab or 2Ag:2Ab, complement is bound by the appropriate classes of antibody, which is sufficient to attract neutrophils when the complexes are deposited in blood vessel walls or other tissues. However, there are only few Fc or C3b moieties to bind to macrophages or neutrophils capable of ingesting the complexes, and therefore such complexes are not removed quickly from the circulation and have the most potential to induce tissue damage. At equivalence of antigen and antibody the maximum amount of complement is fixed for that particular system, and although such complexes are likely to be removed more quickly than those formed in antigen excess they still have much potential for tissue damage. Complexes found in antibody excess of equivalence of antigen fix less complement than those at equivalence but have many more Fc groups to bind to leukocyte receptors. They are therefore quickly removed.

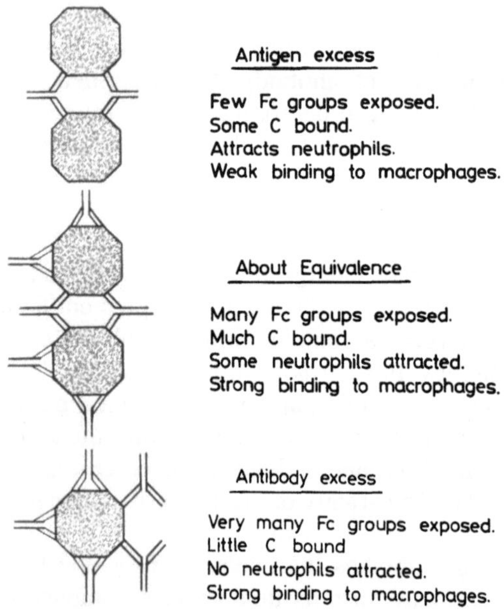

Figure 1. Properties of complexes with varying Ag:Ab ratios.

The tissue-damaging complexes are those in slight to moderate antigen excess of antibody. There is thus inadequate antibody, either because of antigen remaining in excess while the antibody is being first synthesized or because of partial immune deficiency causing the individual to fail to respond adequately to the antigenic stimulus.

Complexes may bind to several types of cell, which results either in release of tissue-damaging pharmacological substances or in their harmless removal. Complexes with IgG_1 IgG_2, IgG_3, and IgG_4 will bind to platelets, causing aggregation and release of lysosomal substances, histamine, and serotonin. The complement determinants C3a and C5a will bind to basophils, mediating release of their vasoactive substances and a platelet activating factor. Neutrophils bind and ingest complexes containing IgG_1 and IgG_3. This may result in some degradation of the complex, but the lysosomal enzymes are released which degrade tissues and also increase vascular permeability directly or by stimulating release of mediators from mast cells. The monocyte phagocytic cell system in the liver and several other organs is most effective at the harmless removal of complexes, but it is possible that C3b reacting with the macrophage receptors stimulates release of more complement and proteolytic enzymes that mediate local tissue damage. This is more likely to occur in macrophages present within lesions rather than in the normal histiocytic macrophages, e.g., Kupffer cells of the liver. Lymphocyte activities are also modified by immune complexes. T-cell functions may be suppressed, and although of possible significance in responses to tumors, the occurrence of such suppression in immune complex disorders is yet to be ascertained. B-cell activity also appears to be decreased for a short time, but the binding of antigen in the complex may also enhance subsequent antibody formation.

The activity of antibody in classical serum sickness is analogous to the precipitation curve with formation of immune complexes from the antigen excess to the antibody excess of equivalence. Antigen that persists in the circulation and stimulates formation of antibody binds with the first-formed antibody, resulting in complexes in antigen excess of equivalence of antibody. With further formation of antibody, complexes contain antibody in excess of antigen, and they are quickly removed. Removal of the complexes and degradation or excretion of the antigen are accompanied by healing of the lesions.

1.3. Increased Vascular Permeability and Deposition of Complexes

As stated in the introduction, immune complexes are being formed continually and may be detected in small amounts in serum of normal persons. These are quickly and harmlessly removed. Vasculitis occurs only when complexes greater than a critical size, in sufficient amount, become deposited beneath the endothelium. For this to occur there must be increased vascular permeability and some separation of the endothelium, permitting penetration of the complexes. Once beneath the endothelium the complexes usually accumulate along the internal elastic lamina or the basement membrane according to the size and type of vessel.

Many mediators or tissue changes may lead to increased vascular permeability predisposing to the deposition of complexes. These include histamine and kinins active in anaphylaxis, complement anaphylatoxin products that also mediate release of pharmacologically active substances from mast cells, bacterial endotoxins that may act directly on the endothelium or activate complement, bacterial exotoxins, lymphocyte products of delayed hypersensitivity, trauma, the postinflammatory state of healed vascular lesions, and several others.

Histamine and other vasoactive amines, anaphylatoxin, and drugs releasing histamine when injected locally, or passive anaphylaxis induced locally, have all been shown to mediate increased vascular permeability and deposition of complexes beneath the endothelium of venules.

Pretreatment with antihistamine prevented the increased vascular permeability, and also deposition of complexes (Manjo and Palade, 1961; Cochrane, 1963a,b). Similarly in the more generalized immune complex disease in rabbits, immune complexes were deposited only if there was a concurrent increased vascular permeability (Kniker and Cochrane, 1968).

Mast cells and basophils contain most of the histamine that is likely to induce vascular changes, and its release is usually associated with an IgE antibody-mediated anaphylactic reaction. This is consistent with the urticarial rashes or occasionally morbilliform or erythematous rashes that occurred in the early stages of serum sickness responses to horse globulins, in which the IgE antibody was specific for an impurity if not the globulin itself. In the generalized reaction such changes were sufficient to prepare vessels for deposition of the circulating complexes in organs at risk. It is possible to find some patients, mainly nonatopic, with noniatrogenic, spontaneous, necrotizing vasculitis whose lesions are associated with urticaria, but in the majority of cases of spontaneous leukocytoclastic vasculitis there is no definite history of urticaria or of anaphylactic sensitivity, although the vasculitis is not infrequently preceded by an erythematous rash.

Anaphylactic sensitivity reactions may be of little consequence in preparing vessels for deposition of complexes leading to vasculitis disorders. In patients with spontaneous vasculitis we found no change in the total IgE; in those whose vasculitis followed bacterial infection, and in whom there was evidence of formation of bacterial antigen–antibody complexes, no antibacterial IgE antibody was found by biological tests (Parish, 1971d). Subsequent tests by RAST or direct tests on leukocytes have shown evidence of such IgE antibodies, but the amounts are considered to be insufficient in most cases to mediate significant anaphylactic changes in blood vessels.

Complement anaphylatoxin products are another potent histamine-releasing stimulus which could well occur in immune complex reactions. Complement activated by antigen–antibody complexes, or in a more specific instance by bacterial endotoxin, has cleaved from it the C3a and C5a anaphylatoxin fragments that release mast cell histamine. From mast cells these fragments are capable of releasing 20–30% of the available histamine, similar to the amount released by an IgE-mediated reaction (Johnson *et al.*, 1975). This occurs *in vitro* when human complement is activated to generate C3a and C5a by the classical or alternative sequences and used to treat human basophils as in an autologous system (Hook *et al.* 1975; Hook and Siraganian, 1977; Grant *et al.*, 1975). Some proteolytic enzymes, particularly chymotrypsin, also release histamine from mast cells, and it is possible that endogenous chymotrypsinlike enzymes have this activity *in vivo*. Examination of histological preparations shows that, in or near edematous exudates, mast cells show metachromasia, dispersion, and even solution of the granules. The infiltrating neutrophils also contribute to the inflammatory process a lysosome cationic polypeptide, designated "band 2," from rabbit cells that degranulates and releases histamine from mast cells. A similar substance has been found in human neutrophils (Kelly and White, 1973).

Initiation of increased vascular permeability by anaphylaxis or anaphylatoxin may be perpetuated by endogenous proteolytic enzymes and products from infiltrating neutrophils. The basophil also enhances vascular permeability indirectly when challenged IgE-sensitized basophils release a platelet-activating factor (PAF) that aggregates platelets, releasing vasoactive amines and generating a substance promoting coagulation (Benveniste *et al.*, 1972; Pinckard and Henson, 1977) and apparently preparing vessels for deposition of immune complexes (Benveniste, 1974). This factor amplifies or enhances the activity of two types of cells by cooperation, although their major activities are independent of each other.

Antigen–antibody complexes aggregate platelets, resulting in release of their vasoactive amines, partly by binding through the C3b receptors (in platelets of animals, although probably not those of man) and interaction with fibrinogen, but evidence is accumulating, as in a human platelet–zymosan complex system that the Fc of IgG, of all four subclasses, may contribute to the binding of the complex to the platelet membrane and its ensuing activation (Martin *et al.*, 1978) which may involve the later-binding complement components. There are at least two processes leading to the release of platelet histamine. One follows the cleavage of C3 during the binding of antigen with antibody which damages the platelet membrane to release histamine without platelet aggregation (Siraganian *et al.*, 1968). The second follows the interaction of preformed complexes and complement, resulting in aggregates that are ingested by the platelets and in release of lysosomal enzymes, ADP, histamine, and serotonin (Henson, 1970). Injection of preformed complexes into rabbits and guinea pigs reduces the number of platelets in the blood, especially when the complexes induce lesions. It has been further found that platelets accumulate in the lungs, with neutrophils and any eosinophils, following injection of complexes into animals which developed no vascular lesions; eventually the leukocytes and some of the platelets are released, while some platelets apparently disintegrate or are ingested by histiocytes. If lesions are induced by the complexes, the platelets accumulate at the sites (Parish, unpublished). This has some similarities with IgE-induced systemic anaphylaxis in rabbits, in which it was shown that platelets aggregated for a short time in vessels of several organs, particularly the lungs (Pinckard *et al.*, 1977). Further investigations are required to relate these findings to immune complex diseases. Apparently, at least in the rabbit, anaphylaxis or complexes result in aggregation of platelets; this is usually associated with release of their vasoactive substances. The aggregation is reversible, and some of the platelets return to the circulation. This may occur without evidence of deposition of immune complexes, and certainly without the onset of vasculitis.

Platelets are also aggregated, and tend to release their pharmacological substances by a variety of other agents that are also the products of inflammation, e.g., thrombin, prostaglandins, and adenosine diphosphate, and by contact with collagen. Some of these undoubtedly promote and exacerbate the changes resulting from the initial stimulus of deposition of complexes and infiltration by neutrophils, contributing to the histological changes observed in vasculitis.

Increased vascular permeability is a feature of delayed hypersensitivity, and that attributable to specific immunological reactivity occurs 6–12 hr after cutaneous antigen challenge and increases to become greatest at 18–24 hr; although declining in amount, it still remains increased above that at the control sites at 48 hr. There is a concomitant increase in the amount of fibrin accumulating at the site, which by 48 hr may show a twentyfold increase above that in the control tissue in guinea pigs (Colvin and Dvorak, 1975).

Another lymphocyte-mediated response increases vascular permeability as in cutaneous basophil hypersensitivity or the "Jones-Mote phenomenon." These erythematous, usually nonindurated lesions are mediated by lymphocytes with antigenic specificity, the activity of which is enhanced by basophils whose attraction and function appear not to be dependent on specific antibody but are controlled by the lymphocytes. In guinea pigs the duration of this type of hypersensitivity is usually considered to be short, and appears to be a transitional phase between a delayed-type lymphocyte-mediated hypersensitivity and formation of specific antibody, because subsequent challenges with antigen elicit a sequence of cutaneous anaphylaxis, Arthus response, and some basophil/lymphocyte participation (Colvin *et al.*, 1973). The dominant late feature is the Arthus response, and on appearance of significant amounts of antibody, cutaneous basophil hypersensitivity wanes. In the absence of formation of antibody, or in the presence of only small amounts, the basophil hypersensitivity may persist. The rate of onset and duration of increased vascular permeability in cutaneous basophil hypersensitivity are similar to those of delayed hypersensitivity, but the deposition of large amount of fibrin does not occur (Colvin and Dvorak, 1975). A phase is likely in which increased vascular permeability may be elicited when small amounts of antibody are free to form complexes with excess of antigen, and then the individual is very susceptible to immune complex disease.

A systemic form of cutaneous basophil hypersensitivity resulted in a maculopapular rash occurring after 6 hr and reaching a maximum intensity at 18–24 hr with the histological features of basophils, lymphocytes, and dilatation of superficial venules of the skin. The skin was much more susceptible than other organs (Dvorak *et al.*, 1977). This type of hypersensitivity could become a model not only of systemic rashes in man but also of the processes, not obviously IgE mediated, by which complexes are deposited to induce vasculitis. The special susceptibility of the skin is very relevant to spontaneous cutaneous vasculitis in man, in whom other organs are not noticeably affected.

There is some evidence that these studies on guinea pigs have a counterpart in man. Transient reactions have frequently been observed during immunization procedures. Human lyphocytes release a chemotactic factor for basophils, although this has not been separated from the factor attracting mononuclear cells (Lett-Brown *et al.*, 1976) or from a product of human mononuclear cell cultures that releases histamine from human basophils (Thueson *et al.*, 1977).

Consideration of mediators of increased vascular permeability should not be confined to endogenous substances, although these are undoubtedly the more frequent and potent. In some instances, however, bacterial exotoxins may also contribute to the vascular permeability, predisposing to deposition of bacterial antigens or to unrelated antigens in complexes. Virus infections may also be associated with such vascular changes. It has been shown that streptolysin O, streptococcal erythrogenic toxin, and diphtheria toxin induce vascular changes permitting deposition of complexes (Parish, 1970), and not all persons infected with organisms releasing the exotoxins form neutralizing antibody (Parish, 1971c). The amount of toxin is critical in experimental studies; a very high concentration permits deposition of complexes but also impedes leukocyte activity or is leukocidal. It is possible that the cutaneous changes in a streptococcal infection, even if clinically inapparent, will result in deposition of whatever complexes are present in the blood.

1.4. Sequence of Changes in Arthus-Type Reactions

The changes occurring in Arthus and immune-complex-mediated reactions have been well reviewed (Dixon, 1971; Cochrane and Koffler, 1973; Cochrane and Janoff, 1974).

The essential features are the formation of complexes of precipitating antibody and antigen, activation of complement, and attraction of neutrophils which release their proteolytic enzymes (Figure 2). In the classical Arthus reaction the antigen is injected. In immune complex disorders the circulating complexes are deposited beneath the endothelium or are formed locally in a prepared, susceptible tissue.

Following deposition beneath the endothelium, the constituents of the complexes can be detected near the internal elastic lamina, or near the basement membrane of small vessels, as fine granules or large aggregates, initially tending to be linear along the margin of the tissue layer, limiting further penetration, but later as irregular deposits probably dispersed by the phagocytes ingesting them and further diffusion following the degradation of the limiting tissues. The products of activated complement, C3a, C5a, and the complex $C\overline{567}$, attract neutrophils to the site, and in experimental animals depletion of complement results in persistence of the complexes for 96 hr or longer without the onset of acute vasculitis. However, mild changes can be induced in animals treated with cobra venom factor to deplete them of C3 to C9 activity, and therefore the full complement sequence is not essential. The infiltrating neutrophils ingest the complexes, resulting in release of their lysosomal enzymes, particularly the acidic proteases and elastase and

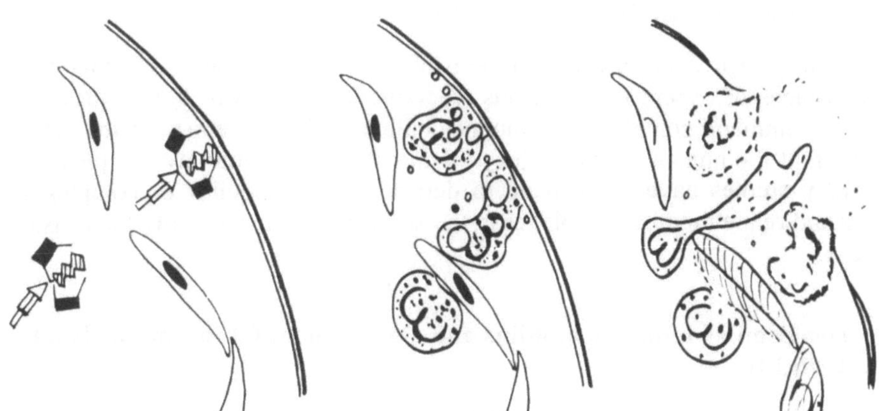

Figure 2. Diagrammatic representation of the Arthus response.

collagenase, at a pH optimum for the enzymes which mediate most of the tissue damage. These enzymes degrade the internal elastic lamina of larger and the basement membrane of smaller vessels. The enzymes deoxyribonuclease and ribonuclease probably contribute to the histological change.

More neutrophils are attracted into the compact tissue of the vessel walls, mediating further change, while the products of degenerated neutrophils accumulate to form the characteristic debris and nuclear "dust" giving rise to the term "leukocytoclastic vasculitis." Platelets continue to adhere to the damaged endothelium, participating in the formation of a thrombus, and degradation products of the vessel wall acquire the staining properties of fibrinoid changes.

Ingestion by neutrophils of protein–antigen–antibody complexes with complement results in their rapid degradation within 8 hr and complete or almost complete removal in 24–48 hr. Removal of this inducing stimulus reduces the neutrophil infiltration, and the infiltration by macrophages previously obscured become apparent. In the later stages of uncomplicated Arthus or immune-complex-induced reactions, the mononuclear cells accumulate, superficially resembling a delayed hypersensitivity reaction except that in the more severe responses there are increased numbers of plasma cells. Other mononuclear cells in the lesion are macrophages, fibroblasts, lymphocytes, and endothelial cells. The relative numbers of each cell type vary with the duration and rate of healing. This mononuclear cell response, according to its severity, regresses and the vessel heals.

The experimental lesion after a single inducing stimulus is transient, as are the Arthus or Arthus-like lesions occurring in man injected with appropriate antigens or in serum sickness resulting from therapy. The spontaneous vascular disorders have lesions with a similar histology to that of experimental lesions but tend to be persistent or show regression and recurrence. Despite the similarity in histology and the evidence of immune complexes in the lesions and blood, other mediators undoubtedly contribute to the spontaneous disease.

Chronic immune complex disease induced by daily injections of antigen sufficient to induce a transient antigen excess over antibody in rabbits results in glomerulonephritis with little involvement of the blood vessels.

2. Investigations of Human Vasculitis

The histological similarities of lesions of spontaneous vasculitis in man to the various stages of experimental Arthus reactions, together with the occurrence of circulating immune complexes, immunoglobulins, and complement in the lesions, indicate that the human vasculitis may be due to antigen–antibody complexes.

Many studies have been made to detect immunoglobulins or complexes in lesions and relate them to complexes in the serum in order to identify the causative antigens.

2.1. Detection of Immunoglobulins and Complement C3 in Various Forms of Vasculitis

There have been several reports over many years on the detection of immunoglobulins and complement C3 in various cutaneous vasculitis disorders (Table 1), which show several inconsistencies. Differences in results may be due to chance presentation of patients, the age and number of lesions examined, the preparation of the tissues, specificity of antisera, the ratio of fluorescein to antibody molecules, and other technical details. During recent years there has been a great improvement in techniques and in specificity of antisera, so it is difficult to compare older with more recent findings.

Some differences may be due to the nature of the stimuli inducing the lesions. An indication of the effects of selecting patients is evident when comparing our two groups of patients. The first group was chosen on the basis of a history of infection or a febrile episode 1–3 months preceding the onset of vasculitis in order

TABLE 1. Reports on the Incidence of Immunoglobulins and C3 in Vasculitis Lesions

	Number with Ig or C3/number tested				
Disorder	IgG	IgA	IgM	C3	Reference
Nodular vasculitis	8/8	nd	0/8	8/8	Stringa *et al.* (1966)
Necrotizing vasculitis[a]	4/4	nd	0/4	4/4	Stringa *et al.* (1967)
Nodular vasculitis	3/4	nd	nd	nd	Parish and Rhodes (1967)
Erythema nodosum leprosum[b]	10/17	nd	nd	10/17	Wemambu *et al.* (1969)
Purpura/cryoglobulins	5/6	4/6	3/6	nd	Cream (1971)
Mononuclear cell vasculitis	3/28	1/28	6/28	1/28	Parish (1971a) (postinfection series)
Necrotizing vasculitis	18/61	0/61	12/61	5/61	
Erythema nodosum	4/5	0/5	3/5	0/5	
Mononuclear cell vasculitis	8/36	1/36	16/36	29/36	Parish (to be published) (random series)
Necrotizing vasculitis	18/93	4/93	26/93	49/93	
Mononuclear cell vasculitis	3/5	0/5	0/5	3/5[d]	Parish (1972) (postinfection series)
Necrotizing vasculitis	1/3	0/3	0/3	3/3	
Polyarteritis nodosa	0/2	nd	2/2	1/2	Gocke *et al.* (1970, 1971)
Necrotizing vasculitis	15/26	0/18	8/18	9/15	
Livedo vasculitis	3/4	0/3	3/3	0/3	Schroeter *et al.* (1971)
Facial granuloma	3/3	3/3	3/3	3/3	
Leukocytoclastic vasculitis[e]	3/3	1/3	3/3	3/3	Braverman and Yen (1975)
Necrotizing vasculitis	4/22	1/22	0/22	5/33[f]	Handel *et al.* (1975)
Palpable purpura	0/13	6/13	6/13	9/13[g]	Sams *et al.* (1975)
Necrotizing vasculitis[a]	0/2	2/2	2/2	2/2	Asghar *et al.* (1975)
Necrotizing vasculitis	1/1	0/1	0/1	1/1	Verrier Jones *et al.* (1976)
Granuloma annulare[h]	0/11	0/11	1/11	1/11	Umbert and Winkelmann (1976)
Granuloma annulare	0/20	0/20	6/20	10/20	Dahl *et al.* (1977)
Leukocytoclastic vasculitis[i]	0/5	1/5	3/5	4/5	Gower *et al.* (1977)
Levamisole induced	0/1	0/1	1/1	1/1	MacFarlane and Bacon (1978)
Allergic vasculitis	3/10	1/10	1/10	6/10	Secher *et al.* (1978)
Systemic lupus erythematosus	0/1	0/1	1/1	1/1	Schocket *et al.* (1978)
Periarteritis nodosa	7/7	0/7	7/7	7/7	Michalak (1978)

[a] Described as "allergic vasculitis" (Gougerot-Ruiter syndrome), but histological features are consistent with term "necrotizing vasculitis."
[b] Examination made in acetone-fixed preparations. This increases the incidence as nonaggregated globulin is retained.
[c] Mainly granulomatous changes, usually with degeneration.
[d] 3/5 for C3 but all 5/5 had complement when tested with antiserum to C3c, C3d, and C4.
[e] Clinical lesions, spontaneous (their Table 2).
[f] Total patients stated as 31, but (p. 849) C3 found in 3 of 11 and 2 of 12.
[g] 9 from sites of lesions, also 7 from uninvolved sites of which 2 persons had none in lesions (their Table 3).
[h] Vessels of only 1 patient involved. Extravascular IgM and C3 present in others.
[i] Data on spontaneous lesions from their Figure 4, last column.

to increase the opportunity of finding bacterial antigens in the lesions. The second group was chosen at random whenever samples were available, irrespective of history. Similar early or small lesions were sampled from all patients. The antiglobulin sera improved over the years, especially when we prepared fluorescein-labeled F $(ab')_2$ reagents (Parish, 1977), but retesting the earlier antiglobulin sera showed no evidence of antigen nonspecific binding. In the series of patients examined after bacterial infection, leukocytoclastic lesions had IgG in 30% and IgM in 20%, whereas in the randomly selected series the lesions contained IgG in 19% and IgM in 28%. The difference between lesions of the selected and random series is even greater when comparing the mainly mononuclear cell lesions; in the selected group IgG was found in 46% and IgM in 21%, whereas in the random group IgG was found in 22% and IgM in 44%. Such differences could reflect differences in the stimuli to vasculitis, and dispersion and deposition of bacterial antigens could give rise to a different response than following viral infection or autologous antigens. The results of tests made on different populations and in different countries could well be influenced by the incidence of bacteremia or by hygiene. Moreover, certain lesions, e.g., granuloma annulare, may be particularly associated with IgM. In our study of mainly mononuclear cell or granulomatous lesions, IgM was found in 44% of the series of randomly selected patients.

Although there are differences in reports on the finding of IgG and IgM, most reports are consistent that IgA is seldom found in vasculitis lesions but occurs in other cutaneous disorders, e.g., dermatitis herpetiformis. IgD and IgE have also been detected within the lesions (Table 2). The significance of the IgD is not known, but considering the small amount present in normal serum it has been detected in a significant number of lesions. It is unlikely to form complexes attracting neutrophils, although in the lesions the IgD deposits have a distribution similar to that of other immunoglobulins, and are not confined to lymphocytes as has been described in contact dermatitis lesions (Cormane *et al.*, 1973). The IgE occurs either as fine granules or on mast cell membranes.

2.2. Comments on the Significance of Immunoglobulins in Lesions

The immunoglobulin and complement found in lesions are frequently assumed to represent antibody of complexes that induced the lesion. In the great majority of investigations, the identity of the antigen is not known. In the few instances in which concomitant double immunofluorescent staining with rhodamine and fluorescein has shown bacterial or candida antigen complexed with immunoglobulin, there has been a strong indication that the globulin is antibody for the antigen (Parish, 1970; 1971a). Attempts to identify the antibodies by eluting the globulin from skin sections or slices were unsuccessful; either too little was yielded for further testing, or the antibody eluted was so similar to that of the serum to indicate natural diffusion into the skin.

In another approach to the problem of antibody specificity, bacterial antigens were labeled by various methods and added to the sections, but there was too much nonspecific adherence to detect bacterial antibody (Parish, 1971a). However, recent improvements in the techniques may enable us to repeat this investigation.

Antibody and complement do not persist long in typical Arthus reactions; in laboratory animals they persist for only 24–48 hr (Cochrane *et al.*, 1959) and in histamine-induced lesions in man they are much reduced in most subjects by 24 hr

TABLE 2. Detection of IgD and IgE in Cutaneous Vasculitis Lesions

Lesion		Number positive/number tested		Reference
		IgD	IgE	
Vasculitis		1/3	nd	Cormane and Giannetti (1971)
Necrotizing vasculitis		2/3	nd	Parish (1972)
Mononuclear cell vasculitis		3/5	nd	
Necrotizing vasculitis		2/4	0/4	Parish (1973)
Mononuclear cell vasculitis		4/7	1/7	
Necrotizing vasculitis[a]		1/1	nd	Cormane *et al.* (1973)
Necrotizing vasculitis[a]		1/1[b]	2/2	Asghar *et al.* (1975)
Necrotizing vasculitis[a]	7	9/12	nd	Weidner (1975)
Necrotizing vasculitis	2			
Periarteritis nodosa	2			
Bechcet's oral lesion	1			
Necrotizing vasculitis		2/4	0/4	Parish (1977)
Mononuclear cell vasculitis		5/10	2/10	

[a]Described as "allergic vasculitis" (Gougerot-Ruiter syndrome).
[b]2 described, but 1 of these is same patient as in Cormane *et al.* (1973).

(Gower *et al.*, 1977). The apparently frequent finding of immunoglobulins in lesions could be due to reduced ability to degrade complexes, but more probably results from deposition of fresh complexes, or in older lesions local synthesis of globulins, possibly rheumatoid factors, as shown in a few patients (Parish, 1976a).

An inflammatory focus containing active phagocytic cells will take up any complexes or aggregated globulins fortuitously deposited from the blood. These complexes may not exacerbate the lesion, particularly if ingested by macrophages (Parish, 1970), but an immunofluorescent examination of a spontaneous lesion does not differentiate between complexes that may contribute to the initiation or exacerbation of the lesion and those that may have been subsequently taken up.

The role of antiglobulin–globulin complexes and the detection of locally synthesized rheumatoid factors in mononuclear cell infiltrated lesions are considered later.

2.3. Partial "Immune Deficiency" and Weak-Affinity Antibodies in Immune Complex Disorders

It is not possible to assess evidence of reduced formation of antibody to a particular antigen in immune-complex-mediated vasculitis unless the identity of the antigen is known and the amounts can be compared to those of persons forming antibody to the same antigen without disease. However, such a comparison became possible in examining persons whose vasculitis followed bacterial infection and the bacterial antigen–antibody complexes were presumed to have induced the initial lesions.

Antibodies to protein and polysaccharide antigens of streptococci in persons with cutaneous vasculitis following streptococcal pharyngeal infection were less able to form tissue-damaging complexes when compared with antibodies from patients without vasculitis although convalescent from similar infection. The antibodies were less effective in fixing complement and in mediating erythrocyte immune adherence, formed complexes releasing less acid phosphatase and acid protease from human neutrophils, and induced smaller vascular lesions in guinea pig skin (Parish, 1971b,c). Furthermore, in assays of neutralizing antibody to streptococcal toxins from the organism infecting the serum donor, persons with vasculitis tended to form little or no antibody to one toxin although forming adequate amounts to others, whereas persons without vasculitis after the streptococcal infection formed neutralizing antibody to all five toxins examined (Parish, 1971c).

The failure to find as much antibody to bacterial somatic antigens in persons with vasculitis as in those without vasculitis could be interpreted as representing the residual antibody after the more firmly binding antibody had penetrated the tissues when inducing the lesions, or as evidence of reduced ability to form antibody capable of eliminating the antigen, i.e., partial immune deficiency.

The failure to form antibody to one of several streptococcal toxins to which the patient had presumably been exposed is indicative of reduced ability of persons susceptible to vasculitis to form adequate amounts of antibody to all exogenous antigens. This failure to neutralize the streptococcal toxins may be important in the etiology of the vasculitis, in that the toxins streptolysin O, streptokinase, hyaluronidase, proteinase, and erythrogenic toxin may impair the integrity of blood vessels, predisposing them to further damage.

Low-affinity antibody, binding weakly to antigen, forms unstable antigen–antibody complexes that would not be readily eliminated. This could result in the persistence of complexes in the blood that, because of weak binding of the antibody, are likely to be in antigen excess of equivalence (Soothill and Steward, 1971). This is further supported in tests in mice immunized with various antigens. There were consistent strain-related variations in antibody affinity (Steward and Petty, 1972a,b), but of further interest in the interpretation of the results of tests on human sera is that the genetic control of antibody affinity in mice differs from that controlling amounts of antibody formed (Steward and Petty, 1976). Moreover, strains of mice with low-affinity antibody response have an associated poor carbon clearance or poor recovery from carbon blockage, indicating impaired macrophage function (Passwell *et al.*, 1974).

Spontaneous murine lupus is associated with DNA–anti-DNA complexes which are thought to contribute to the disease, as also suggested for human lupus. The affinity of anti-DNA antibody for dsDNA in New Zealand mice increases to about 20 weeks of age, but thereafter it decreases, becoming weaker in females than in males, so at the time the disease occurs, especially in the more susceptible sex, the binding properties of the antibodies are much weaker, and potentially harmful antigen and complexes are not cleared by phagocyte monocytes from the circulation and may accumulate with harmful effects in the kidneys (Steward *et al.*, 1975).

2.4. Histamine-Mediated Vasculitis

One procedure by which it is possible to examine the onset of vasculitis in patients with circulatory complexes is to inject histamine intradermally to induce increased vascular permeability, which could lead to deposition of complexes or aggregated globulin. This has been shown in leukocytoclastic vasculitis (Braverman and Yen, 1975; Gower *et al.*, 1977) and in levamisole-induced vasculitis with circulating complexes (McFarland and Bacon, 1978). The amounts of histamine injected were in excess of physiological concentrations, but they established the fact that immunoglobulins and complement were deposited, and vasculitis resulted.

Gower *et al.* (1977) examined their patients at intervals up to 24 hr, and the sequence of immunoglobulin and complement deposition, followed by infiltration by mononuclear cells and neutrophils and accumulation of fibrin, showed the progression of the typical features of leukocytoclastic vasculitis. These changes did not occur when histamine was injected into *normal* persons. Thus it appears established that persons with vasculitis have circulating plasma substances, probably complexes, that become deposited at sites of increased vascular permeability, resulting in inflammation.

3. Identification of Antigens Possibly Forming Immune Complexes in Patients with Cutaneous Vasculitis

The antigens forming the immune complexes in vasculitis have seldom been identified, except for a few reports of bacterial and viral antigens in lesions with immunoglobulin. Some antigen appears to be altered IgG, as in complexes of rheumatoid factors deposited as cryoglobulins or formed locally with IgG reacting with anti-IgG synthesized in the tissue of more chronic lesions. Recent studies on the composition of circulating immune complexes indicate the frequency of occurrence of several antigens. Among those known to form complexes (Table 3), the following have been implicated as agents inducing vasculitis: bacteria, viruses, and fungi, DNA, and IgG in cryoglobulins and other rheumatoid immune complexes.

3.1. Bacterial Antigen in Immune Complexes and Vasculitis Lesions

Bacteria and some yeasts, particularly candida species, are a very probable source of antigen to form complexes. Bacteria and their degradation products are continually entering the body from the intestine, lungs, and skin as harmless, fortuitously encountered substances, or as secondary colonizers of viral infections and damaged tissue, or as primary infecting agents. Antibodies, usually in small amounts, can be found in human serum to a wide range of bacteria either as antibodies specific for a genus or species or cross-reacting with several genera of bacteria or yeasts. As the amounts of these antibodies tend to be small, except in recently infected or immunized persons, it is probable that complexes in antigen excess of equivalence of antibody are frequently formed but appear to be harmlessly removed from the blood or other tissues.

Immune complexes are likely to be formed during or after every bacteremia. Subacute bacterial endocarditis is associated with generalized release of bacterial emboli and circulating immune complexes and the formation of rheumatoid factor (Williams and Kunkel, 1962; Carson *et al.*, 1978). Meningococcal infection is associated with arthritis and cutaneous vasculitis. The presence of circulating antigen, antibody, and reduced amounts of serum C3 indicates the presence of complexes, which is further supported by the finding of meningococcal antigen and C3 in synovial fluid leukocytes and in one of three skin biopsies (Whittle *et al.*, 1973; Greenwood *et al.*, 1973). Immune complexes were reported in children with recurrent upper respiratory tract infection (Delire and Masson, 1977) and in a case of gonococcal septicemia (Danielsson *et al.*, 1975), a disease in which the not infrequent finding of gonococcus organisms in skin and joint lesions would indicate the formation of complexes to be a usual event. In lepromatous leprosy immune complexes probably containing mycobacterial antigen have been found in

TABLE 3. Some Sources of Antigens in Immune Complexes

Exogenous antigens
1. Drugs, e.g., classical serum sickness, antibiotics, chemicals
2. Environmental antigens; substances ingested or inhaled
3. Infections:
a. Bacteria, e.g., streptococci, *Mycobacterium tuberculosis* and *M. leprosum*
b. Viruses, e.g., hepatitis, dengue, Epstein–Barr, herpes simplex
c. Fungi, e.g., *Candida* sp.
d. Protozoa, e.g., malaria, trypanosomes
e. Helminths, e.g., schistosomes, *Onchocerca* sp., ?*Ascaris*
Endogenous antigens
1. Immunoglobulins, aggregates, modified or native monomer
2. Nuclear antigens, various forms of DNA
3. Cell specific, tumors, damaged organs, e.g., heart, autoallergy

the sera, (Bjorvatn *et al.*, 1976) and mycobacterial antigen with immunoglobulin and C3 in the lesions (Wemambu *et al.*, 1969). Staphylococcal or micrococcal antigen was found to penetrate the affected and "normal" skin of eczematous patients (Welbourn *et al.*, 1976), some of whom had complement-activating IgM antibody (Parish *et al.*, 1976) although no examination was made for complexes.

Medical manipulations may induce bacteremia and probably circulation of immune complexes. Okell and Elliott (1935) established the occurrence of bacteremia after tooth extraction. Bacteremia has been reported following barium enema (LeFrock *et al.*, 1975) and sigmoidoscopic examination of the bowel (Le Frock *et al.*, 1973), a large source of bacteria and their products.

In our studies of patients with cutaneous vasculitis following a known bacterial infection, or pyrexia believed to follow bacterial infection (Parish and Rhodes, 1967; Parish, 1970; 1971a), streptococcal, staphylococcal, candidal, or mycobacterial antigens were found in a significant proportion of the cases (Table 4). Streptococcal group A antigen was found most frequently, which must be due to the selection of a large number of the patients with streptococcal tonsillitis or pharyngitis. The candidal antigens may have been derived from the pharynx or intestine, where *Candida albicans* is a common commensal. Precipitins to candida are frequently found in man, even normal persons, and skin tests may induce Arthus reactions in susceptible hosts. The bacterial antigens were usually intracellular and spread diffusely within the cytoplasm of the cell or were finely granular. The diffuse nature of the antigens indicated that they were degraded material and not intact organisms. The immunofluorescent reagents have been shown to distinguish between intact discrete organisms and diffuse antigen in the same histological section.

3.2. Virus as Antigen in Immune Complexes

Viruses are a probable source of antigen in certain immune complex disorders. Not only is man frequently at risk to viral diseases, but also there are subclinical viral infections that could generate sufficient antigen to form complexes in antigen excess of equivalence of antibody. There has been much interest in viral antigen or viral antigen–antibody complexes as possible initiators of nephritis, and some of the findings are likely to be relevant to vasculitis in other tissues.

Despite the initial difficulties in detecting hepatitis (Australia) antigen, some of the more significant findings on viral antigen–antibody complexes have been made in this system. In six of 16 patients with periarteritis (polyarteritis) nodosa, hepatitis antigen was found in the blood, and evidence of complexes by C1q interaction was found in three patients. In two of the patients the antigen and IgM were present in the lesions, which in one of the patients also contained complement (Gocke *et al.*, 1970; 1971). Similar complexes have been found on the glomerular basement membrane in glomerulonephritis (Coombes *et al.*, 1971). Even more conclusive evidence was obtained in a careful postmortem study of seven cases of periarteritis Michalak, 1978). Hepatitis antigen, immunoglobulin, C1q, and C3 were found in the vascular lesions. Furthermore, the amount of antigen was greatest in recent lesions containing fibrinoid, and decreased in amount according to the stage of healing, being absent in healed lesions. Six of the patients had similar complexes in areas of glomerulonephritis. The severity of the hepatic lesions did not correlate

TABLE 4. Bacterial Antigen in Skin: Patients Selected for Examination Whose Vasculitis Followed Infection[a]

Tissue	Total	*Streptococcus* A	*Streptococcus* D	*Staphylococcus aureus*	*Micrococcus*	*Candida*	*Mycobacterium tuberculosis*
Mononuclear cell vasculitis	22	6	0	3	0	2	5
Neutrophil vasculitis group	58	4	4	0	0	6	1
Erythema nodosum	5	2	2	0	0	0	0
Normal	108	0	0	17	38	22	0

[a] From Parish (1971a).

with the severity of the vascular lesions. The evidence naturally lacking from the postmortem examinations was the detection of antigen–antibody complexes in the blood. However, in other studies on blood, complexes of hepatitis B antigen have been found in patients with acute and chronic hepatitis or in chronic hepatitis antigen carriers (Carella *et al.*, 1977; Fye *et al.*, 1977; Lurhuma *et al.*, 1977). Another feature relevant to vasculitis is the ability of immune complexes to aggregate platelets.

As mentioned earlier, aggregation of platelets contributes to increased vascular permeability and formation of thrombi. Hepatitis antigen–antibody complexes formed *in vitro* aggregated platelets, and this property was related to the anticomplementary activity of the sera (Daugharty and Gogel, 1976).

It is likely that any virus whose antigens enter the circulation in sufficient amount could form immune complexes with the appropriate antibodies. Immune complexes that activate complement have been found in association with dengue hemorrhagic fever (Theofilopoulos *et al.*, 1976; Bokisch *et al.*. 1974), adenovirus in seven patients with idiopathic thrombocytopenic purpura (Lurhuma *et al.*, 1977), and Epstein–Barr virus (Wands *et al.*, 1976; Lurhuma *et al.*, 1977).

In experimental studies *in vitro,* Notkins (1971) found that complexes of herpes simplex virus could be formed with specific antibody which did not neutralize the virus, but subsequent incubation of the complexes with antiglobulin for the antiviral antibody, or with complement, neutralised the viral infectivity. Rheumatoid factor bound to the virus–antibody complexes without affecting neutralization but increased the susceptibility of the virus to neutralization by complement. Herpes simplex has other properties which could contribute to the onset or exacerbation of vasculitis by generating chemotactic activity from complement with antibody for both neutrophils and monocytes (Snyderman *et al.*, 1972) and by stimulating formation of Fc receptors on the membranes of infected cells that may bind the antibody of complexes (Costa and Rabson, 1975), thus contributing to the local accumulation of bound and aggregated immunoglobulins.

In recent studies we found herpes simplex antigen with immunoglobulin and complement in chronic vasculitis lesions and circulating complexes of noninfectious herpes antigen, with specific antibody, rheumatoid factor, and complement, in the serum. The complexes could be dissociated and recombined, and bound further complement. They were also shown to be potentially tissue damaging.

Critical techniques for detecting small amounts of complexes in serum are now in use, and when reliable reagents to detect viral antigens are more widely available the importance of viruses in initiating vasculitis and other manifestations of immune complex disease will be ascertainable.

3.3. DNA as Antigen in Immune Complexes

DNA is a potential antigen in complexes with antibody and complement that could be expected to form tissue-damaging immune complexes. Very little has been done to examine the occurrence of these complexes during cutaneous vasculitis, and their possible contribution to the changes should be considered.

DNA may be released from damaged tissues and from bacteria and viruses. Release of DNA occurs in diseases with widespread or severe tissue damage, as in systemic lupus erythematosus and rheumatoid arthritis, but also occurs after surgery or treatment with large doses of corticosteroids and may even occur in small amounts in clinically healthy persons (Barnett, 1968). The DNA, as determined by antinuclear antibodies, may be non-organ-specific or specific for particular cells, e.g., granulocytes or lymphocytes. When considering the frequent opportunities for viral infections it is tempting to attribute viruses as a source of DNA, but viral DNA tends not to be strongly immunogenic compared to protein coat antigens, and DNA may well be released from nuclei damaged by viruses. In mice, bacterial lipopolysaccharide induces release of DNA into the blood followed by formation of anti-DNA antibodies, but the amount of circulating DNA has little influence on the amount of antibody formed and substantial amounts of antibody may occur in animals in which little DNA is found in the blood (Izui *et al.*, 1977c). It is relevant to studies on DNA complexes that the half-life of DNA in the circulation of normal mice is very short.

Antinuclear antibodies occur with various frequencies in many disorders, being common in SLE and rheumatoid arthritis. They may be of immunoglobulin class G, A, or M, and in particular IgG_1 and IgG_3, which like IgM activate complement.

It is not surprising that release of DNA and the presence of antinuclear antibodies result in the formation of immune complexes, some of which contain components of complement (Agnello *et al.*, 1970), and binding of DNA by DNase-treated immune complexes from SLE sera is interpreted as evidence of DNA–anti-DNA complexes, together with an inverse relation between the amounts of such complexes/cryoprecipitates and amounts of some complement components and evidence of complement binding (Harbeck *et al.*, 1973; P. Davis *et al.*, 1977; J. Davis *et al.*, 1978). The existence of such complexes has been questioned when different methods were used for their detection (Izui *et al.*, 1977b).

There is, however, very little evidence that DNA–anti-DNA complexes induce an immune complex disease of vessels, particularly of the Arthus-type. Fluctuations in the amount of complexes, their size, and antibody avidity correlated with exacerbations of SLE may well reflect the sequel to further tissue damage rather than evidence of immune complex mediation. Similarly DNA, anti-DNA, and complement in skin lesions (Landry and Sams, 1973) may be the result of antibody reacting with antigen released from damaged cells, and such reactants in the kidney (Kunkel and Tan, 1964; Koffler *et al.*, 1967) could be due to accumulation of substances filtered from the plasma. In laboratory animals, however, there are indications of pathogenicity. Glomerulonephritis has been induced in rabbits by DNA–anti-DNA complexes (Natali and Tan, 1972) and in mice following injections of lipopolysaccharides when complexes of DNA–anti-DNA were found in the kidneys (Izui *et al.*, 1977a). In the mice the complexes were not found in the serum, similar to the failure to find them in man (Izui *et al.*, 1977b), but they are believed to be formed within the kidney. Much critical work needs to be done before the tissue-damaging effects of DNA–anti-DNA complexes can be considered established.

3.4. Cryoglobulins as Immune Complexes in Vasculitis

Cryoproteins are plasma proteins—e.g., cryofibrinogen, C-reactive protein–albumin complexes, immunoglobulins, or immunoglobulin complexes—forming precipitates or floccular aggregates in the cold which are reversible and disperse again when the serum or fluid is warmed. Cryoproteins are believed to contribute to the signs of Raynaud's phenomenon, vascular purpura, and vascular thrombosis progressing to gangrene in limbs.

Of special relevance to cutaneous vasculitis are the mixed polyclonal cryoglobulins which may be found in serum-sickness-type lesions associated with arthritis, glomerulonephritis, and vasculitis. These are usually complexes of IgM and IgG, and should be regarded as immune complexes with a particular property of being precipitated in the cold.

Patients with vasculitis may have cryoglobulins, usually of mixed immunoglobulins, in the serum (Cream, 1971); an incidence of 33% in 47 patients is reported (Cream, 1973). Some lesions were found to contain immunoglobulins of the same classes as found in the cryoglobulins (Cream, 1971). Although it is tempting to consider such an association as cause and effect, the globulins likely to be found in lesions are IgG and IgM, which are also commonly found in the cryoprecipitates, and their presence in both may be unrelated. The finding of IgA, which in our experience is rare in vasculitis lesions, in both the lesion and the cryoprecipitate is more convincing evidence of deposition of the complex in the lesions.

Cryoprecipitating complexes may be composed only of immunoglobulins, possibly with traces of complement, or may contain DNA or residues of microbial organisms. Complexes of IgM with IgG, or even IgG with IgG, may be dissociated and recombined to show the presence of an autoantiglobulin reacting with immunoglobulin. Immunoglobulins may also react with α- and β-lipoproteins to form cryoprecipitating complexes that activate complement (Linscott and Krane, 1975; Kodama, 1977). If the contention is accepted that immune complex cryoglobulins differ little from other immune complexes, apart from their precipitability in the cold, the discussions above of DNA and microbial antigens in complexes are also applicable to cryoglobulins. Cryoglobulins from rheumatoid arthritis synovial fluid have been found to contain both DNA and antinuclear antibody, and the antinuclear antibody may be non-organ-specific, or specific for some particular cells, e.g., granulocytes (Wiik *et al.*, 1975). Antibodies to bacteria have been detected in cryoglobulins in rabbits immunized with streptococcal vaccine. The cryoglobulins contained both antiglobulins and antibodies to the immunizing streptococcus (Herd, 1973). In man, evidence of cryoglobulins following infectious mononucleosis has long been recognized (Kaplan, 1968). Levo *et al.* (1977) examined the presence of HBs antigen or its antibody in the sera and cryoprecipitates from 19 patients with mixed cryoglobulinemia; 74% of cryoprecipitates were positive for either HBs antigen or its antibody.

Similarity of biological activity of cryoglobulin complexes and non-cold-precipitable immune complexes is evident from the ability of the cryoglobulin complexes to activate complement (Muller *et al.*, 1976) and to induce vasculitis when whole plasma or isolated cryoglobulin was injected into the skin of the donor patient, although in this patient there was no complement in the complex and no anticomplementary activity (Whitsed and Penny, 1971).

4. Possible Contribution of Rheumatoid Factors to Vasculitis

4.1. Serum Rheumatoid Factors

Rheumatoid factors as antiglobulins for denatured or aggregated IgG may be beneficial by facilitating the removal of complexes or harmful by potentiating the tissue-damaging effects. Rheumatoid factors as 19 S or 7 S IgM and 7 S IgG may bind with IgG that is partially denatured to expose "hidden" determinants, or to IgG aggregated as a result of denaturation, or as complexes with antigen. Another form of rheumatoid factor, more frequently found in joint fluid, but also occurring in serum, is self-associating IgG in which the IgG acts as antibody through the $F(ab')_2$ and as antigen in the Fc position to form IgG-IgG complexes in which the molecules are mainly anti-IgG antibodies (Pope *et al.*, 1975; Natvig and Munthe, 1975). Depending on the class or IgG subclass of the rheumatoid antiglobulin, complement may be activated and C3b bind to the complex. The immune complex, therefore, increases in size and has additional IgG Fc, and C3b determinants by which it binds to macrophage cell receptors, thereby facilitating removal of the complex. This is one beneficial property of rheumatoid factors. Another beneficial activity is the contribution to the neutralization of virus by specific antibody and complement, as mentioned in relation to virus as antigen in immune complexes.

The binding of rheumatoid antiglobulins to immune complexes may enhance the pathogenetic properties of complexes by the same process that may aid their more rapid removal. They may

1. Change soluble complexes into larger less soluble aggregates.
2. Increase the size of immune complexes.
3. Increase the amount of complement fixed, or change complexes not binding complement into those that do so.

For example, complexes formed of antigen in great excess of equivalence of antibody fix little or no complement, but IgM or IgG rheumatoid antiglobulins binding to the complexes may make soluble complexes into less soluble larger aggregates, increase the size of preformed complexes, and bind complement (Tesar and Schmid, 1970). The C3b is a potent opsonin increasing phagocytosis by the leukocytes. The large aggregates, when ingested, result in the release of lysosomal enzymes—the larger the aggregates the greater the amounts of enzymes released (Henson, 1971), and therefore the greater likelihood of tissue damage. Other inflammatory phenomena, *viz.* metabolic changes in neutrophils with increased hexose monophosphate shunt activity, and generation of chemotactic factors, could also follow the conversion of soluble complexes to an insoluble form as is induced by rheumatoid factor (Turner *et al.*, 1976a,b).

The greater activation of complement by rheumatoid factors reacting with circulating complexes will also mediate several other inflammatory processes.

Rheumatoid factors occur in a wide range of disorders, particularly those with a chronic course, but detection depends much on the methods used, and very sensitive techniques detect small amounts in the sera of normal healthy persons. It is to be expected to find rheumatoid factors associated with infection, e.g., subacute bacterial endocarditis (Williams and Kunkel, 1962) and viral hepatitis (Abruzzo and Heimer, 1974), in which circulating immune complexes occur at some stage of the disease.

Rheumatoid factors have been detected in sera of patients with leukocytoclastic (necrotizing) vasculitis, and associated with the pathogenesis (Mongan *et al.*, 1969) or as indirect evidence of the occurrence of circulating complexes during or preceding the onset of vasculitis (Parish, 1970, 1971a). In an examination of rheumatoid arthritis Mongan *et al.* (1969) concluded that necrotizing vasculitis occurred exclusively in patients with the greater amounts of rheumatoid factor (latex flocculation tests) and that in these patients the serum complement activity was significantly less than in patients without vasculitis.

Using techniques making available different IgG determinants to examine sera of patients during or after vasculitis, rheumatoid anti-IgG factors detected by sheep cells sensitized with rabbit IgG and by human group O rhesus D positive cells sensitized with complete anti-rhesus D were found in a significant proportion (Parish, 1970, 1971a), and subsequent studies by other techniques have shown over 90% of patients with vasculitis to have some form of antiglobulin activity.

4.2. Tissue-Bound, Possibly Locally Formed, Rheumatoid Factors

The local formation of rheumatoid factors is considered to be a potent stimulus to the chronic inflammation of synovial membranes in rheumatoid arthritis. The antiglobulins binding to complexes or denatured IgG form new complexes, activating complement and exacerbating the lesions (Munthe and Natvig, 1972a,b). This phenomenon is likely to occur in any chronically inflamed tissue, and IgM and possibly IgG rheumatoid factors binding aggregated IgG have been detected in cutaneous vasculitis lesions composed mainly of mononuclear cells (Parish, 1976a) in immunofluorescent tests using $F(ab')_2$ reagents to avoid the participation of the Fc of the fluorescein-conjugated IgG reagent. Lesions containing IgG Fc and Fab were not found to bind aggregated whole IgG or a papain-treatment-derived IgG Fc, whereas lesions containing IgM + Fab or IgG + IgM + Fab did so. No lesion bound aggregated IgM. It is not yet known if the lesions containing mixed IgG + IgM represent IgM antiglobulin with bound IgG as antigen or mixed IgG and IgM antiglobulins. The first findings on a few patients have been enlarged with similar results and the subclasses mainly IgG_1 and IgG_3 identified. In some, complement was detected in the original lesions and could also be bound on subsequent treatment of sections *in vitro*.

These results show that as in rheumatoid arthritis lesions, and probably other chronic disorders, some vasculitis lesions contain rheumatoid antiglobulin factors, and it is probable that these antiglobulins could form complexes perpetuating the inflammation.

5. Role of C-Reactive Protein in Vasculitis

C-reactive protein (C-RP) is an acute-phase protein which appears in increased amounts in sera during infection and tissue damage (Hill, 1951; Hedlund, 1961), being synthesized in the liver and released into the blood. C-RP forms calcium-dependent precipitating complexes with somatic C-polysaccharide of the pneumococcus, and of several other bacteria and fungi. It induces more rapid movement of randomly migrating leukocytes *in vitro* (Wood, 1951), and promotes leukocyte phagocytosis (Kindmark, 1971). C-RP also activates complement through the classical pathway (Kaplan and Volanakis, 1974; Siegal *et al.*, 1975) and induces complement-dependent hemolysis of red cells treated with C-substance (Osmand *et al.*, 1975).

C-RP was found in the serum of patients with vasculitis by precipitation with pneumococcal C-substance and specific anti-C-reactive protein in agar gels, an insensitive technique that detected C-RP in only eight of 108 normal persons (Parish, 1970; 1971a). However, when using anti-C-RP in Mancini radial immunodiffusion plates, or ^{131}I-labeled anti-IgG superimposed on the Mancini test procedure, it was possible to determine the amounts of C-RP in sera and show the greater amounts occurring during vasculitis than in normal sera, as a high proportion of normal persons had small amounts of C-RP (Parish, 1976b) (see Table 5).

Immunofluorescence tests revealed the presence of C-RP in neutrophil-infiltrated and mononuclear cell-infiltrated vascular lesions alone or in the presence of bacterial antigen, or complement as C1 or more frequently C3 (Parish, 1971a; 1976b). The deposits of C-RP and complement in the same lesions, however, rarely coincided unless relatively large amounts were present when they tended to overlap. More than half the lesions contained C-RP (Table 6). The significance of C-RP in vasculitis was examined using C-RP purified from pleural effusions. It was confirmed that C-RP activated human complement when aggregated or when combined with bacterial C-substance, and the complement so activated attracted both human neutrophils and eosinophils. Heating the serum to destroy the complement abrogated the chemotactic activity. The activity of the C-RP by weight was equal to that of IgG. Furthermore, C-RP–complement complexes were ingested by leukocytes to release lysosomal enzymes but not the cytoplasmic enzyme lactic dehydrogenase (Parish, 1977). The potential tissue-damaging activity shown *in vitro* was confirmed by injecting aggregated human C-RP into the skin of guinea pigs and rabbits, resulting in Arthus-like lesions.

It is concluded, therefore, that C-RP, which occurs in serum during vasculitis or other inflammations, and if found in the lesions, has similar biological activities to aggregated IgG and therefore to immune complexes. Increased amounts of C-RP are found fairly quickly after injury and therefore may act as an antigen-nonspecific substance that activates complement and stimulates the activity of leukocytes before specific antibody is formed. In the lesions, it appears to have the properties of an immune complex attracting and activating leukocytes. It may function as a stimulus to the benefit of inflammatory responses to tissue injury, e.g., hasten the removal of damaged tissue, but should also be considered as an agent contributing to the exacerbation and persistence of vasculitis induced by other substances or trauma and other physical damage.

TABLE 5. Amount of C-RP in Sera of Patients with Vasculitis and of Normal Persons Matched for Age and Sex[a]

		C-RP (ng/ml)	
Serum donors	Total	Range[b]	Mean
Normal	12	<200	—
Normal	18	200–1,800	790
Mononuclear cell vasculitis	31	2,500–95,000	28,200
Neutrophil cell vasculitis	39	6,300–160,000	56,400
Indolent ulcer leg	3	209,000–312,000	286,000

[a] From Parish (1976b). Patients with mainly mononuclear cell or mainly neutrophil cell vasculitis.
[b] Concentrations 4000 ng or greater assayed by radial immunodiffusion; at 200–4000 ng by the radioactive antiglobulin procedure.

TABLE 6. C-RP with Complement Components C1 and C3, and IgG in Cutaneous Vasculitis Lesions, after Fixation (to 1974)[a]

		Number of lesions containing					
Tissue	Total	C-RP alone	C-RP +C1	C-RP +C3	C-RP +C1C3	C-RP +C3IgG	Total C-RP
Mononuclear cell vasculitis	32	1	2	7	1	6	17
Neutrophil cell vasculitis	26	1	0	6	5	7	19

[a] From Parish (1976b).

6. Summary of Investigations on Human Vasculitis

Immune complexes are found fairly frequently in persons with acute leukocytoclastic, or necrotizing, vasculitis. They occur in the serum and may be found in the lesions. The serum may also show decreased amounts of complement or contain immunoconglutinin and rheumatoid factors as indirect evidence of immune complexes. Immunoglobulins and complement are found in some lesions, and, in a few, bacterial or viral antigens appear bound to the immunoglobulins as complexes. Exogenous antigens are rarely found, unless the patients have been selected for examination because the vasculitis has followed a known infection. It is probable that after the initial stimulus the antigen of the complexes in serum and the lesions is endogenous IgG, as in the rheumatoid group of disorders. Such complexes are found as mixed polyclonal immunoglobulin cryoglobulins in serum and deposits of the same classes of immunoglobulin in the lesions.

Immunoglobulins and complement do not normally persist for more than 24 hr after injection of immune complexes in experimental animals, so their frequency of detection in the human lesions indicates repeated deposition from the blood or local formation at the site of damaged tissues. It is not certain that the complexes detected are those that initiated the lesions. They have the potential to induce vasculitis, as shown by the complexes formed with patient's antibody *in vitro* which attract neutrophils and stimulate them to release their lysosomal enzymes and induce vasculitis in the skin of animals. The deposition of immunoglobulins and occurrence of vasculitis lesions following injection of histamine into the skin of patients with vasculitis are important evidence of the potential of substances in the blood to induce lesions if deposited in susceptible tissue. Similar injections of histamine in normal persons do not induce vasculitis.

Normal persons not infrequently have immune complexes circulating for a short time. These complexes may differ in amount and properties, e.g., the antigen–antibody ratio, when compared to complexes in persons with vasculitis. There is evidence that persons with vasculitis have a partial immune deficiency and there is insufficient antibody to form complexes in excess of antigen, so the complexes are not quickly removed from the blood. Experimental evidence on animals also indicates the importance of the affinity of the antibodies; weak-binding antibodies predispose to immune complex diseases.

Once the vasculitis is induced, several inflammatory factors probably contribute to the perpetuation of the lesions. One such substance is C-reactive protein, which acts like aggregated IgG in its ability to activate complement, attract neutrophils, and induce vasculitis on injection into skin.

7. References

Abruzzo, J. L., and Heimer, R., 1974, IgG anti-IgG antibodies in rheumatoid arthritis and certain other conditions, *Ann. Rheum. Dis.* **33**:258–261.

Agnello, V., Winchester, R. J. and Kunkel, H. G., 1970, Precipitive reactions of the C1q component of complement with aggregated gamma globulin and immune complexes in gel diffusion, *Immunology* **19**:909–919.

Asghar, S. S., Faber, W. R. and Cormane, R. H., 1975, C1q precipitin in the sera of patients with allergic vasculitis (Gougerot-Ruiter syndrome), *J. Invest. Dermatol.* **64**:113–118.

Barnett, E. V., 1968, Detection of nuclear antigens (DNA) in normal and pathologic human fluids by quantitative complement fixation, *Arthr. Rheum.* **11**:407–417.

Benveniste, J., 1974, Platelet activating factor, a new mediator of anaphylaxis and immune complex deposition from rabbit and human basophils, *Nature (London)* **249**:581–582.

Benveniste, J., Henson, P. M., and Cochrane, C. G., 1972, Release of histamine from rat mast cells by complement peptides C3a and C5a, *J. Immunol.* **28**:1067.

Bjorvatn, B., Barnetson, R. S., Kronvall, G., Zubler, R. H., and Lambert, P. H., 1976, Immune complexes and complement hypercatabolism in patients with leprosy, *Clin. Exp. Immunol.* **26**:388–396.

Bokisch, V. A., Mueller-Eberhard, H. J., and Dixon, F. J., 1974, Complement a potential mediator of the hemorrhagic shock syndrome dengue, in: *Advances in the Biosciences,* Vol. 12, p. 417, Schering Symposium on Immunopathology, Pergamon, New York.

Boonpucknavig, V., Bhamarapravati, N., Boonpucknavig, S., Futrakul, P., and Tanpaichitr, P., 1976, Glomerular changes in dengue hemorrhagic fever, *Arch. Pathol. Lab. Med.* **100(4)**:206–212.

Braverman, I. M., and Yen, A., 1975, Demonstration of immune complexes in spontaneous and histamine-induced lesions and in normal skin of patients with leukocytoclastic angiitis, *J. Invest. Dermatol.* **64**:105–112.

Brown, W. R., and Lee, E. H., 1976, Studies on IgE in human intestinal fluids, *Int. Arch. Allergy Appl. Immunol.* **50**:87–94.

Carella, G., Digeon, M., Feldmann, G., Jungers, P., Drouet, J., and Bach, J. F., 1977, Detection of hepatitis B antigen in circulating immune complexes, *Scand. J. Immunol.* **6**:1297–1304.

Carson, D. A., Bayer, A. S., Eisenberg, R. A., Lawrance, S., and Theofilopoulos, A., 1978, IgG rheumatoid factor in subacute bacterial endocarditis: Relationship to IgM rheumatoid factor and circulating immune complexes, *Clin. Exp. Immunol.* **31**:100–103.

Cochrane, C. G., 1963a, Studies on the localization of circulating antigen-antibody complexes and other macromolecules in vessels. I. Structural studies, *J. Exp. Med.* **118**:489–502.

Cochrane, C. G., 1963b, II. Pathogenetic and pharmacodynamic studies, *J. Exp. Med.* **118**:503–513.

Cochrane, C. G., and Janoff, A., 1974, The Arthus reaction: A model of neutrophil and complement mediated injury, in: *The Inflammatory Process,* 2nd ed., Vol. 3 (B. W. Zweifach, L. Grant, and R. T. McCluskey, eds.), pp. 85–162, Academic, New York.

Cochrane, C. G., and Koffler, D., 1973, Immune complex disease in experimental animals and man, *Adv. Immunol.* **16**:185–264.

Cochrane, C. G., and Weigle, W. O., 1958, The cutaneous reaction to soluble antigen-antibody complexes: A comparison with the Arthus phenomenon, *J. Exp. Med.* **108**:591–604.

Cochrane, C. G., Weigle, W. O., and Dixon, F. J., 1959, The role of polymorphonuclear leucocytes in the initiation and cessation of the Arthus vasculitis, *J. Exp. Med.* **110**:481–494.

Colvin, R. B., and Dvorak, H. F., 1975, Role of the clotting system in cell-mediated hypersensitivity. II. Kinetics of fibrinogen/fibrin accumulation and vascular permeability changes in tuberculin and cutaneous basophil hypersensitivity reactions, *J. Immunol.* **114**:377–386.

Colvin, R. B., Pinn, V. W., Simpson, B. A., and Dvorak, H. F., 1973, Cutaneous basophil hypersensitivity. IV. The "late reaction": Sequel to Jones-Mote type hypersensitivity. Comparison with rabbit Arthus reaction. Effect of passive antibody on induction and expression of Jones-Mote hypersensitivity, *J. Immunol.* **110**:1279–1289.

Coombes, B., Shorey, J., Barrera, A., Stostny, P., Eigenbrodt, E. H., Hull, A. R., and Carter, N.

W., 1971, Glomerulonephritis with deposition of Australia antigen–antibody complexes in glomerular basement membrane, *Lancet* **2**:234–237.

Cormane, R. H., and Giannetti, A., 1971, IgD in various dermatoses; immunofluorescence studies, *Br. J. Dermatol.* **84**:523–533.

Cormane, R. H., Husz, S., and Hammerlinck, F. F., 1973, Immunoglobulin and complement bearing lymphocytes in eczema, *Br. J. Dermatol.* **88**:307–312.

Costa, J. C., and Rabson, A. S., 1975, Role of Fc receptors in herpes simplex virus infection, *Lancet* **2**:77–78.

Cream, J. J., 1971, Immunofluorescent studies of the skin in cryoglobulinaemic vasculitis, *Br. J. Dermatol.* **84**:48–53.

Cream, J. J., 1973, Immune complex disease and mixed cryoglobulinemia, in: *Immunopathology of the Skin: Labelled Antibody Studies* (E. H. Beutner, T. P. Chorzelski, S. F. Beam, and R. E. Jordon, eds.), pp. 137–152, Dowden, Hutchinson and Ross, Philadelphia.

Dahl, M. V., Ullman, S., and Goltz, R. W., 1977, Vasculitis in granuloma annulare: Histopathology and direct immunofluorescence, *Arch. Dermatol.* **113**:463–467.

Danielsson, D., Norbert, R., and Svanbom, M., 1975, Circulating immune complexes in a patient with prolonged gonococcal septicemia, *Acta Dermatovener. (Stockholm)* **55**:301–304.

Daugharty, H., and Gogel, R., 1976, Platelet aggregation by hepatitis B surface antigen-antibody complexes, *Infect. Immun.* **14**:752–758.

Davis, J. S., Godfrey, S. M., and Winfield, J. B., 1978, Direct evidence for circulating DNA/anti-DNA complexes in systemic lupus erythematosus, *Arthr. Rheum.* **621**:17–22.

Davis, P., Cumming, R. H., and Verrier-Jones, J., 1977, Relationship between anti-DNA antibodies complement consumption and circulating immune complexes in systemic lupus erythematosus, *Clin. Exp. Immunol.* **28**:226–232.

Delire, M., and Masson, P. L., 1977, The detection of circulating immune complexes in children with recurrent infections and their treatment with human immunoglobulins, *Clin. Exp. Immunol.* **29**:385–392.

Dixon, F. J., 1971, Experimental serum sickness, in: *Immunological Diseases,* 2nd ed. (M. Samter, ed.), pp. 253–264, Little, Brown, Boston.

Dvorak, H. F., Dvorak, A. M., Simpson, B. A., Richerson, H. B., Leskowitz, S., and Karnovsky, M. J., 1970, Cutaneous basophil hypersensitivity. II. A light and electron microscopic description, *J. Exp. Med.* **132**:558–582.

Dvorak, H. F., Hammond, M. E., Colvin, R. B., Manseau, E. J., and Goodwin, J., 1977, Systemic expression of cutaneous basophil hypersensitivity, *J. Immunol.* **118**:1549–1556.

Fye, K. H., Becker, M. J., Theofilopoulos, A. N., Moutsopoulos, H., Feldman, J. L., and Talal, N., 1977, Immune complexes in hepatitis B antigen-associated periarteritis nodosa: Detection by antibody-dependent cell-mediated cytotoxicity and the Raji cell assay, *Am. J. Med.* **62**:783–791.

Giacovazzo, M., D'errico, G., and Spagna, G., 1976, Adenovirus and rheumatoid arthritis, *Boll. Soc. Ital. Biol. Sper.* **51**:1633–1637.

Gocke, D. J., Hsu, K., Morgan, C., Lockshin, M., Bombardieri, S., and Christian, C. L., 1971, Vasculitis in association with Australia antigen, *J. Exp. Med.* **134**:330s–336s.

Gower, R. G., Sams, W. M., Thorne, E. G., Kohler, P. F., and Claman, H. N., 1977, Leukocytoclastic vasculitis: Sequential appearance of immunoreactants and cellular changes in serial biopsies, *J. Invest. Dermatol.* **69**:477–484.

Grant, J. A., Dupree, E., Goldman, A. S., Schultz, D. R., and Jackson, A. L., 1975, Complement-mediated release of histamine from human leukocytes, *J. Immunol.* **114**:1101–1106.

Greenwood, B. M., Whittle, H. C., and Bryceson, A. D. M., 1973, Allergic complications of meningococcal disease. II. Immunological investigations, *Br. Med. J.* **2**:737–740.

Handel, D. W., Roenigk, H. H., Shainoff, J., and Deodhar, S., 1975, Necrotizing vasculitis: Etiologic aspects of immunology and coagulopathy, *Arch. Dermatol.* **111**:847–852.

Harbeck, R. J., Bardana, E. J., Kohler, P. F., and Cair, R. I., 1973, DNA–anti-DNA complexes, their detection in systemic lupus erythematosis sera, *J. Clin. Invest.* **52**:789.

Hedlund, P., 1961, Clinical and experimental studies on C-reactive protein (acute phase protein), *Acta Med. Scand. Suppl.* **361**:7–71.

Henson, P. M., 1970, Mechanisms of release of constituents from rabbit platelets of antigen–antibody complexes and complement, I. Lytic and nonlytic reactions, *J. Immunol.* **105**:476–489.

Henson, P. M., 1971, The immunologic release of constituents from neutrophil leukocytes. I. The role of antibody and complement on nonphagocytosable surfaces or phagocytosable particles, *J. Immunol.* **107:**1535–1546.

Herd, Z. L., 1973, Antiglobulins and cryoglobulins in rabbits producing homogeneous streptococcal antibodies, *Immunology* **25:**923.

Hill, A. G. S., 1951, C-reactive protein in chronic rheumatic diseases, *Lancet* **2:**807–811.

Hook, W. A., and Siraganian, R. P., 1977, Complement-induced histamine release from human basophils. III. Effect of pharmacologic agents, *J. Immunol.* **118:**679–684.

Hook, W. A., Siranganian, R. P., and Wahl, S. M., 1975, Complement-induced histamine release from human basophils. I. Generation of activity in human serum, *J. Immunol.* **114:**1185–1190.

Hughes, P., and Beck, J. S., 1970, Studies on the pathogenic action of human antinuclear antibodies: Inflammatory skin reactions in mice to immune complexes formed *in vitro* from human antinuclear antibodies and human leucocytes, *J. Pathol.* **101:**27–38.

Ishizaka, K., 1963, Gamma globulin and molecular mechanisms in hypersensitivity reactions, *Progr. Allergy* **7:**32–106.

Izui, S., Lambert, P. H., Fournie, G. J., Turler, H., and Miescher, P. A., 1977a, Features of systemic lupus erythematosus in mice injected with bacterial lipopolysaccharides: Identification of circulating DNA and renal localization of DNA-anti-DNA complexes, *J. Exp. Med.* **145:**1115–1130.

Izui, S., Lambert, P. H., and Miescher, P. A., 1977b, Failure to detect circulating DNA–anti-DNA complexes by four radio immunological methods in patients with systemic lupus erythematosis, *Clin. Exp. Immunol.* **30:**384–392.

Izui, S., Zaldivar, N. M., Scher, I., and Lambert, P., 1977c, Mechanism for induction of anti-DNA antibodies by bacterial lipopolysaccharides in mice, *J. Immunol.* **119(6):**2151–2156.

Johnson, A. R., Hugli, T. E., and Muller-Eberhard, H. J., 1975, Release of histamine from rat mast cells by complement peptides C3a and C5a, *Immunology* **28:**1067–1080.

Jones, J. V., Cumming, R. H., Asplin, C. M., Harman, R. R. M., and Tribe, C. R., 1976, Necrotizing vasculitis: A circulating immune complex producing inflammatory skin lesions, *Br. J. Dermatol.* **94:**123–130.

Kaplan, M. E., 1968, Cryoglobulinemia in infectious mononucleosis: Quantitation and characterization of the cryoproteins, *J. Lab. Clin. Med.* **71:**754–765.

Kaplan, M. H., and Volanakis, J. E., 1974, Interaction of C-reactive protein complexes with the complement system. 1. Consumption of human complement associated with the reaction of C-RP with pneumococcal C-polysaccharide and with the choline phosphatides lecithin, and sphingomyelin, *J. Immunol.* **112:**2135–2147.

Kelly, M. T., and White, A., 1973, Histamine release induced by human leukocyte lysates: Implication of a specific complement independent rencytotoxic reaction, *Infect. Immun.* **8:**8.

Kindmark, C.-O., 1971, Stimulating effect of C-reactive protein on phagocytosis of various species of phagogenic bacteria, *Clin. Exp. Immunol.* **8:**941.

Kodama, H., 1977, Determination of cryoglobulins as lipoprotein–autoantibody immune complexes and antigenic determinants against antilipoprotein autoantibody, *Clin. Exp. Immunol.* **28:**437–444.

Kniker, W. T., and Cochrane, C. G., 1968, The localisation of circulating immune complexes in experimental serum sickness: The role of vasoactive amines and hydrodynamic forces, *J. Exp. Med.* **127:**119–136.

Koffler, D., Schur, P. H., and Kunkel, H. G., 1967, Immunological studies concerning the nephritis of systemic lupus erythematosus, *J. Exp. Med.* **126:**607–624.

Kunkel, H. G., and Tan, E. M., 1964, Auto-antibodies and disease, *Adv. Immunol.* **4:**351–395.

Landry, M., and Sams, W. M., 1973, Systemic lupus erythematosus: Studies of the antibodies bound to skin, *J. Clin. Invest.* **52:**1871–1880.

Le Frock, J. L., Ellis, C. A., Turchik, J. A., and Weinstein, L., 1973, Transient bacteremia associated with sigmoidoscopy, *New Engl. J. Med.* **289:**467–469.

Le Frock, J. Ellis, C. A., Klainer, A. S., and Weinstein, L., 1975, Transient bacteremia associated with barium enema, *Arch. Intern. Med.* **135:**835–837.

Lett-Brown, M. A., Boetcher, D. A., and Leonard, E. J., 1976, Chemotactic responses of normal human basophils to C5a and to lymphocyte-derived chemotactic factor, *J. Immunol.* **117:**246–252.

Levo, Y., Gorevic, P. D., Kassab, H. J., Zucker-Franklin, D., and Franklin, E. C., 1977, Association between hepatitis B virus and essential mixed cryoglobulinemia, *N. Engl. J. Med.* **296:**1501–1504.

Linscott, W. D., and Kane, J. P., 1975, The complement system in cryoglobulinaemia: Interaction with immunoglobulins and lipoproteins, *Clin. Exp. Immunol.* **21:**510–519.

Lurhuma, A. Z., Riccomi, H., and Masson, P. L., 1977, The occurrence of circulating immune complexes and viral antigens in idiopathic thrombocytopenic purpura, *Clin. Exp. Immunol.* **28:**49–55.

Manjo, G., and Palade, G. E., 1961, Studies on inflammation. 1. The effect of histamine and serotonin on vascular permeability; an electron microscope study, *J. Cell Biol.* **11:**571–605.

Martin, S. E., Breckenridge, R. T., Rosenfeld, S. I., and Leddy, J. P., 1978, Responses of human platelets to immunologic stimuli: Independent roles for complement and IgG in zymosan activation, *J. Immunol.* **120:**9–14.

McFarlane, D. G., and Bacon, P. A., 1978, Levamisole-induced vasculitis due to circulating immune complexes, *Br. Med. J.* **1:**407–408.

Michalak, T., 1978, Immune complexes of hepatitis B surface antigen in the pathogenesis of periarteritis nodosa: A study of seven necropsy cases, *Am. J. Pathol.* **90:**619–627.

Mongan, E. S., Cass, R. M., Jacox, R. F., and Vaughan, J. H., 1969, A study of the relation of seronegative and seropositive rheumatoid arthritis to each other and to necrotizing vasculitis, *Am. J. Med.* **47:**23–35.

Muller, S., Rother, U., and Westerhausen, M., 1976, Complement activation by cryoglobulin: Evidence for a pathogenic role of an IgG (kappa) cryoglobulin in cutaneous vasculitis, *Clin. Exp. Immunol.* **23:**233–241.

Munthe, E., and Natvig, J. B., 1972a, Immunoglobulin classes, subclasses and complexes of IgG rheumatoid factor in rheumatoid plasma cells, *Clin. Exp. Immunol.* **12:**55–70.

Munthe, E., and Natvig, J. B., 1972b, Complement-fixing intracellular complexes of IgG rheumatoid factor in rheumatoid plasma cells, *Scand. J. Immunol.* **1:**217–229.

Natali, P. G., and Tan, E. M., 1972, Experimental renal disease induced by DNA–anti-DNA immune complexes, *J. Clin. Invest.* **51:**345–355.

Natvig. J. B., and Munthe, E., 1975, Self-associating IgG rheumatoid factors represents a larger response of plasma cells in rheumatoid tissue, *Ann. N.Y. Acad. Sci.* **256:**88.

Notkins, A. L., 1971, Infectious virus–antibody complexes: Interaction with antiglobulins, complement and rheumatoid factor, *J. Exp. Med.* **134:**41s–51s.

Okell, C. C., and Elliott, S. D., 1935, Bacteremia and oral sepsis with special reference to the aetiology of subacute endocarditis, *Lancet* **2:**869–872.

Osmand, A. P., Mortenson, R. F., Siegal, J., and Gewurz, H., 1975, Interaction of C-reactive protein with the complement system. III. Complement dependent passive haemolysis initiated by CRP, *J. Exp. Med.* **142:**1065–1077.

Parish, W. E., 1970, Complexes of bacterial antigens with IgG or IgM antibodies in cutaneous vasculitis, in: *International Symposium on Immune-Complex Diseases, Spoleto, Italy*, pp. 98–109, Carlo Erba, Milan.

Parish, W. E., 1971a, Studies on vasculitis, I. Immunoglobulins, β1C, C-reactive protein, and bacterial antigens in cutaneous vasculitis lesions, *Clin. Allergy* **1:**97–109.

Parish, W. E., 1971b, Studies on vasculitis. II. Some properties of complexes formed of antibacterial antibodies from persons with or without cutaneous vasculitis, *Clin. Allergy* **1:**111–121.

Parish, W. E., 1971c, Studies on vasculitis. III. Decreased formation of antibody to M protein, group A polysaccharide and to some exotoxins, in persons with cutaneous vasculitis after streptococcal infection, *Clin. Allergy* **1:**295–309.

Parish, W. E., 1971d, Studies on vasculitis. IV. The low incidence of antibacterial anaphylactic antibodies in the sera of persons with cutaneous vasculitis following bacterial infection, *Clin. Allergy* **1:**433–446.

Parish, W. E., 1972, Cutaneous vasculitis: Antigen–antibody complexes and prolonged fibrinolysis, *Proc. R. Soc. Med.* **65:**276–278.

Parish, W. E., 1973, Cutaneous vasculitis: The occurrence of complexes of bacterial antigens with antibody, and of abnormalities associated with chronic inflammation, in: *Immunopathology of the Skin: Labelled Antibody Studies* (E. H. Beutner, T. P. Chorzelski, S. F. Bean, and R. E. Jordon, eds.), pp. 153–169, Dowden Hutchinson and Ross, Philadelphia.

Parish, W. E., 1976a, Studies on vasculitis, VI. Antiglobulins or rheumatoidlike factors in cutaneous vasculitis lesions detected by an improved immunofluorescence procedure, *Clin. Allergy* **6**:533–541.

Parish, W. E., 1976b, Studies on vasculitis. VII. C-reactive protein as a substance perpetuating chronic vasculitis. Occurrence in lesions and concentrations in sera, *Clin. Allergy* **6**:543–550.

Parish, W. E., 1977, Features of human spontaneous vasculitis reproduced experimentally in animals: Effects of antiglobulins, C-reactive protein and fibrin, in: *Bayer Symposium VI,* pp. 117–151, Springer-Verlag, Berlin.

Parish, W. E., and Rhodes, E. L., 1967, Bacterial antigens and aggregated gamma globulin in the lesions of nodular vasculitis, *Br. J. Dermatol.* **79**:131–147.

Parish, W. E., Welbourn, E., and Champion, R. H., 1976, Hypersensitivity to bacteria in eczema. II. Titre and immunoglobulin class of antibodies to staphylococci and micrococci, *Br. J. Dermatol.* **95**:285–293.

Passwell, J. H., Steward, M. W., and Southhill, J. F., 1974, Intermouse strain differences in macrophage function and its relationship to antibody responses, *Clin. Exp. Immunol.* **17**:159–167.

Pinckard, R. N., and Henson, P. M., 1977, Activation of procoagulant activity in rabbit platelets by basophil-derived platelet activating factor (PAF), *Fed. Proc.* **36**:1329.

Pinckard, R. N., Halonen, M., Palmer, J. D., Butler, C., Shaw, J. O., and Henson, P. M., 1977, Intravascular aggregation and pulmonary sequestration of platelets during IgE-induced systemic anaphylaxis in the rabbit: Abrogation of lethal anaphylactic shock by platelet depletion, *J. Immunol.* **119**:2185–2193.

Pope, R. M., Teller, D. C., and Mannik, M., 1975, Intermediate complexes found by self-association of IgG-rheumatoid factors, *Ann. N.Y. Acad. Sci.* **256**:82.

Sams, W. M., Claman, H. N., Kohler, P. F., McIntosh, R. M., Small, P., and Mass, M. F., 1975, Human necrotizing vasculitis: Immunoglobulins and complement in vessel walls of cutaneous lesions and normal skin, *J. Invest. Dermatol.* **64**:441–445.

Schocket, A. L., Lain, D., Kohler, P. F., and Steigerwald, J., 1978, Immune complex vasculitis as a cause of ascites and pleural effusions in systemic lupus erythematosus, *J. Rheumatol.* **5**:33–38.

Schroeter, A. L., Copeman, P. W. M., Jordon, R. E., Sams, W. M., and Winklemann, R. K., 1971, Immunofluorescence of cutaneous vasculitis associated with systemic disease, *Arch. Derm.* **104**:254–259.

Secher, L., Permin, H., and Juhl, F., 1978, Immunofluorescence of the skin in allergic diseases: An investigation of patients with contact dermatitis. Allergic vasculitis and atopic dermatitis, *Acta Dermatovener. (Stockholm)* **58**:117–120.

Siegal, J., Osmand, A. P., Wilson, M. F., and Gewurz, H., 1975, Interactions of C-reactive protein with the complement system. II. C-reactive protein-mediated consumption of complement by poly-L-lysine polymers and other polycations, *J. Exp. Med.* **142**:709–721.

Siraganian, R. P., Secci, A. G., and Osler, A. G., 1968, The allergic response of rabbit platelets. 1. Membrane permeability changes, *J. Immunol.* **101**:1130–1139, 1140–1147, 1148–1153.

Snyderman, R., Wohlenberg, C., and Notkins, A. L., 1972, Inflammation and viral infection: Chemotactic activity resulting from the interaction of antiviral antibody and complement with cells infected with herpes simplex virus, *J. Infect. Dis.* **126**:207–209.

Soothill, J. F., and Steward, M. W., 1971, The immunopathological significance of heterogeneity of antibody affinity, *Clin. Exp. Immunol.* **9**:193.

Steward, M. W., and Petty, R. E., 1972a, The use of ammonium sulphate globulin precipitation for determination of the affinity of anti-protein antibodies in mouse serum, *Immunology* **22**:747–756.

Steward, M. W., and Petty, R. E., 1972b, The antigen binding characteristics of antibody pools of relative affinity, *Immunology* **23**:881–887.

Steward, M. W., and Petty, R. E., 1976, Evidence for the genetic control of antibody affinity from breeding studies with inbred mouse strains producing high and low affinity antibody, *Immunology* **30**:789–797.

Steward, M. W., Katz, F. E., and West, N. J., 1975, The role of low affinity antibody in immune complex disease; the quality of anti-DNA antibodies in NZB/W F_1 hybrid mice, *Clin. Exp. Immunol.* **21**:121–130.

Stringa, S. G., Bianchi, C., and Zingale, S. B., 1966, Nodular vasculitis: Immunofluorescent study, *J. Invest. Dermatol.* **46**:1–5.

Stringa, S. G., Bianchi, C., Casala, A. M., and Bianchi, O., 1967, Allergic vasculitis Gougerot-Ruiter syndrome, *Arch. Dermatol.* **95**:23–27.

Tesar, J. T., and Schmid, F. R., 1970, Conversion of soluble immune complexes into complement-fixing aggregates by IgM-rheumatoid factor, *J. Immunol.* **105:**1206–1214.

Theofilopoulos, A. N., Wilson, C. B., and Dixon, F. J., 1976, The Raji cell radioimmune assay for detecting immune complexes in human sera, *J. Clin. Invest.* **57:**169–182.

Thueson, D. O., Speck, L., and Grant, J. A., 1977, Histamine-releasing activity produced by human mononuclear cells, *Fed. Proc.* **36:**1300 (abstr).

Turner, R., Collins, R., Browner, S. , Kaufmann, J., Schumacher, H. R., Parker, M., and De Chatelet L., 1976a, Neutrophil and rheumatoid factor-immunoglobulin G insoluble complex interactions: Phagocytosis and sequelae, *J. Rheumatoid* **3:**109–117.

Turner, R. A., Mashburn, H., Collins, R., Parker, M., De Chatelet, L., and Schumacher, H. R., 1976b, IgG complex interactions with rheumatoid factor and neutrophils, *Arthr. Rheum.* **19:**827.

Umbert, P., and Winkelmann, R. K., 1976, Granuloma annulare: Direct immunofluorescence study, *Br. J. Dermatol.* **95:**487–492.

Verrier Jones, J., Cumming, R. H., Asplin, C. M., Harman, R. R. M., and Tribe, C. R., 1976, Necrotizing vasculitis: A circulating immune complex producing inflammatory skin lesions, *Br. J. Dermatol.* **94:**123–130.

Wands, J. R., Perrotto, J. L., and Isselbacher, K. J., 1976, Circulating immune complexes and complement sequence activation in infectious mononucleosis, *Am. J. Med.* **60:**269–272.

Weidner, F., 1975, Immunofluorescent investigations in cutaneous vasculitis. II. Histotopical demonstration of IgD and fibrin, *Arch. Dermatol. Res.* **254:**215–224.

Weigle, W. L., 1961, Fate and biological action of antigen–antibody complexes, *Adv. Immunol.* **1:**283.

Welbourn, E., Champion, R. H., and Parish, W. E., 1976, Hypersensitivity to bacteria in eczema. I. Bacterial culture, skin tests and immunofluorescent detection of immunoglobulins and bacterial antigens, *Br. J. Dermatol.* **94:**619–632.

Wemambu, S. N. C., Turk, J. L., Waters, M. F. R., and Rees, R. J. W., 1969, Erythema nodosum leprosum: A clinical manifestation of the Arthus phenomenon, *Lancet* **2:**933–935.

Whitsed, H. M., and Penney, R., 1971, IgA/IgG cryoglobulinaemia with vasculitis, *Clin. Exp. Immunol.* **9:**183–191.

Whittle, H. C., Abdullahi, M. T., Fakunle, F. A., Greenwood, B. M., Bryceson, A. D. M., Parry, E. H. O., and Turk, J. L., 1973, Allergic complications of meningococcal disease. I. Clinical aspects, *Br. Med. J.* **2:**733–737.

Wiik, A., Jensen, E., Friis, J., and Bach-Andersen, R., 1975, Participation of granulocyte-specific antinuclear factors in rheumatoid joint fluid cryoprecipitates, *Acta Pathol. Microbiol. Scand. Sect. C* **83:**265–272.

Williams, R. C., and Kunkel, H. G., 1962, Rheumatoid factor, complement and agglutinin aberrations in patients with subacute bacterial endocarditis, *J. Clin. Invest.* **41:**666–675.

Wood, H. F., 1951, Effect of C-reactive protein on normal human leucocytes, *Proc. Soc. Exp. Biol. Med.* **76:**843–847.

17

Laboratory Diagnosis of Immediate Hypersensitivity Disorders

LARRY L. THOMAS and
LAWRENCE M. LICHTENSTEIN

1. Introduction

1.1. Clinical Indication

The diagnosis of immediate hypersensitivity disorders must necessarily begin with a thorough patient history. Only after the physician has first established a temporal relationship between allergic symptoms and exposure to a specific allergen is further diagnostic evaluation indicated. Once a reasonable suspicion is established, laboratory confirmation can be obtained utilizing a variety of procedures which range from relatively simple to more elaborate and costly immunological methods.

In a sense, laboratory diagnosis of immediate hypersensitivity disorders began in 1967 with the elucidation and description of IgE antibody by Ishizaka and Ishizaka (1967). Their work not only provided insight into the mechanisms of IgE-mediated reactions but also defined IgE as a clinical determinant of diagnostic concern. The measurement of serum IgE content was made possible by the discovery of a patient with IgE myeloma by Johansson and Bennich (1967). With the availability of large quantities of IgE, purification of IgE protein and preparation of monospecific antibodies against IgE became feasible. Together, these advances led to the development of procedures for the measurement of total and allergen-specific IgE levels.

LARRY L. THOMAS and LAWRENCE M. LICHTENSTEIN • Department of Medicine, Division of Clinical Immunology, The Johns Hopkins University School of Medicine, Baltimore, Maryland 21239.

Although a convincing argument can be made that allergic reactions, like all inflammatory reactions, are multicomponent processes, diagnostic tests for the other parameters of inflammatory processes are beyond the scope of this chapter. Accordingly, the focus will be on the diagnosis of IgE antibody-associated disorders, with such diseases as hypersensitivity pneumonitis excluded.

1.2. Standardization of Major Allergens

Before the diagnostic tests themselves can be considered, the problem of allergen standardization, which impairs both the laboratory diagnosis and the treatment of allergic disorders, must be addressed. Currently, the potency of an allergenic extract is most often expressed in "protein nitrogen units" or PNU. This is a measure of the nitrogen content of the extract proteins that are precipitated by phosphotungstic acid. At best, the PNU values are a crude and often misleading indication of potency since the allergen often constitutes only a fraction of the total protein in the extract. With the absolute percentage of allergen varying from preparation to preparation, PNU values have little relevance to the biological potency of allergenic extracts. This problem is further complicated by the frequent discrepancies between the PNU content determined by the manufacturer and that determined in the individual laboratory or by the FDA (Baer *et al.*, 1970, 1974).

This uncertainty is avoided with the identification and isolation of the individual allergens within an extract. Since in most cases the molecular weights of the primary allergens are in the range of 25,000–50,000, these proteins can be quantitated by immunodiffusion or immunoelectrophoresis. The potency of the extract can then be expressed in terms of the content of the primary allergen. The identification and subsequent purification of ragweed antigen E (King *et al.*, 1964) and rye grass group I (Johnson and Marsh, 1965) have permitted standardization of crude ragweed and grass pollen extracts on the basis of these major allergens. Similar standardization of honeybee venom extracts was made possible by the identification of phospholipase A as the major allergen in honeybee venom (Sobotka *et al.*, 1976a). The advantage of standardizing extracts in this manner is demonstrated in Figure 1. While the antigen E content of six commercially prepared ragweed extracts correlated with biological potency, there was no correlation with the PNU content of the extract (Baer *et al.*, 1970), as claimed by the manufacturer or determined by the investigators. Although standardizing extracts in this manner is useful, the requirement for monospecific antibodies restricts application of immunodiffusion to extracts containing known and purified allergens.

The procedure which currently appears to hold the most promise for uniform standardization of allergenic extracts is that of radioallergosorbent (RAST) inhibition (Gleich *et al.*, 1974). The RAST technique for measuring IgE antibody will be discussed in detail below (Section 3.3). In the present context, this technique involves the interaction of allergen-coated beads with a serum pool of IgE antibody; this reaction is inhibited by extracts of unknown potency. All extracts can then be assigned a potency relative to the inhibition obtained with a known standard. Since the allergen extract itself is bound to the beads, the technique of RAST inhibition circumvents the need for purified allergens. Gleich *et al.* (1974) have shown that extracts standardized in this fashion have a highly predictable biological potency.

With its commercial availability and increasingly widespread use, the RAST inhibition technique will likely become the method of choice for standardizing the potency of allergenic extracts. Presently, however, there is no uniform, practical method for the comparison of results obtained in one laboratory with those obtained in another. For this reason, each laboratory must currently establish its own criteria for standardization of allergenic extracts and exercise caution when using new extract preparations. This latter point becomes of obvious importance in skin testing procedures.

2. Skin Testing

2.1. Introduction

Skin testing is the primary test for the diagnosis of allergic disorders. Since the work of Prausnitz and Küstner (1921), it has been known that the wheal and flare which follows local administration of allergen results from specific IgE antibodies against the allergen. The wide acceptance of skin testing is due not only to its controlled mimicry of allergic reactions but also to its simplicity, which allows testing to be done in the physician's office without the need of costly diagnostic equipment. Skin testing offers the additional advantage that a large number of tests can be conducted rapidly and with results available immediately.

A problem in skin testing is that alluded to above, namely, the differing potencies of individual extracts. While physicians and clinics in the past often prepared their own allergen extracts, today the extracts of almost every known allergen are commercially available. Usually obtained in concentrated forms, the extracts are diluted to the appropriate concentrations by the physician, relying on experience and the maxim that it is safer to overestimate rather than underestimate the potency of an extract. As a common practice, results with any new extract preparation should be compared with a preparation of known potency on at least a few patients.

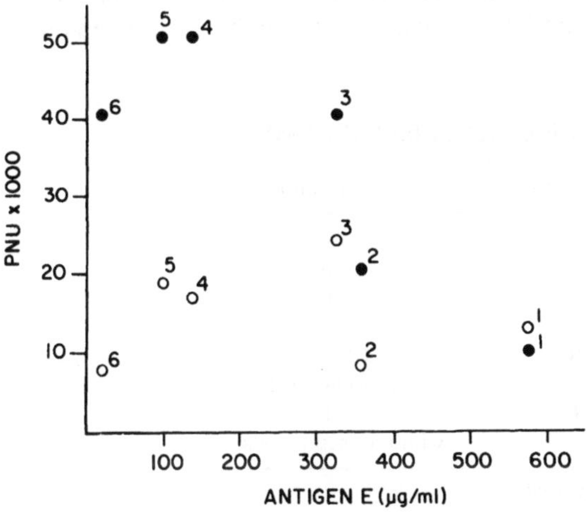

Figure 1. Relationship between PNU and antigen E content of six ragweed extracts. •, PNU claimed by manufacturer; o, PNU measured by the investigators. From Baer *et al.* (1970), *J. Allergy Clin. Immunol.* **45**:347–354.

2.2. Test Procedures

The two methods commonly employed for skin testing are intradermal skin tests and prick tests. Each method utilizes the forearm (or back when a large number of tests are to be done) for the test surface, but the methods differ in the means of administration and scoring of results. In the intradermal procedure, 0.02–0.05 ml of extract is injected; the volume is not crucial since the resultant wheal and erythema are more a function of the extract concentration than the volume, although the latter must be consistent. After 15–20 min, the site is examined for wheal and erythema formation, and the response is quantitated by measuring the mean diameter, calculated from the greatest and smallest diameters. The reactions are then graded according to an arbitrary but consistent scheme, such as that shown in Table 1. In practice, a dilution of extract expected to give a minimal reaction is first tested. If negative, serial tenfold greater concentrations are administered until either a positive reaction is elicited or the highest concentration to be tested is reached without a reaction. Conversely, if the initial dilution is positive, serial tenfold dilutions are tested, with the greatest dilution giving a 2+ reaction considered the end point. For example, highly sensitive ragweed subjects give a 2+ response with 10^{-5} or 10^{-6} μg antigen E/ml, while less sensitive individuals exhibit a 2+ reaction to 10^{-4}–10^{-3} μg/ml (Norman *et al.*, 1973).

In the prick test, a drop of extract is placed on the skin and the skin is punctured (< 1 mm) through the drop with a needle. After about 1 min, the drop is wiped away and the site is examined 15 min later. The wheal and flare produced by the prick test is smaller than that observed with the intradermal test, and, consequently, the response is often expressed in terms of the dimensions of the reaction without subsequent grading. To obtain reactions of equal dimensions with the two techniques, an approximate thousandfold greater concentration must be used in the prick test. With this adjustment, the results obtained by each technique correlate well (Belin and Norman, 1977).

2.3. Clinical Interpretation

There is no clear indication for employing one test over the other, although the prick test may be more convenient for the pediatric patient and somewhat faster overall for the adult patient. The best indication for which test to use is that

TABLE 1. Grading System for Skin Test[a]

Grade	Erythema (mm)	Wheal (mm)
0	<5	<5
±	5–10	5–10
1+	11–20	5–10
2+	21–30	5–10
3+	31–40	10–15 with pseudopods
4+	>40	>15 without pseudopods

[a] From King and Norman (1962).

one with which the laboratory or physician has the greatest experience. The same considerations apply to interpretation of both the intradermal and prick test results. In this regard, the major problem is to distinguish truly positive and negative reactions from false positive and negative reactions. An apparently positive response can, in some cases, be induced by the testing procedure itself. Some individuals may react to the needle trauma alone or, more often, to the diluent itself. For this reason, a diluent control is routinely included in any series of tests. False positives may also result following administration of extracts at the upper concentration ranges since most proteins in concentrated form can promote local irritation. Accordingly, positive reactions obtained with the less concentrated extracts have the greatest clinical significance.

Apparently negative reactions can result from poor injection or pricking technique (i.e., subdermal rather than intradermal) as well as reduced sensitivity to the tests, such as may occur when the patient is on medication. Most medications used to treat allergic conditions (steroids, theophylline, β-agonists) do not interfere with the tests (Chipps *et al.*, 1978); antihistamines, however, may reduce sensitivity (Perper *et al.*, 1973). To be certain that the patient's skin is responsive, most physicians test skin reactivity to a histamine solution as a positive control. False-negative reactions also result from the use of deteriorating or inappropriate extracts. An important consideration in food and drug allergies is that an individual may be sensitive to a metabolic product of the allergen rather than to the intact allergen. In some cases, sensitivity arises only after the metabolic product has become bound to a circulating macromolecule. With the exception of penicillin skin testing reagents, which contain both penicillin and its metabolic products, skin testing is of little value in these cases; consequently, diagnoses must be made on the basis of the patient's history alone.

Within these limitations, skin testing is a valid and useful diagnostic tool. Although the precision of both skin testing procedures is, at best, ±300%, it is possible to distinguish between individuals of lesser and greater sensitivity on the basis of the 2+ end point. This is illustrated in Figure 2.

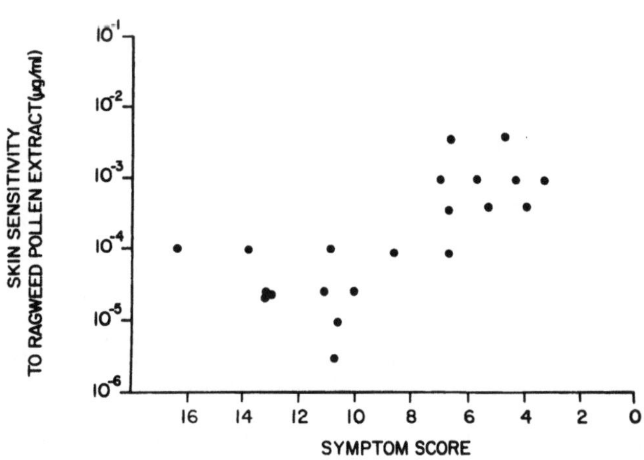

Figure 2. Correlation between skin test sensitivity to ragweed pollen extract and symptom score of patients during ragweed season. From Norman *et al.* (1973), *J. Allergy Clin. Immunol.* **52**:210–224.

3. Determination of Total and Specific IgE

3.1. Introduction

Since the early demonstration by Prausnitz and Küstner (1921) that reaginic sensitivity accompanied the transfer of serum from an allergic to a normal individual, the role of serum components in allergic reactions has been recognized. As noted, however, it was not until 1967 that the responsible "reagins" were identified as IgE antibodies. With its participation in allergic mechanisms established, the measurement of serum level IgE became of clinical interest. Although the cell-fixed IgE is probably the more clinically relevant, its quantitation is presently done only within the realm of the research laboratory. The finding in many systems (Bazaral *et al.*, 1973; Hamburger *et al.*, 1974; Conroy *et al.*, 1977) of a strong correlation between the amounts of cell-fixed and circulating IgE, however, suggests a dynamic equilibrium between the two pools (Figure 3).

Initial efforts to determine IgE antibody levels with the standard methods used for measurement of other serum immunoglobulins proved unsuccessful because of their limited sensitivity. Unlike the other classes of immunoglobulins which circulate in microgram and milligram per milliliter concentrations, IgE is present at nanogram per milliliter levels. Thus, the serum IgE concentration is below the lower limits of sensitivity of the radial immunodiffusion technique (≥ 1 μg/ml) routinely used for the determination of other classes of serum immunoglobulin levels (Mancini *et al.*, 1965). As stated above, the development of procedures with greater sensitivity became possible following the discovery by Johansson and Bennich (1967) of a patient with E myeloma. Since that initial report, about ten additional patients have been discovered with E myeloma, providing a continuous source for pure human IgE. There are currently three procedures available for the measurement of total serum IgE. Two of the methods are classified as solid-phase radioimmunoassays while the third is a double antibody technique.

Of further diagnostic importance was the development of a solid-phase

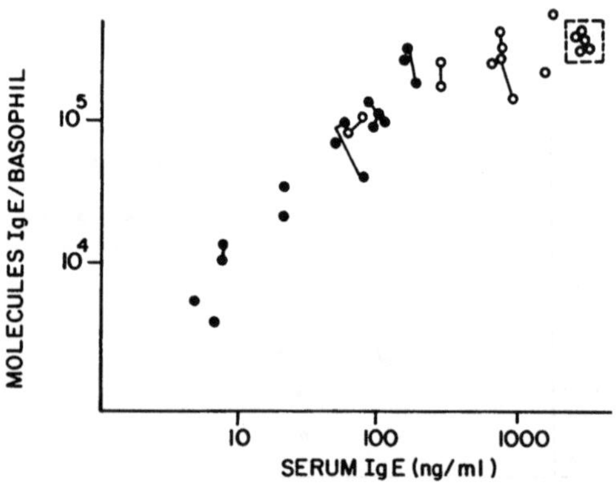

Figure 3. Correlation between cell-bound and serum IgE. ○, Allergic individuals; •, nonallergic individuals. Lines connect values determined for the same individual at separate times. The points contained within the square represent multiple determinations for a single individual. From Conroy *et al.* (1977), *J. Immunol.* **113**:1317–1321. © 1977, The Williams and Wilkins Co., Baltimore.

radioimmunoassay for the determination of allergen-specific IgE (Wide *et al.*, 1967). Although, as already noted, the specific IgE molecules fixed to the basophil and mast cell membranes would be of primary diagnostic interest, quantitation of this IgE is not feasible. Measurement of specific IgE in the serum by the RAST test, however, has proven useful in the diagnosis of allergic disorders (Wide, 1973; Berg and Johansson, 1974).

3.2. Measurement of Total IgE

3.2.1. Competitive Radioimmunosorbent Test (Competitive RIST)

The competitive RIST assay, first described by Wide (1971), is a competitive binding assay in which sample IgE competes with added [^{125}I]-IgE for a limited number of anti-IgE molecules covalently linked to cellulose or Sephadex particles (Figure 4A). After an overnight incubation and subsequent wash, the radioactivity of the particles is measured, with the sample IgE content inversely proportional to the measured radioactivity. The absolute IgE levels are obtained from a standard curve constructed with sera of known IgE content which are also carried through

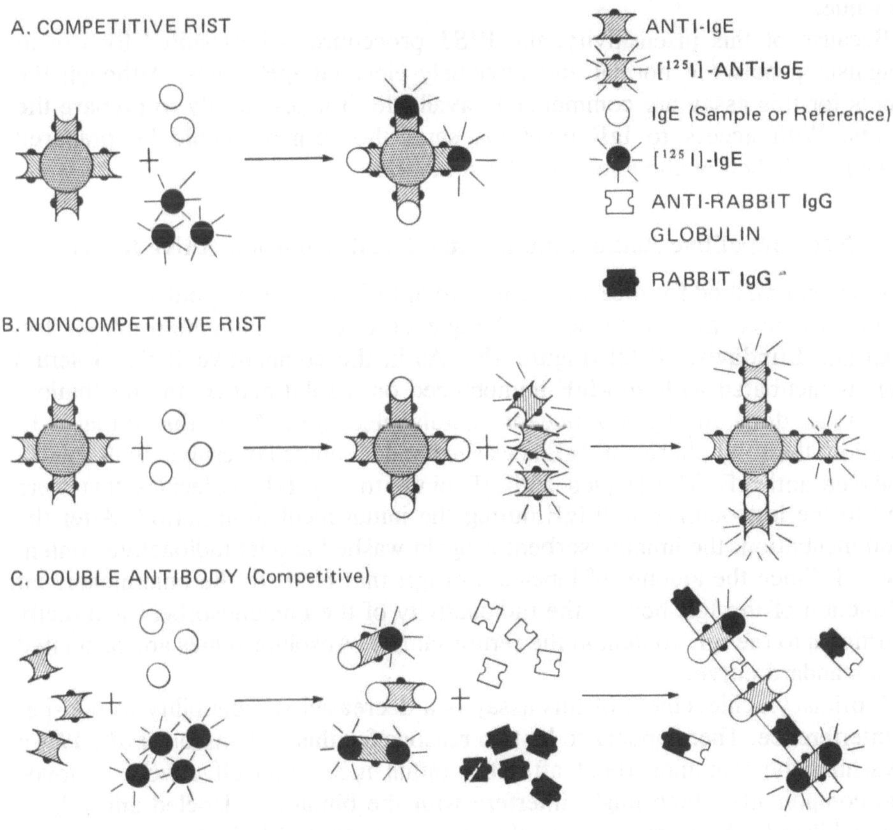

Figure 4. Procedures for measurement of serum total IgE level.

Figure 4. Procedures for measurement of serum total IgE level.

the assay procedure. In practice, the standard curve includes an IgE concentration range of approximately 2–1000 ng/ml. Although IgE levels are currently expressed in either International Units per milliliter, based on a World Health Organization reference serum, or nanograms per milliliter, the latter designation will be utilized here. Conversion between the two values is done using the accepted equivalency of 2.4 ng IgE per International Unit. To express its results in these units, the individual laboratory can standardize its own reference serum against an international reference serum.

The major disadvantage to the RIST technique are a limited sensitivity and a significant variability (15–20%). The precision is particularly poor in samples having less than 100 ng IgE/ml (Johansson *et al.*, 1976). To optimize the sensitivity as much as possible, the assay mixture routinely contains a quantity of anti-IgE that can bind maximally only about 20% of the added [^{125}I]-IgE. In addition, nonspecific interference to which the technique is subject is minimized. The anti-IgE employed is prepared from immune rabbit sera to avoid the possibility of antibodies in the sample cross-reacting with the anti-IgE (Foucard *et al.*, 1975). To reduce interference from other serum components, both the sample and standard sera are diluted (e.g., 1:5 and 1:10) prior to the assay; assaying the IgE content of each sample at two dilutions also provides an internal control for the accuracy of each value.

Because of this insensitivity, the RIST procedure is best suited for use in distinguishing between normal and obviously elevated IgE levels. Although the reagents for this assay are commercially available, it is less costly to prepare the reagents. With access to IgE myeloma sera, the reagents could be prepared following published methodology (Adkinson, 1976).

3.2.2. Noncompetitive Radioimmunosorbent Test (Noncompetitive RIST)

A second method for measurement of total IgE is a noncompetitive assay that may be described as a sandwich technique or direct radioimmunosorbent test (Ceska and Lundqvist, 1972) (Figure 4B). As in the competitive RIST, a serum sample is incubated with anti-IgE immobilized on a solid matrix; the incubation, however, is done in the absence of radiolabeled IgE. After this initial 3-hr incubation, the solid-phase anti-IgE is washed and incubated overnight with soluble ^{125}I-labeled anti-IgE. The labeled anti-IgE binds to any IgE molecules that were bound to the immobilized anti-IgE during the initial incubation period. After the second incubation, the immunosorbent is again washed and its radioactive content measured. Since the amount of labeled anti-IgE that binds to the immunosorbent is a function of the IgE bound, the radioactivity of the immunosorbent is directly proportional to the IgE content in the serum sample. Absolute values are calculated from a standard curve.

A primary achievement of this assay is a decreased susceptibility to nonspecific interference. There appear to be two reasons for this (Johansson *et al.*, 1976): (1) washing the immunosorbent after the initial incubation effectively removes serum components which might interfere with the binding of labeled anti-IgE to the immobilized IgE molecules; (2) unlike the competitive RIST procedure, excess anti-IgE is coupled to the insoluble matrix. Thus, antibodies in the serum sample directed against the anti-IgE itself will have less influence on IgE binding. As a result, anti-IgE purified from immunized goat or sheep serum can be employed for the immunosorbent. The labeled anti-IgE, however, must be purified from immune rabbit sera. Since nonspecific interference does occur with undiluted serum samples, samples are diluted prior to the assay as described above for the competitive RIST. Optimally, the samples are diluted such that the values fall in the midrange of the standard curve.

The second major achievement of this assay is the increased sensitivity and greatly improved reproducibility. Unlike the competitive RIST, this technique can measure ≧ 1 ng/ml of IgE with precision; the variability over the entire range of the standard curve (1–1000 ng/ml) is less than 5%. This method is clearly indicated for IgE determinations in samples expected to have a low IgE content, such as serum from infants (Orgel *et al.*, 1975), and when maximal accuracy is required.

Other advantages also contribute to making this technique a method of choice. Purified IgE is required only for antibody production and avoids the expense of iodinated E myeloma protein. Of importance to laboratories routinely measuring both total and specific IgE levels, the labeled anti-IgE employed in this procedure is the same as that used in the RAST measurement of specific IgE (see below). As for the competitive RIST, reagents for this method are also commercially available. Since the commercial kit uses paper disks as the immunosorbent, this method is sometimes referred to as "PRIST" (for paper-RIST). The reagents can also be prepared according to published methodology (Adkinson, 1976).

3.2.3. Double Antibody Radioimmunoassay

The third method available for the measurement of total IgE is the double antibody radioimmunoassay developed by Gleich *et al.* (1971) (Figure 4C). Similar in principle to the competitive RIST, it exhibits the high degree of sensitivity characteristic of the noncompetitive RIST. The serum sample is incubated together with anti-IgE and added [^{125}I]-IgE, but, unlike in the solid-phase procedures, the anti-IgE is not immobilized on an insoluble matrix. Rather, after an initial 4-hr incubation, anti-rabbit IgG, together with rabbit IgG, is added, and the sample is incubated overnight. With the rabbit IgG serving as a carrier protein, the anti-rabbit IgG precipitates the soluble immune complexes of anti-IgE and bound sample or labeled IgE. The amount of sample IgE that is bound is inversely proportional to the radioactivity of the precipitate; absolute IgE levels are calculated using a standard curve.

Although the double antibody technique avoids the need for immobilized anti-IgE, it does require the second precipitating antibody. The anti-IgE must be purified from immune rabbit serum as in the other procedures, while the anti-rabbit IgG is produced in sheep or goats. The latter antibody need not be highly purified, but a precipitin curve must be run to establish the serum dilution required for optimal precipitation. The reagents for the double antibody procedure are also commercially available, but at considerable expense. For this reason, preparation of the reagents according to published methodology (Gleich *et al.*, 1971; Adkinson, 1976) is recommended.

Although the double antibody method is subject to nonspecific interference, this is much less of a problem than with the competitive RIST, probably because of use of a soluble rather than immobilized antibody. The practice of measuring

IgE content in diluted serum samples essentially eliminates nonspecific interference. The sensitivity of this method is excellent over the entire standard curve of 1–1000 ng/ml, with a precision equal to that of the noncompetitive RIST. Gleich and Dunnette (1977) have in fact shown that the double antibody and noncompetitive RIST yield the same results for sera and body fluids such as saliva and colostrum having IgE contents ranging from 2–25,000 ng/ml. These procedures therefore represent dual methods of choice with regard to precision, reliability, and consistency.

3.2.4. Significance of Total IgE Antibody Levels

Although IgE antibody levels were defined as a dianostic parameter in 1967 (Ishizaka and Ishizaka, 1967), routine methods for antibody quantitation were not applicable. With the development of the methods presented above, measurement of serum IgE content became possible. The diagnostic interpretation of IgE levels, however, still requires caution. Contributing significantly to this need for caution is the rather large overlap in serum IgE levels of atopic and nonatopic individuals (Table 2). With such overlap, discriminating between allergic and nonallergic individuals on the basis of total IgE is clearly difficult. This problem has been reduced somewhat by the establishment of the normal range of IgE values in nonatopic individuals. Determinations of IgE content in sera of rigorously selected nonatopic populations have yielded geometric means of 50–120 ng IgE/ml (Waldmann *et al.,* 1972; Nye *et al.,* 1975). Although mean values in the random adult population would be higher, Nye *et al.* (1975) reported an IgE level of approximately 800 ng/ml as the 95% confidence limit for an elevated serum content.

Distinguishing between elevated and normal IgE levels is complicated further by age, genetic, and parasite-related influences on IgE levels. The age-related influence is of particular importance in the pediatric patient. In neonates, the mean IgE level is approximately 5 ng/ml, with over 50% having no detectable IgE (Orgel *et al.,* 1975). This level increases with age, although there is a discrepancy at which age adult values are reached (Gerrard *et al.,* 1974; Kjellman *et al.,* 1976). Consequently, establishing criteria for elevated levels in children is more difficult (Berg and Johansson, 1969; Kjellman *et al.,* 1976). Important in both pediatric and adult evaluation is the documented genetic control of basal IgE levels (Marsh *et al.,* 1974; Gerrard *et al.,* 1976). The likelihood of high IgE levels and incidence of allergic disease is greater in individuals of families with a positive atopic history.

TABLE 2. Total Serum IgE Levels in Atopic and Nonatopic Adults[a]

Population	*N*	Range	Mean	95% interval	Reference
Nonatopic	98	1–2,700	179[b]	6–780[c]	Gleich *et al.* (1971)
	73	6–5,000	105[d]	5–2,045	Waldmann *et al.* (1972)
	102	2.5–9,178	309[b]	2.5–1,241	Nye *et al.* (1975)
Atopic	133	55–12,750	—	—	Gleich *et al.* (1971)

[a] Adapted from Adkinson (1976).
[b] Arithmetic mean.
[c] 94% interval.
[d] Geometric mean.

Although a link between IgE and other nonallergic diseases has not clearly been established, the association of high IgE levels with many parasitic infections is well recognized (Johansson *et al.*, 1968; Kojima *et al.*, 1972). This is of obvious importance in environments where parasitism is prevalent.

With the broad overlap in IgE values of atopic and nonatopic individuals, the likelihood of allergic disease is greatest with a highly elevated IgE level. The wide range in serum IgE levels of atopic individuals, however, indicates that some highly sensitive patients may have a low total IgE content. This apparent disparity is reconciled by findings which demonstrate that IgE specific for a single allergen may constitute up to 40% of the total IgE (Schellenberg and Adkinson, 1975; Gleich and Jacobs, 1975). Thus, although total IgE is low, a significant percentage of that IgE may be specific for the relevant allergen. This is underscored by the results of Conroy *et al.* (1977) which suggest that only minimal occupation of basophil IgE receptors is sufficient to sensitize the cell.

3.3. Measurement of Specific IgE

3.3.1. Radioallergosorbent Test (RAST)

The radioallergosorbent test (RAST) (Wide *et al.*, 1967) is quite similar to the noncompetitive RIST, but the allergen or allergenic extract, rather than anti-IgE, is immobilized on the solid-phase matrix (Figure 5). The allergosorbent is incubated first for 4 hr with dilutions of the serum sample to bind IgE antibodies for the immobilized allergen. After washing to remove adherent serum components, the allergosorbent is incubated overnight with radiolabeled anti-IgE, the same as employed in the noncompetitive RIST. With labeled anti-IgE binding to the bound IgE molecules, the radioactivity of the allergosorbent is directly proportional to the amount of bound, and thus sample, allergen-specific IgE.

Although the RAST is a highly sensitive and precise (< 5% intraassay variability) technique, its application is limited by a number of inherent problems. Primary among these is that the method, as currently done, yields results in relative antibody titers based on a reference serum. A standard curve is constructed from a series of dilutions of a reference serum, and the activity of each sample is

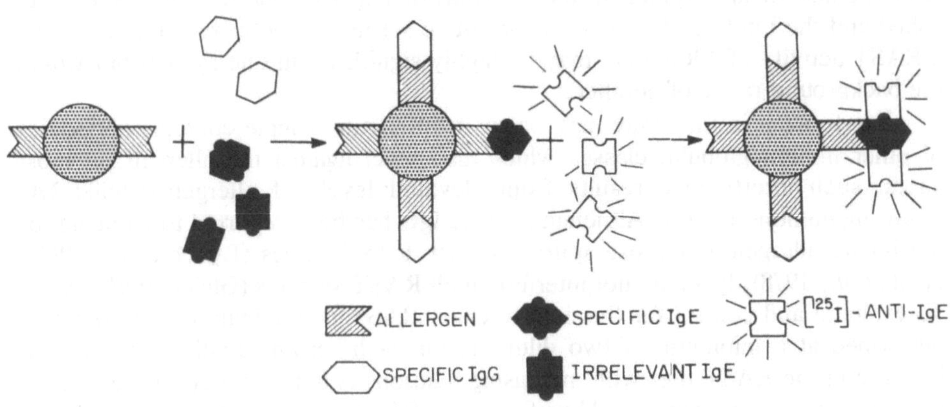

Figure 5. RAST technique.

expressed as the corresponding dilution of the reference serum. Thus, if the reference serum is arbitrarily defined as containing 1000 RAST units, a sample with radioactivity corresponding to a 1:5 dilution of the reference serum would contain 200 RAST units (0.2 × 1000). Reporting results in this manner, with no internationally recognized standard, makes comparison of results from different laboratories almost impossible. This, however, should be reversed with the development of techniques (Schellenberg and Adkinson, 1975; Gleich and Jacob, 1975) which permit quantitation of absolute amounts of IgE antibody against a variety of purified allergens. Although not in general use, sera standardized with these techniques can be used as the reference sera and the routine RAST results then expressed in nanograms of IgE per milliliter.

With no standardized reference sera, it is necessary for each laboratory to establish criteria for defining positive and negative RAST values. The nonspecific binding, that is, activity obtained with sera from nonatopic individuals or from patients sensitive to an unrelated allergen, must be critically evaluated for each RAST sorbent. This is of particular relevance in RAST systems which utilize allergosorbents prepared with allergen extracts. As indicated above, the relevant allergens frequently constitute only a small percentage of the total protein in the extract. Consequently, RAST sorbents prepared from these mixtures can contain multiple allergens. Because many people, including nonatopic individuals, may have low levels of antibodies against common allergens, sorbents containing multiple allergens increase the nonspecific binding or background activity. For this reason, it is necessary to identify which components of an extract are bound to the sorbent and to verify that the relevant allergens are in fact included. In addition, it must be demonstrated that the allergosorbent removes all of the antibodies specific for the allergen(s) from a high-titer serum. This is evaluated using P-K testing or leukocyte passive sensitization (see below).

Since the background activity, as well as the total binding capacity, varies with the allergosorbent, each RAST system requires its own blank and high-titer, specific reference serum. Unfortunately, this requirement is currently disregarded in commercially available RAST procedures. These systems utilize a single allergosorbent and reference serum specific for other allergens. The deficiencies in this approach should be evident. RAST results can be interpreted intelligently only after the statistical variation in background, or negative, values had been established and the binding of a high-titer, positive serum characterized. For example, a RAST activity of 1000 units may be highly significant in one system but within the background range of another.

Interference in the assay may occur if the serum sample contains antibodies of other immunoglobulin classes which also react against the allergen. In most cases, such interference results from elevated levels of allergen-specific IgG following immunotherapy. Although specific IgG has been reported to compete for the bound allergen and cause spuriously low RAST values (Lynch *et al.*, 1975; Paull *et al.*, 1978), IgG may not interfere in all RAST systems (Gleich *et al.*, 1977). To evaluate and control for this interference, RAST determinations are routinely performed at a minimum of two dilutions for each serum sample. An apparent increase in the RAST titer with increasing dilutions is indicative of interference in the minimally diluted samples. Therefore, a RAST value is accepted if two dilutions yield the same RAST titer.

3.3.2. Interpretation of RAST values

Although allergen-specific IgE is of greater clinical relevance than total IgE, RAST technology as it presently exists provides only a semiquantitative index of specific IgE levels. Only in limited instances when the IgE content of the reference serum has been quantitated in absolute units (Schellenberg and Adkinson, 1975; Gleich and Jacobs, 1975) does the RAST assay yield more than relative antibody titers. Still, RAST values, when appropriately determined, have proven to be of diagnostic use (Wide, 1973; Berg and Johansson, 1974) and have been found to correlate rather well with skin test sensitivity (Norman *et al.*, 1973; Lichtenstein *et al.*, 1973), as shown in Figure 6. This correlation is strongest for highly sensitive individuals.

The uncertainty in interpretation of RAST results, however, becomes apparent with values that are less than highly elevated. As for total IgE levels, there is a considerable spectrum of values in which it is difficult to distinguish between control and elevated RAST values. This leads to a significant proportion of false-positive and false-negative results. During the evaluation of two RAST systems for the diagnosis of venom hypersensitivity, Sobotka *et al.* (1978) found 15–20% each of false positives and false negatives, based on a positive history and skin test response to the appropriate venom. The prevalence of false values was similar for determinations made using a RAST sorbent prepared with purified allergen and a sorbent prepared with an allergen extract. The primary reason for the frequent occurrence of false values was the wide overlap in the RAST values obtained for

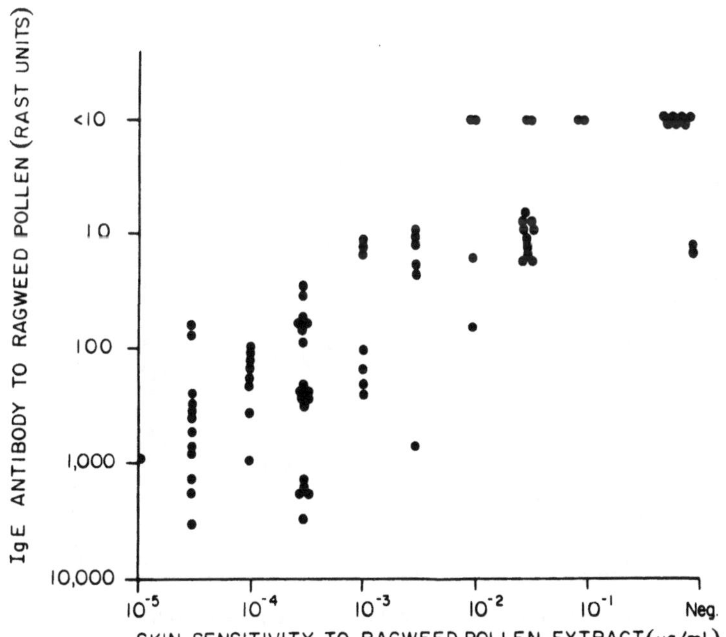

Figure 6. Correlation between IgE antibody to antigen E (in arbitrary RAST units) and skin test sensitivity (2+ endpoint). From Norman *et al.* (1973), *J. Allergy Clin. Immunol.* **52**:210–224.

control and sensitive individuals. This is illustrated in Figure 7. Although sera of three control populations were utilized to define the background activity, sera of a significant number of history and skin test positive patients gave background, or negative, RAST values. Most false-negative values occur with atopic individuals who have an extremely low total IgE level. Although the specific IgE level in such patients may represent a significant percentage of their total IgE, the absolute quantity of antibody yields a RAST value only marginally elevated above the control level. Concomitant measurement of total IgE will help identify false negatives of this nature. As alluded to already, false-negative values may also arise with patients having a high level of specific IgG (Lynch *et al.*, 1975; Paull *et al.*, 1978). This is an obvious consideration in patients undergoing immunotherapy.

Because of this rather large overlap in RAST values, together with the manner in which RAST results are reported, the RAST technique must currently be considered a semiquantitative diagnostic screen. A high RAST value, appropriately determined, will likely indicate allergic sensitivity, but the inherent uncertainties in RAST methodology cloud the interpretation of lesser values. In these instances, skin test sensitivity is of greater diagnostic use.

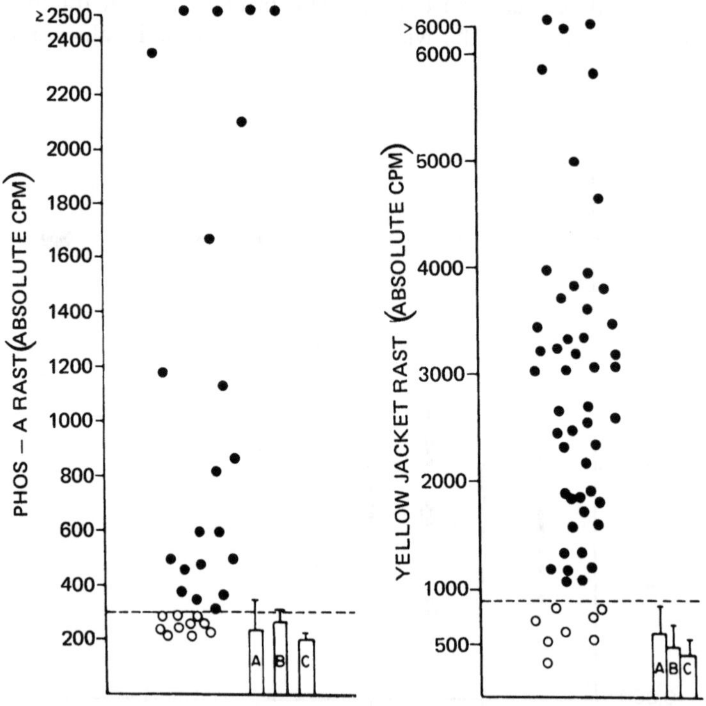

Figure 7. Comparison of RAST values for skin test positive patients to background activity. Patients were sensitive to either honeybee venom (phospholipase A) or yellow jacket venom; RAST values are given as cpm [^{125}I]-anti-IgE bound. Nonspecific binding ± SD by sera from three control populations is represented by bar graphs. •, Positive RAST values; ○, negative RAST values. From Sobotka *et al.* (1978), *J. Immunol.* **121**:2477–2484. © 1978, The Williams and Wilkins Co., Baltimore.

4. Measurement of Specific IgG

4.1. Double Antibody Technique

Immunotherapy has long been recognized to provide symptomatic relief in pollen-sensitive individuals. Since 1935 (Cooke *et al.*, 1935), the clinical improvement following immunotherapy has been attributed to the existence of a class of antibodies termed "blocking antibodies." These antibodies were found to inhibit both skin test reactivity (Loveless, 1943) and *in vitro* histamine release from human leukocytes (Lichtenstein and Osler, 1966). Using the latter system, it was shown that essentially all of the blocking antibodies were of the IgG class (Lichtenstein *et al.*, 1968a); furthermore, a significant correlation between blocking antibody levels and clinical improvement was demonstrated in ragweed-sensitive patients (Lichtenstein *et al.*, 1968b). These studies suggested, therefore, that quantitation of allergen-specific IgG levels might provide a means to assess the clinical protection provided by immunotherapy.

Initially, inhibition of *in vitro* histamine release constituted the best method for the quantitation of specific IgG levels. This procedure, however, has now been replaced by two radioimmunoassays (Yunginger and Gleich, 1973; Sobotka *et al.*, 1976b; Gleich *et al.*, 1977). Although the two methods are similar in that each is a double antibody technique, that of Sobotka *et al.* (1976b) is described because of its increased sensitivity.

An allergen or allergen extract radiolabeled with ^{125}I is incubated for 4 hr with dilutions of the serum sample (Figure 8). Goat anti-IgG is then added, and the incubation is continued overnight. To maintain the amount of total IgG (carrier protein) constant, sample dilutions greater than 1:40 are made using a 1:40 dilution of a control serum. The resultant precipitate is washed and the radioactive content quantitated, with the amount of IgG bound directly proportional to the amount of radioactivity. Maximal antigen binding is established in each assay, using a standard serum prepared by pooling several high-titer sera of individuals treated with the relevant allergen or extract. The IgG titer of each sample is then expressed as the reciprocal of the serum dilution giving 50% maximal binding. For purified allergens, the technique has been further extended to permit quantitation of the IgG content

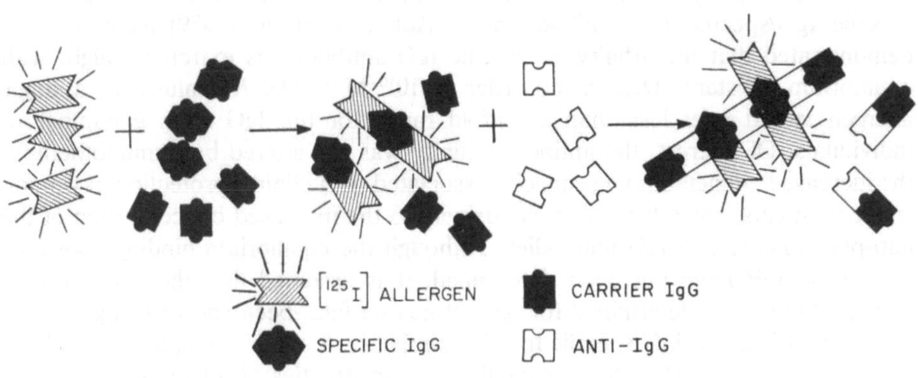

Figure 8. Radioimmunoassay for measurement of specific IgG.

in absolute units (Adkinson *et al.*, 1979). With the IgG concentration in the standard or reference serum determined by saturation analysis (Mulligan *et al.*, 1966), the IgG content of the samples can be interpolated from a standard curve constructed from a series of dilutions of the reference serum. In this manner, IgG levels of 0.5 μg/ml or greater can be detected with a coefficient of variation of approximately 7%. Further sensitivity, although not routinely required, can be achieved with appropriate modifications (Adkinson *et al.*, 1979). Background activity with either purified allergen or with an allergen extract constitutes only 1–2% of the total radioactivity added.

4.2. Clinical Significance

The suppression of seasonal increases in IgE levels by immunotherapy was first suggested by studies measuring P-K sensitivity (Sherman *et al.*, 1940) and leukocyte sensitivity *in vitro* (Levy and Osler, 1967). The development of RAST methodology led to confirmation of this observation in ragweed-sensitive patients (Lichtenstein *et al.*, 1973; Gleich *et al.*, 1977). Furthermore, RAST determinations showed that the postseasonal level of IgE antibodies to antigen E was lower after immunotherapy (Lichtenstein *et al.*, 1973; Evans *et al.*, 1976; Gleich *et al.*, 1977). Of diagnostic importance, these declines in specific IgE levels were apparently unrelated to clinical symptoms (Lichtenstein *et al.*, 1973). In two of the studies, however, coincident increases in the specific IgG titer were observed with the decline in IgE antibody level (Lichtenstein *et al.*, 1973; Evans *et al.*, 1976).

Although statistically significant correlations between increases in specific IgG levels and clinical protection were thus established, it was not known if the association was one of cause and effect. A cause-and-effect relationship, however, has been suggested for the protection provided by immunotherapy for Hymenoptera venom sensitive patients (Lessof *et al.*, 1978). Treatment with whole body extract provided no clinical protection, while complete protection was afforded by venom treatment; this correlated with the finding that only venom treatment increased the specific IgG content. Still, it has not proven possible to predict the extent of clinical protection with a single IgG value. This implies that the relationship between specific IgG and clinical protection is more subtle than originally believed.

One possibility is that the degree of protection may be a function of the specific IgG/specific IgE antibody ratio. Adkinson *et al.* (1979) have recently demonstrated that the affinity of specific IgG antibodies is extremely high, with equilibrium constants (K_0) in the order of 10^{10} M^{-1}. The K_0 values for a single allergen varied over less than a tenfold range for the IgG from a number of individuals. Of interest, the antibody affinity was not altered by immunotherapy; the increased antigen-binding capacity associated with clinical protection in venom-treated patients was attributable exclusively to the increased concentration of the anti-phospholipase A IgG antibodies. Although the equilibrium binding constants of specific IgE have not been determined, it is assumed that the K_0 of IgE is comparable to that determined for IgG. It has, in fact, been shown using another system that IgE and IgG specific for phospholipase A exhibit comparable avidities (Paull *et al.*, 1978). Thus the potentially similar affinities of allergen-specific IgG and IgE emphasizes the significance of the relative antibody concentrations.

Other contributing factors to the clinical protection must still be considered. The finding that minimal amounts of antibody are sufficient to sensitize basophils to release by anti-IgE (Conroy *et al.*, 1977) suggests that cell reactivity may be an important parameter. A genetic influence on antibody production similarly cannot be excluded. The positive correlation between IgE and IgG antibody levels (Yunginger and Gleich, 1973; Platts-Mills *et al.*, 1978) is consistent with a common genetic influence governing the response of each antibody to the allergen. Thus, although the level of specific IgG antibody has been found to correlate significantly with clinical protection, it cannot be stated that it is the only determinant of protection.

5. Auxiliary Procedures

Although the methods discussed above represent the procedures routinely used in the diagnosis of allergic disorders, they do not constitute all of the available tests. One reason for the acceptability of the diagnostic tests already described is their commercial availability and relatively straightforward assay protocols. Additional methods, however, do exist, and some find extensive use in the research laboratory. Since these tests can be of diagnostic use in some instances, accessibility to such resources should be exploited whenever possible.

5.1. Histamine Release from Leukocytes *in Vitro*

This procedure mimics one of the primary components of the allergic reaction, the IgE-mediated release of histamine from human basophils (Lichtenstein and Osler, 1964). Basophils comprise less than 1% of the circulating leukocytes but are the only bloodborne cells to contain histamine and to have cell-fixed IgE antibody molecules (Ishizaka *et al.*, 1972). Accordingly, human leukocytes can be used without need for further purification. Leukocytes isolated by dextran sedimentation are incubated in a calcium-containing buffer with the allergen, in concentrations of nanogram to microgram per milliliter, at 37°C for 30–60 min. Allergen extracts can also be used. The histamine released is quantitated and expressed as a percentage of the total cellular histamine content. A typical histamine release curve for an individual allergic to ragweed antigen E is shown in Figure 9. Leukocyte sensitivity is often expressed as the antigen concentration yielding 30% release. The limiting factor until recently has been measurement of histamine. Early methods were time consuming and limited to measuring the content in a relatively few samples. These restrictions have been overcome by the development of an automated method for the fluorometric determination of histamine content (Siraganian, 1975). With this system, histamine concentrations as low as 1 ng/ml can be measured with precision and a large number of samples can be analyzed rapidly. A current limitation to the automated system is cost.

Because histamine release is a function of antigen–IgE antibody interaction, this represents a sensitive method for the detection of allergen-specific IgE molecules on the basophil surface. In addition, this technique provides an index of cellular "releasability," which may be altered in some allergic disorders (Kern and Lichtenstein, 1976). Cell sensitivity by histamine release has been shown to correlate well with skin test results and RAST determinations (Lichtenstein *et al.*, 1973; Norman *et al.*, 1973; Sobotka *et al.*, 1976b). Results with this technique have also been found to correlate with symptom severity in pollenosis (Figure 10). For diagnostic uses, absence of histamine release with a particular antigen or extract implies a lack of sensitivity to the allergens in question. There are, however, individuals who are history and skin test positive to a particular allergen but fail to release histamine when leukocytes are challenged with the allergen. The ability of the cells to release can then be evaluated using anti-IgE as the stimulus (Lichtenstein *et al.*, 1970).

5.2. Passive Sensitization

The detection of allergen-specific IgE was historically performed using the Prausnitz–Küstner (Prausnitz and Küstner, 1921), or P-K, test of passive sensitization. The test is based on the prolonged retention of IgE at the site of injection and the ability of IgE to bind to receptors on mast cells. The P-K test is now obsolete, although there is still a limited use of monkeys as the recipients for passive sensitization. They are the only heterologous species in which human IgE will fix to the mast cells, but even they are tenfold less sensitive. With the allergen injected intravenously after sensitization of the skin, the test is analogous to the passive cutaneous anaphylaxis (PCA) reaction in other species. Ethical considerations and the expense of monkeys will soon make this last vestige of the P-K reaction similarly obsolete.

Another method for passive sensitization, and the method of choice, is the passive sensitization of leukocytes from a normal donor with an allergic serum (Levy and Osler, 1966). In this way, the basophils are made sensitive to the allergen and histamine release can be evaluated as discussed above. Although this technique has been proven valuable in research, it is too cumbersome for routine

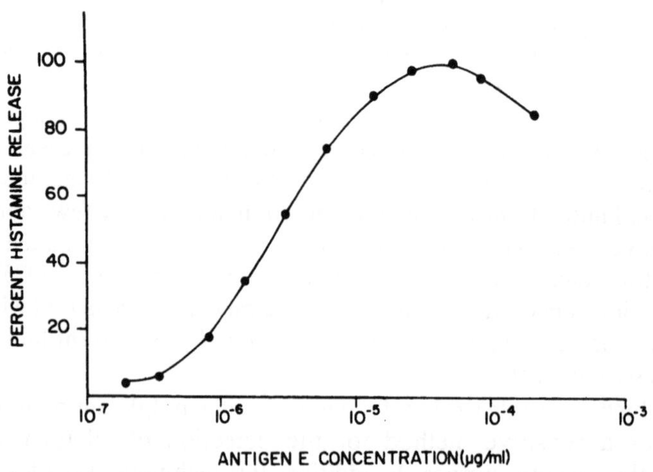

Figure 9. Dose response for histamine release with antigen E from leukocytes of a ragweed allergic individual. From Lichtenstein (1971), *Ann. N.Y. Acad. Sci.* **185**:403–412.

diagnostic use and is limited by the number of normal donors who are good passive recipients. It is of value, however, as the only method available to evaluate a parameter of potential importance, the ability of IgE antibody to fix to the basophil and mast cell receptors. The serological methods for IgE quantitation provide a measure of the antibody-combining sites only; leukocyte passive sensitization evaluates both that and the Fc function of IgE. Although the finding that sera from different donors vary in their ability to sensitize leukocytes from a single donor (Conroy and Lichtenstein, 1976) suggests heterogeneity with respect to the function of the Fc portion of IgE, the diagnostic importance of this parameter is not yet defined.

5.3. Bronchial and Conjunctival Challenge

Localized administration of allergens into bronchial, conjunctival, or nasal mucosa has been occasionally employed to measure allergic sensitivity, with the rationale that the procedures permit evaluation of sensitivity at the sites of clinical symptoms. Such provocation techniques have been utilized most often to measure sensitivity to pollens and other airborne allergens. These procedures in general are, however, not particularly suited for diagnostic evaluation because of difficulties in quantitating results. Responses generally can be graded only as either positive or negative, while proper controls often cannot be included. One test which is

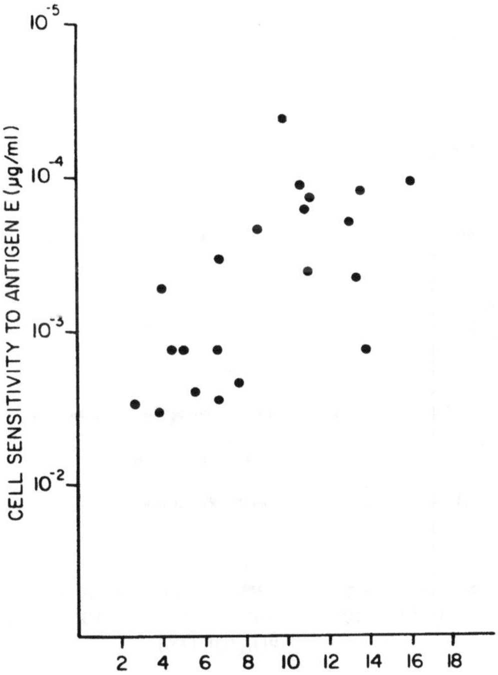

Figure 10. Correlation between leukocyte sensitivity to antigen E and symptom score of patients during ragweed season. Cell sensitivity is expressed as allergen concentration giving 50% release. From Lichtenstein *et al.* (1973), *J. Clin. Invest.* **52**:472–482.

semiquantitative is inhalation challenge, or bronchoprovocation. In this technique, reduction in specific airway conductance or an increase in resistance is determined following inhalation of known concentrations of aerosolized allergen. Although this procedure has been advocated for use in the diagnosis of allergic asthma, the benfit-to-risk ratio limits diagnostic use of this test. Further, a study of ragweed-sensitive individuals indicated that bronchoprovocation and skin testing provided similar quantitative indications of allergic sensitivity (Bruce *et al.*, 1975) (Figure 11). Other provocative techniques have likewise not proven superior to skin testing.

6. Summary

With the description of IgE antibody and the development of methodology for its measurement, laboratory diagnosis of allergic disorders began to emerge. Initially beset by insensitive procedures, discriminating between normal and elevated serum IgE levels has become increasingly reliable with the advent of techniques such as the direct RIST. This diagnostic capability is further enhanced by the concomitant measurement of specific IgE with the RAST procedure. The importance of determining both total and specific IgE levels is illustrated by atopic individuals who have a relatively low total IgE content, which nevertheless consists of a high percentage of specific IgE. The diagnostic value of these determinations, however, is not without limitations. These limitations are particularly evident in

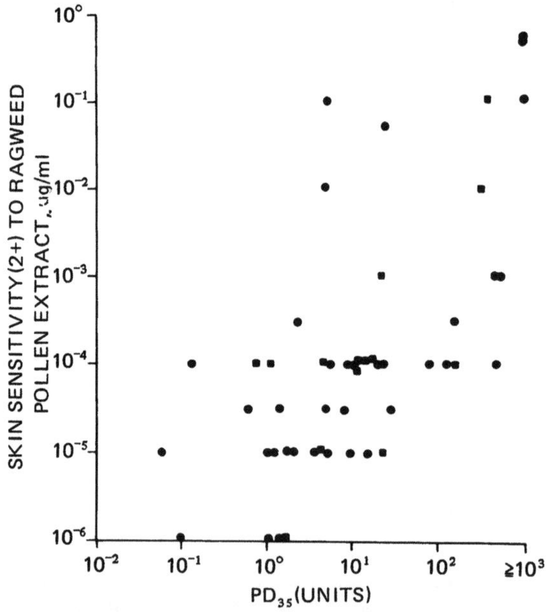

Figure 11. Correlation between provocation dose (PD_{35}) of ragweed extract causing 35% decrease in airway conductance (in arbitrary units) and skin test sensitivity (2+ end point) to ragweed pollen extract. •, Ragweed asthmatic patients; ▪, ragweed-sensitive, nonasthmatic donors. From Bruce *et al.* (1975), *J. Allergy Clin. Immunol.* **56**:331–337.

RAST measurements because of the rather wide spectrum of ambiguous RAST values.

The present uncertainty in the interpretation of IgE measurements ensures the continuation of end-point skin testing as the best single criterion for diagnosis of allergic disease. None of the other procedures has yet surpassed skin testing in diagnostic usefulness. Further contributing to the popularity of skin testing are the minimal expense and simplicity as compared to the other techniques. Still, some uncertainty is introduced by the current lack of standardization among allergenic extracts. For this reason, it is recommended that no single procedure be used exclusively in the diagnosis of allergic disease. Rather, information obtained by both skin testing and measurement of total and specific IgE levels provides the most reliable basis for an accurate diagnosis.

7. References

Adkinson, N. F., Jr., 1976, Measurement of total serum IgE and allergen specific IgE antibody, in: *Manual of Clinical Immunology* (N. Rose and H. Friedman, eds.), pp. 590–602, American Society for Microbiology, Washington, D. C.

Adkinson, N. F., Jr., Sobotka, A. K., and Lichtenstein, L. M., 1979, Evaluation of the quantity and affinity of human IgG "blocking" antibodies, *J. Immunol.* **122:**965–972.

Baer, H., Godfrey, H., Maloney, C. J., Norman, P. S., and Lichtenstein, L. M., 1970, The potency and antigen E content of commercially prepared ragweed extracts, *J. Allergy* **45:**347–354.

Baer H., Maloney, C. J., Norman, P. S., and Marsh, D. G., 1974, The potency and group I antigen content of six commercially prepared grass pollen extracts, *J. Allergy Clin. Immunol.* **54:**157–164.

Bazaral, M., Orgel, H. A., and Hamburger, R. N., 1973, The influence of serum IgE levels of selected recipients, including patients with allergy helminthiasis and tuberculosis, on the apparent P-K titre of a reaginic serum, *Clin. Exp. Immunol.* **14:**117–125.

Belin, L. G., and Norman, P. S., 1977, Diagnostic test in the skin and serum of workers sensitized to *Bacillus subtillus* enzyme, *Clin. Allergy* **7:**55–68.

Berg, T., and Johansson, S. G. O., 1969, IgE concentrations in children with atopic diseases: A clinical study, *Int. Arch. Allergy* **36:**219–232.

Berg, T. L. O., and Johansson, S. G. O., 1974, Allergy diagnosis with the radioallergosorbent test, *J. Allergy Clin. Immunol.* **54:**209–221.

Bruce, C. A., Rosenthal, R. R., Lichtenstein, L. M., and Norman, P. S., 1975, Quantitative inhalation bronchial challenge in ragweed hay fever patients: A comparison with ragweed-allergic asthmatics, *J. Allergy Clin. Immunol.* **56:**338–346.

Ceska, M., and Lundqvist, U., 1972, A new and simple radioimmunoassay method for the determination of IgE, *Immunochemistry* **9:**1021–1030.

Chipps, B. E., Teets, K. C., Sanders, J. P., Sobotka, A. K., Norman, P. S., and Lichtenstein, L. M., 1978, The effects of theophylline and terbutaline on immediate skin tests and basophil histamine release, *J. Allergy Clin. Immunol.* **61:**171–172 (Abstr.).

Conroy, M. C., and Lichtenstein, L. M., 1976, Measurement of IgE binding to human leukocytes, *Fed. Proc.* **35:**898.

Conroy, M. C., Adkinson, N. F., Jr., and Lichtenstein, L. M., 1977, Measurement of IgE on human basophils: Relation to serum IgE and anti-IgE induced histamine release, *J. Immunol.* **118:**1317–1321.

Cooke, R. A., Barnard, J. H., and Stull, A., 1935, Serological evidence of immunity with co-existing sensitization in a type of human allergy (hay fever), *J. Exp. Med.* **62:**733–750.

Evans, R., Pence, H., Caplan, H., and Rocklin, R. E., 1976, The effect of immunotherapy on humoral and cellular responses in ragweed hay fever, *J. Clin. Invest.* **57:**1378–1385.

Foucard, T., Bennich, H., Johansson, S. G. O., and Lundqvist, U., 1975, Human antibodies to bovine gamma globulin: Occurrence in immunological disorders and influence on allergy and radioimmunoassays, *Int. Arch. Allergy Appl. Immunol.* **48:**812–823.

Gerrard, J. W., Horne, S., Vickers, P., Mackenzie, J. W. A., Goluboff, N., Garson, J. Z., and Maningas, C. S., 1974, Serum IgE levels in parents and children, *J. Pediatr.* **85:**660–663.

Gerrard, J. W., Ko, M., Vickers, P., and Gerrard, C. D., 1976, The familial incidence of allergic disease, *Ann. of Allergy* **36:**10–15.

Gleich, G. J., and Dunnette, S. L., 1977, Comparison of procedures for measurement of IgE protein in serum and secretions *J. Allergy Clin. Immunol.* **59:**377–382.

Gleich, G. J., and Jacob, G. L., 1975, Immunoglobulin E antibodies to pollen allergens account for high percentages of total immunoglobulin E protein, *Science* **190:**1106–1108.

Gleich, G. J., Averback, A. K., and Svedlund, H. A., 1971, Measurement of IgE in normal and allergic serum by radioimmunoassay, *J. Lab. Clin. Med.* **77:**690–698.

Gleich, G. J., Larson, J. B., Jones, R. T. and Baer, H., 1974, Measurement of the potency of allergy extracts by their inhibitory capacities in the radioallergosorbent test, *J. Allergy Clin. Immunol.* **53:**158–169.

Gleich, G. J., Jacob, G. L., Yunginger, J. W., and Henderson, L. L., 1977, Measurement of the absolute levels of IgE antibodies in patients with ragweed hay fever: Effect of immunotherapy on seasonal changes and relationship to IgG antibodies *J. Allergy Clin. Immunol.* **60:**188–198.

Hamburger, R. N., Fernandez-Cruz, E., Arnaiz, A., Perez, B., and Bootello, A., 1974, The relationship of the P-K titre to the serum IgE levels in patients with leprosy, *Clin. Exp. Immunol.* **17:**253–260.

Ishizaka, K., and Ishizaka, T., 1967, Identification of γE antibodies as a carrier of reaginic activity, *J. Immunol.* **99:**1187–1198.

Ishizaka, T., DeBernardo, R., Tomioka, H., Lichtenstein, L. M., and Ishizaka, K., 1972, Identification of basophil granulocytes as a site of allergic histamine release, *J. Immunol.* **108:**1000–1008.

Johansson, S. G. O., and Bennich, H., 1967, Immunological studies of an atypical (myeloma) immunoglobulin, *Immunology* **13:**381–394.

Johansson, S. G. O., Mellbin, T., and Vahlquist, B., 1968, Immunoglobulin levels in Ethiopian preschool children with special reference to high concentrations of immunoglobulin E (IgND), *Lancet* **1:**1118–1121.

Johansson, S. G. O., Bergland, A., and Kjellman, N.-I. M., 1976, Comparison of IgE values as determined by different solid phase radioimmunoassay methods, *Clin. Allergy* **6:**91–98.

Johnson, P. and Marsh, D. G., 1965, "Isoallergens" from rye grass pollen, *Nature (London)* **206:**935–937.

Kern, F., and Lichtenstein, L. M., 1976, Defective histamine in release in chronic urticaria, *J. Clin. Invest.* **57:**1369–1377.

King, T. P., and Norman, P. S., 1962, Isolation studies of allergens from ragweed pollen, *Biochemistry* **1:**709–711.

King, T. P., Norman, P. S., and Connell, J. T., 1964, Isolation and characterization of allergens from ragweed pollen. II, *Biochemistry* **3:**458–468.

Kjellman, N.-I. M., Johansson, S. G. O., and Roth, A., 1976, Serum IgE levels in healthy children quantified by a sandwich technique (PRIST), *Clin. Allergy* **6:**51–59.

Kojima, S., Yokogawa, M., and Tada, T., 1972, Raised levels of serum IgE in human helminthiases, *Am. J. Trop. Med. Hyg.* **21:**913–918.

Lessof, M. H., Sobotka, A. K., and Lichtenstein, L. M., 1978, Effects of passive antibody in bee venom anaphylaxis, *Johns Hopkins Med. J.* **142:**1–7.

Levy, D. A., and Osler, A. G., 1966, Studies on the mechanisms of hypersensitivity phenomena. XIV. Passive sensitization *in vitro* of human leukocytes to ragweed pollen antigen, *J. Immunol* **97:**203–212.

Levy, D. A., and Osler, A. G., 1967, Studies on the mechanisms of hypersensitivity phenomena. XVI. *In vitro* assays of reaginic activity in human sera: Effect of therapeutic immunization on seasonal titer changes, *J. Immunol.* **99:**1068–1077.

Lichtenstein, L. M., 1971, The role of cyclic AMP in inhibiting the IgE-mediated release of histamine, *Ann. N. Y. Acad. Sci.* **185:**403–412.

Lichtenstein, L. M., and Osler, A. G., 1964, Studies on the mechanisms of hypersensitivity phenomena. IX. Histamine release from human leukocytes by ragweed pollen antigen, *J. Exp. Med.* **120:**507–530.

Lichtenstein, L. M., and Osler, A. G., 1966, Studies on the mechanisms of hypersensitivity phenomena. XII. An *in vitro* study of the reaction between ragweed pollen antigen, allergic human serum and ragweed sensitive cells, *J. Immunol.* **96**:169–179.

Lichtenstein, L. M., Holtzman, N. A., and Burnett, L. S., 1968a, A quantitative *in vitro* study of the chromatographic distribution and immunoglobulin characteristics of human blocking antibody, *J. Immunol.* **101**:317–324.

Lichtenstein, L. M., Norman, P. S., and Winkenwerder, W. L., 1968b, Clinical and *in vitro* studies on the role of immunotherapy in ragweed hay fever, *Am. J. Med.* **44**:514–524.

Lichtenstein, L. M., Levy, D. A., and Ishizaka, K., 1970, *In vitro* reversed anaphylaxis: Characteristics of anti-IgE mediated histamine release, *Immunology* **19**:831–842.

Lichtenstein, L. M., Ishizaka, K., Norman, P. S., Sobotka, A. K., and Hill, B. M., 1973, IgE antibody measurements in ragweed hay fever: Relationship to clinical severity and the results of immunotherapy, *J. Clin. Invest.* **52**:472–482.

Loveless, M. H., 1943, Immunological studies of pollinosis. IV. The relationship between thermostable antibody in the circulation and clinical immunity, *J. Immunol.* **47**:165–180.

Lynch, N. R., Durand, P., Newcomb, R. W., Chai, H., and Bigley, J., 1975, Influence of IgG antibody and glycopeptide allergens on the correlation between the radioallergosorbent test (RAST) and skin testing or bronchial challenge with *Alternaria*, *Clin. Exp. Immunol.* **22**:35–46.

Mancini, G., Carbonara, A. O., and Heremans, J. F., 1965, Immunochemical quantitation of antigens by single radial immunodiffusion, *Immunochemistry* **2**:235–254.

Marsh, D. G., Bias, W. B., and Ishizaka, K., 1974, Genetic control of basal serum immunoglobulin E level and its effect on specific reaginic sensitivity, *Proc. Natl. Acad. Sci. USA* **71**:3588–3592.

Mulligan, J. J., Osler, A. G., and Rodriguez, E., 1966, Weight estimates of rabbit anti-human serum albumin based on antigen binding capacity, *J. Immunol.* **96**:324–333.

Norman, P. S., Lichtenstein, L. M., and Ishizaka, K., 1973, Diagnostic tests in ragweed hay fever, *J. Allergy Clin. Immunol* **52**:210–224.

Nyl, L., Merratt, T. G., Landon, J., and White, R. J., 1975, A detailed investigation of circulating IgE in a normal population, *Clin. Allergy* **5**:13–24.

Orgel, H. A., Hamburger, R. N., Bazarel, M., Gorrin, H., Groshong, T., Lenoir, M., Miller, J. R., and Wallace, W., 1975, Development of IgE and allergy in infancy, *J. Allergy Clin. Immunol.* **65**:296–307.

Paull, B., Jacob, G. L., Yunginger, J. W., and Gleich, G. J., 1978, Comparison of binding of IgE and IgG antibodies to honeybee venom phospholipase-A, *J. Immunol.* **120**:1917–1923.

Perper, R. J., Sanda, M., and Lichtenstein, L. M., 1973, The relationship of *in vitro* and *in vivo* allergic histamine release: Inhibition in primates by cAMP active agonists, *Intl. Arch. Allergy Appl. Immunol.* **43**:837–844.

Platts-Mills, T. A. E., Snajdr, M. J., Ishizaka, K., and Frankland, A. W., 1978, Measurement of IgE antibody by an antigen binding assay: Correlation with PK activity and IgG and IgA antibodies to allergens, *J. Immunol.* **120**:1201–1210.

Prausnitz, C., and Küstner, H., 1921, Studien über Überempfindlichkeit, *Centralbl. Bakteriol. Abt. I Orig.* **86**:160–169.

Schellenberg, R. R., and Adkinson, N. F., Jr., 1975, Measurement of absolute amounts of antigen-specific human IgE by a radioallergosorbent test (RAST) elution technique, *J. Immunol.* **115**:1577–1583.

Sherman, W. B., Stull, A., and Cooke, R. A., 1940, Serologic changes in hay fever cases treated over a period of years, *J. Allergy* **11**:225–240.

Siraganian, R. P., 1975, Refinements in the automated fluorometric histamine analysis system, *J. Immunol. Methods* **7**:283–290.

Sobotka, A. K., Franklin, R. M., Adkinson, N. F., Jr., Valentine, M. D., Baer, H., and Lichtenstein, L. M., 1976a, Allergy to insect stings. II. Phospholipase A: The major allergen in honeybee venom, *J. Allergy Clin. Immunol.* **57**:29–40.

Sobotka, A. K., Valentine, M. D., Ishizaka, K., and Lichtenstein, L. M., 1976b, Measurement of IgG-blocking antibodies: Development and application of a radioimmunoassay, *J. Immunol.* **117**:84–90.

Sobotka, A. K., Adkinson, N. F., Jr., Valentine, M. D., and Lichtenstein, L. M., 1978, Allergy to insect sting. IV. Diagnosis by radioallergosorbent test (RAST), *J. Immunol.* **121**:2477–2484.

Waldmann, T. A., Stober, W., Polmar, S. H., and Terry, W. D., 1972, IgE levels and metabolism in immune deficiency diseases, in: *The Biological Role of the Immunoglobulin E Systems* (K. Ishizaka and D. H. Dayton, eds.), pp. 247–258, USPHS, Washington, D.C.

Wide, L., 1971, Solid-phase antigen-antibody systems, in: *Radioimmunoassay Methods* (K. E. Kirkham and W. M. Hunter, eds.), pp. 405–412, E. and S. Livingstone, Edinburgh.

Wide, L., 1973, Clinical significance of measurements of reaginic (IgE) antibody by RAST, *Clin. Allergy Suppl.* **3**:583–595.

Wide, L., Bennich, H., and Johansson, S. G. O., 1967, Diagnosis of allergy by an *in vitro* test for allergen antibodies, *Lancet* **2**:1105–1107.

Yunginger, J. W., and Gleich, G. J., 1973, Seasonal changes in IgE antibodies and their relationship to IgG antibodies during immunotherapy for ragweed hay fever, *J. Clin. Invest.* **52**:1268–1275.

18

Immunological and Pharmacological Management of Allergic Diseases

ROY PATTERSON

1. Allergic Rhinitis

Allergic rhinitis is an immediate-type, IgE-mediated reaction involving the nasal mucosa. It is usually associated with a similar type involvement of the conjunctiva, and often of the mucosa of the oropharynx. Symptoms consist of rhinorrhea, sneezing, nasal congestion, pruritis of the nose and conjunctiva, lacrimation, and pruritis of the oropharynx. Physical examination usually shows edematous nasal mucosa which is often pale and bluish in appearance, in contrast to the normal pink appearance of the mucosa. The conjunctiva is erythematous. A major diagnostic aid in allergic rhinitis is a history of seasonal occurrence or the occurrence of symptoms in relation to an identified exposure to allergen such as animals. The diagnosis is primarily made by such a history and confirmed by demonstration of the presence of IgE antibodies by cutaneous testing which demonstrates an immediate-type, wheal-and-flare reaction. *In vitro* laboratory tests, demonstrating serum IgE antibody, may provide equivalent information with certain allergens. A typical case of allergic rhinitis usually does not provide a difficult diagnostic problem when there is a clear seasonal and geographic or environmental relation of the symptoms. Perennial allergic rhinitis may be more difficult to define, particularly if the cause of the nasal symptoms is nonallergic rhinitis occurring in the subject who has IgE antibodies against common inhalant antigens.

The etiological agents in allergic rhinitis are almost always inhalant antigens.

ROY PATTERSON • Allergy Section, Department of Medicine, Northwestern University Medical School, Chicago, Illinois 60611.

Rarely, food antigens can induce similar symptoms. In the latter case, the correlation of food ingestion with the onset of symptoms is almost always readily apparent to an observant patient. Prior to initiation of long-term immunological management, it is important that adequate diagnosis be made since appropriate immunological management may result in disruption of the patient's environment or a lengthy, expensive, and tedious program of treatment.

1.1. Immunological Management

1.1.1. Avoidance Therapy

The preferred management of any allergic condition is avoidance of the antigen responsible for inducing the reaction. In the management of allergic rhinitis this can be accomplished with great success with certain antigens. The animal danders that are of major importance in the causation of the nasal symptoms should be avoided. If cat or dog dander is the major inciting antigen a "cure" of chronic symptoms may result from elimination of the household pet. This solution is often considered unsatisfactory by patients but nevertheless is the therapy of choice for significant symptoms. In the case of house dust allergy, control of exposure to house dust can often result in marked amelioration of symptoms. The measures of control of house dust exposure need not be excessively rigid. Particular attention to control of house dust in the patient's bedroom by enclosing mattresses, box springs, and pillows in plastic casings will often have a significant beneficial effect achieved with minimal cost and effort.

Avoidance of other common causes of inhalant-induced rhinitis may be very difficult. The airborne pollens, which travel for considerable distances, cannot be successfully avoided even by geographic moves with rare exceptions. Even in these cases, geographic moves are often economically and socially unfeasible. In those cases where symptoms are of sufficient duration and are uncontrolled by safe and benign medications, a more intense form of immunotherapeutic approach may be indicated. This includes the use of allergen injection therapy (allergen immunotherapy).

1.1.2. Immunotherapy

Allergen immunotherapy is the systemic administration of the antigens which are the etiological agents in the individual case of allergic rhinitis. Such therapy began after the recognition that pollen was capable of inducing the symptoms of allergic rhinitis. One theoretical basis for its initial use was an attempt to immunize individuals against a presumed grass pollen toxin (Noon and Cantab, 1911). The apparent success with the injection of pollen antigens and the gradually increasing understanding that the etiological mechanism of allergic rhinitis was a hypersensitivity or allergic phenomenon based on immunological mechanisms rather than a toxic phenomenon led to a shift in the concept of the mechanism of action of allergen therapy. The shift was toward the idea that desensitization was produced by administration of the offending antigen. This concept subsequently required reevaluation because later observations indicated that a complete loss of sensitivity does not usually occur (as demonstrated by continued skin reactivity), and the term "hyposensitization" was introduced to denote the state of reduced reactivity, without the total loss of allergic reactivity. Both terms, "desensitization" and "hyposensitization," continue to be used by some practitioners for inhalant immunotherapy. In the usual procedure for allergen immunotherapy, rarely does complete loss of sensitivity or true desensitization occur. Under certain conditions—for example, the rapid administration of penicillin, insulin, or horse serum—true desensitization does occur in IgE-mediated sensitivity.

Thus the clinical program of allergen immunotherapy, which began with the wrong hypothesis, has continued for about seven decades with much of the current methods of treatment primarily derived from empirical clinical trials. Recent rapid advances in immunology have led to methods of analyses of alterations produced by the therapy which should provide a more clear-cut understanding of the mechanisms of action, and thus more rational applications for clinical use.

Because the use of allergen immunotherapy arose through empirical clinical trials, there are variations in clinical methodology as carried out by different practitioners of allergy. One relatively standard method will be reviewed. Those inhalant allergens that cannot be avoided and provide significant morbidity are used for allergic immunotherapy. Except in rare circumstances (such as in a veterinary physician), injection therapy for animal danders is not used because the injection of animal proteins and the presence of high environmental antigen concentrations usually do not result in significant benefit.

Also, such therapy with animal proteins in highly sensitive individuals is often accompanied by local and systemic reactions which are, at least, uncomfortable. There is the more serious risk of the induction of anaphylaxis due to the animal protein. Similarly, food allergens are not used for injection therapy in the rare case in which they cause allergic rhinitis. Under unusual circumstances, such as baker's asthma, where a serious socioeconomic problem exists, immunotherapy with the appropriate antigen may be considered. The common inhalant allergens used for immunotherapy in the United States include ragweed, grass, and tree pollen allergens. Antigens from mold spores and house dust compose the other two major inhalant groups. Selection of the appropriate allergens for injection therapy is dependent on the careful diagnosis of the patient's disease and the etiological allergens involved as described above.

A common method of antigen administration is to begin with small doses of antigen, for example, 0.05 ml of a 1:10,000 weight/volume of pollen antigen. This is approximately 2.5 protein nitrogen units (0.15 μg protein). The protein nitrogen unit is a common reference term for pollen antigen content, although it does not clearly define the content of the individual pollen antigens. The dose of antigen is increased weekly in a subcutaneous injection, often by increments of 0.05 ml. This procedure is followed until a maintenance dose of 0.5 ml of a 1:100 weight/volume dose is achieved. Such a maintenance dose of approximately 2500 protein nitrogen units (0.15 mg protein) is considered desirable by many clinicians. After such a maintenance dose is achieved, the treatment intervals are progressively changed to every 2 weeks, every 3 weeks, and finally every 4 weeks. The rate of achieving the maintenance dose and the maximal interval between doses depend on the tolerance of the individual patient. General duration of therapy is between 3 and 4 years. Again, the length of therapy may vary with the individual patient and include such factors as the length of time required to reach maintenance therapy and the clinical response of the patient. This allergen immunotherapy is a course of perennial therapy. Other methods of immunotherapy have included coseasonal or preseasonal therapy. In coseasonal therapy, injections are given weekly or biweekly during the pollen season. In preseasonal therapy, therapy begins several months before the pollen season and is continued through the pollen season and terminates at the end of the pollen season. Objections to the latter two forms of therapy have been based on the fact that a high maintenance dose is often not achieved by the time of the pollen season and studies of efficacy of pollen immunotherapy have shown that efficacy is dependent on total dose of antigen administered (Johnstone and Dutton, 1968; Sadan *et al.*, 1969).

For many years, the efficacy of allergen immunotherapy was founded on clinical anecdotal information. More recently, controlled clinical studies have demonstrated efficacy of this type of therapy. For details of a number of such studies, the following reviews are available: Patterson *et al.* (1978a), Lieberman and Patterson (1974), and Irons *et al.* (1975). Ragweed pollenosis, because of its well-defined seasonal component and the usual severity of the clinical problem, has been a useful clinical condition for clinical research in the evaluation of the efficacy of immunotherapy.

Throughout the years a number of studies of the immunological effects of immunotherapy have been carried out. The results of such studies will not be reviewed in detail, but are summarized as follows. In ragweed pollenosis there is a postseasonal rise in IgE antibodies directed against ragweed antigen. Ragweed pollen immunotherapy has been shown to suppress this rise in IgE antibodies in some patients. Pollen immunotherapy has been shown to produce a rise in IgG antibodies against ragweed pollen antigens. This IgG antibody, which does not fix to mast cells, is considered to be protective and is the "blocking" antibody described in the 1930s (Cooke *et al.*, 1935) and postulated as a major therapeutic effect of pollen immunotherapy. Other studies have shown that there can be a decrease in reaginic antibodies (IgE antibody) with prolonged immunotherapy. Further, certain patients who have received prolonged, intensive immunotherapy may show a decrease in the ability of their peripheral blood basophils to release histamine to allergen challenge. These indices of immune response vary from patient to patient and are most easily demonstrated in groups of patients. It is possible that different immunological mechanisms may account for clinical improvement in different subjects. The immunological assessments described thus provide research tools rather than methods of assessing the immunological course for the patient. Details of immunological effects are described in reviews of the studies (Patterson *et al.* 1978a; Lieberman and Patterson, 1974; Irons *et al.*, 1975).

1.1.3. Problems of Immunotherapy

Probably the major problem of immunotherapy is the cost-benefit ratio. Because the major clinical problem numerically is allergic rhinitis, this is the major disease for which allergen immunotherapy is used. Allergic rhinitis, although of high incidence and a source of significant discomfort for many patients, does not constitute an incapacitating or lethal problem. Allergen injection therapy is a procedure requiring multiple visits to physician offices, with the resultant physician costs and additional expenses related to work loss and transportation cost. This has resulted in utilization of the therapy by the populations most able to afford the cost for increased comfort from symptoms of a relatively benign disease state. A second problem is the risk of allergen injection therapy. A common side effect of therapy is a local reaction at the site of injection. Far more uncommonly, a patient may have symptoms of malaise and fatigue following the treatment and occasionally nasal symptoms or asthma. The major hazard of therapy is anaphylaxis. Often termed a systemic or generalized allergic reaction, this is potentially a fatal reaction, although rarely so. In the hands of trained and experienced clinical allergists, the risk of a serious generalized allergic reaction is remote, but always a possibility.

It is obvious that the administration of a protein antigen which produces an IgG antibody response should receive attention as a potential inducer of circulating immune complexes and immune complex disease. Seven decades of experience with immunotherapy have not shown an association of immunotherapy with any disease classified or tentatively classified as an immune complex disease. Some studies have suggested the possibility of immune complex formation, but a recent extensive study indicates an absence of immunological abnormalities following immunotherapy, including immune complex formation (Levinson *et al.*, 1978). An explanation for this is likely to be that the amount of protein antigen used in immunotherapy is far less than that capable of inducing immune complex disease in experimental animals. Indeed, in the average allergic individual the risk of anaphylaxis prohibits the administration of amounts of protein that could produce immune complex disease. Thus while suggested as a potential hazard, in reality, conclusive evidence in support of such a problem is not apparent.

Finally, a problem with allergen immunotherapy is that patients' response to therapy varies. A marked control of symptoms may occur in some patients, diminution of symptoms in others, and occasionally no apparent therapeutic response in still others. At times, in some cases a response may occur but the expectations of patients are not satisfied and they report a treatment failure because they have not received adequate prior explanation that complete disappearance of symptoms rarely occurs. Evaluation of the progress of the perennial rhinitis patient should be done at 12 and 18 months after starting treatment to determine degree of effect, and, if no benefit has occurred, possibly therapy should be discontinued. The explanation for complete treatment failures is unknown. Individuals who have nonallergic rhinitis of the vasomotor type with coincidentally positive skin tests would not be expected to benefit from immunotherapy.

1.1.4. Newer Forms of Immunotherapy

Over many years, attempts have been made to improve allergen immunotherapy by reducing the number of injections required and retaining efficacy. These procedures have been reviewed in detail elsewhere (Patterson *et al.*, 1978a). For example, pollen antigens have been administered in an emulsion of water in oil. This resulted in a form of repository therapy with slow release of antigen from the water-in-oil emulsion. Such therapy was terminated for general investigational use because of the question of safety of the hydrocarbon oil constituent of the emulsion. Alum-precipitated allergens as used in alum-precipitated tetanus toxoid to provide a more prolonged antigen stimulus are currently in use and under continuing investigation. In other experimental approaches, attempts have been made to modify allergens by chemical treatment. Formaldehyde treatment of allergen has been used to produce an allergoid presumptively based on the concept that allergenicity may be reduced while immunogenicity is retained (Haddad *et al.*, 1972). In a different approach, allergens have been treated to construct higher-molecular-weight polymers (Metzger *et al.*, 1976). The latter have reduced allergenicity with retained immunogenicity because of molecular sieve fractionation exclusion of low molecular weight antigens, reduced ability of the polymers to react with IgE bound to mast cells, but retention of antigenic determinants by the larger molecules.

Based on animal experimentation, it is reasonable to expect that in the future methodology will be developed for controlled stimulation in humans of T-suppressor lymphocytes capable of reducing or terminating production of IgE antibodies against specific allergens. The application of these basic research studies on lymphocyte control mechanisms to the clinical practice of allergy will likely take considerable time.

1.2. Pharmacological Management

1.2.1. Antihistamines

The primary pharmacological management of allergic rhinitis is based on the use of antihistamine therapy. These agents may completely control minimal symptoms, and are safe. The limitations of this therapy are only the inability of antihistamines to control severe rhinitis and drug side effects. General principles of use of antihistamines include the regular administration of the antihistamines at appropriate intervals, up to four times daily. The antihistamines will be more effective when used regularly in prevention of onset of symptoms rather than in relief of symptoms after their onset. Because of the large number of antihistamines available, it is recommended that physicians become highly experienced in the use of a limited number of these agents so that both effectiveness and side effects can be easily evaluated in the individual patient.

The antihistamines utilized for allergic rhinitis are now recognized as blockers of the histamine-1 receptor sites on cells. There are three major types of compounds: ethanolamines, ethylenediamines, and alkylamines. Examples of effective agents of these three groups are diphenhydramine, tripelennamine, and chlorpheniramine, respectively. The first is a very effective antihistamine but is commonly not used routinely for daytime therapy because of its soporific side effect. The other antihistamines listed are somewhat less effective but significantly less soporific than diphenhydramine. The soporific effect of these drugs may decrease or disappear after regular use. Occasionally, subjects taking antihistamines chronically appear to become refractory to the therapeutic benefit also, and this may be corrected by switching to an antihistamine of a different therapeutic class, for example, from chloropheniramine to tripelennamine. The antihistamines listed are by no means the only effective agents and are cited here merely as useful examples. Patients initiating an antihistamine regimen should be warned about the soporific side effects and cautioned regarding their use while driving or in conjunction with alcohol until the medication has been used for a trial period. Antihistamines are often used as delayed-release preparations, at times in combination with nasal decongestants. Selection of such preparations should be based on physician experience and on patient acceptance.

1.2.2. Sympathomimetic Agents

Sympathomimetic agents with combined β and α-stimulatory effects, such as ephedrine, may have some benefit in control of nasal symptoms. α-Adrenergic agents such as phenylephrine, particularly when applied topically, will have a definite transient vasoconstrictive action with transient relief of nasal congestion. These agents are often used in combination preparations with antihistamines or may be used singly in subjects unable to tolerate the side effects of antihistamines. Their use as oral agents often has limited efficacy in allergic rhinitis. The chronic topical application of vasoconstricting agents to the nasal mucosa in allergic rhinitis is inappropriate. Short use (2–3 days) during upper respiratory infections or to promote drainage during sinus infections may provide a therapeutic adjunct. Persistent and frequent use beyond a several-day period may result in a rebound-type phenomenon with nasal congestion termed "rhinitis medicamentosa." It is simply an intense nasal response to misuse of vasoconstricting agents.

1.2.3. Corticosteroids

Corticosteroids have a dramatic effect in the control of symptoms of allergic rhinitis. The mechanisms by which such actions occur are unknown except for the broad antiinflammatory action of these agents. Injectable corticosteroids, oral agents, or topical agents all will control the nasal symptoms. In severe cases of seasonal allergic rhinitis, uncontrolled by antihistamines and with a limited period of duration of symptoms, corticosteroids become an appropriate therapeutic consideration. For example, during the 6-week ragweed season of the midwestern United States, the use of corticosteroids during the 4 weeks that pollen concentration is highest would be an appropriate form of treatment. The prolonged use of corticosteroids for multiseasonal or perennial rhinitis must be considered cautiously in that potent corticosteroids with known side effects would be required for long-term use for control of symptoms which are uncomfortable but not life threatening or incapacitating. When indicated for control of seasonal rhinitis, the order of preference of the corticosteroids is as follows: Topical dexamethasone, initially at a higher dose to control symptoms and then reduced to the minimal dose to maintain remission, is the first drug of choice. A topical nasal corticosteroid rarely controls the associated allergic conjunctivitis, and systemic steroids may then be indicated. In this case, oral prednisone on an alternate-day regimen is used. The dose of about 0.6 mg/kg on alternate days usually controls symptoms and is then tapered to a lower dose once the rhinitis has responded to initial therapy. Single injections of depot corticosteroids are efficacious, but the use of this form of therapy results in sustained levels of corticosteroids and probably a more prolonged suppression of adrenal cortical function than low-dose alternate-day prednisone or minimal-dose topical dexamethasone.

In summary, the appropriate use of pharmacological agents as required by the severity of the individual patient's symptoms will control many if not a majority of cases of seasonal rhinitis. When duration of symptoms is throughout a significant portion of the year, and these symptoms are uncontrolled with benign (noncorticosteroid) agents, allergen immunotherapy should be considered.

2. Asthma

2.1. Definition

Asthma is a complex respiratory disease probably best characterized as the presence of a hyperreactive airway. It is characterized by physiologically reversible obstructive airway disease and execessive production of respiratory mucus. The clinical presentation is intermittent wheezing dyspnea which varies markedly from patient to patient and even within the same patient at different times. There are a variety of forms, ranging from mild low-grade wheezing, requiring no medication, to very severe asthma resulting in recurrent episodes of status asthmaticus, a potentially lethal state of uncontrolled asthma. Mixtures of reversible and irreversible obstructive lung disease may occur in the same patient, and asthma induced only by exercise occurs in a few patients. A variety of stimuli including immunologically specific and nonspecific (smoke, cold air, exercise) may stimulate the hyperreactive airway of the asthmatic.

2.2. IgE-Triggered Asthma

Although the characteristic of asthma is an airway hyperreactive to multiple irritant stimuli, there is a broad group of asthmatics who have an antigen/antibody-mediated reaction as one of the primary triggers of an airway response. These individuals have IgE antibodies against antigens which are inhaled and which can result in the release of multiple factors from IgE-sensitized mast cells.

A major hypothesis of the mechanism of asthma stimulated by inhaled allergens has been that the sequence of antigen reacting with IgE fixed to mast cells with resultant mediator release. The release of biologically active mediators presumptively results in an immediate-type obstruction in the airway. Experimental evidence in support of this hypothesis has recently been obtained in an animal model of asthma (Patterson *et al.*, 1978b), which demonstrated that sensitized bronchial lumen mast cells from asthmatic monkeys can transfer antigen reactivity to airways of recipient animals.

There are many patients with asthma who have no apparent IgE antibodies to inhalant antigens. These "intrinsic" asthmatics often have an onset of the disease in the postchildhood period and in general may have more severe asthma than inhalant-triggered asthma. In the "intrinsic" asthmatic there is a frequent relation of exacerbations of asthma with respiratory infections. A small group of asthmatics have a curious triad of aspirin reactivity (which produces an acute onset of severe, possibly fatal asthma), nasal polyps, and chronic asthma. The explanation for the aspirin response is unknown, although there is no good evidence that it is an immunological response to aspirin. It has been suggested that aspirin acting as a partial prostaglandin synthetase inhibitor in these patients results in an abnormal shift of prostaglandin formation to those prostaglandins or intermediates which act as bronchoconstricting agents. Evidence for such a hypothesis is supported by the occurrence of acute asthma in some aspirin reactors to other drugs which are inhibitors of prostaglandin synthetase.

2.2.1. Immunological Management

Immunological management of asthma is restricted to IgE-triggered asthma; no immunological management will alter the course of non-IgE-related asthma. An exception is influenza immunization, which is indicated for all patients with asthma because asthma can be made dramatically worse by influenza. Routine annual influenza immunization should be a part of the chronic preventive medical care of the asthmatic.

a. Avoidance Therapy. The same principles of avoidance therapy described for allergic rhinitis are applicable for IgE-mediated asthma. It is even more important to consider such factors in the asthmatic because what may produce symptomatic discomfort in rhinitis could result in severe asthma with emergency room visits or hospitalization for status asthmaticus in the asthmatic. This is particularly true for animal or even bird sensitivity. Cat asthma, in particular, may exist as a chronic condition of limited severity, but when coupled with respiratory infection may lead to severe asthma requiring hospitalization. It is essential that the role of animal sensitivity be excluded as a component of the patient's disease when these sources of antigens are present in the patient's environment. Avoidance of nonspecific irritants such as paint fumes or occupational dusts may be of benefit. *Under no circumstances should an asthmatic smoke cigarettes.*

b. Immunotherapy. Immunotherapy for those antigens identified as important factors in IgE-triggered asthma has been standard practice for many years. Controlled studies of the efficacy of immunotherapy described above have been less extensive and may be less conclusive in asthma. Reviews of immunotherapy listed in the section on allergic rhinitis in this chapter may be examined for detailed reports. Such studies are more difficult to conduct in asthma because of the complexity of the clinical evaluation of the long-term progress of the disease. Further, the use of a controlled, double-blind placebo study raises possible questions of the ethics of withholding therapy. Two opinions exist regarding immunotherapy in asthma. One opinion is that immunotherapy is unproved for IgE-mediated asthma and should be considered an experimental approach. The other opinion is that the IgE-mediated component of inhalant asthma is the result of immunological, cellular, and biochemically mediated mechanisms similar to those in allergic rhinitis. Since immunotherapy has been demonstrated to be efficacious in allergic rhinitis through immunological actions not completely understood, it is reasonable to use immunotherapy in inhalant-induced asthma, particularly because the latter constitutes a disease of greater morbidity. Clinicians using immunotherapy for inhalant asthma associated with allergic rhinitis have observed, anecdotally, subsidence of the asthma prior to improvement of the rhinitis. Many clinical allergists believe that a proper attitude toward immunotherapy for asthma is that it should be standard (for the reasons described above) until and unless further double-blind controlled studies show that such therapy is not efficacious.

2.2.2. Pharmacological Management of Asthma

a. Acute Asthma. An acute asthmatic attack sufficiently severe that the patient requires emergency room evaluation is treated with epinephrine. Generally, 0.3 ml of 1:1000 epinephrine subcutaneously will manage acute asthma of most adults. This may be repeated two or three times at intervals of 10–15 min. If a response has not occurred after such therapy, the use of intravenous aminophylline may reverse an acute asthmatic attack. This is given as 500 mg of aminophylline intravenously in a rapid 100-ml intravenous drip to an adult. Aminophylline has been given as a direct intravenous medication, and 250 mg may be administered no more rapidly than 25 mg/min. This provides an alternative method of acute administration. However, the direct administration of undiluted aminophylline is hazardous, and the drip method described above is strongly recommended as the safest procedure. The use of epinephrine or epinephrine with aminophylline will reverse most acute episodes of asthma. Following clinical improvement, the physician supplying emergency care should look for precipitating factors such as infections and treat such associated conditions as indicated. Further, the patient should have guidance regarding follow-up management to prevent a recurrence of acute asthma. The continued management should include establishing physician contact for chronic care, initiating regular oral bronchodilators, and increasing the dose of corticosteroids if the patient is a corticosteroid-dependent (CSD) asthmatic.

b. Status Asthmaticus. Status asthmaticus is a state of asthma which is unresponsive to epinephrine and aminophylline utilized as described above. It is a medical emergency requiring hospitalization and very close observation in order to prevent a fatality from respiratory failure. Routine epinephrine or other β-agonist treatment will have little effect in status asthmaticus because, by definition, status asthmaticus is unresponsive to epinephrine. The principles of management of status asthmaticus include intravenous aminophylline as a loading dose and maintenance of the blood level of 10–20 μg/ml as determined in institutions where theophylline measurements can be obtained. Oxygen therapy, hydration, treatment of respiratory infection, or treatment of heart failure or other illnesses or associated complications is essential. If these approaches are used, the patient may be expected to gradually improve. Close observation of the patient clinically and with blood gas and pH determinations is essential, and the managing physician must be prepared to provide intubation and respiratory assistance at any time. An essential component of therapy is the use of corticosteroid therapy. Although often withheld in the past to observe the response in the patient to the regimen just described, the immediate use of corticosteroids appears indicated in status asthmaticus, not only in the CSD asthmatic but also in asthmatics who have not required corticosteroids in the past. The early use of corticosteroids will reduce the risk of status asthmaticus progressing to respiratory failure and will shorten the period of hospitalization. The latter reduces complications that may occur with prolonged hospitalizations, especially in the aged and obese. Two hundred milligrams of hydrocortisone sodium succinate as an intravenous drip every 4–6 hr is a satisfactory regimen. The earlier the high-dose corticosteroids are administered at the onset of significant asthma, the more effective this therapy will be. Thus the CSD asthmatic who has prednisone at home and has acute asthma should be told to take an oral dose before leaving for the emergency room. Similarly, corticosteroids should be started in the emergency room prior to transfer to the medical floor because of possible delays in receiving the first dose during the hospital admission process.

Following control of the patient's asthma, as evidenced by blood gas determinations and physical examination, the patient's regimen may be changed to oral prednisone, oral bronchodilators, and termination of oxygen therapy for continued observation prior to discharge. Essential to the long-term satisfactory management of asthma is evaluation of the reason for occurrence of the status asthmaticus and the establishment of a regimen of outpatient management which will prevent a recurrence of asthma of such severity that hospitalization is required.

c. Chronic Asthma. The pharmacological management of chronic asthma is dependent on the physician classifying the type of asthma (IgE-triggered, aspirin sensitive, etc.) and the state of severity of the asthma. Such evaluation requires information regarding previous emergency room visits, hospitalizations, previous use of corticosteroids, missed school or work days, and the past medications used and the apparent degree of success of these in control of the disease. The goal of therapy should be functional patients who are performing daily activities without significant restriction and are satisfied with the quality of their life pattern. This management is achieved through close contact with the physician while a satisfactory regimen is established. This control of asthma is accomplished by pharmacological agents which will control asthma, using the minimum amount of therapy that will be effective and that has the least potential for untoward side effects over a long period of time. The therapy is graded from oral bronchodilators to cromolyn sodium and, if necessary, topical and systemic corticosteroids.

2.2.3. β-Adrenergic Agonists

β-Adrenergic agonists stimulate β-receptors and elevate intracellular cAMP. These agents will relax smooth muscle constriction and stimulate cardiac receptors. More specific β-agonists which will primarily stimulate either the β_1- or β_2-receptors have been identified. Specific β_2-stimuli probably will come into increasing clinical use in the future in the management of asthma. The β_2-agonists stimulate smooth muscle receptors with relaxation with less effect on the cardiac receptors and produce less cardiac stimulatory effect. Their clinical use has demonstrated an increase in a different type of side effect. This adverse effect is muscle tremor which some patients may consider a significant deterrent to their use. A common β-adrenergic drug in use for many years has been ephedrine sulfate. Used in adult doses of 25 mg three or four times daily, ephedrine sulfate will result in control of mild asthma. Side effects consist of central nervous system stimulaton and cardiac stimulation, primarily tachycardia. These side effects may be minimal in some patients and often decline with continuous regular use of ephedrine. In clinical practice, it is often advisable to initiate therapy at one-half the maintenance dose and increase slowly to maintenance as tolerance to the side effects occurs.

β-Agonists have been used by inhalation for many years. The inhalation of these agents, such as isoproterenol, results in immediate subjective relief and improvement in pulmonary function. At times they may provide a useful adjunct to control of acute asthma by the patient. This must be balanced against the tendency of some patients to abuse the inhalation of β-agonists by excessive use. Many clinicians regard the control of asthma by systemic bronchodilators as the preferred method of therapy.

2.2.4. Phosphodiesterase Inhibitors

Phosphodiesterase inhibitors increase the level of intracellular cAMP by inhibition of the action of phosphodiesterase, which catalyzes the degradation of cAMP. Thus both β-adrenergic agonists and phosphodiesterase inhibitors increase intracellular levels of cAMP by different mechanisms. Both types of agents are presumed to have a bronchodilatory activity based on this effect of increasing intracellular cAMP. The methylxanthines are phosphodiesterase inhibitors. Aminophylline (theophylline ethylenediamine) is one commonly used drug. A variety of other forms are available. These drugs serve as effective bronchodilators when given acutely as intravenous medication, rectally as a rectal suppository, or orally. Sustained action is achieved by regular, oral administration or use of newer sustained-action preparations. Aminophylline can be administered orally as 100 to 200 mg four times daily to an adult. The lower dose is often initiated with a gradual increase to tolerance or followed by obtaining theophylline blood levels. Aminophylline may act as a significant gastric irritant, and this gastric irritation may prohibit the attainment of the desired dosage. Other side effects include nervousness, headache, and tachycardia. Convulsions may occur at toxic levels, particularly in children.

It has been common practice for physicians to use combinations of β-agonists and phosphodiesterase inhibitors such as ephedrine and aminophylline often with a mild sedative, available in a large variety of available preparations. Although criticized as polypharmacy, combined preparations have had long acceptance in clinical use with control of many cases of chronic asthma with relatively few side effects. An easy and common method of managing chronic asthma consists of the administration of one of these combinations of ephedrine and aminophylline four times daily. In many mild cases of asthma this regimen will satisfactorily control asthma and even prevent nocturnal episodes of asthma when this is a particular problem. When this program does not control a patient's symptoms satisfactorily, additional aminophylline may be added to the regimen initially at 100 mg four times daily, increasing to 200 mg four times daily, depending on control of asthma and the side effects induced by these drugs.

Although the β-adrenergic agonists and phosphodiesterase inhibitors singly or in combination are effective bronchodilating agents in acute or chronic asthma, they do not satisfactorily control asthma in many patients. In these cases, other drug therapy, as described below, must be considered. A more detailed review of these bronchodilators has been published (Van Arsdel and Paul, 1977).

2.2.5. Cromolyn Sodium

Cromolyn sodium has been available for use in asthma for several years, particularly outside the United States. It has been available for use in the United States for a sufficient period of time to evaluate its general role in the therapy of asthma. It is presumed to react by inhibition of the antigen-induced release of mediators from IgE-sensitized mast cells. It does not interfere with antigen-antibody reactions, appearing to act by a poorly defined mechanism inhibiting mediator release from these cells. Efficacy has been shown in chronic asthma by double-blind controlled studies. Cromolyn must reach the bronchial mucosa by inhalation of a powder in a somewhat complex delivery system at a dose of 20 mg four times daily. The oral route is not effective because of poor gastrointestinal absorption. Cromolyn sodium should be tried in asthmatics poorly controlled by the oral bronchodilators described above, particularly if the asthma appears to be triggered by inhalant allergens. Cromolyn should be tried for 2–3 months with careful clinical monitoring of the patient to determine whether improved control of the asthma has occurred. It appears to be effective in only some patients. Patients responsive to cromolyn are more likely to be children and are generally individuals with IgE-stimulated asthma. In some patients relatively dramatic control of asthma may be observed. In other cases no effect may be observed, and in still others there may be an initial apparent successful response (possibly a "placebo" effect) but no long-term benefit. Because cromolyn sodium must be delivered as a powder to the hyperreactive airway of the asthmatic, some patients may not be able to tolerate initial trials with the drug. In these cases, a short course of oral prednisone (5–7 days) may be required to provide sufficient control of asthma so that cromolyn sodium can be initiated. The oral steroids may then be terminated and the efficacy of cromolyn sodium judged over the next few months. The current expense of the medication is such that if it is not providing significant benefit after a 2–3 month trial it should be terminated. Cromolyn sodium is under investigation as a topical ophthalmic and topical nasal therapeutic agent for allergic conjunctivitis and allergic rhinitis, respectively. The development of cromolyn has led to a dramatic stimulation of research for similar agents which are absorbed after oral administration. These drugs are under clinical trial at the current time.

2.2.6. Corticosteroids

a. Systemic. Corticosteroids have a dramatic effect on the control of asthma. Their use in the hospitalized asthmatic has been described above. Mechanism of action in asthma is unknown. Proposals of the method of action include the general potent antiinflammatory action of these agents and possibly the inhibition of action of prostaglandin activities in the airway. The corticosteroid which is most generally used is prednisone. The use of prednisone rather than other corticosteroids is based on its short duration of action, efficacy, and cost. Dramatic control of asthma with prednisone will occur in almost all cases, and when properly used it can provide enormous benefit for the severe asthmatic. When the dramatic effect of corticosteroids in asthma was observed about 30 years ago, corticosteroids were excessively used. This resulted in the clinical side effects of corticosteroids and led to an excessively negative attitude by both some patients and some physicians. The consequence is that some patients have not received adequate control of asthma with prednisone in spite of asthma which is incapacitating and even life threatening. Corticosteroids are still overused in some cases. It must be emphasized that they are the most potent agents available and their use should be restricted to those cases which are uncontrolled by other modalities of immunological and pharmacological management. At the same time, it must be emphasized that withholding prednisone when indicated for asthma is not appropriate care. The result may be a respiratory cripple instead of a functional person, and inadequate use of prednisone may even result in fatalities. The numerous side effects of prednisone should be well known to any physicians using them for therapy. These side effects are dose related. Usually, it is found that a relatively moderate to low dose of prednisone can provide satisfactory control of asthma. These doses of prednisone are at levels which do not provide significant complications in a great majority of patients. If prednisone is required, it is given at a dose of approximately 0.5 mg/kg of body weight per day for an ambulatory patient or at least twice that dose for asthma of sufficient severity to require hospitalization. After clearing of the asthma, the prednisone is converted to a single alternate-day morning dose. Generally, about 0.75 mg/kg body weight as a single alternate-day morning dose will completely control asthma, and when this has been demonstrated reduction of the dosage can begin. This must be done by the physician. Tapering of dosage at increments of 5 mg/dose every 2–4 weeks to a level of 30 mg on alternate days is followed by a slower reduction at increasing intervals. In chronic asthma, a dose of prednisone will be found below which the patient will begin to have acute or chronic episodes of asthma. At that point, determined by close contact between physician and patient, the dose is stabilized. There should be periodic attempts to determine whether a lower dose of prednisone will suffice. At the lowest dose of maintenance prednisone there may be periods when sharp increases are required for exacerbations of asthma. These can result from respiratory infections, particularly viral infections, seasonal climatic changes, or unknown causes. The above are general guidelines, and care of each patient must be individualized.

The patient with chronic corticosteroid-dependent asthma requiring surgical procedures should have complete control of asthma established by prednisone as a daily dose prior to the surgical procedure and a cortisone acetate preparation (100 mg intramuscularly) every 8 hr beginning 24 hr before and continuing until oral prednisone may be resumed (Oh and Patterson, 1974).

The hypoxemia of significant asthma is considered to be a risk during pregnancy, and the use of prednisone, when indicated, should be continued during pregnancy (Schatz *et al.*, 1975).

Patients on chronic prednisone should receive adequate instructions about control of asthma with increased prednisone when traveling, particularly in foreign countries. They should have the availability of immediate contact with their physician for early treatment of exacerbations. Most corticosteroid-dependent asthmatics who require hospitalization do so because they have not had therapy with an adequate amount of prednisone early in the course of exacerbations of asthma.

b. Topical. A significant advance in the management of severe asthma has been the availability of topical corticosteroids. Several preparations are under study. One agent available for use is beclomethasone diproprionate. Beclomethasone has permitted the discontinuation of systemic prednisone in some CSD asthmatics and resulted in a marked reduction in prednisone requirement in others. Maximal use is four inhalations four times daily. After asthma is well controlled, the amount subsequently required may be determined by slow reduction in dose in the stable asthmatic. Corticosteroid-dependent asthmatics who have been successfully converted to inhaled beclomethasone may require short periodic courses of oral prednisone (30–40 mg per day) when there is an exacerbation of asthma, particularly during a respiratory infection. Beclomethasone by inhalation is not indicated as the agent of choice for acute asthma or for a hospitalized asthmatic for whom systemic corticosteroids are required to establish control. Beclomethasone is a rapidly catabolized agent with primarily topical action, but systemic absorption with adrenal cortical suppression at higher doses must be considered in its use. Complications include oral candidiasis, which has not constituted a major problem in most cases. A recurrent problem of this type may be controlled by reduction in the dose and improvement of oral hygiene. In some ambulatory asthmatics, in whom bronchodilators have not established control and where the use of steroids has become obviously necessary, inhaled beclomethasone is the drug of choice if they are not so ill that prednisone is required. In some of these patients, the inhalation of beclomethasone may stimulate the hyperirritable airway and temporary use of oral prednisone will control asthma to the point where beclomethasone may be initiated and the prednisone reduced and discontinued.

In all patients in whom steroids have been used topically or systemically for control of asthma, the problem of adrenal cortical suppression must be considered even months after these have been discontinued. Replacement therapy for acute stress situations is essential for these patients.

2.2.7. Other Modalities of Therapy

As in any chronic disease state, a variety of therapies have been suggested and tried with variable degrees of success reported. Inhaled anticholinergic agents are under study and may be beneficial in selected patients. Periodically, a variety of other modalities of therapy, including hypnosis, psychotherapy, exercise programs, and various other approaches, are described. Except for transient placebo effect, these are of no benefit. Psychiatric care is indicated if individuals with asthma have complicating psychiatric problems or if they are unable to accept the presence of a chronic disease. Because the primary cause of asthma is not of psychiatric origin, this type of therapy is not indicated as a primary role in care.

3. Anaphylaxis

Anaphylaxis is the generalized immediate-type IgE-mediated reaction that occurs following the introduction of a sufficient amount of antigen into sensitized individuals. The reaction is believed to occur from the release of histamine and possibly other biologically active mediators from IgE-sensitized mast cells. Anaphylaxis constitutes one of the most immediate of the medical emergencies, requiring understanding of therapy so that fatal occurrences may be avoided by immediate use of appropriate drugs.

3.1. Immunological Management

Essential to the prevention of anaphylaxis is identification of causative agents. These may be drugs acting through IgE-mediated mechanisms such as penicillin. A careful history of drug allergy is essential to avoid drug-induced anaphylaxis. Ingestants which are not drugs can produce anaphylaxis, with the most frequent causes being seafoods and nuts. A wide variety of common foods may be causes of food anaphylaxis in individual patients. Again, historical information and physician guidance are necessary to prevent recurrences of the systemic allergic reaction. Certain agents, such as radiographic contrast media, will produce a generalized reaction which simulates an anaphylactic reaction in symptomatology but have not been demonstrated to be IgE mediated in mechanism. The question of readministration of radiographic contrast media, as indicated for diagnostic tests for individuals who have had a previous reaction, has now been managed by appropriate prophylaxis with prednisone and diphenhydramine (Kelly *et al.*, 1978). Anaphylaxis from hymenoptera insect stings has been managed in the past by a program of immunotherapy with whole body extracts of hymenoptera. Such therapy is now under challenge. Specific therapy with appropriate hymenoptera venoms is being currently developed as an appropriate modality for hymenoptera hypersensitivity. Fire ant hypersensitivity is treated by a regimen appropriate for that type of insect.

Anaphylaxis has occurred from a variety of protein substances that are used medicinally, including ACTH, insulin, and heterologous serum used as antitoxins. In these cases, desensitization can be done using increasing concentrations of the protein in subjects requiring the drug medically. This program is particularly successful for patients with a history of insulin anaphylaxis. Such therapy should be given by physicians experienced in managing the potentially severe reactions which may occur during the course of such desensitization.

3.2. Pharmacological Management

Immediate therapy indicated for anaphylaxis is the systemic injection of epinephrine, 0.3 ml of a 1:1000 solution. The earlier this is administered, the more effective the treatment will be in preventing the progression and reversing the reaction. Epinephrine may be given intramuscularly for more rapid absorption in severe cases and, in potentially fatal cases, intravenously, but here the epinephrine must be diluted and 1 ml of a 1:10,000 solution given intravenously. Epinephrine should be carried and self-administered by patients with a history of hymenoptera or fire ant sensitivity when they have a repeat challenge by the insect sting or bite.

Following the initial treatment of anaphylaxis with epinephrine, further pharmacological therapy is based on the severity and the degree of control established by the epinephrine. If epinephrine has not completely controlled the reaction, it may be repeated every 10–15 min and 50 mg of diphenhydramine should be given intravenously. When there is significant bronchospasm, 500 mg of aminophylline should be administered rapidly in a 100-mg intravenous drip. In the absence of bronchospasm, aminophylline should not be used because it may potentiate hypotension. When hypotension occurs and is not reversed by the administration of epinephrine as described above, vasopressor agents are indicated. Because of the loss of fluids from the intravascular compartment due to a generalized increase in vascular permeability, vasopressor agents may not be effective and must then be accompanied by volume repletion with available saline solution or preferably plasma. Laryngeal obstruction should be treated with a tracheostomy and oxygen, if this is a component of the anaphylaxis. Occurrence of cardiac arrest requires all methods now standard for cardiopulmonary resuscitation.

Corticosteroids will not reverse anaphylactic reactions and are not the first choice of therapy. Their use prior to epinephrine is contraindicated in that they delay the administration of the first drug of choice: epinephrine. In any case where the initial pharmacological therapy has been initiated and symptoms of anaphylaxis persist, corticosteroids should be initiated (200 mg of hydrocortisone sodium hemisuccinate intravenously) as an immediate dose and followed by continuous drip of 200 mg every 4 hr. The use of corticosteroids may have a beneficial effect in therapy of prolonged anaphylaxis.

4. Urticaria and Angioedema

4.1. Immunological Management

Urticaria and angioedema can occur separately or together. They may occur as IgE-mediated responses at times associated with system involvement other than the skin (urticaria), and subcutaneously (angioedema). Urticaria and angioedema may occur as a result of IgE-mediated food allergy, and potentially serious reactions may occur if a sufficient amount of food is ingested in a highly sensitive subject. Certain foods, such as strawberries, are thought to produce urticaria through nonimmunological mechanisms. The time relationship between the ingestion of food and the onset of urticaria is usually such that the patient is able to identify the causative agent. Occasionally, food allergy may result from a common ingestant (wheat, eggs, or dairy products) eaten daily and the cause may not be readily apparent. In these patients, a diet diary or a trial of a highly restricted diet such as a synthetic diet or a lamb and rice diet may be used as a diagnostic procedure. These diets are used until the urticaria disappears, and then these foods are added sequentially on different days to determine if they will produce urticaria. An obvious treatment for food allergy is the avoidance of that food. Occasionally, patients can tolerate a well-cooked food when they cannot tolerate a raw food or partially cooked food. This is presumably due to denaturation of the protein antigens by heat.

A second major cause of urticaria and angioedema is drug allergy. Symptoms may be explosive, or a mild case of urticaria may occur. The diagnostic approach to urticaria is careful history of drug ingestants and elimination of unnecessary drugs or substitution of other agents for those suspected of being the etiological agent. In taking a drug history, it is important to remember that patients may not consider certain commonly used medications as drugs and report them as such. Thus the patient should be specifically asked about the ingestion of aspirin, laxatives, and the variety of vitamin preparations available. When a drug is identified as the etiological agent, the therapy is avoidance. When a drug is essential for the management of another medical problem, a desensitization program may be attempted, but this must be done with great caution in order to avoid an anaphylactic reaction and is often unsuccessful.

A variety of infectious diseases may have urticaria as an initial manifestation, even before other systemic symptoms of the infection are present. Virus disease such as hepatitis is an example. Urticaria may be one of the initial physical manifestations of neoplastic disease. In angioedema, particularly in those cases where swelling involves the mucosal surfaces, hereditary angioedema should be excluded by appropriate complement studies. Urticaria and angioedema may be presenting symptoms of collagen-vascular disease, such as lupus erythematosus. In uncommon cases, urticaria may be associated with abnormalities of the complement system.

A variety of cases of urticaria result from physical stimuli such as cold urticaria, solar urticaria, and pressure urticaria. Urticaria may occur from insect bites. The management of these cases depends primarily on identification of cause and avoidance of the stimulus as much as possible. One type of urticaria which often follows exercise and cooling of the body is known as cholinergic urticaria and is managed with explanation, reassurance, and medication described below.

There are many cases of chronic urticaria in which no food or drug allergen, physical stimulus, or underlying disease can be identified. These cases of chronic idiopathic urticaria most often occur in adults. They can provide considerable discomfort to the patient because of the pruritis and the cosmetic abnormality. Although these cases are of an unknown etiology, the patient, and at times physicians, can be involved in a lengthy and unrewarding search for a causative allergen. Such patients may begin to follow bizarre diets because they exclude an additional food each time there is a recurrence of their urticaria due to coincidental relation to a meal. The management of these patients should include exclusion of etiological agents or associated diseases to the greatest extent possible. Then the patient should have his problem explained and managed by the regimens described below.

4.2. Pharmacological Management

4.2.1. Acute Management

Acute, severe urticaria with or without angioedema due to an ingestant will respond to epinephrine (0.3 ml of a 1:1000 solution); this may be followed with an antihistamine such as chlorpheniramine, 4 mg four times daily. Symptoms are usually of short duration, and 24–48 hr of therapy will often suffice.

4.2.2. Chronic Management

The management of chronic idiopathic urticaria is conducted in a graded fashion to establish control of the patient's symptoms. The first drug to be tried is an antihistamine with minimal side effects, such as chlorpheniramine given 4 mg four times daily. If there is only partial control, a second agent, such as ephedrine, 25 mg three times daily, can be added. The combined antihistamine and sympathomimetic agents may be effective together. Occasional patients with chronic idiopathic urticaria will have a dramatic response to therapy with hydroxyzine hydrochloride at a dose of 25 mg three times daily. At times, this dose can be increased gradually as the patient becomes tolerant of the soporific effect of the hydroxyzine. An occasional patient will be managed by as little as 25 mg of hydroxyzine on alternate days. Explanation for this striking effect of hydroxyzine in certain cases of chronic urticaria is unknown. In some cases of chronic idiopathic urticaria, hydroxyzine will have no apparent effect. In cases of chronic urticaria where pruritis is extreme, cyproheptadine may establish significant control.

Corticosteroids topically have little effect in the management of acute or chronic urticaria. Their use as a systemic agent must be considered with caution in chronic urticaria that is uncomfortable but not life threatening. However, in certain cases, the manifestations of urticaria and angioedema are so severe and uncomfortable that control with steroids is required. This is accomplished by a brief course of daily prednisone (e.g., 40 mg daily in an adult), followed by conversion to a single, alternate-day morning dose and gradually tapering of the prednisone to a minimal amount that will control the urticaria and angioedema. It is not uncommon for patients with chronic urticaria to have spontaneous remissions, and the therapies described should periodically be discontinued to determine whether they are still necessary. Treatment of hereditary angioedema is a complex problem, undergoing continual investigation by centers studying this problem.

5. Allergic Bronchopulmonary Aspergillosis (ABPA)

5.1. Diagnosis

The current status of allergic bronchopulmonary aspergillosis (ABPA) is that it is being recognized with increased frequency, particularly in children and younger adults (Rosenberg *et al.*, 1977). Important in early diagnosis is a high index of suspicion of the physician. Patients with asthma and a positive prick test to aspergillus antigen should be considered suspects for ABPA. A history of pulmonary infiltrates, marked eosinophilia, positive sputum cultures for aspergillus, and elevated serum IgE and precipitating antibodies against aspergillus antigen all increase the likelihood of the presence of ABPA. A certain diagnosis can be made by demonstration of hyphae in the sputum, but many patients with ABPA do not produce sputum. Demonstration of central bronchiectasis by bronchography will almost certainly diagnose the disease. However, not all patients with ABPA have central bronchiectasis. Current attempts to improve the serological diagnosis of ABPA by demonstration of elevated IgE and IgG antibody activity against *Aspergillus fumigatus* provide a potentially useful serological approach. It is important that diagnosis be established early as it might be possible to prevent the progressive destruction of bronchial tissue and the fibrosis that may occur in longstanding or recurrent ABPA.

5.2. Management

Corticosteroids are indicated for ABPA. The use of prednisone, at 0.5 mg/kg body weight per day, until all chest X-ray abnormalities have disappeared is indicated. The prednisone may then be converted to alternate-day therapy and the patient observed by periodic chest X-ray examinations. The use of prednisone in ABPA will be followed by a decline of total serum of IgE, which is elevated in all cases of typical ABPA. The prednisone is continued for approximately 3 months. Exacerbations of ABPA should be similarly treated, but these exacerbations may be very difficult to detect and can occur in an almost asymptomatic patient. Long-term studies to attempt to predict early serological changes indicative of a flare of ABPA are currently under way.

6. Hypersensitivity Pneumonitis

6.1. Recognition

In hypersensitivity pneumonitis, again, a high index of suspicion is indicated. Failure to identify hypersensitivity pneumonitis may result in progressive destruction of lung tissue ending in pulmonary fibrosis. Thus a careful environmental and occupational history is indicated for patients with chronic or recurrent pulmonary disease of unknown etiology. Environment or occupational exposures are followed by serological tests against presumptive antigens from humidifiers or antigens from such sources as moldy hay. Pulmonary function studies are done to demonstrate the restrictive type of pulmonary function abnormality. At times, bronchial challenge is indicated to establish the presence of this important disease.

6.2. Management

When a diagnosis of hypersensitivity pneumonitis is established, the principal method of management is avoidance of antigen. This will be dependent on the type of antigen involved and may include elimination of humidifiers, control of occupational dust exposure by appropriate filters and environmental changes, and perhaps a change in occupation. The patient can then be treated with prednisone while studies are repeated until the maximal improvement in pulmonary functions is obtained. Prednisone is then tapered off and discontinued.

7. References

Cooke, R. A., Barnard, J. H., Hebald, S., and Stull, A., 1935, Serologic evidence of immunity with coexisting sensitization in a type of human allergy (hay fever), *J. Exp. Med.* **62:**733–751.

Haddad, Z. H., Marsh, D. G., and Campbell, D. H., 1972, Studies on "allergoids" prepared from naturally occurring allergens, *J. Allergy Clin. Immunol.* **49:**197–209.

Irons, J. S., Pruzansky, J. J., and Patterson, R., 1975, Immunotherapy: Mechanisms of action suggested by measurements of immunologic and cellular parameters, *J. Allergy Clin. Immunol.* **56:**64–77.

Johnstone, D. E., and Dutton, A., 1968, The value of hyposensitization therapy for bronchial asthma of children—A 14-year study, *Pediatrics* **42:**793–802.

Kelly, J. F., Patterson, R., Lieberman, P., Mathison, D. A., and Stevenson, D. D., 1978, Radiographic contrast media studies in high risk patients, *J. Allergy Clin. Immunol.* **62:**181–184.

Levinson, A. I., Summers, R. J., Lawley, T. J., Evans, R., and Frank, M. M., 1978, Evaluation of the adverse effects of long term hyposensitization, *J. Allergy Clin. Immunol.* **62:**109–114.

Lieberman. P., and Patterson, R., 1974, Immunotherapy for atopic disease, *Adv. Intern. Med.* **19:**391–394.

Metzger, W. J., Patterson, R., Zeiss, C. R., Irons, J., Pruzansky, J., Suszko, I., and Levitz, D., 1976, Polymerized ragweed antigen E. V. Clinical and immunological studies, *N. Engl. J. Med.* **295:**1160–1164.

Noon, L., and Cantab, B. C., 1911, Prophylactic innoculation against hay fever, *Lancet* **1:**1572–1573.

Oh, S. H., and Patterson, R., 1974, Surgery in corticosteroid dependent asthmatics, *J. Allergy Clin. Immunol.* **53:**345–351.

Patterson, R., Lieberman, P., Irons, J. S., Pruzansky, J. J., Melam, H., Metzger, W. J., and Zeiss, C. R., 1978a, Immunotherapy, in: *Allergy: Principles and Practices* (E. Middleton, C. Reed, and E. Ellis, eds.), pp. 877–898, Mosby, St. Louis.

Patterson, R., Suszko, I. M., and Harris, K. E., 1978b, The *in vivo* transfer of antigen induced airway reactions by bronchial lumen mast cells, *J. Clin. Invest.* **62:**519–524.

Rosenberg, M., Patterson, R., Mintzer, R., Cooper, B. J., Roberts, M., and Harris, K. E., 1977, Clinical and immunologic criteria for the diagnosis of allergic bronchopulmonary aspergillosis, *Ann. Intern. Med.* **86:**405–414.

Sadan, N., Rhyne, M. B., Mellits, E. D., Goldstein, E. O., Levy, D. A., and Lichtenstein, L. M., 1969, Immunotherapy of pollenosis in children, *N. Engl. J. Med.* **280:**623–627.

Schatz, M., Patterson, R., Zeitz, S., O'Rourke, J., and Melam, H., 1975, Corticosteroid therapy in the pregnant asthmatic patient, *J. Am. Med. Assoc.* **233:**804–806.

Van Arsdel, P. P., Jr., and Paul, G. H., 1977, Drug therapy in the management of asthma, *Ann. Intern. Med.* **87:**68–74.

Index

MIX
Papier aus verantwortungsvollen Quellen
Paper from responsible sources
FSC® C105338

If you have any concerns about our products,
you can contact us on
ProductSafety@springernature.com

In case Publisher is established outside the EU,
the EU authorized representative is:
Springer Nature Customer Service Center GmbH
Europaplatz 3, 69115 Heidelberg, Germany

Printed by Libri Plureos GmbH
in Hamburg, Germany